Precision Pathology of Cancer

Precision pathology of cancer is a new frontier—a systemic diagnostic approach to provide specific therapeutic targets and genetic and metabolic information for the treatment of patients. Not only are cancers extremely diverse, but there is also heterogenetic variation among patients with the same cancer; owing to differences in genetic makeup and metabolic levels, a drug may work in one patient but be toxic in another. This text covers both basic concepts (the role of the precision pathologist, ethical issues, molecular basis, tools used in precision pathology, and specimen procurement) and clinical practice (the precise genes/pathways, ongoing clinical trials, therapeutics, pharmacogenomics, pharmacoproteomics, and pharmacometabolomics) in precision pathology of cancer.

To
our families and friends
for
their love and support

Precision Pathology of Cancer
From Basic Concept to Clinical Practice

Edited by
Xianfeng F. Zhao and Shiyong Li

CRC Press
Taylor & Francis Group
Boca Raton London New York

CRC Press is an imprint of the
Taylor & Francis Group, an **informa** business

Designed cover image: Editors

First edition published 2025
by CRC Press
2385 NW Executive Center Drive, Suite 320, Boca Raton FL 33431

and by CRC Press
4 Park Square, Milton Park, Abingdon, Oxon, OX14 4RN

CRC Press is an imprint of Taylor & Francis Group, LLC

ISBN: 9781032844862 (hbk)
ISBN: 9781032844886 (pbk)
ISBN: 9781003513469 (ebk)

DOI: 10.1201/9781003513469

Typeset in Times
by Apex CoVantage, LLC

Contents

Preface

Precision medicine marks a new milestone in the history of modern medicine. Instead of the traditional "one size fits all" method, this new approach for patient care allows physicians to systemically select treatments that take individual variabilities into account (1). Precision medicine is also referred to by some as "personalized medicine" or "individualized medicine". Although these different terms reflect different aspirations and interpretations of the systemic approach to future patient care, they generally include two major aspects: 1) specific treatment of diseases based on the defined therapeutic targets and 2) tailored management of patients according to the individual's genetic and metabolic makeup. With the emergence of precision medicine, healthcare is becoming more and more *precise.*

Unlike the definition of "precision medicine" that might have ethical indications and concerns over possibly inequitable access (2), the definition of precision pathology is more straightforward, since pathology is the basis of medicine and thus precision medicine must be based on precision pathology. Then how do we define precision pathology? Precision pathology is a systemic diagnostic approach to provide specific therapeutic targets for diseases and genetic and metabolic information for patients. Traditionally, pathologists provide a diagnosis and classification of a disease based on morphology and other ancillary studies; clinicians manage patients based on their experience in clinical trials in treating the diagnosed disease. However, more and more evidence shows that diseases are extremely diverse, and so are individual patients. Utilization of chemotherapeutic drugs does not always cure cancer but often leads to new malignancies due to their nonspecific cytotoxic properties. Due to the different genetic makeups and enzymatic levels in the metabolism, one drug may work in one individual but not in another. Every drug has side effects which will vary among different individuals; one dose of drug may not be enough for one individual but may be toxic for a different patient. To solve these issues, 1) we need to dissect each disease thoroughly via genetic analysis and molecular studies to identify the driving forces of the disease and specifically target them, and 2) we need to understand the genomics and metabolism of each patient to craft a specific regimen to treat the disease with minimal side effects.

To reach the goals of precision pathology, pathologists must utilize all the molecular tools to identify the genomic aberrations, genetic mutations, aberrant expressions and posttranslational modifications of abnormal cells, and genetic makeup and metabolic profile of the patient. These molecular tools include cytogenetics, PCR sequencing, next-generation sequencing, mass spectrometry, and biosensor technology, integrated with artificial intelligence (AI). The new generation of pathologists should embrace knowledge of molecular pathology and the new concept of precision pathology and apply the knowledge and concepts to their clinical practice.

This book will present readers with comprehensive knowledge of precision pathology based on the organs and systems. It consists of two integral parts: the first will familiarize the readers with the concept of precision pathology, and the second will focus on identification of therapeutic targets of various cancers by pathologists and the application of these targets in targeted therapy. Due to limited progress in some organs/systems, this edition will focus on the organs and systems that have seen the most advancement in precision medicine; more organs/systems will be added in future editions.

REFERENCES

1. Collins FS, Varmus H. A New Initiative on Precision Medicine. N Engl J Med. 2015; 372(9):793–795.
2. Chan S, Erikainen S. What's in a name? The politics of 'precision medicine'. Am J Bioethics. 2018;18(4):50–52.

Editors

Xianfeng F. Zhao, MD PhD MBA, is Professor and Chair, Department of Pathology and Laboratory Medicine at the University of Tennessee Health Science Center College of Medicine, Memphis, Tennessee.

Shiyong Li, MD PhD, is the Professor and Director of Hematopathology, Department of Pathology and Laboratory Medicine at the Emory University School of Medicine, Atlanta, Georgia.

Contributors

Maher Albitar, MD
Chief Executive Officer
Genomic Testing Cooperative
Irvine, CA

Armita Bahrami, MD
Professor
Department of Pathology and Laboratory Medicine
Emory University School of Medicine
Atlanta, GA

Andrew B. Boucher, MD
Assistant Professor
Department of Neurosurgery
University of Tennessee Health Science Center College of Medicine
Memphis, TN

Yingbei Chen, MD PhD
Associate Attending Pathologist
Department of Pathology
Memorial Sloan Kettering Cancer Center
New York, NY

Eunice Chou, MD
Resident
Department of Pathology and Laboratory Medicine
Emory University School of edicine
Atlanta, GA

George Deeb, MD
Associate Professor
Department of Pathology and Laboratory Medicine
Emory University School of Medicine
Atlanta, GA

Fatemeh Derakhshan, MD, PhD
Assistant Professor
Department of Pathology and Cell Biology
Columbia University
New York, NY

Maria Diab, MD
Assistant Professor
Department of Hematology and Medical Oncology
Emory University School of Medicine
Atlanta, GA

Krisztina Hanley, MD
Professor
Department of Pathology and Laboratory Medicine
Emory University School of Medicine
Atlanta, GA

Lara Harik, MD
Associate Professor
Department of Pathology and Laboratory Medicine
Emory University School of Medicine
Atlanta, GA

Richard B. Hessler, MD
Chief of Pathology
Erlanger Health System
Chattanooga, TN

Wen-Yu Hsiao, MD PhD
Resident
Department of Pathology and Laboratory Medicine
Emory University School of Medicine
Atlanta, GA

Jian Jing, MD PhD
Assistant Professor
Department of Pathology and Laboratory Medicine
University of Colorado Anschutz Medical Center
Denver, CO

Rebecca Leibowitz
Fourth Year Medical Student
Emory University School of Medicine
Atlanta, GA

Emal Lesha, MD
Resident
Department of Neurosurgery
University of Tennessee Health Science Center
College of Medicine
Memphis, TN

Xia Li, PhD
Associate Professor
Department of Pathology
University of Arizona College of Medicine-Phoenix
Phoenix, AZ

Guang Liu, MD
Assistant Professor
Department of Pathology
University of Arizona College of Medicine-Phoenix
Phoenix, AZ

Zaid Mahdi, MD
Assistant Professor
Department of Pathology and Laboratory Medicine
Emory University School of Medicine
Atlanta, GA

Jane L. Meisel, MD
Associate Professor
Department of Hematology and Medical Oncology
Emory University School of Medicine
Atlanta, GA

Haider A. Mejbel, MD
Assistant Professor
Department of Pathology and Laboratory Medicine
Emory University School of Medicine
Atlanta, GA

Mustafa Motiwala, MD
Resident
Department of Neurosurgery
University of Tennessee Health Science Center
College of Medicine
Memphis, TN

Doreen N. Palsgrove, MD
Assistant Professor
Department of Pathology
The University of Texas Southwestern Medical Center
Dallas, TX

Fresia Pareja Zea, MD PhD
Assistant Attending Pathologist
Department of Pathology
Memorial Sloan Kettering Cancer Center
New York, NY

Lawrence M. Pfeffer, PhD
Professor
Department of Pathology and Laboratory Medicine
University of Tennessee Health Science Center
College of Medicine
Memphis, TN

Dara Ross, MD
Assistant Attending Pathologist
Department of Pathology and Laboratory Medicine
Memorial Sloan Kettering Cancer Center
New York, NY

Faisal Saeed, MD
Assistant Professor
Department of Pathology and Laboratory Medicine
Emory University School of Medicine
Atlanta, GA

Arron Sohn, MD
Surgical Pathologist
Hackensack Pathology Associates, LLC
Hackensack, NJ

Benjamin K. Stoff, MD MA
Associate Professor
Department of Pathology and Laboratory Medicine
Emory University School of Medicine
Atlanta, GA

Gulisa Turashvili, MD, PhD
Associate Professor
Department of Pathology and Laboratory Medicine
Emory University School of Medicine
Atlanta, GA

Sara Wobker, MD MPH
Associate Professor
Department of Pathology and Laboratory Medicine
University of North Carolina at Chapel Hill
Chapel Hill, NC

Zachary Wolner, MD
Assistant Professor
Department of Dermatology
Emory University School of Medicine
Atlanta, GA

Sarah J. Wood, MD
Chief Fellow
Department of Medical Oncology
Emory University School of Medicine
Atlanta, GA

Wei Zheng, MD PhD
Assistant Professor
Department of Pathology and Laboratory Medicine
Emory University School of Medicine
Atlanta, GA

1

Precision Pathology

Xianfeng F. Zhao

1.1 Precision Pathology as a New Frontier

Precision medicine, the approach to disease treatment and prevention that considers the individual genes, environment, and lifestyle of each patient, depends on precision pathology. But what exactly is precision pathology? Unlike traditional pathology which applies pattern recognition, precision pathology is a systemic approach to employ cutting-edge technology to identify the etiological factors of a disease and optimize treatment by focusing on the disease's therapeutic targets and patient's metabolism. Precision pathology has two main tasks: 1) to define the treatment goal and therapeutic target and 2) to optimize treatment specific to each individual patient. Thus, to succeed in treatment, pathologists must first determine the causative agents of the disease and proper therapeutic targets, then tailor treatment according to an expected physiological and pathological response based on the patient's metabolism. Therefore, precision pathology is defined as a systemic approach in determining the overall pathology of the disease and providing complete objective evidence for clinicians to manage patients for optimal clinical outcomes. It requires all the genomic, proteomic, metabolomic, and pharmacomic information of the disease and the host for the precision pathologist, with the assistance of artificial intelligence (AI), to provide the most appropriate evidence for clinicians and patients to design their optimal therapeutic plans.

1.2 Why Should Pathology Go Precision?

Pathologists traditionally diagnose diseases from specimens harvested by clinicians; clinicians collect patient specimens and send them to pathology laboratories. Pathologists in the laboratories examine the specimens first with naked eyes. Some preliminary diagnoses can be made by an experienced pathologist in the grossing room based on the color, shape, and texture of the lesions. The specimens are then submitted for histological examination to confirm and fine-tune the diagnoses. Diagnoses made by pathologists are very straightforward—they call what they see. Because of this, people often consider pathological diagnosis the most objective since they believe pathologists make diagnoses based solely on what they see in tissues. In fact, pathologists always integrate all the clinical information and radiologic findings into their diagnoses. Afterwards, treatment options are largely left with clinicians.

I used to explain to medical students the pathologist's role in patient care using the process of criminal investigation as an analogy. If we take disease as the "crime", primary care physicians often get the first report of the "crime", radiologists help to locate the "crime scene", and surgeons help to collect evidence from the "crime scene". With the collected evidence from the different investigators (blood from primary care physicians, fine needle aspirations/core needle biopsies from radiologists, and excisional biopsies from surgeons), pathologists, as "judges", analyze all the evidence (sometimes even conflicting) to rule in or rule out the "suspect(s)" and reach the verdict (final pathological diagnosis). The "suspects" will be either "released" (free of disease), "sentenced" (treated with medication), or "executed" (excised, radiated, and/or chemolyzed).

Traditional pattern recognition approach has been used by pathologists for diagnosis and classification of diseases; this tradition has dictated pathology for centuries and guided the diagnosis, classification, and treatment of diseases. Clinical trials based on cancer classification led to the development of numerous new drugs for cancer therapy. However, except for a handful of outstanding examples of targeted therapies, most cancers are still managed by surgical resection, radiation, and/or chemotherapy. As radiation and chemotherapy often lead to secondary malignancies, precision therapy with agents targeting specific oncogenic drivers achieved promising clinical outcomes and is more desirable. As a result, demand for detection and interpretation of oncogenic drivers lies on the shoulder of pathologists. To deal with the vast amount of laboratory data, precision pathology with the assistance of AI must be implemented. As seen in hematopathology, integrated approaches have already greatly improved pathological diagnosis and classification of diseases (Figure 1.1, left). Even this approach still relies on pattern recognition; the popular molecular classification with gene profiling uses mostly tissue-specific genes and only a handful of oncogenic drivers that are relevant to oncogenesis (1). Furthermore, this approach could lead us astray. For example, one algorithm of Burkitt lymphoma (BL) classification employing 196 genes, most of which are tissue specific, lymphocyte specific, B cell specific, and germinal center cell specific (2, 3), identified a provisional BL with 11q aberration, irrespective of the absence of *MYC* aberration (4). However, this approach remains widely accepted as part of the mainstream diagnostic strategy simply because there is a lack of an alternative.

DOI: 10.1201/9781003513469-1

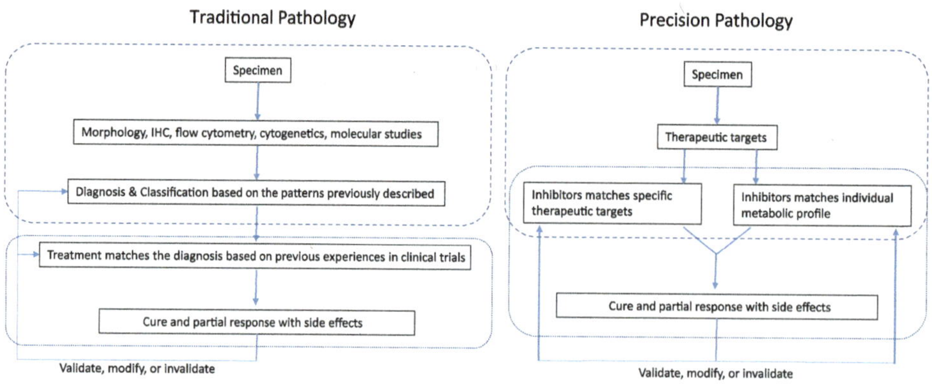

FIGURE 1.1 Comparison of traditional pathology (left) and precision pathology (right). The procedures inside the rough broken lines are within the scope of pathologists; the procedures inside the fine broken lines are within the scope of clinicians. Some overlaps exist between pathologist and clinician duties in precision pathology, suggesting more involvement in clinical decision making by pathologists.

Precision pathology analyzes diseases as a whole in every individual to provide "ideal" therapeutic targets and treatment plans (Figure 1.1, right). With the evolution of precision pathology, neither traditional diagnosis nor classification may even be necessary. For example, when *JAK2* mutations are identified in myeloproliferative neoplasm and B-cell acute lymphoblastic leukemia, treatment may be alike—to target the mutated JAK2 (5, 6). Similarly, when overexpressed *MYC* is detected in a lymphoma, MYC inhibition may be a reasonable strategy, regardless of a BL, diffuse large B-cell lymphoma (DLBCL) or something in between (7). Under this approach, is it still necessary to devote limited resources and efforts to determining the germinal center origin simply because of CD10 expression or mantle zone origin due to its CD5 positivity? Furthermore, cyclin D-driven mantle cell lymphomas may require a different treatment from cyclin D-negative mantle cell lymphomas (8). The same principle also applies to tumors of different lineages with the same *ALK* aberration, such as in non-small cell lung cancer (NSCLC) and ALK-positive anaplastic large cell lymphoma (ALCL). As more therapeutic targets are defined by molecular assays with decreasing costs and increasing availabilities, traditional morphologic reviews, immunophenotypic studies, cytogenetic analyses, and molecular profiling may not always be indispensable (8). These saved resources will be essential for identifying more molecular therapeutic targets, delineating pathway interactions, or evaluating individuals' responses to treatments. Such a change will revolutionize pathology practice; pathology textbooks may have to be rewritten and the standard of pathology practice updated. By employing AI, precision pathology will be a somewhat automated process with well-trained pathologists overseeing the performance of the diagnostic process.

1.3 Precision Pathology vs. Molecular Pathology

Since both utilize molecular techniques, many people cannot differentiate precision pathology from molecular pathology. To understand the differences between these two, let's make a comparison. Molecular pathology is also known as molecular diagnostics, which refers to the process of utilizing molecular techniques and molecular information to diagnose or assist in the diagnosis of diseases, such as diagnosis of COVID-19 infection by detecting the SARS-CoV2 viral RNA, detection of *IGH* or *TCR* rearrangement in supporting the diagnosis of malignant lymphomas, and detection of *JAK2* mutations in confirming the diagnosis of myeloproliferative neoplasms. Since information for precision therapies, such as *BCR::ABL1* fusion, *ALK* rearrangement, and *EGFR* mutations, is also produced from molecular diagnostic laboratories, it is easy to think precision pathology is identical or similar to molecular pathology. On the contrary, precision pathology uses a systemic approach which employs whole genome analysis, whole proteomic and metabolomic analyses, pharmacomic analysis, and AI to craft a therapeutic plan to guide clinical therapeutics. All in all, molecular pathology focuses on providing molecular information for diagnosis, whereas precision pathology focuses on providing molecular information for therapy.

1.4 Precision Pathology of Cancer

Cancer is a genetic disease. All cancers harbor genetic abnormalities that drive the oncological process. Cancer is heterogeneous and evolves from time to time, so the molecular targets are dynamic and constantly undergo changes. In another word, the oncogenic targets are not fixed, and they keep changing their directions and dimensions during the clinical course and with treatment. To precisely manage cancer, the therapeutic targets should be constantly evaluated; recurrent cancer cannot be managed the same as primary cancer, and cancer in one host is different from cancer (even with the same diagnosis) in another. One part of cancer is different from other parts of cancer (due to cancer heterogeneity). Even cancer cells might be different from each other within the same mass, carrying different genetic abnormalities. Whenever possible, all the genes in cancer should be analyzed to identify all the driver mutations so that no cancer cells are left behind after each round of therapy.

1.5 Precision Pathologists

With the development of various biological techniques and AI, pathologists know patients much better from the laboratories, sometimes even better than physically seeing the patients, since most of the genetic makeup and metabolomics would not show at the patient's interviews and/or on physical examinations. With big data and machine learning, pathologists would be able to collect and process tons of information from patients. The information will not only be related to the patient's disease but also the patient's physiology, the interactions between the disease and the patient, the interactions between the disease and treatment, and the interactions between the treatment and the patient. Since the information can be accumulated with time all through the patient's life, constant interactions with clinicians will be the norm. With first-hand material and derived data, pathologists could guide clinicians with treatment plans (9).

There may be disagreement among physicians of different specialties as to their roles in precision medicine, but pathologists have the following major advantages in precision medicine:

1) Pathologists have direct access to patient specimens. Evidence-based medicine relies on objective data produced in the clinical laboratories. Whether surgical specimens, cytological specimens, body fluids (including blood), or a patient's normal or abnormal discharges, they will be sent to clinical laboratories and analyzed by various assays. Since pathologists are well-trained experts in analyzing these data, they have an advantage in using these patient specimens in the clinical diagnosis, treatment, and prognosis of diseases.
2) Pathologists have access to cutting-edge diagnostic technologies. Molecular profiling, next-generation sequencing, omics, machine learning, and AI are more and more widely used in clinical laboratories. Although these advanced technologies can be available in any laboratory, only the laboratories certified by Clinical Laboratory Improvement Amendments (CLIA of 1988) are qualified to make clinical diagnoses for patient care, and only pathologists have access to these diagnostic tools.
3) Pathologists have first-hand laboratory data on therapeutic targets of disease and patients' pharmacogenomics, pharmacoproteomics, and pharmacometabolomics (10). With the help of AI analysis, they can integrate all these data and design therapeutic plans for managing patients. Under the guidance of precision pathologists, clinicians (and/or pharmacists) will use these therapeutic plans to manage patients.
4) With direct access to patient specimens, pathologists have an advantage in carrying out translational research, such as biomarker discovery, identification of novel therapeutic targets, and pharmacometabolomics-informed pharmacogenomics (11). The research discoveries can be translated directly into clinical practice.
5) Since precision medicine considers individual variability, clinician-led population-based clinical trials to generalize a therapeutic regimen will eventually give way to target-based and individualized therapeutic plans designed by precision pathologists and precision clinicians.

Both involved in diagnostic science, pathologists and radiologists play unique roles in precision medicine. As AI will be heavily employed in radiology, image interpretation will be accelerated and promptly reported with almost no delays, which will make it possible to skip image interpretation to immediately perform tissue biopsy if a malignancy is suspected. Effective collaboration of radiologists and pathologists is already happening between interventional radiologists and cytopathologists. With various molecular tools available, a limited amount of tumor cells/tissues obtained by fine-needle aspiration (FNA)/core needle biopsy (CNB) might be able to provide therapeutic targets for treatment of patients prior to a pathological diagnosis. To expedite diagnostic studies, radiology might be combined with pathology in providing diagnostic service to clinicians. A proposal to establish Human Diagnostic Medicine is currently under discussion, and cross-disciplinary diagnostics may be an emerging but challenging practice in the future.

As critical members of the precision medicine team, precision pathologists will be more actively involved in devising therapeutic strategies in managing patients due to the advantages they have in obtaining the firsthand materials and information required for the effective management of patients (Figure 1.2). Instead of the current horizontally organized departmental teaming, vertical teams with a primary care provider, radiologist/surgeon, pathologist, omics expert, and hematologist/oncologist are needed to provide care to an individual patient with a diagnosed malignancy. In contrast to clinicians who should be familiar with drug efficacy and adverse effects, precision pathologists should be familiar with the therapeutic targets and pharmacomics of those agents so that they can provide information for clinicians to optimally manage patients. Although at the current stage, ordering molecular tests remains largely clinician driven, with the decreasing costs of molecular testing, increasing availability of FDA-approved therapeutic agents, and application of AI, molecular testing will be more and more the responsibility of precision pathologists.

Traditional pathologists are consultants to clinicians and passively provide advice and suggestions to clinicians, who directly take care of patients. These roles may change in the future of precision medicine. According to one vision, if a healthcare system is likened to an airplane (12), within the patient care team, the pathologist is the pilot, with the radiologist being the co-pilot and the omics expert the flight engineer. The radiologist, like radar, will identify the accurate location of lesions, and the omics expert will provide the landscape for the route, whereas the pathologist will fly the healthcare team (surgeons and oncologists) to the destination—optimal care of the patient. Although it remains controversial whether this comparison is accurate, this vision stresses the critical role of precision pathologists in future precision medicine.

Thanks to the inherited advantages of precision pathologists, they will lead the duty-bound advancement of precision

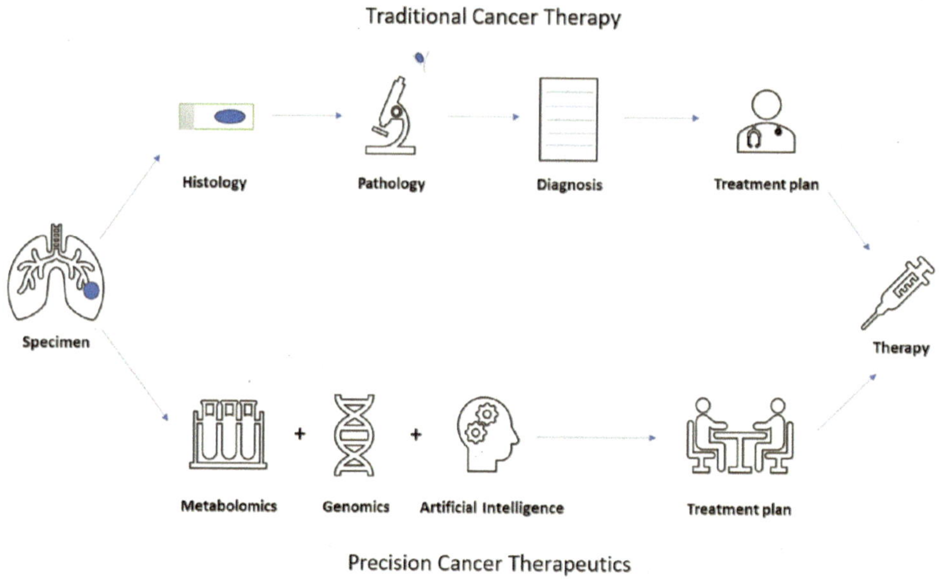

FIGURE 1.2 Change of patient care practice. Traditional procedure flow of cancer diagnosis and treatment (upper) vs. future precision cancer therapeutics (lower) with precision pathology guiding the treatment plan.

medicine, and thus precision pathology will not only be the basis of precision medicine but also guide its direction. The important role of pathologists in precision medicine cannot be overstressed and will be further elaborated upon in the next chapter.

1.6 Challenges and Opportunities

As a yet-to-be-explored frontier, precision pathology also faces many challenges. For example, whole genome/exome sequencing (WGS/WES) remains expensive and unaffordable to most patients, the clinical significance of most genetic variants remains unknown, and FDA-approved targeted molecular agents are only available to a handful of oncogenic drivers. All these will restrict the full potential of precision pathology in clinical practice. Precision pathology is also limited by current issues in molecular diagnostics. For examples, most genetic tests in molecular pathology laboratories have not been standardized, the sources of reference materials remain undetermined, omics is still a dream for most of the clinical laboratories, and AI has just been utilized in analyzing histology images. There is a lack of the current procedural terminology (CPT) codes for reimbursement of significant numbers of molecular tests. All these challenges are hurdles hindering the advancement of precision pathology, while they also provide new opportunities for it.

1.7 Summary

Precision pathology, as an exciting new concept, will have a strong impact on precision medicine. With inherited advantages, precision pathologists should take on leadership roles in the direction of precision medicine. As a new frontier, bumps and bends do exist in the path. Even with those challenges, precision pathology will become routine in future pathology laboratories, and every pathologist should be familiar with precision pathology and eventually become a precision pathologist. The concept of precision pathology should be integrated into the curriculum of pathology courses in the medical schools, residency programs, and fellowship training. All these will be discussed in depth in later chapters.

REFERENCES

1. Golub TR, Slonim DK, Tamayo P, et al. Molecular classification of cancer: Class discovery and class prediction by gene expression monitoring. Science. 1999; 286(5439): 531–537.
2. Hummel M, Bentink S, Berger H, et al. A biologic definition of Burkitt's lymphoma from transcriptional and genomic profiling. N Engl J Med. 2006; 354(23): 2419–2430.
3. Dave SS, Fu K, Wright GW. Molecular diagnosis of Burkitt's lymphoma. N Engl J Med. 2006; 354(23): 2431–2442.
4. Salaverria I, Martin-Guerrero I, Wagener R, et al. A recurrent 11q aberration pattern characterizes a subset of MYC-negative high-grade B-cell lymphomas resembling Burkitt lymphoma. Blood. 2014; 123(8): 1187–1198.
5. Meyer SC, Keller MD, Chiu S, et al. CHZ868, a Type II JAK2 inhibitor, reverses Type I JAK inhibitor persistence and demonstrates efficacy in myeloproliferative neoplasms. Cancer Cell. 2015; 28(1): 15–28.
6. Wu SC, Li LS, Kopp N, et al. Activity of the Type II JAK2 inhibitor CHZ868 in B cell acute lymphoblastic leukemia. Cancer Cell. 2015; 28(1): 29–41.

7. Zhao XF, Hassan A, Perry A, et al. C-MYC rearrangements are frequent in aggressive mature B-Cell lymphoma with atypical morphology. Int J Clin Exp Pathol. 2008; 1(1): 65–74.
8. Jares P, Colomer D, Campo E. Molecular pathogenesis of mantle cell lymphoma. J Clin Invest. 2012; 122(10): 3416–3423.
9. Zhao XF. Precision pathology—A new frontier. Hematopathology. 2018; 3(2): 24–25.
10. Neavin D, Kaddurah-Daouk R, Weinshilboum R. Pharmacometabolomics informs pharmacogenomics. Metabolomics. 2016; 12(7): 121.
11. Ji Y, Hebbring S, Zhu H, et al. Glycine and a glycine dehydrogenase (GLDC) SNP as citalopram/escitalopram response biomarkers in depression: Pharmacometabolomics-informed pharmacogenomics. Clin Pharmacol Ther. 2011; 89(1): 97–104.
12. Seltzer S. The diagnostic cockpit of the future: A unified vision of data output. Presentation at the APC 2019 Annual Meeting, Boston, MA.

2

The Role of Precision Pathologists

Maher Albitar and Xianfeng F. Zhao

2.1 Introduction

Precision medicine requires precision pathology (1). While companion diagnostic testing is one part of precision pathology delivering information on a specific biomarker, pathologists are also required to deliver a precise diagnosis, determine the underlying biological and molecular abnormalities, define the potential clinical course and prognosis, and point out the targetable abnormalities for therapy selection. Furthermore, pathologists can play a major role in monitoring the efficacy of therapy, determining response, and predicting relapse.

The old concept of the pathologist as the physician who looks through the microscope and makes a diagnosis is no longer acceptable. Pathologists must be involved in all aspects of patient care, and pathologists' role is becoming more difficult and demanding. A modern pathologist must be a scientist, diagnostician, and, to some degree, a clinician. Furthermore, pathologists must have proper familiarity with the financial implications of reimbursement for clinical decisions. This broadening role of pathologists represents a significant challenge for pathology practices and departments as well as hospitals. These challenges must be addressed in training programs and the workflow in pathology departments.

New drugs and therapeutic approaches are being developed at a faster pace than ever before, and this is helping in changing the practice of medicine. The state of the science behind the practice of medicine is very exciting in this fast-paced expansion in our knowledge of diseases. Moreover, a tremendous array of tools and technology is now available for pathologists to use and explore in daily practice. Keeping up with all these changes requires hard work and continuous focus on education and learning. Pathologists must take the lead in adapting and implementing the new changes. In this chapter, we will attempt to define the changes in the practice of pathology, define the challenges in our practice, and propose some ideas to address them.

2.2 Precision Medicine and Precision Pathology

The promise of precision medicine is to provide medical care that is individualized for the specific disease for the specific patient (2). While pathologists were the first to point out the variation between patients in qualifiable fashion, now it is also important to quantify this variation. For example, pathologists have pointed out for many years that not all adenocarcinomas of the colon are the same; now it is important to point out the specific differences, like the presence or absence of mutations in *KRAS*, *BRAF*, *APC*, or others (3). Furthermore, it is becoming important to designate differences in the host constitution and corresponding response to their disease. A patient with a germline specific polymorphism or mutation may require a specific treatment, as the outcome might be different from those patients without this specific germline abnormality (4). Additionally, the host immune response to the disease might be different between patients. For example, solid tumors with lymphoid cells infiltrating the tumor may dictate an outcome that is different from that in patients with a less active tumor microenvironment (5).

The pathologist's evaluation of the disease must consider and report all these variations and explain their clinical implications. This is particularly relevant in cancer diagnosis and treatment but can be expanded to other non-neoplastic diseases.

2.3 Pathologist as a Member of Multidisciplinary Team

Precision medicine requires a precise understanding of the patient's status and the exact features of the disease. This requires a multidisciplinary team, including an internist, oncologist, pathologist, pharmacist, radiologist, and frequently radiotherapist and surgeon. The interaction between various members of the team is very important for the delivery of proper therapy carefully tailored for the specific patient. Pathologists' workflow and pathology departments must be structured to accommodate such interaction.

With patient-centered care, the patient can order molecular tests directly through commercial labs. Except for oncologists in academic institutions (approximately 20%), most community oncologists (approximately 80%) have limited knowledge of cancer genetics/genomics, proteomics, metabolomics, and pharmacomics. A huge amount of genetic/genomic, proteomic, metabolomic, and pharmacomic data generated in molecular diagnostic laboratories need to be interpreted, and community oncologists need to be educated by precision pathologists for them to design optimal care plans for precision therapy of their patients.

DOI: 10.1201/9781003513469-2

2.4 Pathologists as the Keepers of Tissue Samples and Biological Sample Repositories

Samples are extremely important in the age of biomarkers. Pathologists should be responsible for determining what type of samples need to be collected, as well as dictating their quantity and quality. Furthermore, they should be very careful in using these samples. They should pay careful attention to all needed tests and how tissue can accommodate all needed tests, not only at that moment but also potentially in the future. This is particularly important since core or needle biopsy is frequently used to obtain samples. Residual samples should be carefully logged, categorized, and stored. Pathologists should be responsible for maintaining and updating a database that clearly characterizes the samples and provides protocols and tools for de-identification. The database must be easily searchable and should be updated for any change in inventory. This should not only be limited to tissue samples collected for the purpose of establishing diagnosis but also include samples collected proactively for potential future research and innovation. Samples should be collected with flexibility and an open mind to allow for future development helpful to individual patients, to pure research, and to the development of new assays. For example, plasma, serum, urine, and even saliva might be appropriate samples for certain tests. Pathologists should be familiar with and responsible for the proper process for protecting patients' rights and confidentiality and making sure that proper consent and institutional review board approval are obtained.

2.5 Pathologists and Tumor Heterogeneity

With targeted therapy, it is important to distinguish between founding or trunk mutation and progressor or secondary mutations. Targeted therapy, when used to eliminate cancer, should target the founding mutation. Heterogeneity within the tumor sample and the co-presence of multiple subclones in a tumor should be noted by the pathologist using various technologies, including morphology, immunohistochemistry, and molecular diagnostics. It is imperative that this heterogeneity be studied fully and described and explained to the treating physician, so therapy decisions are tailored to target all subclones.

2.6 Pathologists and Clinical Trials

Pathologists are frequently asked to be involved in clinical trials not only to confirm diagnosis and evaluate response but also to design and test biomarkers that can be used for selecting patients or for correlative exploratory research. The pathologist must be engaged in the entire process and should give full advice on proper testing for confirming diagnosis or response as well as on the practicality and robustness of the methodology employed in the test. Selecting the proper technology to be used in the companion testing may make a huge difference in determining the robustness and accuracy of the companion test, and as such, the pathologist should guide development of companion testing with a practical scientific approach and consideration of potential commercial issues or problems that may arise.

The focus of pharmaceutical companies is usually to get approval for a drug, and a consulted pathologist must balance the interest of the pharmaceutical company and selection of the proper companion test that is reliable and cost effective and can be easily adapted in various laboratories.

2.7 Pathology Reports

Due to an exponential expansion of knowledge in biology and medicine, pathology reports should not only be comprehensive but also provide basic and practical information on the findings, as well as recommendations for therapeutic approaches. Pathology reports should provide a general discussion of the clinical relevance and implications of the morphologic, immunophenotypic, and genomic findings. This information will help the treating physician to make more educated decisions about the patient and course of action.

Keeping up with scientific developments and individual patient data and having them available to pathologists frequently requires help from databases and algorithms that should be developed by pathology practices as dictated by specialization. Pathologists should take advantage of artificial intelligence and computer-aided decision making in their daily practice.

Furthermore, patients currently have the right to request and read their own pathology reports, and, in our opinion, pathology reports should incorporate a section that describes and summarizes the findings in simple terms for a lay person.

2.8 Pathologists and Commercial Diagnostic Companies

With the advent of highly sophisticated technology requiring specialized skill and expensive instruments, diagnostic pathology is becoming more dependent on reference laboratories that have the volume to justify investing in expensive instruments and recruitment of highly specialized and skilled individuals. However, this creates a new challenge for pathologists, both the pathologists referring samples to commercial laboratories and the pathologists recruited to work for those commercial laboratories. While commercial diagnostic companies and hospital-based laboratories are expected to generate profits, pathologists must play a significant role in preserving the integrity of pathology practice and offer the most reliable services for their patients with the concept of "do no harm, medically or financially".

Selecting and ordering the appropriate medically necessary and cost-effective tests in current medical practice is becoming very difficult and complex. Practicing clinicians need the pathologist's advice in selecting the proper and cost-effective tests, and it is the duty of the pathologists to be current and knowledgeable about the various technologies and tests offered on the market.

Furthermore, pathologists employed by commercial companies should insist on being the ones who approve clinical tests, resist the pressure of the business, and not approve or offer tests that are not robust or reliable. Unfortunately, some commercial companies are driven by market pressure and offer tests that are unreliable or provide tests that are not supported by proper clinical data. On the other hand, some tests provide important information that should be considered with other clinical and laboratory findings but are not covered by the Centers for Medicare and Medicaid Services (CMS) or insurance companies, and these tests can be very valuable for patient care. Pathologists should order the best and most accurate tests when needed, irrespective of the coverage by insurance companies or CMS. Not all clinical laboratory tests give a binary result, and many provide information in gray zones that, when considered with other findings, may give highly important information. For example, a patient with a mutation in exon 18 of the *EGFR* gene may respond to EGFR tyrosine kinase inhibitors (TKIs) even though most such inhibitors are not clinically tested against mutations in exon 18 (6). When a pathologist is faced with selecting a test that includes mutations in exon 18 of *EGFR* in addition to standard testing (exons 19, 20 and 21) vs. a test that includes exon 18, the pathologist should select the more comprehensive test and explain the lack of confirmation of response data for mutation in exon 18. Commercial companies may choose the test that is reimbursable, but pathologists should order and approve the most comprehensive and reliable test. Pathologists should not accept offering a test that may deprive the patient of receiving potentially effective therapy.

Most commercial companies evaluate pathologists based on productivity and exert pressure to do more and generate more revenue. While productivity should be the pathologist's goal, it should not compromise patient care. Some cases may require significantly more time than others, and each case should be given the proper attention and time to be fully evaluated.

2.9 Challenges for Pathologists

Recently, the FDA announced its interest in regulating laboratory testing and laboratory-developed tests (LDTs). While the intention of the FDA is to ensure that clinical laboratories are offering safe and reliable testing, considering the rate of advances in the field of testing, the extra level of complexity needed in going through FDA approval may hamper the rate of progress in testing. Further, by the time a test is approved by the FDA, the technology or the principle of such testing may be obsolete. Pathologists practice medicine when they invent a new test, but they do not manufacture devices. Tests must take advantage of state-of-the art technology and the most updated scientific knowledge. Pathologists are trained and should be continuously educated to perform this job and functionality.

Unfortunately, some tests being offered by commercial companies are not well developed, and these companies may make statements that are not well supported by evidence. Such a practice is forcing regulatory agencies such as the FDA to interfere and regulate those tests. Therefore, it is necessary for pathologists to be more vocal and active in regulating diagnostics and not allow a few commercial companies and willing pathologists to compromise the integrity of clinical testing.

2.10 Summary

It is a very exciting time to be a practicing pathologist. There is more than ever a need for laboratory testing and biomarkers to guide clinicians in their clinical decisions. Diagnoses and disease classifications are becoming more dependent on solid molecular and immunophenotypic markers and less dependent on subjective morphologic features. Biomarkers are becoming the cornerstone for most of the new therapeutic approaches in precision medicine. However, pathologists must adapt to the rapid changes in medicine, biology, technology, and informatics. They must be deeply involved in molecular advances, and they must lead in integrating the new knowledge and technology into everyday medicine. Accepting and implementing machine learning and artificial intelligence might be necessary to keep up with every field of medicine and pathology.

REFERENCES

1. Dietel M. Molecular pathology: A requirement for precision medicine in cancer. Oncol Res Treat. 2016;39(12):804–810.
2. Schork NJ. Personalized medicine: Time for one-person trials. Nature. 2015;520(7549):609–611.
3. Rodriguez-Salas N, Dominguez G, Barderas R, et al. Clinical relevance of colorectal cancer molecular subtypes. Crit Rev Oncol Hematol. 2017;109:9–19.
4. Smith SA, French T, Hollingsworth SJ. The impact of germline mutations on targeted therapy. J Pathol. 2014;232(2):230–243.
5. Zito Marino F, Ascierto PA, Rossi G, et al. Are tumor-infiltrating lymphocytes protagonists or background actors in patient selection for cancer immunotherapy? Expert Opin Biol Ther. 2017;17(6):735–746.
6. Ma W, Brodie S, Agersborg S, et al. Significant improvement in detecting BRAF, KRAS, and EGFR mutations using next-generation sequencing as compared with FDA-cleared kits. Mol Diagn Ther. 2017;21(5):571–579.

3

Ethical Issues in Precision Pathology

Xianfeng F. Zhao

3.1 Introduction

Since its inception in 2011, precision medicine has been rife with bioethical controversy (1). Numerous research initiatives have proposed to address the bioethical issues, such as the health disparity, privacy, and security (2, 3). The last decade has also seen hot debates over the bioethics of precision medicine (4) that spill over to precision pathology.

Traditionally, pathologists assume few ethical responsibilities other than reporting laboratory results without violating patient privacy and confidentiality. They usually leave the difficult clinical decisions to clinicians. However, as their involvement in clinical decision-making processes grows, and more patients order genetic tests directly from laboratories, pathologists will become involuntarily involved in ethical conundrums due to reporting genetic results of unknown clinical, social, and economic significance and reporting to stakeholders other than the patient.

3.2 Autonomy vs. Social Responsibility

Beauchamp enumerated four principles of health care ethics (5): *beneficence*, *maleficence*, *autonomy*, and *justice*. Principles of patient autonomy and new regulations (6, 7) enable patients to order genetic tests directly from laboratories without prescription by primary care providers. With enormous marketing efforts on TV, print advertisement, and the Internet by booming direct-to-consumer genetic testing (DTC-GT) laboratories, genetic testing has become a commodity rather than just a diagnostic tool. Testing results are commonly used for predictions about health, providing information about common traits, and offering clues for a person's ancestry. But it is not as simple as getting a flu shot. There are far more serious implications. Interpretation of the testing results is not always straightforward since the functions of many genes are still yet to be defined; genetic results affect not only the subject who orders the test but also the subject's closest relatives, such as siblings and children who may or may not want to know the genetic results. Certain genetic diseases may also lead to increased premiums for health and life insurance. Certain genetic abnormalities may be utilized for legal defense of certain crimes. If disclosed, genetic information may also affect the subject's employment.

3.3 Reporting Genes with Unknown Functions

Remarkable technological advancements such as next-generation sequencing (NGS) can generate large amounts of data and identify numerous variant mutations in a matter of days, but our current knowledge of the clinical significance of some variants is lagging far behind. These variants of uncertain significance (VUS) can be identified in genes with known or unknown functions. Some VUS may be relevant to sequencing for the original rationale for sequencing the patient, whereas others may be unrelated. Some unknown VUS may have clinical significance and deserve further investigation, while others might just reflect polymorphism of little significance. Vears et al. surveyed 27 laboratory personnel, representing 24 laboratories in Europe, Canada, and Australia, and they found variation in the reporting practices of VUS across the laboratories within the study (8). To avoid this reporting dilemma, many commercial laboratories choose to sequence limited numbers of genes in their panels, which largely consist of genes with well-known functions. Although there is no consensus as to which VUS should or should not be on their reports, standards and guidelines have been established by a joint effort by the American College of Medical Genetics and Genomics and the Association for Molecular Pathology for interpreting VUS (9). However, large variations in reporting policies still exist between laboratories in the world (10).

3.4 Who Should Know the Results or Be Tested?

Almost all diseases are caused by two factors: 1) an intrinsic cause from the human body or 2) extrinsic environmental factor(s), including radiation, toxicity, and biohazard pathogens. Although lifestyle can change the condition of our bodies to some extent, what we cannot change is the genetic makeup we inherited from our parents. As we are aware that we are sick because we are genetically liable to diseases, genetic information will always have some implications, particularly for some diseases with serious disability and fatality. One extreme example is prion disease. When a *PRNP* variant has been detected in an index case, should the relatives be informed and/or tested as well?

A small study showed that anxiety rates were high and similar between noncarriers and untested subjects when they were told the risk of a devastating genetic disease. Whether the relatives were informed and/or tested did not seem to make a difference (11).

DOI: 10.1201/9781003513469-3

Amyotrophic lateral sclerosis (ALS) is another devastating genetic disease. Since its familiar forms and the sporadic forms are clinically indistinguishable and over 30 genetic mutations have been linked to the familial forms and rarely the sporadic forms, identification of a mutation in one family member will lead to requests for testing from relatives who are eager to know their own individual risk of developing ALS (12).

Cancer is a genetic malignancy, and *BRCA1*, *BRCA2*, and *TP53* mutations have been implicated in lifetime high risk of breast cancer development (13). Although it is well accepted in the Western world that mastectomy and salpingo-oophorectomy are used to lower the risk of breast cancer and ovarian cancer in patients with mutations in those genes (14), in Asian countries, family members may hesitate to be genetically tested for those mutations for the following reasons: high costs of tests, perceived lack of ability to cope with test results, and insufficient information about genetic testing (15).

3.5 Healthcare Disparity

Owing to the innovations in NGS, we have seen a marked decrease in the costs of genetic testing. As compared to routine chemistry and hematology tests, genetic tests remain expensive. Most insurance companies either entirely or partially cover the costs of genetic testing if the tests are requested by the health care providers. Medicare and Medicaid usually also cover medically indicated genetic tests. However, DTC genetic tests are usually paid for by patients out of their own pockets.

Because of this, genetic tests are a luxury of the rich, and low-income families cannot afford expensive genetic tests unless it is medically indicated. When a mutation variant is identified in a rich person, the poor relatives will not be able to access their own genetic information even though they may have huge anxiety. Inequality and injustice become the ethical issues of precision pathology.

Whole genome sequencing (WGS) is no longer a dream and can be performed for $100 (16). Laboratory developed tests (LDTs) will play an important role in this endeavor and become a target for regulation by US Food and Drug Administration (FDA), Congress, and other stakeholders (17). Whether WGS routinely performed on all newborns should be a standard of care will be the next challenge facing regulatory agencies. Changes of coding and coverage which lead to lower reimbursement may also impose a financial burden on clinical testing laboratories and thus hinder patient access to genetic tests (18).

3.6 Standard Care

On September 18, 2019, Congressman Eric Swalwell reintroduced the bipartisan bill Advancing Access to Precision Medicine Act (19), which would pilot-test whether Medicaid coverage of a variety of types of genetic and genomic sequencing for children can help settle their diagnostic challenges, improve clinical outcomes, and ultimately reduce program expenditures. On January 27, 2020, the Centers for Medicare & Medicaid Services (CMS) announced that NGS for beneficiaries with inherited ovarian or breast cancer will be covered by Medicare (20). Currently only genetic tests for certain diseases have become the standard of care and can be reimbursed by Medicare and Medicaid. One universal genetic test should be the WGS for all newborns whether they have insurance coverage or not. This approach will identify all the harmful mutations at the beginning of life, and many diseases can be prevented and treated early. For example, glucose-6-phosphate dehydrogenase (G6PD) deficiency disease, if detected early, can be prevented by avoiding oxidative stressors (21) or corrected by CRISPR as in sickle cell disease (22). Similar approaches can be used for other hemoglobinopathies, such as hemoglobin S/C disease and hemoglobin S/β+ thalassemia. Gene mutations with the ability to cause cardiovascular diseases and hypertension can be prevented by adopting a healthy lifestyle in early life. Detection of mutations in oncogenes and tumor suppressor genes may also enable us to start surveillance early, manage tumors properly, and prolong the patient's life expectancy.

3.7 Prenatal Tests and the Fetus's Rights

There are lots of debates over fetal rights (23). Prenatal genetic tests are currently utilized to identify fetuses with genetic defects and prevent the birth of unhealthy children such as those with Down syndrome and other overt inherited genetic diseases. With booming DTC-GT services, parent(s) may request WGS directly from laboratories to look for certain genetic diseases in order to make a decision on abortion (23). Then the fetus's right will be challenged. Genetic tests could also be used to identify a fetus as a result of adultery and cause tensions between legal partners (24). Prenatal genetic tests have also been used by parents in some cultures to select male fetuses (25), leading to imbalanced gender distribution in the population.

3.8 Genetic Discrimination and Eugenics

There are no "good" or "bad" genes, but some genes may be associated with more desirable features or healthy traits, whereas other genes may be associated with health risks. If disclosed, individuals with "undesirable" genes may be discriminated against, find it hard to have a relationship, experience more difficulty finding a job, and be declined for health and life insurances. Although genetic information can be utilized to improve the health and quality of life of individuals and is being used to select embryos when employing *in vitro* fertilization (26), this information could also be used by some people to control "undesirable" populations (27) and provide a ground for racists and Nazis (28). Eugenics for "desirable" features will eventually abolish genetic diversity, which is entirely undesirable for humankind.

3.9 Summary

With more involvement in clinical decision making, precision pathologists will share more ethical responsibilities with their clinical partners. They will seek informed consent from patients for molecular tests, select tissue sources for diagnostic studies, choose gene panels and analysis methodologies, recommend drugs and dosages for therapy, monitor therapeutic efficacy and adverse effects, and evaluate clinical outcomes and document any undesirable reactions. Since medicine is individualized, each individual patient will have a unique pathological analysis and therapy. New medical and ethical standards need to be established to apply to this newly emerging discipline.

REFERENCES

1. National Research Council (US) Committee on a Framework for Developing a New Taxonomy of Disease. Toward Precision Medicine: Building a Knowledge Network for Biomedical Research and a New Taxonomy of Disease. Washington, DC: National Academies Press; 2011.
2. Sankar PL, Parker LS. The precision medicine initiative's all of us research program: An agenda for research on its ethical, legal, and social issues. Genet Med. 2017; 19(7): 743–750.
3. Korngiebel DM, Thummel KE, Burke W. Implementing precision medicine: The ethical challenges. Trends Pharmacol Sci. 2017; 38(1): 8–14.
4. Roberts JS, Ostergren J. Direct-to-consumer genetic testing and personal genomics services: A review of recent empirical studies. Curr Genet Med Rep. 2013; 1(3): 182–200.
5. Beauchamp TL. The 'four principles' approach to health care ethics. In: Ashcroft RE, Dawson A, Draper H, et al. eds. Principles of Health Care Ethics. 2. West Sussex: John Wiley & Sons, Inc; 2007: 3–10.
6. Direct access testing from concept to reality. AACC/ASCLS Healthcare Forum. July 23, 2003, Philadelphia, PA.
7. Institute of Medicine (US) Committee on Quality of Healthcare in America. Crossing the Quality Chasm: A New Health System for the 21st Century. Washington, DC: National Academy Press; 2001.
8. Veers DF, Senekal K, Berry P. Reporting practices for variants of uncertain significance from next generation sequencing technologies. Eur J Med Genet. 2017: 60(10): 553–558.
9. Richards S, Aziz N, Bale S, et al. Standards and guidelines for the interpretation of sequence variants: A joint consensus recommendation of the American College of Medical Genetics and Genomics and the Association for Molecular Pathology. Genet Med. 2015; 17(5): 405–424.
10. Vears DF, Niemiec E, Howard HC, et al. Analysis of VUS reporting, variant reinterpretation and recontact policies in clinical genomic sequencing consent forms. Eur J Hum Genet. 2018; 26(12): 1743–1751.
11. Schwartz M, Brandel JP, Babonneau ML, et al. Genetic testing in prion disease: Psychological consequences of the decisions to know or not to know. Front Genet. 2019; 10: 895.
12. Corcia P, Lumbroso S, Cazeneuve C, et al. Pre-symptomatic diagnosis in ALS. Rev Neurol (Paris). 2020; 176(3): 166–169.
13. Lalloo F, Evans DG. Familial breast cancer. Clin Genet. 2012; 82(2): 105–114.
14. Domchek SM, Friebel TM, Singer CF, et al. Association of risk-reducing surgery in BRCA1 or BRCA2 mutation carriers with cancer risk and mortality. JAMA. 2010; 304(9): 967–975.
15. Sun S, Li ST, Ngeow J. Factors shaping at-risk individuals' decisions to undergo genetic testing for cancer in Asia. Health Soc Care Commun. 2020; 28(5): 1569–1577.
16. Neville S. Cheaper DNA sequencing unlocks secrets of rare diseases. Financial Times. 5 March 2018. Retrieved 30 September 2020. https://www.ft.com/content/017a3a50-f6f1-11e7-a4c9-bbdefa4f210b
17. Klein RD. Current policy challenges in genomic medicine. Clin Chem. 2020; 66(1): 61–67.
18. Hsiao SJ, Mansukhani MM, Carter MC, et al. The history and impact of molecular coding changes on coverage and reimbursement of molecular diagnostic tests: Transition from stacking codes to the current molecular code set including genomic sequencing procedures. J Mol Diagn. 2018; 20(2): 177–183.
19. Swalwell reintroduced the bipartisan bill advancing personalized medicine. Press Release. 18 September 2019. Retrieved 31 August 2020. https://swalwell.house.gov/media-center/press-releases/swalwell-reintroduces-bipartisan-bill-advancing-personalized-medicine
20. Waddill K. CMS: Medicare will cover genetic diagnostics for certain cancers. HealthPayerIntelligence. xtelligent Healthcare Media. 2012–2020. Retrieved 31 August 2020. https://healthpayerintelligence.com/news/cms-medicare-will-cover-genetic-diagnostics-for-certain-cancers
21. Bubp J, Jen M, Matuszewski K. Caring for glucose-6-phosphate dehydrogenase (G6PD)-deficient patients: Implications for pharmacy. P T. 2015; 40(9): 572–574.
22. Hoban MD, Lumaquin D, Kuo CY, et al. CRISPR/Cas9-mediated correction of the sickle mutation in human CD34+ cells. Mol Ther. 2016; 24(9): 1561–1569.
23. Paul A. Controversial conceptions: The unborn and the American Convention on Human Rights. Loyola Univ Chi Int Law Rev. 2012; 9: 208–247. Retrieved 31 August 2020. https://lawecommons.luc.edu/cgi/viewcontent.cgi?article=1001&context=lucilr
24. Kass LR. Toward a More Natural Science: Biology and Human Affairs. New York: Free Press; 1985: 80.
25. Oomman N, Ganatra BR. Sex selection: The systematic elimination of girls. Reprod Health Matters. 2002; 10(19): 184–188.
26. Sevulescu J. Procreative beneficence: Why we should select the best children. Bioethics. 2001; 15(5-6): 413–426.
27. DenHoed A. The forgotten lessons of the American eugenics movement. The New Yorker. 27 April 2016. Retrieved 30 August 2020. https://www.newyorker.com/books/page-turner/the-forgotten-lessons-of-the-american-eugenics-movement
28. Black E. War against the Weak: Eugenics and America's Campaign to Create a Master Race. New York: Four Walls Eight Windows; 2003: 438.

4

Molecular Basis of Precision Pathology

Xianfeng F. Zhao

4.1 Introduction

Precision medicine rests on advanced knowledge of the molecular mechanisms of cancer and other human diseases and molecular evidence provided by pathology laboratories. Molecular evidence includes biomarkers and therapeutic targets to be utilized in precision therapy. Among millions of genetic, genomic, proteomic, and metabolomic variations, only a small number have been well defined with clear clinical significance. This chapter will discuss the recent advances in molecular cancer biology and cutting-edge technologies to define the molecular basis for the practice of precision pathology.

4.2 Drivers vs. Riders

Genotype determines phenotype, and we have long believed that cancer develops owing to mutated "driver" genes (1, 2). Genetic alterations are common in cancer cells, but not all genetic alterations are important for cancer development (3); some genetic alterations cause cancer and thus are considered "drivers", whereas other alterations just happened to be carried by cancer cells; their presence is less relevant to cancer development, and thus they are called "riders" or "passengers". By using next-generation sequencing (NGS), we can easily detect hundreds and thousands of mutations in a cancer specimen, but how do we know which is a driver mutation and which is a rider mutation? Using structured, transparent, accessible reporting (STAR) methods, the Cancer Genome Atlas (TCGA) project has analyzed 9,079 tumor samples across 33 cancer types with 1,457,702 total mutations using seven algorithms and finally identified 299 unique genes (2). These so-called cancer driver genes harbor >3,400 putative missense driver mutations implied in anatomical sites and cancer/cell types. The authors believe that 299 genes is are still too many. To design 299 drugs to target all these mutations is not only infeasible but also cost ineffective.

By definition, the "driver" genes are usually activated oncogenes, for their mutations lead to tumor development; most of the oncogene products are components of signal transduction cascades, including growth factors; hormone receptors; G proteins; protein kinases; or transcription factors that regulate fundamental cellular processes such as growth, proliferation, differentiation, metabolism, and apoptosis. Classical oncogenes include *ABL1*, *JAK2*, *KRAS*, *MYC*, and *BRAF* (Table 4.1), and they are the most legitimate therapeutic targets for precision medicine (4). Some oncogene products are well-defined therapeutic targets for non-small cell lung cancer (NSCLC), such as EGFR, ALK, KRAS, MET, ROS, and RET. They are routinely analyzed for mutations by laboratories, and a family of small molecules and humanized antibodies are available for clinical use (5). Herceptin, a humanized antibody, has been used for years in the treatment of human epidermal growth factor receptor 2 (Her-2)–positive early breast cancer (6) and improved the survival of patients. Testing for *BRAF* mutations has been utilized to guide the treatment of melanomas with various inhibitors (7).

In contrast, tumor suppressor genes, when they have lost their normal functions by either deletions or missense mutations, will permit cancer development (8). *TP53* is the most well-known and classical tumor suppressor gene, and its abnormality is present in the vast majority of cancer types (9). Other tumor suppressor genes include *RB*, *APC*, and many genetic stability and DNA repair genes (Table 4.2) (10). Their normal function is to safeguard cells from neoplastic changes due to genetic damage, but they themselves can also be liable to genetic damage and thus lose their normal surveillance functions. When this happens, the cells will undergo uncontrollable growth, dedifferentiation, or immortality, and tumors will develop. An enormous amount of work has been done in targeting tumor suppressor genes, but correcting the function of tumor suppressor genes remains a challenge to precision therapeutics (11).

If both oncogenes and tumor suppressor genes are considered "driver" genes since changes in both kinds of genes lead to tumorigenesis, then what genes are considered "rider" genes? "Rider" genes refer to the genes that usually are present in cancer cells but do not cause neoplasia. They are usually biomarkers of end-stage differentiation or lineage determination. For example, pancytokeratin is a marker of epithelial cell differentiation and useful for classifying cancers into carcinomas, but it is at least now not considered a tumorigenic molecule. Leukocyte common antigen (LCA)/CD45 is a marker for white blood cells (WBCs), and if negative, it excludes hematopoietic origin. However, loss of CD45 suggests dedifferentiation of WBC and neoplastic change (12). Similar markers commonly used by pathologists are S100 and vimentin, which indicate neuroendocrine or mesenchymal origin of tumors. Several reactive biomarkers, though nonspecific, can be hallmarks for certain neoplastic process. For example, Hodgkin lymphoma is often associated with eosinophilia

DOI: 10.1201/9781003513469-4

TABLE 4.1

List of Oncogenes

Oncogene	Function/Activation	Cancer*
ABL1	Promotes cell growth through tyrosine kinase activity	Chronic myeloid leukemia
AFF4::MLLT11	Fusion affects the MLLT11 transcription factor/ methyltransferase MLLT11 is also called HRX, ALL1, and HTRX1	Acute leukemias
AKT2	Encodes a protein-serine/threonine kinase	Ovarian cancer
ALK	Encodes a receptor tyrosine kinase	Lymphomas
ALK::NPM	Translocation creates fusion protein with nucleophosmin (NPM)	Large cell lymphomas
RUNX1 (AML1)	Encodes a transcription factor	Acute myeloid leukemia
RUNX1::MTG8	New fusion protein created by translocation	Acute leukemias
AXL	Encodes a receptor tyrosine kinase	Hematopoietic cancers
BCL-2, 3, 6	Blocks apoptosis (programmed cell death)	B-cell lymphomas and leukemias
BCR::ABL1	New protein created by fusion of BCR and ABL triggers unregulated cell growth	Chronic myeloid and acute lymphoblastic leukemia
MYC	Transcription factor that promotes cell proliferation and DNA synthesis	Leukemia; breast, stomach, lung, cervical, and colon carcinomas; neuroblastomas and glioblastomas
MCF2 (DBL)	Guanine nucleotide exchange factor	Diffuse large B-cell lymphoma
DEK/NUP214	New protein created by fusion	Acute myeloid leukemia
TCF3::PBX1	New protein created by fusion TCF3 also called E2A	B-lymphoblastic leukemia
EGFR	Cell surface receptor that triggers cell growth through tyrosine kinase activity	Squamous cell carcinoma, glioblastomas, lung cancer
MLLT11	Fusion protein created by a translocation t(11;19)	Acute leukemias
ERG::FUS	Fusion protein created by t(16:21) translocation. The ERG protein is a transcription factor	Myeloid leukemia
ERBB2	Cell surface receptor that triggers cell growth through tyrosine kinase activity, a.k.a. HER2 or neu	Breast, salivary gland, and ovarian carcinomas
ETS1	Transcription factor	Lymphoma
EWSR1::FLI1	Fusion protein created by t(11:22) translocation.	Ewing sarcoma
CSF1R	Tyrosine kinase	Sarcoma
FOS	Transcription factor for API	Osteosarcoma
FES	Tyrosine kinase	Sarcoma
GLI1	Transcription factor	Glioblastoma
GNAS (GSP)	Membrane-associated G protein	Thyroid carcinoma
HER2/neu	Overexpression of signaling kinase due to gene amplification	Breast and cervical carcinomas
TLX1	Transcription factor, a.k.a. HOX11	T-lymphoblastic leukemia
FGF4	Encodes fibroblast growth factor, a.k.a. HST1	Breast and squamous cell carcinomas
IL3	Cell signaling molecule	B-lymphoblastic leukemia
FGF3 (INT-2)	Encodes a fibroblast growth factor	Breast and squamous cell carcinomas
JUN	Transcription factor for API	Sarcoma
KIT	Tyrosine kinase	Sarcoma
FGF4 (KS3)	Herpes virus-encoded growth factor	Kaposi sarcoma
K-SAM	Fibroblast growth factor receptor	Stomach carcinomas
AKAP13	Guanine nucleotide exchange factor, a.k.a. LBC	Myeloid leukemias
LCK	Tyrosine kinase	T-cell lymphoma
LMO1, LMO2	Transcription factors	T-cell lymphoma
MYCL	Transcription factor	Lung carcinomas
LYL1	Transcription factor	T-lymphoblastic leukemia
NFKB2	Transcription factor. Also called LYT-10	B-cell lymphoma

(Continued)

TABLE 4.1 (Continued)

Oncogene	Function/Activation	Cancer*
NFKB2/C±1	Fusion protein formed by the (10;14)(q24;q32) translocation of NFKB2 next to the C alpha 1 immunoglobulin locus	
MAS1	Angiotensin receptor	Mammary carcinoma
MDM2	Encodes a protein that inhibits and leads to the degradation of p53	Sarcomas
MLLT11	Transcription factor/methyltransferase (also called HRX and ALL1)	Acute myeloid leukemia
MOS	Serine/threonine kinase	Lung cancer
RUNX1T1	Fusion of transcription repressor to factor to a transcription factor. A.k.a. MTG8 and AML1-MTG8	Acute leukemias
MYB	Transcription factor	Colon carcinoma and leukemias
MYH11::CBFB	New protein created by fusion of transcription factors via an inversion in chromosome 16.	Acute myeloid leukemia
NEU	Tyrosine kinase. Also called ERBB2 or HER2	Glioblastomas and squamous cell carcinomas
MYCN	Cell proliferation and DNA synthesis	Neuroblastomas, retinoblastomas, and lung carcinomas
MCF2L (OST)	Guanine nucleotide exchange factor	Osteosarcomas
PAX5	Transcription factor	Lympho-plasmacytoid B-cell lymphoma
PBX1::E2A	Fusion protein formed via t(1:19) translocation. Transcription factor	B-lymphoblastic leukemia
PIM1	Serine/threonine kinase	T-cell lymphoma
CCND1	Encodes cyclin D1. Involved in cell cycle regulation. Also called PRAD1	Breast and squamous cell carcinomas
RAF1	Serine/threonine kinase	Many cancer types
RARA::PML	Fusion protein caused by t(15:17) translocation. Retinoic acid receptor	Acute promyelocytic leukemia
HRAS	G-protein. Signal transduction	Bladder carcinoma
KRAS	G-protein. Signal transduction	Lung, ovarian, and bladder carcinoma
NRAS	G-protein. Signal transduction	Breast carcinoma
REL::NRG	Fusion protein formed by deletion in chromosome 2. Transcription factor	B-cell lymphoma
RET	Cell surface receptor. Tyrosine kinase	Thyroid carcinomas, multiple endocrine neoplasia type 2
RHOM1, RHOM2	Transcription factors a.k.a. LMO1 and LMO2	T-lymphoblastic leukemia
ROS1	Tyrosine kinase	Sarcoma
SKI	Transcription factor	Carcinomas
SIS (a.k.a. *PDGFB*)	Growth factor	Glioma, fibrosarcoma
SET::CAN	Fusion protein formed by rearrangement of chromosome 9. Protein localization	Acute myeloid leukemia
SRC	Tyrosine kinase	Sarcomas
TAL1, TAL2	Transcription factor. TAL1 is also called SCL	T-lymphoblastic leukemia
NOTCH1 (TAN1)	Altered form of Notch (cellular receptor) formed by t(7:9) translocation	T-lymphoblastic leukemia
TIAM1	Guanine nucleotide exchange factor	T-cell lymphoma
TSC2	GTPase activator	Renal and brain tumors
NTRK1	Receptor tyrosine kinase	Colon and thyroid carcinomas

Source: modified from ref. 4

Note: * The cancer types listed in this column are those that are predominantly associated with each oncogene, but this is not a complete list.

TABLE 4.2

List of Tumor Suppressor Genes

Tumor Suppressor Gene	Product Function/Activation	Cancer*
APC	Protein that associates with beta-catenin	Colon/rectum carcinoma
BRCA1	Protein that is involved in repair damaged DNA	Breast and ovarian carcinomas
BRCA2	Protein that is involved in repair damaged DNA	Breast carcinoma

(Continued)

TABLE 4.2 (Continued)

Tumor Suppressor Gene	Product Function/Activation	Cancer*
DPC4/SMAD4	Protein that transduces TGF-ß signals from cell surface to nucleus	Pancreatic carcinoma
INK4	Inhibitors of CDK4: p16[INK4a], p15[INK4b], p18[INK4c], and p19[INK4d]	Melanoma, lung carcinoma, brain tumors, leukemias, lymphomas
MADR2	MAD-related protein 2 that regulates TGF-ß signaling	Colon/rectum carcinoma
NF1	Neurofibromin that helps regulate cell growth	Neurofibrosarcoma
NF2	Merlin, also known as schwannomin, that regulates several key signal transduction pathways controlling cell shape, growth, and adhesion	Meningioma
TP53	Transcription factor that plays complex roles in cell cycle checkpoints, senescence, autophagy, and apoptosis	Brain tumors; breast, colon/rectum, esophageal, liver, and lung carcinomas; sarcomas; leukemias and lymphomas
PTC/PTCH	Receptor for the secreted hedgehog ligands	Basal cell carcinoma
PTEN	A dual specificity protein and lipid phosphatase that blocks PI3K signaling	Brain tumors; melanoma; prostate, endometrial, kidney, and lung carcinomas
RB	Protein that inhibits cell cycle progression exerted through repression of the E2F1 transcription factor	Retinoblastoma; sarcomas; bladder, breast, and lung carcinomas
VHL	E3 ubiquitin ligase that negatively regulates the hypoxia inducible factor (HIF)	Renal cell carcinoma
WT1	Protein that plays a role in cell growth, differentiation and apoptosis	Wilms tumor

Source: modified from ref. 10

* The cancer types listed in this column are those that are predominantly associated with each tumor suppressor gene, but this is not a complete list.

and fibrosis due to IL-5 and TGF-β (13, 14) secreted by the lymphoma cells. Marrow fibrosis in myeloproliferative neoplasm (MPN) always indicates the release of platelet-derived growth factor (PDGF) by the dysplastic megakaryocytes (15). Some of the biomarkers, such as CD19, CD20, and CD79a in B cells and CD3 in T cells, not only indicate the lineages but also are components of signal transduction pathways (16–19). Although these biomarkers are currently not considered oncogene products, they have been targeted by various antibodies to suppress the growth of those cells (16–19) and even been proven effective.

4.3 Signal Transduction Cascades

Signals are transferred from the external environment to the cell nucleus via three steps: reception, transduction, and response. The first step involves the receptors embedded in the cell membrane. Activation of the receptor will trigger the signal transduction cascade all the way to the transcription factors in cell nucleus. As any of these three steps can go wrong and lead to malignancies, the components are usually encoded by the so-called proto-oncogenes (20), genes with potential to become oncogenes. Many of these oncogene products are biomarkers for pathological diagnosis of cancers and potential therapeutic targets for precision medicine (Table 4.3). Pan-Cancer analyses show that focal adhesion pathways, mitogen-activated protein kinase (MAPK) signaling, phosphatidylinositol-3-OH kinase (PI3K) signaling, Notch signaling, and Wnt/β-catenin signaling are the most commonly activated signal transduction pathways in cancers (21–23), and PI3K is the most common molecule that is involved in the interaction with these pathways (21), suggesting that crosstalk between different cancer pathways are universally present in cancers and targeting crosstalk is a reasonable strategy in precision oncology.

4.4 Oncogenic Network and Node Theory

Genes function via their products, such as RNA and proteins. Most oncogenes produce proteins that are components of signal transduction pathways, including growth factors, hormone receptors, G proteins, protein kinases, or transcription factors regulating fundamental cellular processes such as growth, proliferation, differentiation, metabolism, and apoptosis (20). More and more evidence indicates that external signals are transduced via networks rather than pathways (24). Crosstalk between pathways is not random and occurs at certain molecules (junctions) between different pathways. Signal transduction is not unidirectional, and frequent feedback and reflex arcs are present at many levels of the cascade (24).

The concept of functional "nodes" originated in 2009 (25) when the interactions between different signal transduction pathways were being investigated (Figure 4.1). A "node" refers to a junctional molecule that relays signals from one functional unit to another in a living cell. Although nodes can be any molecules that form an integral part of a functional network, here I focus on proteins. These proteins function as switches by phosphorylation (on) and dephosphorylation (off) to control the signal flows in the cells. Due to their critical roles in controlling cell information flow, nodes are important for both cancer cells and precision pathologists. Cancer develops by activation of oncogene products and depends on constitutive activation of the proto-oncogene products (26) and constant stimulus flow to the nucleus. The signals might be blocked by certain events, such as spontaneous mutation of the downstream molecules or deliberately targeting the molecules in the pathway. In order to keep the signal flow to the nucleus, cells will mobilize their reserve mechanism by shunting signals to a different pathway via the junctional "node" (24). Precision pathologists should pay special attention and make every effort to identify these "nodes".

TABLE 4.3
Signal Transduction Pathway Oncoproteins

Step	Component	Pathway	Cancer
Reception	EGFR	EGFR-ERB	Breast, lung
	PDGFRa	PI3K/AKT/mTOR	Bladder, breast, colon, lung, gastrointestinal stromal tumor
	PDGFRb	PI3K/AKT, RAS/ERK	Lung, colon, melanoma, etc.
	FGF1	PI3K/AKT, RAS/ERK	Breast
Transduction	PI3K	PI3K/AKT/mTOR	Lymphoma, prostate
	AKT	PI3K/AKT	Breast, prostate
	BRAF	RAS/RAF/MEK/ERK	Melanoma, papillary thyroid, ovary, colon
	mTOR	PI3K/AKT/mTOR	Breast, lymphoma
	RAS	RAS/MEK/ERK	Pancreatic, colon
	MEK	RAS/MEK/ERK	Various
	ERK	RAS/MEK/ERK	Various
Response	MYC	MYC pathway	Leukemia, lymphoma
	MYB		Leukemia, lymphoma

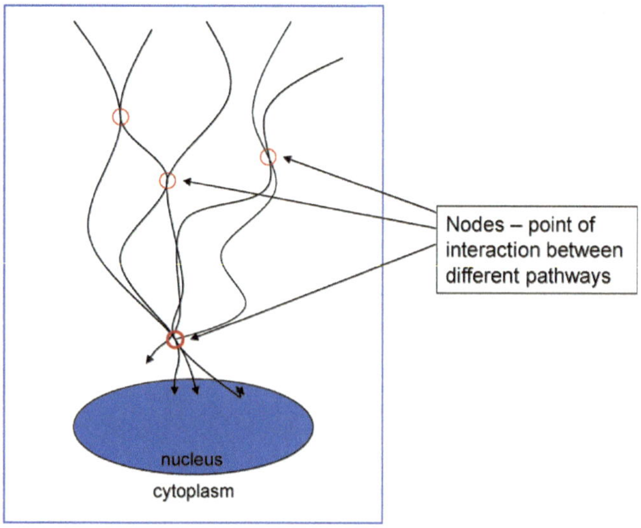

FIGURE 4.1 Crosstalk between different pathways occurs at the node (from ref. 25 with permission). The signal of one pathway can be shunted to a different pathway at the upstream node when there is a blockage (either by null mutation or inhibition) of signal transduction downstream. The more pathways crosstalk there, the more important the node is to the cellular function.

Cancer evolves and advances during its progression. One survival strategy is to gain novel function by mutations to adapt to the new environment and become resistant to specific therapy. Node theory provides an alternative mechanism of survival and drug resistance to cancer cells. The drug resistance I refer to here is resistance to targeted therapy towards certain oncogene products (24), not resistance to traditional cytotoxic chemotherapeutic agents. To optimize the efficacy of targeted therapeutic agents, identification of the "shunting" nodes is important for precision oncologists because their patients will receive the optimal therapeutic effects and clinical outcomes. Understanding the functional equilibrium of nodes will help us decrease the risk of secondary malignancies when treating primary cancers.

4.5 Cancer Epigenetics

Epigenetics, a term originally coined by Conrad Waddington to describe heritable changes in a cellular phenotype that were independent of alterations in the DNA sequence, refers to the process of changing the cellular function by chromatin modification (27). Epigenetics is one of the major drivers of myeloid neoplasms and thus the ideal target for precision therapy (28). Oncogenic transformation parallels the induced pluripotent reprogramming of stem cells (29). This process involves transcription factor and chromatin regulators. Transcription factors play roles as either facilitators or barriers depending on whether they are oncogenes or tumor suppressor genes. Similarly, chromatin regulators function as effectors and modulators of reprogramming and oncogenesis (29). Chromatin regulators are enzymes that regulate methylation of cytosines on DNA and posttranslational modification of histones (30). Post-translational modifications of lysine-rich N-terminal histone "tails" include acetylation and methylation, as well as ubiquitination, phosphorylation, and sumoylation. There are over 700 proteins that regulate chromatin function, and based on their effects, they have been categorized as writers, erasers, readers, movers, shapers, and insulators (30). Currently these molecules are considered ideal therapeutic targets for cancer therapy.

4.6 Cancer Cell Cycle Checkpoints

One of the malignant features of cancer is its growth advantage via rapid cell cycle progression that is directly related to its aggressiveness. For example, Burkitt lymphoma and small cell lung cancer (SCLC) are respectively the most aggressive B-cell lymphoma and lung cancer due to their high proliferation indices. Cancer cells proliferate through the cell cycle in several phases: G1, S, G2, and M phases. Every phase is regulated by several factors, including oncogene products and tumor suppressors. Cancer cells cycle even in quiescence (G0), with p53-induced DNA repair to correct any genetic errors that have been introduced in the previous cell cycle (31). When a cell enters G1 to prepare for DNA synthesis, p53 and other tumor suppressors keep G1 as long as possible to make sure no genetic variants are propagated to the progeny cells (32), which explains why non-malignant cells usually have longer G1 phase than their malignant counterparts. Cancer cells have lost this checkpoint by the loss-of-function mutations in p53 with a shortened G1 phase. The rapid transition from G1 to S phase is assisted by several cyclin-dependent kinases (CDKs), such as CDK4 and CDK6. Cyclin D1, overexpressed in mantle cell lymphoma, binds CDK4/6 to phosphorylate Rb, which releases its suppression on E2F that promotes cells to progress to S phase (33). After the DNA duplication in the S phase, CDK1 (cdc2 in yeast) assisted by cyclin B1 promotes cells to mitosis (M phase) (Figure 4.2). Targeting CDK1 leads to cancer cell cycle arrest and apoptosis (34). Several highly selective CDK4/6 inhibitors have been developed in treating metastatic breast cancers (35).

4.7 PD-1 and PD-L1 Immune Checkpoint Pathway

Programmed cell death protein-1 (PD-1, or CD279) is expressed on T cells, B cells, NK cells, histiocytes, and antigen-presenting dendritic cells to maintain peripheral immune tolerance (36), but this mechanism is hijacked by some cancer cells to escape immune surveillance. By expressing PD-L1, the ligand for PD-1, the tumor cells interact with the CD8+ cytotoxic T cells to decrease their ability in killing tumor cells (37). Through PD-1/PD-L1 ligation, the tumor cells increase the immunosuppression of CD4+ Treg cells and thus decrease the immune responses of B cells and macrophages (38). Taking advantage of this mechanism, the tumor cells present themselves as "friends" rather than "foes" to the immune system and camouflage them into a favorable environment that assists the tumor development and growth.

Identification of the PD-1/PD-L1 pathway marks a milestone in the history of tumor immunology and immunotherapy. Since

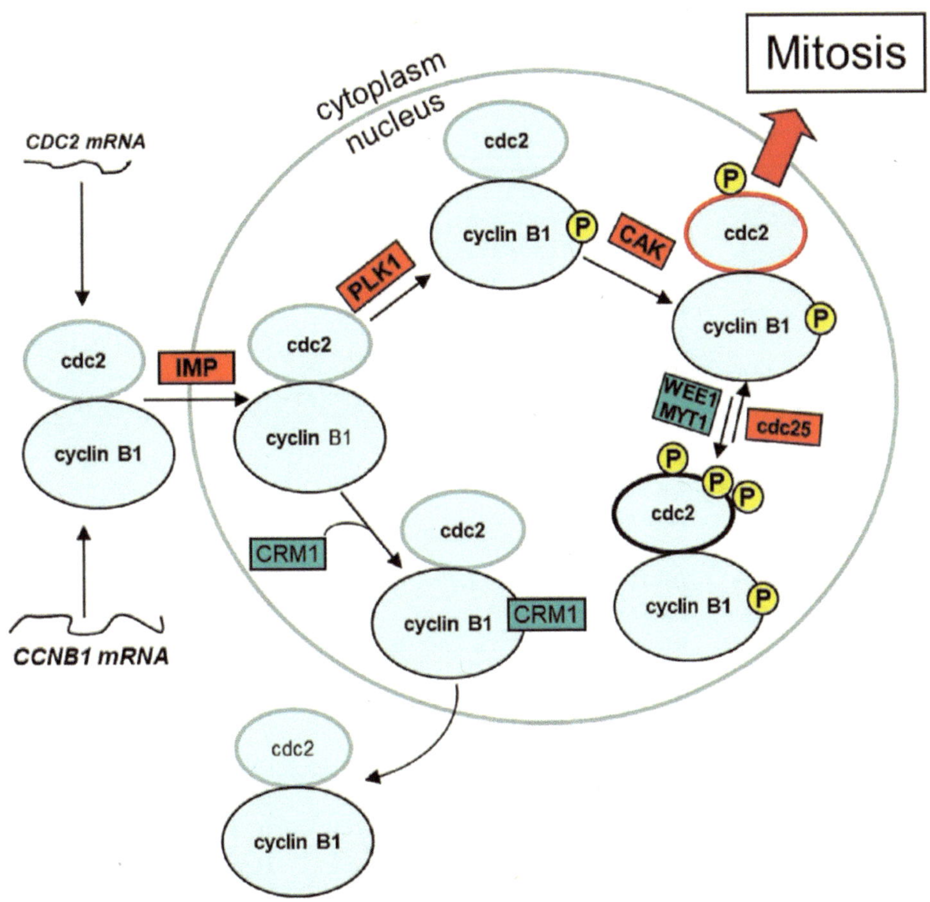

FIGURE 4.2 Functions of CDK1 (cdc2) and cyclin B1 in cell cycle progression. The oncoproteins are in red, whereas the tumor suppressors are in green. CAK, CDK-activating kinase; CRM1, chromosomal maintenance 1, also known as exportin 1; IMP, importin; PLK1, polo like kinase 1; WEE1/MYT1, Ser/Thr kinases inhibiting CDK1 by hyperphosphorylation of Y15 and T14 of CDK1.

tumor cells utilize this pathway to escape immune surveillance, blockage of this pathway is a rationale for treating cancers with PD-L1 expression (39). Humanized monoclonal antibodies against PD-1 and/or PD-L1 are being utilized in managing patients with various cancers (40), and preliminary results are very promising. Table 4.4 shows several ongoing clinical trials targeting the PD-1/PD-L1 immunomodulatory checkpoint pathway.

4.8 Cancer Is *Cancer* Indeed

According to the most updated data from the National Cancer Institute, there are 13 major cancer types and hundreds of well-defined cancers named after their origin of organs or tissues (41). These tumors look different, behave differently, and carry different biomarkers, but they all share similar properties—uncontrolled growth and immortality. Every cancer harbors at least one affected oncogene and/or tumor suppressor gene, particularly *PI3K* and *TP53* genes (9). Just one recent study has identified 299 driver genes (2), but how can we target all the driver oncogenes to slow down the impulse of cancer growth? It is neither practical nor cost-effective to develop drugs for each of the driver genes. The Pan-Cancer studies show that the vast majority of cancers utilize only several signal transduction pathways for their growth and survival (22, 42). Although cancers frequently develop drug resistance, they are highly dependent on the activation of oncogenes for survival (43), and targeting the activated oncogenes would be a fatal blow to cancer cells. Targeting the nodes at multiple levels of the signal transduction network is an effective strategy to overcome drug resistance of cancer cells (24). Pathologists should identify the most critical nodes and provide the information to the clinical oncologists, while drug companies should focus on developing agents targeting the most common oncogene products in all cancers, which will make effective use of our resources and markedly decrease the cost of precision oncology.

It is well known that cancer is quite heterogeneous (44)—the same cancer is different in different individuals; the same cancer is different in different organs and tissues of the same individual; the same cancer is different when it occurs at different times; the same cancer has different cancer cells in the same mass. These differences are at the genetic and molecular levels that are beyond the capacity of our microscope, and thus the cancer should be well sampled for molecular studies. An excisional biopsy is always preferred, but a well-sampled tumor by image-guided core needle biopsy is also acceptable for precision analysis.

4.9 Pharmacomics

Sir William Osler (1849–1919) once said, "It is much more important to know what sort of a patient has a disease than what

TABLE 4.4
Clinical Trials of PD-1/PD-L1 Inhibitors

Agents	Tumors	PD-L1 IHC Platforms	Cells Scored by IHC	Clinical Trial
Pembrolizumab	Urothelial cancer	Dako 22C3 pharmDx Assay	Combined score of TC and IC	Keynote-052
	Melanoma	Dako 22C3 pharmDx Assay	Combined score of TC and IC	Keynote-041
	HNSCC	Dako 22C3 pharmDx Assay	Combined score of TC and IC	Keynote-055
	NSCLC	Dako 22C3 pharmDx Assay	TC	Keynote-001
	Melanoma	Dako 22C3 pharmDx Assay	Combined score of TC and IC	Keynote-001
Nivolumab	Squamous NSCLC	Dako 28–8 pharmDx Assay	TC	Checkmate-017
	Non-squamous NSCLC	Dako 28–8 pharmDx Assay	TC	Checkmate-057
	Urothelial cancer	Dako 28–8 pharmDx Assay	TC	Checkmate-275
	Urothelial cancer	Dako 28–8 pharmDx Assay	TC	Checkmate-032
	Renal cell cancer	Dako Assayc	TC	Checkmate-025
	Squamous NSCLC	Dako Assayc	TC	Checkmate-063
	Renal cell cancer	Dako 28–8 pharmDx Assay	TC	NCT01354431.
	Melanoma	Dako Assayc	TC	Checkmate-066
	Multiple cancers	IHC staining with anti-PD-L1 mAb 5H1	TC	NCT00730639
Atezolizumab	NSCLC	Ventana SP142 assay	TC or IC	OAK
	Urothelial cancer	Ventana SP142 assay	IC	NCT02108652
	Renal cell cancer	Ventana SP142 assay	IC	NCT01375842
	Multiple cancers	Ventana SP142 assay	IC	NCT01375842
	NSCLC	Ventana SP142 assay	TC or IC	POPLAR
Durvalumab	Urothelial cancer	Ventana SP263 assay	TC or IC	NCT01693562
Avelumab	Urothelial cancer	Dako assay	TC	NCT01772004

Source: modified from ref. 36

Abbreviations: CI confidence interval, HNSCC head and neck squamous cell carcinoma, IC tumor infiltrating immune cell, mAb monoclonal antibody, TC tumor cell

Dako Assay: anti-PD-L1 antibody is not given.

sort of a disease a patient has." When a patient is treated with a drug, what we want is the optimal clinical outcome: to achieve the highest possible efficacy of the drug for the disease and the lowest toxicity for the patient. Unfortunately, higher drug levels are often required to attain a better efficacy and in turn often lead to drug toxicity. It is a challenge to find the balance between efficacy and toxicity.

Modern medicine has seen enormous progress in clinical therapeutics thanks to the innovation of the drug industry and numerous clinical trials. Most clinical trials are population-based studies of nonspecific toxins that follow the majority rule. Although body weight/body surface and other factors may be weighed in the trials, the subjects in the trials are largely treated the same to standardize the trials, ignoring the fact that every individual is unique. Each is unique at the gene levels, protein levels, and other metabolite levels in interacting with, metabolizing, detoxicating, and excreting various drugs and agents (45).

4.9.1 Pharmacokinetics

Once a drug is ingested, its effects depend largely on the pharmacokinetics of the drug (46), how well it is absorbed in the gastrointestinal tract, how it is distributed in the blood and tissue compartments, how it is metabolized and what is the efficacy of each of the metabolic intermediates, and how soon it is inactivated and excreted into stool and urine and out of the body. All these steps are also directly or indirectly determined by the metabolism, which differs among different individuals. A simple example is drinking a small cup of hard liquor. Alcohol can be absorbed faster in one person than in others. After absorption, ethanol will circulate in the blood and be distributed to various parts of the body. Since ethanol is fat soluble, individuals with more body fat will store the extra ethanol in their adipose tissue and thus decrease the bioavailability and dampen the effects. The ethanol molecule can be broken down by alcohol dehydrogenase (ADH) in the liver into acetaldehyde, which is further broken down rapidly by acetaldehyde dehydrogenase (ALDH) into acetate. Since ADH and ALDH levels vary from individual to individual, ethanol effects differ between individuals, and the ADH and ALDH alleles determine the risk of alcoholism (47).

4.9.2 Pharmacodynamics

Once a drug has reached its target organs and cells, pharmacodynamics will determine its efficacy on the cells. The drug can bind to its receptors with different affinities, and the receptors will trigger a series of signals transduced into the nucleus to turn on or shut off gene expressions (48). Some drugs instead of targeting the extracellular receptors can be internalized with or without modifications to bind their intracellular target molecules (particularly proteins and enzymes), either activating and/or augmenting the molecular function or inhibiting and/or inactivating molecular activities (49). Receptors, transduction pathways, transcription factors and the ligand receptors may differ from one individual to another, and the difference may be determined at the genetic level. These differences will account for the different drug effects in different individuals even with the same drug levels.

4.9.3 Pharmacogenomics

Both pharmacokinetics and pharmacodynamics of a drug are determined at the gene level by its pharmacogenomics. Pharmacogenomics is dealing with the genetic factors that affect reaction to drugs. The most important genetic factor is cytochrome (*CYP*) P450 polymorphism (50). The human P450 superfamily consists of 57 genes and over 59 pseudogenes encoding 18 families and 44 subfamilies of P450 proteins. P450s are universally present in nature, and they can inactivate as well as activate drugs and xenobiotics (51). Although over 100 variants have been identified, 10 members of the families *CYP1*, *CYP2*, and *CYP3* account for almost all the drug metabolism by P450 (52) (Table 4.5). Genetic variations lead to either gain or loss of the *CYP* P450 functions (53). The former increases drug clearance and lowers concentrations, whereas the latter reduces drug clearance and increases plasma concentrations, leading to great

TABLE 4.5

Most Common CYP P450 in Pharmacogenetics

CYPs	Function	Clinical Significance
1A1	Metabolism of carcinogens	Most important xenobiotic
1A2	Drug metabolism and synthesis of cholesterol	Determinant of clozapine dosage
2B6	Synthesis of cholesterol and steroids	Metabolize nicotine, bupropion, cyclophosphamide
2C8	Metabolism of xenobiotics	Primarily responsible for the hydroxylation and N-demethylation of rosiglitazone
2C9	Metabolism of xenobiotics, steroids and fatty acids	Metabolic elimination of phenytoin and S warfarin
2C19	Metabolism of xenobiotics	Conversion of clopidogrel to its active form
2D6	Metabolism of xenobiotics and drug-drug interactions	Metabolism of ~20% of the commonly used drugs
2E1	Metabolism of acetone, fatty acids, and xenobiotics	Metabolism of anesthetics, ethanol, nicotine, etc.
3A4	Oxidize foreign organic molecules (xenobiotics)	Metabolism of many drugs; detoxifying bile acids
3A5	Drug and steroid metabolism	Influencing tacrolimus blood levels

Source: (modified from ref. 52)

TABLE 4.6

Types of Metabolizers

Type	Genetic Variation	Enzyme Activities	Clinical Significance
Poor metabolizer (PM)	Homozygous variant mutation/ complete deletion of the genes	Markedly reduced/ none	Adverse reaction to usual dose of drugs; lack of therapeutic efficacy for prodrug
Intermediate metabolizer (IM)	Heterozygous variant mutation	Half or decreased	Lower than usual doses; low efficacy for prodrug expected
Extensive metabolizer (EM)	No variation	Functional level	Normal
Ultrarapid metabolizer (UM)	Duplication of functional genes/ SNPs with activating mutations	Increased	Lack of efficacy with usual dose of drug; enhanced prodrug effects

Source: Modified from refs. 54 & 55.

variations on drug effects in different individuals. Almost all genetic mechanisms can cause genetic variations in P450 (54, 55), which result in four major phenotypic changes in the *CYP* P450 enzyme activities (Table 4.6). Various susceptibilities to environmental agents due to *CYP* polymorphism also determine the risk of developing malignancies (56, 57).

4.9.4 Pharmacoproteomics and Pharmacometabolomics

Although the human genome encodes only ~20,000 proteins, there are probably millions of actual functional proteins, considering the posttranslational modifications that exponentially enrich the diversity of the human proteome (58). These functional proteins (mostly enzymes) interact with drugs in a dynamic state that goes well beyond the genomic analysis. Most of the therapeutic targets for oncogenes are actual proteins, and therefore pharmacoproteomics occupies an important position in pharmacomics and precision pathology. As a drug can be inactivated or activated by metabolism, analysis of the pharmacometabolomics of the patient will also help us understand the overall metabolism of the subjects and the fates of drugs and thus tailor the most appropriate dosage to everyone. This strategy will achieve the greatest effectiveness of medication and keep adverse effects to a minimum.

4.10 Summary

Precision medicine depends on the molecular evidence provided by precision pathology. From the cell membrane to the nucleus, every component and organelle of the cell can be altered by driver mutations and various other mechanisms, as illustrated, and they may serve as therapeutic targets for precision treatment. While considering its high heterogenicity, we should also invest in developing drugs that target common cancer pathways/ oncogenic mechanisms. The medications and dosage should be tailored to each subject even with the same so-called disease due to population polymorphism and posttranslational modification of the metabolism. Advanced molecular assays and artificial intelligence are indispensable tools for the detection of these abnormalities.

REFERENCES

1. Watson IR, Takahashi K, Futreal PA, et al. Emerging patterns of somatic mutations in cancer. Nat Rev Genet. 2013;14(10):703–718.
2. Bailey MH, Tokheim C, Porta-Pardo E, et al. Comprehensive characterization of cancer driver genes and mutations. Cell. 2018;173(2):371–385.
3. Adouda Adjiri. DNA mutations may not be the cause of cancer. Oncol Ther. 2017;5(1):85–101.
4. Cancer Genes. *Cancer Quest*. Emory University; 2020. www.cancerquest.org/cancer-biology/cancer-genes
5. Lindeman NI, Cagle PT, Beasley MB, et al. Molecular testing guideline for selection of lung cancer patients for EGFR and ALK tyrosine kinase inhibitors: Guideline from the College of American Pathologists, International Association for the Study of Lung Cancer, and Association for Molecular Pathology. Arch Pathol Lab Med. 2013;137(6):828–860.
6. Baselga J, Tripathy D, Mendelsohn J, et al. Phase II study of weekly intravenous trastuzumab (Herceptin) in patients with HER2/neu-overexpressing metastatic breast cancer. Semin Oncol. 1999;26(4 Suppl. 12):78–83.
7. Cheng L, Lopez-Beltran A, Massari, F et al. Molecular testing for BRAF mutations to inform melanoma treatment decisions: A move toward precision medicine. Mod Pathol. 2018;31(1):24–38.
8. Tumor Suppressor Gene. National Cancer Institute; 2020. www.cancer.gov/publications/dictionaries/cancer-terms/def/tumor-suppressor-gene
9. Soussi T, Wiman KG. TP53: An oncogene in disguise. Cell Death Differ. 2015;22(8):1239–1249.
10. Cooper GM. Tumor suppressor genes. In *The Cell: A Molecular Approach*. 2nd edition. Sunderland, MA: Sinauer Associates; 2000.
11. Liu Y, Hu X, Han C, et al. Targeting tumor suppressor genes for cancer therapy. Bioessays. 2015;37(12):1277–1286.
12. Behm FG, Raimondi SC, Schell MJ, et al. Lack of CD45 antigen on blast cells in childhood acute lymphoblastic leukemia is associated with chromosomal hyperdiploidy and other favorable prognostic features. Blood. 1992;79(4):1011–1016.
13. Di Biagio E, Sánchez-Borges M, Desenne JJ, et al. Eosinophilia in Hodgkin's disease: A role for interleukin 5. Int Arch Allergy Immunol. 1996;110(3):244–251.

14. Nakayama S, Yokote T, Hiraoka N, et al. Role of mast cells in fibrosis of classical Hodgkin lymphoma. Int J Immunopathol Pharmacol. 2016;29(4):603–611.
15. Kuter DJ, Bain B, Mufti G, et al. Bone marrow fibrosis: Pathophysiology and clinical significance of increased bone marrow stromal fibres. Br J Haematol. 2007;139(3): 351–362.
16. Hekman A, Honselaar A, Vuist WMJ, et al. Initial experience with treatment of human B cell lymphoma with anti-CD19 monoclonal antibody. Cancer Immunol Immunother. 1991;32(6):364–372.
17. Leget GA, Czuczman MS. Use of rituximab, the new FDA-approved antibody. Curr Opin Oncol. 1998;10(6):548–551.
18. Polson AG, Yu S-F, Elkins K, et al. Antibody-drug conjugates targeted to CD79 for the treatment of non-Hodgkin lymphoma. Blood. 2007;110(2):616–623.
19. Kuhn C, Weiner HL. Therapeutic anti-CD3 monoclonal antibodies: From bench to bedside. Immunotherapy. 2016;8(8):889–906.
20. Hartl M, Bister K. Oncogenes. In *Brenner's Encyclopedia of Genetics*. 2nd edition. San Diego, CA: Academic Press; 2013. pp. 164–166.
21. Neapolitan R, Horvath CM, Jiang X. Pan-cancer analysis of TCGA data reveals notable signaling pathways. BMC Cancer. 2015;15:516.
22. Kandoth C, McLellan MD, Vandin F, et al. Mutational landscape and significance across 12 major cancer types. Nature. 2013;502(7471):333–339.
23. Leiserson MDM, Vandin F, Wu H-T, et al. Pan-cancer network analysis identifies combinations of rare somatic mutations across pathways and protein complexes. Nat Genet. 2015;47(2):106–114.
24. Zhao XF. Gene, life and cancer—A node theory. Hematopathology. 2017;2(1):1–13.
25. Zhao XF, Gartenhaus R. Phospho-p70S6K and cdc2/cdk1 as therapeutic targets for diffuse large B-cell lymphoma. Expert Opin Ther Targets. 2009;13(9):1085–1093.
26. Kubota Y, Ohnishi H, Kitanaka A, et al. Constitutive activation of PI3K is involved in the spontaneous proliferation of primary acute myeloid leukemia cells: Direct evidence of PI3K activation. Leukemia. 2004;18(8):1438–1440.
27. Dawson MA, Kouzarides T. Cancer epigenetics: From mechanism to therapy. Cell. 2012;150(1):12–27.
28. Fenaux P, Mufti GJ, Hellstrom-Lindberg E, et al. Efficacy of azacitidine compared with that of conventional care regimens in the treatment of higher-risk myelodysplastic syndromes: A randomised, open-label, phase III study. Lancet Oncol. 2009;10(3):223–232.
29. Suvà ML, Riggi N, Bernstein BE. Epigenetic reprogramming in cancer. Science. 2013;339(6127):1567–1570.
30. Bates SE. Epigenetic therapies for cancer. N Engl J Med. 2020;383(7):650–663.
31. Linke SP, Clarkin KC, Di Leonardo A, et al. A reversible, p53-dependent G0/G1 cell cycle arrest induced by ribonucleotide depletion in the absence of detectable DNA damage. Genes Dev. 1996;10(8):934–947.
32. Pellegata NS, Antoniono RJ, Redpath JL, et al. DNA damage and p53-mediated cell cycle arrest: A reevaluation. Proc Natl Acad Sci. 1996;93(26):15209–15214.
33. Müller H, Moroni MC, Vigo E, et al. Induction of S-phase entry by E2F transcription factors depends on their nuclear localization. Mol Cell Biol. 1997;17(9):5508–5520.
34. Zhao MY, Auerbach A, D'Costa AM, et al. Phospho-p70S6K/p85S6K and cdc2/cdk1 are novel targets for diffuse large B-cell lymphoma combination therapy. Clin Cancer Res. 2009;15(5):1708–1720.
35. Bilgin B, Sendur MAN, Şener Dede D, et al. A current and comprehensive review of cyclin-dependent kinase inhibitors for the treatment of metastatic breast cancer. Curr Med Res Opin. 2017;33(9):1559–1569.
36. Yi M, Jiao D, Xu H, et al. Biomarkers for predicting efficacy of PD-1/PD-L1 inhibitors. Mol Cancer. 2018;17(1):129.
37. Ishida Y, Agata Y, Shibahara K, et al. Induced expression of PD-1, a novel member of the immunoglobulin gene superfamily, upon programmed cell death. EMBO J. 1992;11(11):3887–3895.
38. Ohaegbulam KC, Assal A, Lazar-Molnar E, et al. Human cancer immunotherapy with antibodies to the PD-1 and PD-L1 pathway. Trends Mol Med. 2015;21(1):24–33.
39. Postow MA, Callahan MK, Wolchok JD. Immune checkpoint blockade in cancer therapy. J Clin Oncol. 2015;33(17):1974–1982.
40. Alsaab HO, Sau S, Alzhrani R. PD-1 and PD-L1 checkpoint signaling inhibition for cancer immunotherapy: Mechanism, combinations, and clinical outcome. Front Pharmacol. 2017;8:561.
41. *Cancer Types*. National Cancer Institute; 2020. www.cancer.gov/types
42. Iorio F, Knijnenburg TA, Vis DJ, et al. A landscape of pharmacogenomic interactions in cancer. Cell. 2016; 166(3):740–754.
43. Weinstein IB, Joe A. Oncogene addiction. Cancer Res. 2008;68(9):3077–3080.
44. Vogelstein B, Papadopoulos N, Velculescu VE, et al. Cancer genome landscapes. Science. 2013;339(6127):1546–1558.
45. Goldstein DB, Need AC, Singh R, et al. Potential genetic causes of heterogeneity of treatment effects. Am J Med. 2007;120(4 Suppl 1):S21–S25.
46. Kester M, Karpa KD, Vrana KE. Pharmacokinetics. In *Elsevier's Integrated Review Pharmacology*. 2nd edition. Amsterdam, The Netherlands: Elsevier; 2012. pp. 1–15.
47. Edenberg HJ. The genetics of alcohol metabolism: Role of alcohol dehydrogenase and aldehyde dehydrogenase variants. Alcohol Res Health. 2007;30(1):5–13.
48. Litalien C, Beaulieu P. Molecular mechanisms of drug actions: From receptors to effectors. Pediatr Crit Care. 2011;1553–1568.
49. Rudraiah S, Zhang X, Wang L. Nuclear receptors as therapeutic targets in liver disease: Are we there yet? Annu Rev Pharmacol Toxicol. 2016;56:605–626.
50. Agundez JAG. Cytochrome P450 gene polymorphism and cancer. Curr Drug Metab. 2004;5(3):211–224.
51. Guengerich FP. Cytochrome p450 and chemical toxicology. Chem Res Toxicol. 2008;21(1):70–83.
52. Guengerich FP. Cytochrome P450s and other enzymes in drug metabolism and toxicity. AAPS J. 2006;8(1):E101–111.

53. Manikandan P, Nagini S. Cytochrome P450 structure, function and clinical significance: A review. Curr Drug Targets. 2018;19(1):38–54.
54. Ingelman-Sundberg M, Sim SC, Gomez A, et al. Influence of cytochrome P450 polymorphisms on drug therapies: Pharmacogenetic, pharmacoepigenetic and clinical aspects. Pharmacol Ther. 2007;116(3):496–526.
55. Ingelman-Sundberg M. Pharmacogenetics of cytochrome P450 and its applications in drug therapy: The past, present and future. Trends Pharmacol Sci. 2004;25(4):193–200.
56. Johani FH, Majid MSA, Azme MH, et al. Cytochrome P450 2A6 whole-gene deletion (CYP2A6*4) polymorphism reduces risk of lung cancer: A meta-analysis. Tob Induc Dis. 2020;18:50.
57. Meng Li, Anqi Li, Ruiqing He, et al. Gene polymorphism of cytochrome P450 significantly affects lung cancer susceptibility. Cancer Med. 2019;8(10):4892–4905.
58. Chambliss AB, Chan DW. Precision medicine: From pharmacogenomics to pharmacoproteomics. Clin Proteomics. 2016;13:25.

5

Tools in Precision Pathology

Xia Li and Xianfeng F. Zhao

5.1 Introduction

Precision pathology relies heavily on the molecular techniques developed in the last several decades. It mainly differs from molecular pathology by the fact that the former focuses on targeted therapy, while the latter focuses on diagnosis. Therefore, molecular pathology is considered another milestone of traditional modern pathology, but precision pathology should be regarded as a new frontier and the pathology of the 21st century.

Clinical applications of molecular assays became available as the methods matured in the research laboratories. The earliest examples are the application of Southern blot in the clonal determination of B cells and T cells (1) and polymerase chain reaction (PCR) assay in detecting viruses in clinical specimens (2). With the emergence of next-generation sequencing (NGS) and mass spectrometry (MS), cells are becoming more and more transparent to our pathologists.

5.2 Grossing

Grossing may be considered a primitive procedure in a pathology lab, but it is the first critical step for pathologists to make a diagnosis of a disease (3). It requires a well-trained pathologist with great skills to sample the specimen properly. Although we are in an era with many advanced technologies and molecular tools which can be utilized for the diagnosis of diseases, it is still possible to miss an important finding due to sampling errors. Unfortunately, more and more pathologists do not like to do grossing because they have not been trained properly in their residency programs, which sounds is a concern for residency programs.

The advancement of imaging also poses a challenge for pathologists. Accurate identification of a lesion with high resolution makes specimen sampling easier than before. Excisional biopsies have been replaced more and more by core needle biopsies and even fine-needle aspirations. With the limited amount of tissue, the pathologists have little option in specimen sampling. With multiple small tissue cores in front of them, they often must prioritize assays with a small amount of tissues. With even better artificial intelligence (AI)–assisted imaging and a movement toward less and less invasive procedures, collaboration between interventional radiologists and pathologists is so critical that combined grossing training is no longer a daunting idea.

The future grossing room may be in interventional radiology (IR) rather than pathology, and the radiologist and pathologist will work side by side or even be the same physician.

5.3 Histology

Histology is the basis of traditional pathology. It is the first step in morphologically identifying and classifying diseases. Once received in a pathology laboratory, the specimen will be properly grossed and sampled, formalin-fixed, paraffin-embedded, and sectioned on a microtome to 3–5-µm-thick tissue sections. The tissue sections are then fixed on a glass slide and stained with hematoxylin (H) and eosin (E) buffers. The cell structures will be displayed under the microscope based on the acidophilic and basophilic properties of each cell organelle (4). A well-trained pathologist will be able to distinguish the normal samples from the diseased ones and submit the proper specimen for precision pathology analysis.

5.4 Immunohistochemistry

Immunohistochemistry (IHC) (5) revolutionized traditional pathology with the identification of cell lineages and the classification of tumors. IHC remains critically useful in precision pathology for its simple and seemingly straightforward technology and fast turnaround time. It provides the most visual evidence for antigen detection and gene expression. It is most useful for aberrant gene expression and gene deletion. It may be more useful than gene sequencing because it shows the production of proteins that are the functional units of genes. IHC is currently used for identifying BCL2 and MYC aberrant expression in lymphomas, p53 overexpression or deletion in various tumors, and microsatellite instability (MSI) gene deletions in colon cancers.

5.5 PCR and Sanger Sequencing

Both PCR and Sanger sequencing were awarded the Nobel prize for their revolutionary contribution to the advancement of bioscience and biotechnologies. The former makes the harvest of a sufficient amount of genetic material in a short time a reality, whereas the latter decodes the secret genetic information at one's fingertips. These

DOI: 10.1201/9781003513469-5

two technologies are not only basic molecular tools mostly applied in precision pathology but also broadly used in either the development of downstream technologies or as part of the protocol.

PCR was designed with two short DNA primers flanking a DNA segment (or a gene) and Taq DNA polymerase to amplify the DNA fragment hundreds- and thousands-fold in a short period. The amplified DNA is then subjected to sequencing on an automated DNA sequencer (Figure 5.1). Most of the point mutations, insertions, deletions, and translocations are detected with combined PCR and automated DNA sequencing. Currently, *BCR::ABL1* fusion genes and *JAK2* mutations are detected by PCR and sequencing. Table 5.1 lists examples of genetic abnormalities detected by PCR-Sanger sequencing.

This PCR-sequencing assay is mostly utilized to identify point mutations within a known gene or certain chimeric (fusion) site between two different genes. The assay is useful for low-throughput sequencing of individual genes.

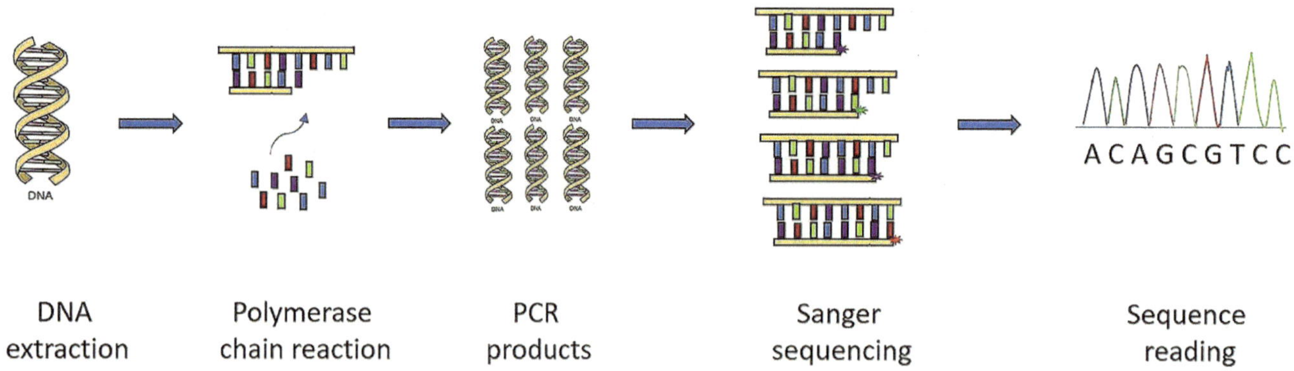

FIGURE 5.1 Workflow of combined PCR and Sanger sequencing.

TABLE 5.1

List of Commonly Used Biomarkers in Cancer Treatment

Biomarker/Gene	Therapeutic Target	Assay	Cancer Type	Drug
BCR::ABL1 (translocation)	ABL1	FISH, NGS, PCR	Chronic myeloid leukaemia	Imatinib, nilotinib
BCR::ABL1 (translocation)	ABL1	FISH, NGS, PCR	Chronic myeloid leukaemia (imatinib-resistant)	Dasatinib
EML4::ALK (translocation)	ALK	FISH, NGS, PCR	Lung adenocarcinoma	Crizotinib, ceritinib
EML4::ALK (translocation)	ALK	FISH, NGS, PCR	Non-small cell lung cancer	Crizotinib, alectinib, ceritinib
BCL2 (mutation)	BCL2	NGS, PCR	Chronic lymphocytic leukemia, acute myeloid leukemia	Venetoclax
BRAF (mutation)	BRAF	NGS, PCR	Lung adenocarcinoma	AZD6244
BRAF (mutation)	BRAF	NGS, PCR	Melanoma	Vemurafenib, dabrafenib, trametinib, cobimetinib
BRCA	BRCA1/2	NGS, PCR	Breast and ovarian cancer	Rucaparib
Germline *BRCA1/2*	BRCA1/2	NGS, PCR	Ovarian cancer	Olaparib
KRAS and *NRAS* wild-type	EGFR	NGS, PCR	Colorectal cancer	Panitumumab, cetuximab
EGFR	EGFR	NGS, PCR	Lung adenocarcinoma	Erlotinib, gefitinib, afatinib, cetuximab
EGFR (mutation)	EGFR	NGS, PCR	Non-small cell lung cancer	Erlotinib, gefitinib, osiertinib
EGFR (amplification)	EGFR	FISH, NGS, PCR	Non-small cell lung cancer	Vandetanib
EGFR (mutation)	EGFRT790M	NGS, PCR	Non-small cell lung cancer	Osiertinib (AZD9291)
EGFR (mutation)	EGFR/ERBB2	NGS, PCR	Non-small cell lung cancer	Afatinib
HER2/neu (amplification)	ERBB2	FISH, NGS, IHC	Breast cancer	Trastuzumab, ado-trastuzumab-entansine, pertuzumab
EZH2 (mutation)	EZH2	NGS, PCR	Follicular lymphoma	Tazemetostat
FGFR2 (translocation)	FEGR2	FISH, NGS, PCR	Cholangiocarcinoma	Pemigatinib
FLT3 ITD/TKD (mutation)	FLT3	NGS, PCR	Acute myelogenous leukemia	Midostaurin, sorafenib
HER2/neu (amplification)	HER2	FISH, NGS	Lung adenocarcinoma	Decinutubub, neratinib, lapatinib, trastuzumab
IDH1 (mutation)	IDH1	NGS, PCR	Acute myeloid leukemia	Ivosidenib, AG-881
IDH2 (mutation)	IDH2	NGS, PCR	Acute myeloid leukemia	Cytarabine, enasidenib, AG-881

(Continued)

TABLE 5.1 (Continued)

Biomarker/Gene	Therapeutic Target	Assay	Cancer Type	Drug
KIT (mutation)	KIT	NGS, PCR	Gastrointestinal stromal tumor	Imatinib
KRAS (mutation)	KRAS	NGS, PCR	Lung adenocarcinoma	Erlotinib, tivantinib, everolimus, ridaforalimus, AZD6244
MET (mutation)	MET	NGS, PCR	Lung adenocarcinoma	Crizotinib
MET (amplification/Exon 14 skipping mutation)	MET	NGS	Non-small cell lung cancer	Crizotinib
NTRK (translocation)	NTRK1/2/3	FISH, NGS, PCR	Multiple solid tumors	Larotrectinib
PDGFRA (mutation)	PDGFRA	NGS, PCR	Gastrointestinal stromal tumor	Imatinib
MSI-H/dMMR	PD-1	IHC	Multiple solid tumors	Pembrolizumab
PIK3CA (mutation)	PIK3CA	NGS, PCR	Breast cancer	Alpelisib
PML::RARA (translocation)	PML/RARA	FISH, NGS, PCR	Acute promyelocytic leukemia	All-trans retinoic acid
RET (rearrangements)	RET	FISH, NGS, PCR	Non-small cell lung cancer	Cabozantinib
ROS1 (translocation)	ROS1	FISH, NGS, PCR	Non-small cell lung cancer	Ceritinib, crizotinob
HRR (mutation)	(BRCA1, BRCA2, ATM, BARD1, BRIP1, CDK12, CHEK1, CHEK2, FANCL, PALB2, RAD51B, RAD51C, RAD51D and RAD54L)	NGS, PCR	Prostate cancer	Olaparib
JAK2 (mutation)	JAK2	NGS, PCR	Polycythemia vera	Ruxolitinib
CBFB/MYH11 (translocation)	CBFB	FISH, NGS, PCR	Acute myeloid leukemia	Gemtuzumab ozogamicin + chemotherapy

Note: (data from NCI, www.cancer.gov/about-cancer/treatment/types/targeted-therapies/targeted-therapies-fact-sheet)

5.6 Fluorescence *In Situ* Hybridization

Fluorescence *in situ* hybridization (FISH) is a molecular cytogenetic technique that uses DNA or mRNA sequences labeled with fluorescent dyes to hybridize with the homologous nucleic acid sequences on the chromosomes so that the chromosome aberrations can be detected (6). These genetic aberrations include characteristic gene fusions or translocations, gene rearrangements, deletions, and duplications/amplifications, all of which are known to be associated with genetic diseases, specific types of cancer, or biomarker genes. In the last few decades, FISH testing has been widely used in clinical oncology practice to guide diagnostics and prognostics. In addition, FISH can facilitate the monitoring of disease progression, the success of bone marrow transplantation, and prognostication outcomes during treatment and function as a predictive tool to stratify cancer patients (7–9). Some of the most common genetic abnormalities identified by FISH in precision pathology can be seen in Table 5.1.

There are many advantages of FISH in molecular diagnostics. First, the assay is highly sensitive and specific, and the resolution is between DNA sequencing and chromosome karyotyping. Second, the turnaround time is 2–4 days, although it can be shortened to 1 day for urgent cases such as acute promyelocytic leukemia (APL). Finally, the scoring and reporting are relatively straightforward. FISH technology has been the gold standard for several companion diagnostic tests (e.g., *ALK* and *ROS1* rearrangements, *HER2* amplification, and UroVysion assays).

With these advantages, FISH assays are widely used in oncology testing. For instance, the National Comprehensive Cancer Network (NCCN) guidelines for non-small cell lung cancer (NSCLC) require molecular diagnostic studies for detecting mutations from *EGFR* and *BRAF*; translocations from *ALK*, *ROS1*, and *RET*; and *MET* exon 14 skipping. Among these genes, *ALK*, *ROS1*, and *RET* rearrangements are mostly detected by FISH, although NGS, real-time PCR, and IHC are also available for identifying these genetic alterations. If a specific rearrangement is positive, then targeted therapy can be used for treating patients.

5.7 Karyotyping

Chromosome analysis, also known as karyotyping, is the process by which photographs of chromosomes are taken to determine the chromosome complement of an individual. Thus, the number of chromosomes and any abnormalities can be identified. "Karyotype" also refers to the complete set of chromosomes in an individual. To visualize the chromosomes, several chromosome banding techniques can be used for distinguishing normal and abnormal chromosomes for clinical and research purposes. For instance, Giemsa (G)-, reverse

(R)-, and centromere (C)-bandings are the most common dye-based chromosome-banding techniques. G-banding involves the staining of trypsin-treated chromosomes. R-banding involves denaturing in hot acidic saline followed by Giemsa staining, and it is the reverse of G-banding. C-banding is specifically used for identifying constitutive heterochromatin by denaturing chromosomes in a saturated alkaline solution followed by Giemsa staining. Different banding techniques may be selected for various purposes of identification of chromosome alterations (10).

The G-banding technique is the most common technology used in cytogenetics laboratories to produce a visible karyotype by staining condensed chromosomes. The metaphase chromosomes are treated with trypsin to partially digest the chromosomes. Then they are stained with Giemsa stain. Heterochromatic regions, which are rich with adenine and thymine (AT-rich) and are relatively gene poor, are stained darker in G-banding. In contrast, less condensed chromatin (euchromatin)-which are rich with guanine and cytosine (GC-rich) and more transcriptionally active-incorporates less Giemsa stain, and these regions appear as light bands in G-banding. From the pattern of bands, the chromosome abnormalities, including numerical and structural aberrations, can be identified by experienced cytogenetics technologists.

In the last few decades, karyotypes have increasingly become a source of diagnostic information. They have helped predict birth defects and diagnose genetic disorders and cancers. Cancer cells are typically characterized by complex karyotypes, including both structural and numerical alterations with predominant karyotypic patterns (11). In routine oncology practice, karyotyping remains the gold standard for identifying aneuploidy, typical or atypical chromosome translocations, and clonal evolution (12–14). As an example, myelodysplastic neoplasms (MDSs) are a heterogeneous group of clonal hematopoietic stem cell disorders. They are characterized by ineffective and dysplastic hematopoiesis and increased risk of transformation into acute myeloid leukemia (AML) (15). Chromosomal abnormalities can be detected in over 50% of patients with *de novo* MDS and in up to 80% of patients with therapy-related MDS (16–18). A complex karyotype, defined as at least three clonal aberrations, is detected in approximately 10% to 15% of MDS patients and is associated with a very short median survival of less than 12 months and a high risk of transformation into AML (19). Therefore, karyotyping has played an essential role in clinical diagnosis, predicting prognosis, and selection of treatment for cancer patients.

5.8 Next-Generation Sequencing

Next-generation sequencing (NGS), also known as massively parallel or deep sequencing, is one of the most significant advancements in biotechnology in the last two decades (20, 21). Compared to first-generation Sanger sequencing using capillary electrophoresis, NGS can generate millions of sequencing reads and provide more accurate results with a high depth of coverage (22, 23). The sensitivity of NGS can be very high, and the lower limit of detection can reach 0.001% vs. 20% for allele frequency in Sanger sequencing. This technique markedly decreased the turnaround time of sequencing. As an example, the first human genome sequencing project started in 1990 and was completed after 13 years (24), while nowadays an entire human genome can be sequenced within a single day. Therefore, NGS has become the most effective tool in the clinical molecular diagnostics field, especially in oncology practice to help guide genetic diagnosis, cancer classification, predictive biomarkers, and personalized medicine (25).

Besides the turnaround time, NGS has also reduced the cost of sequencing substantially. The cost of the first human draft sequence was about $2.7 billion; the cost to sequence a human genome or a Megabase in 2022 is well below $1,000.

There are many different NGS panels used in clinical diagnostics, ranging from small, targeted gene panels to whole-exome or whole-genome sequencing (WGS). For cancer genomics testing, a targeted NGS panel with cancer driver genes is preferred, such as a hereditary cancer panel, *BRCA* panel, lung caner panel, or melanoma panel. There is also a huge economic impact of NGS vs. single-gene testing in clinical practice. Sequential molecular testing of individual genes costs more and takes longer and does not meet the guidelines for oncology practice. For instance, the NCCN guideline for acute myeloid leukemia recommends that molecular testing be performed on AML patients for mutation status of *c-KIT, FLT3* [ITD and TKD], *NPM1, CEBPA* (biallelic), *IDH1, IDH2, TP53,* and other mutations in 3–5 days. Because NGS allows for rapid processing of DNA/RNA simultaneously and detects multiple types of clinically actionable variants, including single nucleotide variants (SNVs), insertions/deletions (INDELs), and gene fusions, in a single workflow within a few days, more and more physicians prefer NGS over single gene testing. A study from Pennell et al. demonstrated that the use of upfront NGS testing in patients with metastatic NSCLC was beneficial with substantial cost savings and shorter time-to-test results for both Centers for Medicare & Medicaid Services (CMS) and commercial payers (26).

NGS also has the advantage of using formalin-fixed paraffin-embedded (FFPE) specimens for solid tumor testing and allowing small amounts of the sample to be processed to generate results. The starting material for NGS testing can be as low as 10 ng DNA, and this is especially important for lung cancer patients because most of the sample types are small biopsies such as fine-needle aspirates. Limited tissue becomes an issue in 70% of lung cancers. While all patients with lung adenocarcinoma must be considered potentially eligible for targeted tyrosine kinase inhibitor (TKI) therapy or immunotherapy, NGS becomes the best approach for patients to get maximized chances with targeted therapy and maximum use of minimal tissue (27).

With the emergence of NGS technologies, precision or personalized medicine has been introduced to public health to implement tailored therapy for patients based on their genomic profiling, replacing the "one size fits all" or single drug-regimen approach (25, 28). Furthermore, a deeper understanding of cancer biology resulted in the discovery of biomarkers and targeted therapy (Table 5.1) (www.cancer.gov/about-cancer/treatment/types/targeted-therapies/targeted-therapies-fact-sheet). By the end of 2018, more than 30 drugs had been developed with companion diagnostic assays for cancer treatment (29, 30). The low costs and easy access to NGS testing made a huge impact on precision medicine. Clinicians rely largely on the molecular profile for risk assessment, early diagnosis, prognosis, and treatment.

5.9 Optical Genome Mapping

Various genetic diseases, including developmental disorders and cancers, are caused by large copy number and structural variations. Optical genome mapping (OGM) is an advanced technology that analyzes ultra-high molecular weight DNA molecules and provides a high-resolution genome-wide analysis highlighting copy numbers and structural alterations. In detail, OGM detects structural variations ranging from 500 bp to Megabase pairs in length and offers assembly and discovery algorithms that far outperform sequencing-based technologies in sensitivity. For detection of mosaicisms or heterogeneous cancer samples, OGM can detect all types of structural variants down to 1% variant allele fraction and calls repeats and complex rearrangements. The structural abnormalities identified by OGM include homozygous insertions/deletions (> 500bp), balanced and unbalanced translocations (> 50 kb), inversions and duplications (> 30 kb), and copy number variations (> 500 kb).

Numerous research studies using OGM have been published as compared to standard techniques (karyotyping, FISH, SNP-array, and reverse transcription multiplex ligation-dependent probe amplification). The outcome of these studies has shown robust performances of OGM in clinical diagnostic practice. A study by Lestringant et al. demonstrated that OGM detected chromosome abnormalities from 72 out of 80 cases of acute lymphoblastic leukemias (ALLs), and these findings were concordant with those previously identified by standard techniques; 8 out of 80 samples showed additional abnormalities by OGM (31). Another study by Goldrich et al. showed that somatic structural variants including insertions, deletions, inversions, duplications, and translocations were also detected by OGM from 20 clinical samples with various tumor types (32).

Overall, OGM has outperformed the standard-of-care tests in many studies and demonstrated its potential as a first-tier cytogenomic test for hematologic malignancies and solid tumors (31–37).

5.10 Pharmacogenomics

Every human being has a different genetic makeup. These differences in genetics along with heterogeneities of disease presentation and environment all contribute to the variability in drug response. Pharmacogenomics refers to the study of the genomic influence on drug response, also known as individual gene–drug interactions in terms of efficacy and toxicity. It has been widely applied in the field of genomics to guide therapeutic interventions and new drug development, which is also a part of the mission of personalized medicine (38).

The goals of pharmacogenomics are to maximize drug efficacy, minimize drug toxicity, predict which patients will respond to intervention, and aid in new drug development. Most importantly, pharmacogenomics has a huge impact on the quality of patients' lives and a reduction in healthcare expenditure.

Hundreds of genes are involved in pharmacogenomics. These genes are either drug targets (e.g., receptors, ion channels, enzymes, immune molecules), drug transporters, or drug-metabolizing enzymes (39). The genotypes of these genes determine the phenotypic variability in response to drugs such as poor metabolizers, intermediate metabolizers, extensive or normal metabolizers, and ultra-rapid metabolizers. The genetic variations relevant to drug metabolism include DNA insertions, deletions, single-nucleotide polymorphisms (SNPs), and copy number variations. With the implementation of high-throughput sequencing technologies, genotyping these genes has become feasible in clinical labs. Currently, SNP genotyping can be done by PCR, SNP microarray, or NGS, though the last is more expensive. A single gene or a panel of genes (e.g., cardiology, psychology, pain management, oncology panel, etc.) can be tested by a single assay. The report will be generated according to the guidelines from the Clinical Pharmacogenetics Implementation Consortium (CPIC) and the Dutch Pharmacogenetics Working Group (DPWG) (40). Then the results will be transferred into the patient's electronic medical records so that physicians can prescribe the right medication with the right dosage to patients based on the reports.

In oncology practice, many drugs are prescribed based on genetic alterations. For example, one of the drugs, gefitinib, is used to target mutation or amplification of epidermal growth factor receptor (*EGFR*) in the treatment of NSCLC patients. This drug is an EGFR inhibitor, which interrupts signaling through the EGFR in target cells. Only ~10% of patients with mutations (e.g., G6719C, delE746-A750, delL747-T751insS, delL747-P753insS, L858R and L861Q) have tumor responses to the drug. This subgroup of patients with NSCLC has specific mutations in the *EGFR* gene that constitutively activate the receptor and confer sensitivity to gefitinib (41, 42).

The goal of personalized medicine is to match each therapeutic regimen with the patient's molecular profile. With the implementation of pharmacogenomics in clinical practice, precision therapy, improvement of public health, and reduction of the cost of healthcare and patients will become a reality.

5.11 Mass Spectrometry

In contrast to cancer genomics to identify and target the genetic alterations associated with cancer, mass spectrometry (MS)–based proteomics are utilized to identify the abnormalities in the proteome that cannot be discerned by genetic studies due to the "expression infidelity" of genes (43). Due to alternative splicing of

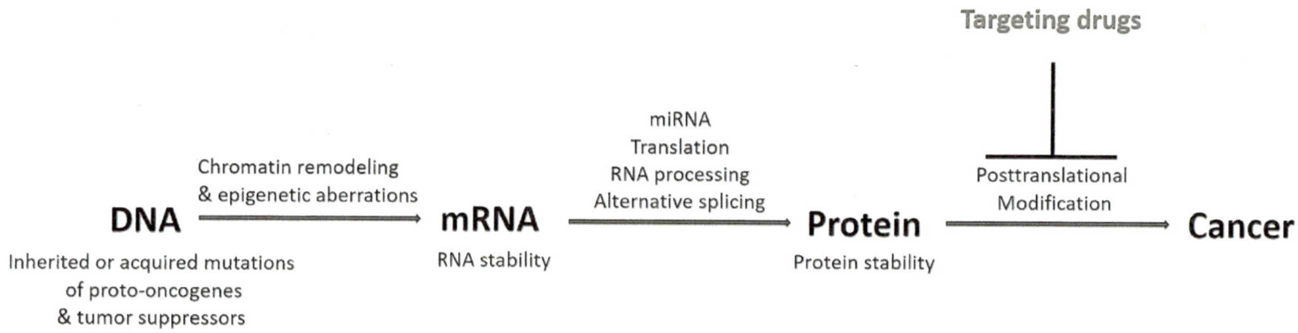

FIGURE 5.2 Central dogma-guided cancer development. "Genetic infidelity" makes proteins the most important molecules to be detected by precision pathology (modified from ref. 43).

primary transcripts, sequence polymorphisms, post-translational modifications, and other protein processing mechanisms, one gene can generate multiple distinct proteins. Therefore, the proteome is much more diverse and complex than the genome. Furthermore, although numerous genetic alterations happen in cancer cells, cancer phenotypes are represented by various proteins, which are the molecular targets for most of the commercially available precision oncology drugs (Figure 5.2).

MS is an analytical tool useful for measuring the mass-to-charge ratio (m/z) of the molecules present in a clinical sample. First designed in the early 20th century by Arthur Jeffrey Dempster and F.W. Aston (44), MS technology has become an integral part of precision pathology. Although varying greatly, a typical mass spectrometer consists of at least three components: an ionization source, a mass analyzer, and a detector. The ionization source (or ionizer) converts the molecules in the clinical samples into ions. The ions can be converted to gas-phase ions, liquid-phase ions, or solid-phase ions depending on different platforms. Once ionized, the ions are sorted and separated according to m/z ratios on a mass analyzer. There are several commercial mass spectrometry analyzers currently available, each of which has trade-offs relating to the speed of operation, resolution of separation, and other operational requirements. The separated ions are then measured and analyzed for identity, quantity, or spatiality using established algorithms (45). Each peak in a mass spectrum shows a component of unique m/z in the sample, and the heights of the peaks connote the relative abundance of the various components in the sample.

MS plays a central role in proteomics, a systemic analysis of all the proteins in a tissue section or a cell. Owing to the high diversity and complexity, proteomics is more daunting and challenging than genomics. Currently, MS is utilized in identifying certain proteins or peptides in a clinical sample (46), but its wide use in clinical laboratories still faces hurdles to full automation.

5.12 Biosensor Assays

A biosensor is defined as a highly sensitive apparatus or device that can "sense" a bioactive molecule or its activity both qualitatively and quantitatively (47). Biosensor technology is widely used in various fields and particularly in medicine (Figure 5.3). The advantages of biosensors are that they are highly sensitive, highly specific, and highly reliable and detect the target molecules in a wide range of concentrations (48). The most important feature of biosensors is that they can be easily automated. Most of the current automated analyzers in clinical laboratories use biosensors, which are also being developed into various point-of-care devices. Current biosensor assays are largely used to detect single molecules or substances. Using different mechanisms, engineers have invented numerous biosensors; each has its pros and cons. Based on the differences in bio-receptors and transducers, biosensors can be classified as: 1) enzyme-based biosensors, 2) tissue-based biosensors, 3) immunosensors, 4) DNA biosensors, 5) magnetic biosensors, 6) thermal biosensors, 7) optical biosensors, and 8) piezoelectric biosensors.

The use of magnetic sensors is relatively new in the field of diagnostics. The first reported use of magnetic biosensors utilized a superconducting quantum interference device (SQUID) to detect binding events of antibodies labeled with magnetic tags. Later, Baselt demonstrated the detection of magnetic nanoparticles using giant magnetoresistive (GMR) sensors (49). GMR sensors have the advantage of room-temperature operation and simpler instrumentation. These sensors are the same sensors used in nearly every hard disk drive from 1994–2004. Since then, magnetic biosensors have followed the hard disk and drive industry moving towards smaller and increasingly sensitive magnetoresistive sensors (50). Using identical antibodies, Hall et al. showed that magnetic biosensors are three orders of magnitude more sensitive than conventional optical techniques due to the lower background (51). Biological samples with autofluorescence and optical labels are susceptible to bleaching, ultimately limiting the sensitivity of optical measurements. However, there is no magnetic background in biological samples, providing a fundamentally cleaner sensing environment. Furthermore, magnetic sensors can be arrayed and multiplexed to perform complex biomarker analysis in a single assay without resorting to bulky optical scanning. Last, magnetic tags can be manipulated with magnetic fields to speed up the reaction (52) and/or remove unbound tags (53).

Magnetic biosensors have been successfully used to detect magnetically labeled biomarkers (proteins, nucleic acids, and even whole cells). This assay strongly resembles the enzyme-linked immunosorbent assay (ELISA), except that the label has been changed from an enzyme or colorimetric tag to a magnetic

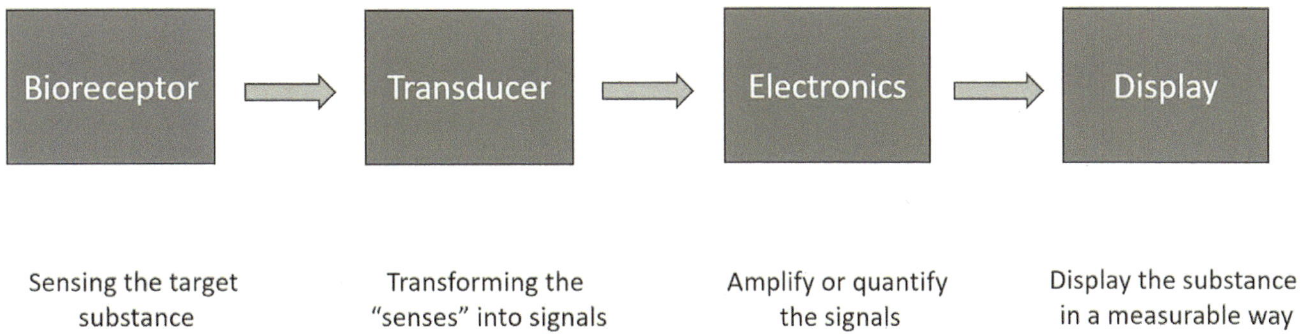

FIGURE 5.3 Components of a biosensor detector. Four components: 1) bioreceptor, 2) transducer, 3) electronics, and 4) display constitute an effective biosensor, which serves as an important tool to convert molecular interactions into electric signals.

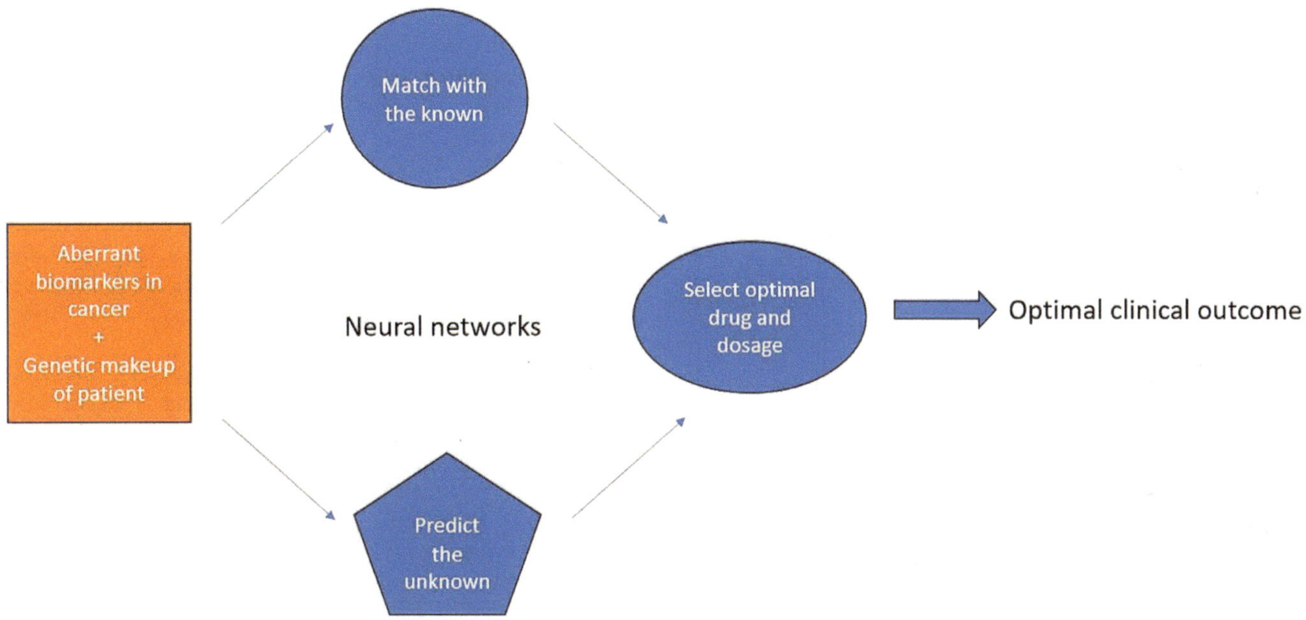

FIGURE 5.4 General workflow of deep learning–based artificial intelligence in precision pathology. First, cancer biomarkers and patient genetic information are collected and entered into the neural networks to screen and match with known information in Big Data; if there are no matches, the AI will provide the best guesstimate according to past experiences. Finally, the drugs and dosages are selected based on the modeled optimal clinical outcomes.

nanotag (MNT). The magnetic immunoassay (MIA) is implemented as follows: 1) a capture antibody, highly specific to a molecule (such as a protein kinase), is immobilized on the surface of the sensor through covalent attachment chemistry. 2) Upon introduction of the sample, which can contain hundreds to thousands of different molecules in vastly different concentrations, the capture antibody selectively binds only to the targeted protein molecule. 3) A biotinylated detection antibody is added and binds to a different site on the captured protein molecule. 4) Finally, MNTs are added and attached to the detection antibody through a high-affinity biotin-streptavidin bond to complete the MIA. The number of MNTs tethered to the surface is quantified by the underlying magnetic sensors. Using this assay, phosphorylated PI3K was captured in a large B-cell lymphoma (Toledo) cell lysates and detected with antibodies against the phospho-PI3K.

5.13 AI and Deep Learning

The application of artificial intelligence in pathology is currently limited to digital pathology (54–60). Diagnostic features are collected with whole slide imaging (WSI) from many similar cases with the same diagnosis. Two strategies are generally used for the applications: 1) hand-crafted or machine learning (ML) and 2) deep learning (DL) with neural networks. Several studies have shown promising results with melanoma lymphocyte infiltration (58), Gleason scoring of prostate cancer (59), quantitative counting of mitotic figures of breast cancer (60), and PD-L1 scoring for lung cancers (61). In some instances, AI performed better than pathologists (62). Despite the limitations, AI will be able to decrease the burden of repetitive work such as scoring that is liable to subjective variations.

AI combined with digital pathology remains limited to the diagnosis and classification of tumors based on traditional morphology. Our perspective about AI application in precision pathology is to analyze the activated pathways using the levels of activated kinases and detect potential signal shunting to identify drug resistance to targeted therapeutic agents (Figure 5.4). With more and more active biomarkers detected, DL could calculate the levels of cellular activity and even estimate accurate doses of drugs that could suppress the tumorigenic activity of cancer cells.

REFERENCES

1. Beishuizen A, Verhoeven MA, Mol EJ, et al. Detection of immunoglobulin heavy-chain gene rearrangements by Southern blot analysis: Recommendations for optimal results. Leukemia. 1993; 7(12): 2045–53.
2. DeBiasi RL, Tyler KL. Polymerase chain reaction in the diagnosis and management of central nervous system infections. Arch Neurol. 1999; 56(10): 1215–9.
3. Huang T, Hughes KT, Myers JL. Go gross or go home: The importance of gross examination in lung cancer staging and diagnosis of nonneoplastic diseases. AJSP Rev Rep. 2020; 25(4): 156–60.
4. Wright JH. A rapid method for the differential staining of blood films and malarial parasites. J Med Res. 1902; 7(1): 138–44.
5. Coons A. The demonstration of pneumococcal antigen in tissues by the use of fluorescent antibody. J Immunol. 1942; 45(3): 159–70.
6. Rudkin GT, Stollar BD. High resolution detection of DNA-RNA hybrids in situ by indirect immunofluorescence. Nature. 1977; 265(5593): 472–3.
7. O'Connor C. Fluorescence in situ hybridization (FISH). Nat Educ. 2008; 1(1): 171.
8. Chrzanowska NM, Kowalewski J, Lewandowska MA. Use of fluorescence in situ hybridization (FISH) in diagnosis and tailored therapies in solid tumors. Molecules. 2020; 25(8): 1864.
9. Sreekantaiah C. FISH panels for hematologic malignancies. Cytogenet Genome Res. 2007; 118(2–4): 284–96.
10. Huang H, Chen J. Chromosome bandings. Methods Mol Biol. 2017; 1541: 59–66.
11. Nicholson JM, Cimini D. Cancer karyotypes: Survival of the fittest. Front Oncol. 2013; 3: 148.
12. Wan TS. Cancer cytogenetics: Methodology revisited. Ann Lab Med. 2014; 34(6): 413–25.
13. Lobo I. Chromosome abnormalities and cancer cytogenetics. Nature. 2008; 1(1).
14. Moorman AV, Harrison CJ, Buck GAN, et al. Karyotype is an independent prognostic factor in adult acute lymphoblastic leukemia (ALL): Analysis of cytogenetic data from patients treated on the Medical Research Council (MRC) UKALLXII/Eastern Cooperative Oncology Group (ECOG) 2993 trial. Blood. 2007; 109(8): 3189–97.
15. Arber DA, Orazi A, Hasserjian RP, et al. International consensus classification of myeloid neoplasms and acute leukemias: Integrating morphologic, clinical, and genomic data. Blood. 2022; 140(11): 1200–28.
16. Fenaux P, Haase D, Sanz GF, et al. Myelodysplastic syndromes: ESMO clinical practice guidelines for diagnosis, treatment and follow-up. Ann Oncol. 2014; 25(Suppl 3): iii57–69.
17. Haase D, Germing U, Schanz J, et al. New insights into the prognostic impact of the karyotype in MDS and correlation with subtypes: Evidence from a core dataset of 2124 patients. Blood. 2007; 110(13): 4385–95.
18. Ding L, Ley TJ, Larson DE, et al. Clonal evolution in relapsed acute myeloid leukaemia revealed by whole-genome sequencing. Nature. 2012; 481(7382): 506–10.
19. Feurstein S, Thomay K, Hofmann W, et al. Routes of clonal evolution into complex karyotypes in myelodysplastic syndrome patients with 5q deletion. Int J Mol Sci. 2018; 19(10): 3269.
20. Wu W, Choudhry H. Next generation sequencing in cancer research. volume 1. New York: Springer; 2013.
21. Shyr D, Liu Q. Next generation sequencing in cancer research and clinical application. Biol Proced Online. 2013; 15(1): 4.
22. Shendure J, Ji H. Next-generation DNA sequencing. Nat Biotechnol. 2008; 26(10): 1135–45.
23. Metzker ML. Sequencing technologies—the next generation. Nat Rev Genet. 2010; 11(1): 31–46.
24. International Human Genome Sequencing Consortium. Finishing the euchromatic sequence of the human genome. Nature. 2004; 431(7011): 931–45.
25. Shabani Azim F, Houri H, Ghalavand Z, et al. Next generation sequencing in clinical oncology: Applications, challenges and promises: A review article. Iran J Public Health. 2018; 47(10): 1453–57.
26. Pennell NA, Mutebi A, Zhou Z-Y, et al. Economic impact of next-generation sequencing versus single-gene testing to detect genomic alterations in metastatic non-small-cell lung cancer using a decision analytic model. JCO Precis Oncol. 2019; 3: 1–9.
27. Lindeman NI, Cagle PT, Aisner DL, et al. Updated molecular testing guideline for the selection of lung cancer patients for treatment with targeted tyrosine kinase inhibitors: Guideline from the College of American Pathologists, the International Association for the Study of Lung Cancer, and the Association for Molecular Pathology. Arch Pathol Lab Med. 2018; 142(3): 321–46.
28. McDermott U. Next-generation sequencing and empowering personalised cancer medicine. Drug Discov Today. 2015; 20(12): 1470–5.
29. Gromova M, Vaggelas A, Dallmann G, et al. Biomarkers: Opportunities and challenges for drug development in the current regulatory landscape. Biomark Insights. 2020; 15: 1177271920974652.
30. Jorgensen JT. A paradigm shift in biomarker guided oncology drug development. Ann Transl Med. 2019; 7(7): 148.
31. Lestringant V, Duployez N, Penther D, et al. Optical genome mapping, a promising alternative to gold standard cytogenetic approaches in a series of acute lymphoblastic leukemias. Genes Chromosomes Cancer. 2021; 60(10): 657–67.
32. Goldrich DY, LaBarge B, Chartrand S, et al. Identification of somatic structural variants in solid tumors by optical genome mapping. J Pers Med. 2021; 11(2): 142.
33. Levy B, Baughn LB, Akkari Y, et al. Optical genome mapping in acute myeloid leukemia: A multicenter evaluation. Blood Adv. 2023; 7(7): 1297–307.
34. Sahajpal NS, Jill Lai CY, Hastie A, et al. Optical genome mapping identifies rare structural variations as predisposition factors associated with severe COVID-19. iScience. 2022; 25(2): 103760.

35. Sahajpal NS, Mondal AK, Ananth S, et al. Optical genome mapping and single nucleotide polymorphism microarray: An integrated approach for investigating products of conception. Genes (Basel). 2022; 13(4): 643.
36. Sahajpal NS, Mondal AK, Tvrdik T, et al. Clinical validation and diagnostic utility of optical genome mapping for enhanced cytogenomic analysis of hematological neoplasms. J Mol Diagn. 2022; 24(12): 1279–91.
37. Shim Y, Lee J, Seo J, et al. Optical genome mapping identifies clinically relevant genomic rearrangements in prostate cancer biopsy sample. Cancer Cell Int. 2022; 22(1): 306.
38. Chambliss AB, Chan DW. Precision medicine: From pharmacogenomics to pharmacoproteomics. Clin Proteomics. 2016; 13: 25.
39. Mroziewicz M, Tyndale RF. Pharmacogenetics: A tool for identifying genetic factors in drug dependence and response to treatment. Addict Sci Clin Pract. 2010; 5(2): 17–29.
40. Cecchin E, Stocco G. Pharmacogenomics and personalized medicine. Genes (Basel). 2020; 11(6): 679.
41. Lynch TJ, Bell DW, Sordella R, et al. Activating mutations in the epidermal growth factor receptor underlying responsiveness of non-small-cell lung cancer to gefitinib. N Engl J Med. 2004; 350(21): 2129–39.
42. Paez JG, Jänne PA, Lee JC, et al. EGFR mutations in lung cancer: Correlation with clinical response to gefitinib therapy. Science. 2004; 304(5676): 1497–500.
43. Zhang B, Whiteaker JR, Hoofnagle AN, et al. Clinical potential of mass spectrometry-based proteogenomics. Nat Rev Clin Oncol. 2019; 16(4): 256–68.
44. Chen G, Fan M, Liu Y, et al. Advances in MS based strategies for probing ligand-target interactions: Focus on soft ionization mass spectrometric techniques. Front Chem. 2019; 7: 703.
45. Geer LY, Markey SP, Kowalak JA, et al. Open mass spectrometry search algorithm. J Proteome Res. 2004; 3(5): 958–64.
46. Domon B, Aebersold R. Mass spectrometry and protein analysis. Science. 2006; 312(5771): 212–7.
47. Bhalla N, Jolly P, Formisano N, et al. Introduction to biosensors. Essays Biochem. 2016; 60(1): 1–8.
48. Mehrotra P. Biosensors and their applications—A review. J Oral Biol Craniofac Res. 2016; 6(2): 153–9.
49. Baselt DR, Lee GU, Natesan M, et al. A biosensor based on magnetoresistance technology. Biosens Bioelectron. 1998; 13(7–8): 731–9.
50. Childress J. Magnetic recording read head sensor technology. Comptes Rendus Phys. 2005; 6(9): 997–1012.
51. Gaster RS, Hall DA, Nielsen CH, et al. Matrix-insensitive protein assays push the limits of biosensors in medicine. Nat Med. 2009; 15(11): 1327–32.
52. Bruls DM, Evers TH, Kahlman JA, et al. Rapid integrated biosensor for multiplexed immunoassays based on actuated magnetic nanoparticles. Lab Chip. 2009; 9(24): 3504–10.
53. Aytur T, Foley J, Anwar M, et al. A novel magnetic bead bioassay platform using a microchip-based sensor for infectious disease diagnosis. J Immunol Methods. 2006; 314(1–2): 21–9.
54. Jiang Y, Yang M, Wang S, et al. Emerging role of deep learning-based artificial intelligence in tumor pathology. Cancer Commun (Lond). 2020; 40(4): 154–66.
55. Niazi MKK, Parwani AV, Gurcan MN. Digital pathology and artificial intelligence. Lancet Oncol. 2019; 20(5): e253–61.
56. Bera K, Schalper KA, Rimm DL, et al. Artificial intelligence in digital pathology—new tools for diagnosis and precision oncology. Nat Rev Clin Oncol. 2019; 16(11): 703–15.
57. Yao K, Singh A, Sridhar K, et al. Artificial intelligence in pathology: A simple and practical guide. Adv Anat Pathol. 2020; 27(6): 385–93.
58. Acs B, Rantalainen M, Hartman J. Artificial intelligence as the next step towards precision pathology. J Intern Med. 2020; 288(1): 62–81.
59. Nagpal K, Foote D, Liu Y, et al. Development and validation of a deep learning algorithm for improving Gleason scoring of prostate cancer. NPJ Digit Med. 2019; 2: 48.
60. Ibrahim A, Gamble P, Jaroensri R, et al. Artificial intelligence in digital breast pathology: Techniques and applications. Breast. 2020; 49: 267–73.
61. Liu J, Zheng Q, Mu X, et al. Automated tumor proportion score analysis for PD-L1 (22C3) expression in lung squamous cell carcinoma. Sci Rep. 2021; 11(1): 15907.
62. Stålhammar G, Fuentes Martinez N, Lippert M, et al. Digital image analysis outperforms manual biomarker assessment in breast cancer. Mod Pathol. 2016; 29(4): 318–29.

6

Specimen Acquisition

Xianfeng F. Zhao and Guang Liu

6.1 Introduction

Precision pathology identifies biomarkers and therapeutic targets from patient samples. Due to tumor heterogeneity, specimen preparation is critical in obtaining the information needed for precision therapy. Patient specimens can be received fresh or formalin-fixed paraffin-embedded (FFPE). They can be from blood, bone marrow aspirate, excised tissues, small core needle biopsies, and even cytology specimens. Whatever the sources are, the volume of the specimen and the number of cells should be sufficient to obtain enough DNA, RNA, or proteins for analysis. Different testing platforms have different specimen requirements, but this chapter will focus on the standard requirement of specimens to be tested.

6.2 Tumor Specimens

6.2.1 Blood and Bone Marrow

Blood and bone marrow specimens are usually acquired for diagnosing hematopoietic and lymphoid tumors. They are collected in either heparinized or ethylenediaminetetraacetic acid (EDTA) vacutainers. Generally, 2–3 mL of blood or bone marrow will yield enough high-quality DNA or RNA for genetic analysis. Specimens collected in both EDTA and acid citrate dextrose (ACD) tubes provide good yields of nucleic acid appropriate for molecular testing. Heparin, however, adsorbs to nucleic acid and is not completely removed by standard extraction techniques. Residual heparin in a DNA or RNA sample can inhibit restriction digests, polymerase chain reaction (PCR), and other enzyme-based molecular biology assays. Therefore, trisodium EDTA or ACD tubes are recommended for most molecular testing (1). However, a recent comparative study of DNA extracted from blood collected in heparin and EDTA tubes showed a similar quality of DNA for PCR analysis (2).

6.2.2 Fresh Tissue

Fresh tissue for precision pathology testing should be delivered to molecular labs as soon as possible or frozen immediately after collection if testing delays are unavoidable, to prevent DNA, RNA, or protein degradation (Table 6.1). If not frozen, it can be placed in a holding media (such as RPMI) and stored at 4°C for a maximum of 48 h. It is generally believed that 10^6 cells are adequate for the extraction of high-quality DNA for genetic analysis. Fresh tissue can be harvested from tumors or obtained via interventional radiology and submitted in RPMI or as frozen sections. On average 1 cm^3 will generate 10^8 tumor cells (3). Touch prep and/or frozen section should be performed to confirm the presence of tumor tissues in the specimen before submission (4).

Specimens harvested from excised tumors by surgery are usually adequate for precision pathology analysis. In contrast, core needle biopsies obtained from interventional radiology are often considered limited for pathological analysis due to the small size and lack of histological architecture. However, if the tissue suffices the minimal volume for analysis (Table 6.2), they are adequate in isolation of DNA or RNA for genetic analysis. More and more recent studies reported successes with this tissue source (4, 5).

6.2.3 FFPE Specimens

Since most tumor specimens are submitted for precision pathological analysis after diagnosis and not every tumor has the defined molecular targets for precision therapy at the time of diagnosis, most specimens to be analyzed are FFPE specimens. More procedures are utilized to prepare the specimen for molecular studies, and therefore the yield of DNA, RNA, and proteins is usually lower than from fresh tissues, and a larger amount of tissue is required to obtain useful results (6).

To ensure the quality of FFPE specimens for molecular analysis (7, 8), the following procedures are recommended:

Collection: The surgically resected specimen is promptly stored under refrigeration at ≤ 4°C and fixed within 1 h after resection, or within 3 h at the latest. Keeping it at room temperature for more than 30 min after resection should be avoided as much as possible. Tissue collected by biopsy is promptly fixed. Cell samples can also be embedded in paraffin after formalin fixation. In this case, fixation is performed as soon as possible after the necessary pretreatment is performed.

Fixation: Fixation is performed at room temperature for 6–48 h, using 10% neutral buffered formalin solution at a volume at least tenfold greater than the tissue volume. EDTA decalcification is preferred, and acid decalcification is avoided.

DOI: 10.1201/9781003513469-6

TABLE 6.1

Freshness of Tissues for Precision Pathology

Tissue	Time from Harvest to Analysis
Blood	24–48 h (at 4°C)
Bone marrow	24–48 h (at 4°C)
Fresh tissue	Within 1 h (at RT) from procedure to RPMI
	Within 24 h (at 4°C) from RPMI to analysis
Frozen tissue	Within 1 h (at RT) from procedure to frozen
	Within 24 h (at –20°C) from frozen to analysis
FFPE Tissue	Within 1 h (at RT) from procedure to formalin fixation
	Within 24 h (at 4–20°C) to analysis

Abbreviations: RPMI, most commonly used cell culture media; RT, room temperature

TABLE 6.2

Recommended Quantity of Tissues Required for Precision Pathology

Tissue	Volume	Cells
Blood	3 mL	$13\text{~}30 \times 10^9$
Bone marrow	3 mL	$\sim 48 \times 10^9$
Fresh tissue	1 mm^3	$\sim 10 \times 10^5$
Frozen tissue	1 mm^3	$\sim 10 \times 10^5$
FFPE Tissue	5 μm (×10) curls	$\sim 10 \times 10^6$

Source: compiled from refs. 3 and 6

Storage: The FFPE block is stored in a cool, dark place (room temperature permissible), avoiding humidity. Storage as unstained FFPE slides is avoided. When the tissue is provided for genomic analysis, sectioning is performed, and it is preferable to use an FFPE block within 3 years after it is prepared. Cross-contamination should be avoided by changing blades when sectioning different samples.

Adequacy and quality: When specimens are provided for genomic study, an FFPE block with the tumor load required for the analysis is selected by a pathologist based on the H&E slide of the specimen prepared during pathological diagnosis and information in the pathology report. Blocks with bleeding, necrosis, or many non-tumor cells, such as inflammatory cells, are avoided to the extent possible. A tumor content percentage of ≥ 30% in a section is desirable, and a minimum of 20% is required. If the tumor content percentage is low, the non-tumor portion is removed by microdissection to increase the content percentage. With tissue sections of 5 × 5 mm in size and a tumor content percentage of 30%, a minimum of ten sections of 4–5-μm slices are needed (Table 6.2). If the tissue is smaller, additional sections are required.

FFTE specimen–derived genomic DNA: Genomic DNA is typically extracted and analyzed in a molecular laboratory, and the quantity and quality of the DNA must meet pre-determined requirements. When analysis is performed on low-quality DNA, special precautions must be taken in interpreting the data.

6.3 Normal (Reference) Control

A major limitation of tumor-only sequencing is its inability to distinguish germline from somatic mutations, and therefore matched tumor-normal sequencing has emerged as a comprehensive analysis for both hereditary cancer predisposition and somatic profiling (9). Paired analysis of tumor and patient normal samples enables unambiguous detection of somatic mutations to guide treatment decisions and allows one to accurately report both germline variants related to hereditary cancer predisposition and somatic mutations in the tumor. Mutations called in the tumor that are not present in the paired normal sample are annotated and reported as somatic.

To define a germline variant, we need a normal reference. But defining the "normal" gene or sequence can be controversial. Normal reference is usually defined as the DNA/RNA sequence or protein level in majority of a healthy population. This "normal" reference can vary among populations of different genetic backgrounds. Therefore, paired tumor/normal sequencing can overcome racial differences in tumor mutational burden (TMB) (10).

A reference sequence is a sequence representing the reference genome, and an alternate sequence is a sequence that differs from the reference sequence. A variant is defined as a combination of a reference and at least one alternate sequence. It is used to refer to a specific region of the genome which differs from a normal genome, and it can be used to describe an alteration that may be benign, pathogenic, or of unknown significance. Variants are used to refer to alterations in DNA, RNA, and protein sequences (and sometimes called mutations or polymorphisms) when compared with a normal reference sequence (11).

A human genome reference sequence is an accepted representation of the human genome sequence that is used by researchers as a standard for comparison to DNA sequences generated in their studies. The scientists responsible for assembling and updating such reference sequences aim to provide the highest-quality, best possible consensus representations of the sequence and structural diversity found in the human genome among populations. The genome reference sequence provides a general framework and is not the DNA sequence of a single person (12).

6.3.1 Blood Samples

Matched normal blood is often used to obtain DNA/RNA as normal reference for analyzing solid tumors without metastasis. Mutations identified in both the blood and the solid tumor are considered germline variants, whereas mutations detected only in the tumor will be reported as somatic variants. Since covert metastasis is hard to detect, caution should be used if any of the tumor-specific mutations are detected in the matched blood samples, which indicates covert metastasis and invalidates the blood sample as a normal reference (13). Another pitfall in using blood as a normal reference is the possibility of detecting somatic mutations derived from a covert clonal hematopoiesis (14).

6.3.2 Buccal Swab, Saliva, and Nails

For hematologic malignancies, one distinct challenge is the lack of easily implementable sources of patient-matched normal controls to confidently identify variants as distinctly somatic. The presence of leukemic contamination in whole blood, buccal swabs, and saliva; poor yield of DNA from hair follicles or nails; and the extensive work required to sort normal cells or grow fibroblast cultures are all well-known challenges in clinical practice.

Both saliva and nails have been used by Sloan Kettering Memorial Cancer Center as normal controls in genomic profiling of hematological malignancies (15). However, this study showed that saliva controls contained high levels of contaminating tumor DNA (up to 38% variant allele frequency (VAF)), which suggests a limited role for saliva as a germline control in hematological malignancies. Although somatic tumor mutations were also observed in nails, nail DNA was most often purely germline (with a high tumor/nail VAF ratio), supporting the utility of nail controls towards deciphering the germline vs. somatic nature of variants detected in neoplastic patient samples.

6.3.3 GM12878 FFPE Scrolls

To standardize the control for FFPE tumor specimen analysis, GM12878 homogeneous cell pellet FFPE scrolls were proposed to be the standard control for molecular analysis of FFPE samples (16) and commercially available at the Coriell Institute for Medical Research. The GM12878 cell line (Repository ID: FF12878) is an Epstein-Barr virus transformed B lymphocyte cell line currently deposited at the NIGMS Human Genetic Cell Repository. It harbors a single bp (G-to-A) transition at nucleotide 681 in exon 5 of the CYP2C19 gene (CYP2C19*2), which creates an aberrant splice site, resulting in a catalytically inactive truncated protein.

6.4 Preanalytical Quality Control

Molecular studies are the most expensive tests in laboratories, and thus strict preanalytical quality control will decrease the amount of testing repetition and save unnecessary costs. Preanalytical variables, such as sample collection, handling, transport, and storage, may affect testing results. The number of errors in the preanalytical phase can be reduced by following standardized procedures. Preanalytical variables also include appropriateness of test request, proper patient identification and preparation, accurate sample collection, and handling and transport to the laboratory. Furthermore, the preanalytical procedures including centrifugation, pipetting, aliquoting, and sorting are all required to get a sample into a condition suitable for analysis. Indicators and quality specifications for requests, sampling, transport, and receiving samples have been recently identified and proposed to laboratory professionals to control and improve all steps included in the preanalytical phase (Table 6.3) (17).

6.4.1 Nucleic Acid

To ensure the reliability of the molecular genetic results, the quantity and quality of nucleic acids (DNA or RNA) must be measured prior to use in a procedure whose success depends on accurately determining the quantity, concentration, integrity, and/or purity of the nucleic acids. Techniques commonly used to assess nucleic acid quantity and/or quality include electrophoresis, UV/VIS spectrophotometry, and fluorescence spectroscopy (18).

Using agarose gel electrophoresis, the nucleic acid concentration can only be roughly estimated by comparing the intensity of the sample nucleic acid band with the corresponding band of the size marker. Gel electrophoresis can also help to check nucleic acid purity and integrity. The standard measurement for nucleic acid quantity and quality is UV spectrophotometry. UV absorbance at 260 nm (A260) is used to measure nucleic acid, and A280 is used to measure contaminating protein in the sample. The intensity of A260 is proportional to the concentration of nucleic acid, and the A260/A280 ratio indicates the purity of the nucleic acids. To convert UV absorption to nucleic concentration, one unit of absorption at 260 nm is equivalent to 50 mg/L of double-stranded DNA or 40 mg/L of RNA. Furthermore, the A260 reading in conjunction with the specific equations can be used to determine the concentration of DNA present in the solution more accurately (19). The standard measure for DNA purity is an A260/280 ratio of 1.8 to 2.0. Values less than 1.8 are indicative of protein contamination, and values of > 2.0 are indicative of RNA contamination. RNA should have A260/280 ratio of 2.0 to 2.3. A ratio below 1.8 indicates protein contamination in the DNA samples and a need for further purification.

TABLE 6.3

Quality Indicators in the Pre-Analytic Phase

QI-1: Appropriateness of test request	Number of requests with clinical question (%)
QI-2: Appropriateness of test request	Number of appropriate tests with respect to the clinical question (%)
QI-3: Examination requisition	Number of requests without physician's identification (%)
QI-4: Examination requisition	Number of unintelligible requests (%)
QI-5: Identification	Number of requests with erroneous patient identification (%)
QI-6: Identification	Number of requests with erroneous identification of physician (%)
QI-7: Test request	Number of requests with errors concerning test input (%)
QI-8: Samples	Number of samples lost/not received (%)
QI-9: Samples	Number of samples collected in inappropriate containers (%)
QI-10: Samples	Number of samples hemolyzed (hematology, chemistry) (%)
QI-11: Samples	Number of samples clotted (hematology, chemistry) (%)
QI-12: Samples	Number of samples with insufficient volumes (%)
QI-13: Samples	Number of samples with inadequate sample-anticoagulant ratio (%)
QI-14: Samples	Number of samples damaged in transport (%)
QI-15: Samples	Number of improperly labeled samples (%)
QI-16: Samples	Number of improperly stored samples (%)

RNA integrity assessments should be determined if such a quality indicator would exclude samples from specific downstream methodologies. RNA in specimens is highly labile because RNase is ubiquitous and difficult to inhibit. For human RNA targets, RNA quality must be assessed. However, depending on the target, it may not be necessary for all specimens to be assessed for RNA quality. RNA quality is not assessed, for example, for many types of viral RNA targets; however, the false negative rate must be documented (20). Guidelines for nucleic acid quality control for NGS assays were jointly recommended by both Association of Molecular Pathology (AMP) and College of American Pathologists (CAP) (21).

The A260/A230 ratio is another key measure of relative purity. The absorption at 230 nm (A230) represents a wavelength range that can identify the presence of several chemical contaminants. For instance, residual chaotropic salts, which can inhibit PCR, particularly multiplex PCR, are known to absorb in the 230 nm and lower wavelengths. The A260/A230 ratio should generally be greater than 1.4 on a scale of 2.0 in order to maximize multiplex PCR methods. It is a critical measurement to assess samples when high purity is required for the assay.

The fluorometric quantitation method is widely regarded as among the most sensitive methods of nucleic acid measurement (22). Although nucleic acid is naturally colorless, certain dyes can intercalate and bind nucleic acid grooves nonspecifically or selectively bind certain types of nucleic acid, and after binding to nucleic acids, the dyes are excited at one wavelength of light and emit another wavelength of light. Therefore, different nucleic acid concentrations will show different light intensities. Differences in spectral characteristics of nucleic acid-bound fluorophores allow sample concentrations to be determined. Evidence indicates that spectrophotometric methods overestimate DNA yield compared to fluorometric methods (Table 6.4) for FFPE specimens, although this may be confounded by different levels of variability among quantification methods (22).

6.4.2 Proteins

Quantitation and qualification are required before submitting protein samples for chromatographic, electrophoretic, and immunochemical separation or analysis. The simplest and most direct assay for protein concentration determination in solution is to measure the UV absorbance at 280 nm. Amino acids containing aromatic side chains (i.e., tyrosine, tryptophan, and phenylalanine) exhibit strong UV-light absorption. Proteins and peptides absorb UV light in proportion to their aromatic amino acid content and total concentration. Another method, traditionally used in amino acid analysis by high-performance liquid chromatography (HPLC), is to label all primary amines (i.e., N-terminus and side chain of lysine residues) with a colored or fluorescent dye such as ninhydrin or o-phthalaldehyde (OPA).

Direct UV-light absorbance and HPLC-reagent approaches have disadvantages that make these methods impractical for use with typical protein samples in proteomics workflows. The UV absorption method is not ideal for protein mixtures, as different proteins have differing aromatic amino acid contents. In addition, any non-protein content that absorbs UV-light will interfere with measurements (23).

To overcome these disadvantages, several colorimetric and fluorescent protein assay techniques have been developed that are used by nearly every laboratory involved in protein research. Protein samples are added to the reagent, producing a color change or increased fluorescence in proportion to the amount added. Protein concentration is determined by reference to a standard curve consisting of known concentrations of a purified reference protein. Types, advantages, and disadvantages of protein assay methods are listed in Table 6.5 (24).

TABLE 6.4

Advantages and Disadvantages of UV Spectrophotometry and Fluorometric Methods

Quantitation Method	Advantages	Disadvantages
UV spectrophotometry	* Quick and simple * Does not require any reagents	* Limited low-end sensitivity * Inaccuracies introduced by contaminants
Fluorescence	* Quick and simple * Highly sensitive for low-level samples * Contaminants pose minimal effect on results	* Requires calibration with standard(s) * Not sequence specific * Does not measure amplifiability

TABLE 6.5

Types, Advantages, and Disadvantages of Protein Assay Methods

Method	Advantages	Disadvantages
UV absorption	* Simple, does not require any assay reagents	* Highly error prone with protein mixtures or complex samples (e.g. cell lysates)
Biuret methods: Protein-copper chelation and secondary detection of reduced copper	* Compatibility with most surfactants (detergents) * Linear response curve ($R2 > 0.95$) * Less protein–protein variation than Coomassie dye–based assays	* Incompatibility with substances that reduce copper * Incompatibility with common reducing agents such as DTT
Colorimetric dye based methods: Protein-dye binding and direct detection of the color change	* Fast and easy to perform * Performed at room temperature * Compatible with most salts, solvents, buffers, thiols, reducing substances, and metal-chelating agents	* Incompatibility with surfactants (detergents) * High protein–protein variation when compared to copper-based assays
Fluorescent dye methods: Protein-dye binding and direct detection of increase in fluorescence associated with the bound dye	* Excellent sensitivity, requiring less protein sample for quantitation * Timing is not a critical factor, so the assays can be adapted for automated handling in high-throughput applications	* Requires specialized equipment

6.5 Standardization

There are many different molecular tests in use across the United States and the world. Some of these are commercially available, while others are developed by testing laboratories. It has become apparent that some of these tests vary widely in their clinical performance. Therefore, standardization is critical in the area of molecular testing. AMP and CAP jointly recommended guidelines on standardized validation of NGS testing (Figure 6.1) (21).

Variable biospecimen collection, processing, and storage practices may introduce variability in biospecimen quality and analytical results. This risk can be minimized within a facility using standardized procedures; however, analysis of biospecimens from different facilities may be confounded by differences in procedures and inferred biospecimen quality. Thus, a global approach to standardization of biospecimen handling procedures and their validation is needed, for example, the series of documents known as NCI Biospecimen Evidence-Based Practices, or BEBPs (25). The detailed and adaptable format of the document is intended to support the development and execution of evidence-based standard operating procedures (SOPs) for human biospecimen collection, processing, and storage operations. To decrease the variability and ensure high quality of collected specimens, CAP recommended a biospecimen kit for the standardized specimen collection to be used in all molecular diagnostic laboratories (26).

Standardization for molecular testing relies on the use of written standards, reference measurement procedures, and reference materials. Standardization of processes will result in high-quality human specimens and genetic materials that can be used to support precision pathology.

6.6 Biorepository

Establishment of a molecular diagnostics laboratory is not only costly but also demands effective management skills. Therefore, small medical centers and private practice pathology groups prefer to send their molecular studies to large academic or commercial diagnostic laboratories. With the rapid progress of genomic profiling, NGS, and various omics, novel targeted therapies unavailable today may emerge tomorrow. Prospective collection of patient specimens will prepare patients and oncologists to embrace future novel therapies.

A biorepository is defined as an entity or facility that collects, receives, processes, catalogs, stores, manages, and/or distributes biospecimens, their derivatives, and relevant data, as needed. It encompasses the physical location as well as the full range of activities associated with its operation (27). The term laboratory may also be used in the checklist to generically refer to a biorepository participating in the CAP's Biorepository Accreditation Program (20)

High-quality biospecimens are needed to improve patient outcomes. As a result of unprecedented research in precision medicine, demand for fit-for-purpose biospecimens is growing rapidly. According to a US survey of National Cancer Institute (NCI)–funded cancer researchers, lack of quality biospecimens resulted in 60% of researchers questioning their findings and 81% limiting the scope of their work (27).

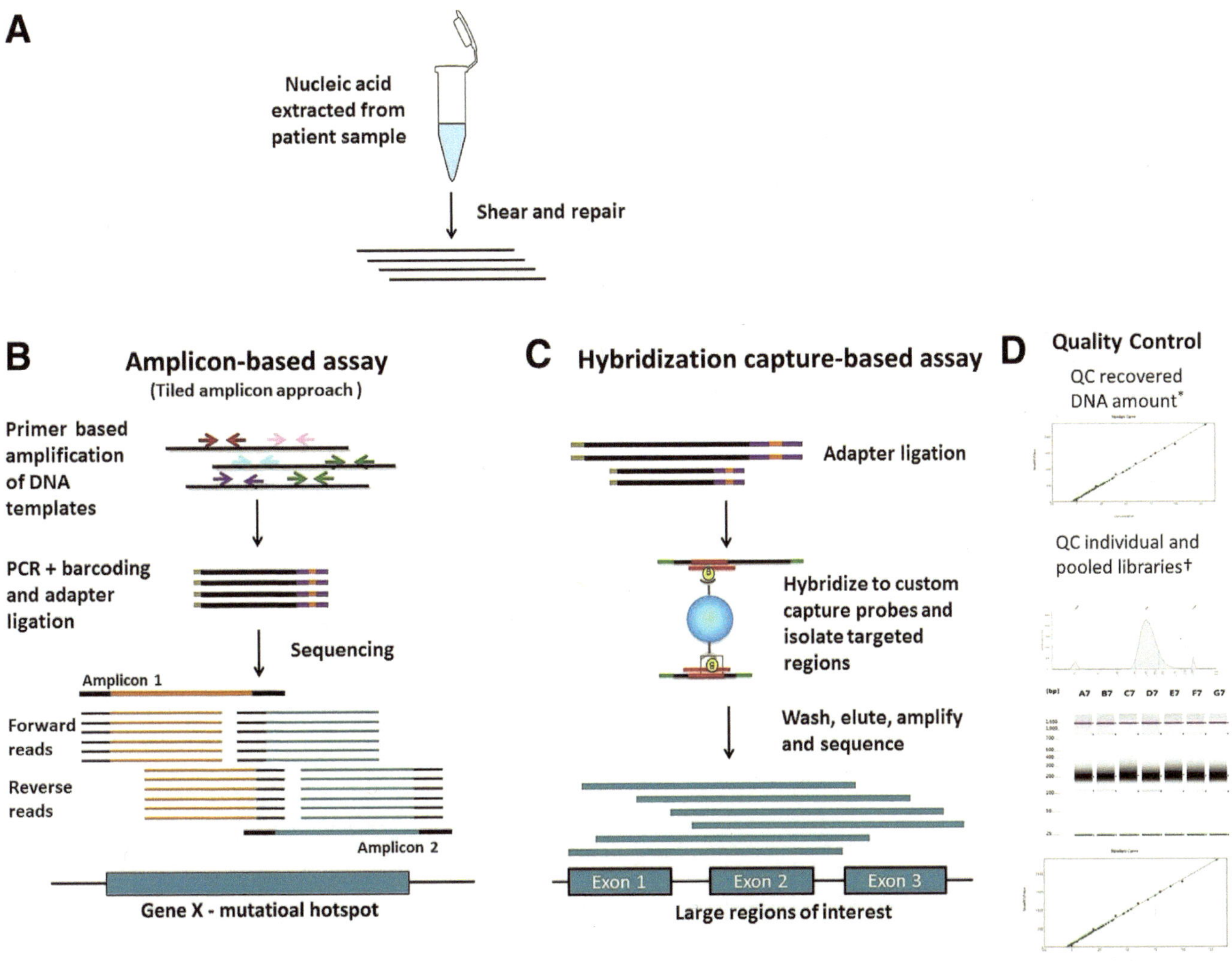

FIGURE 6.1 Standardized validation for NGS assays (from ref. 21 with permission). (A) Nucleic acid is extracted and quantified. The DNA is sheared and repaired to generate fragments of uniform size distribution, and the fragment size can be monitored by gel electrophoresis or Agilent Bioanalyzer. (B) Amplification-based assays: Target enrichment in amplification-based assays consists of PCR amplification of the desired region using primers. A tiled amplicon approach is depicted in which primers are designed to generate multiple overlapping amplicons of the same region to avoid allele dropout. The sequencing reads generated will have the same start and stop coordinates dictated by the primer design. (C) Hybridization capture–based assays: Target enrichment in hybridization capture–based assays uses long biotinylated oligonucleotide probes complementary to a region of interest. Probes hybridize to target regions contained within larger fragments of DNA. As a result, regions flanking the target will also be isolated and sequenced. The sequencing reads from these molecules will have unique start and stop coordinates when aligned to a reference, allowing identification and removal of PCR duplicates. (D) Quality control: The size distribution pattern of the individual and pooled libraries is quality controlled using Agilent TapeStation and quantified using a Spectramax microplate reader. Example images as visualized using an Agilent Bioanalyzer and Spectramax microplate reader are shown. QC, quality control.

6.6.1 Specimen Collection

Working with the pathology assistant, a surgically resected specimen is promptly grossed, and a small portion (more than minimally required for molecular studies) of the sample is harvested, snap frozen in optimal cutting temperature (OCT) compound on a chunk in liquid nitrogen, and stored immediately at –80°C. A standardized procedure for fresh specimen collection should be followed, as stated in earlier sections (Tables 6.1 and 6.2). The specimen is stored in a gridded cabinet and assigned a unique code.

6.6.2 Specimen Coding

After being assigned a unique code in a separate document, the coded specimen will be linked to its clinical information, including the patient's demographics, diagnosis and treatment history, family history, and any other genetic and biochemical studies. All this information should be linked to the Cancer Registry of the medical institution.

A biorepository is a bank as well as a library, and a coding system is required to accurately index the biospecimens deposited in the biobank. Every biorepository may have its own coding system for the banked biospecimens. To manage the traceability of biospecimen preanalytical variations and to provide effective and efficient interconnectivity and interoperability between biobanks, in 2010 the International Society for Biological and Environmental Repositories (ISBER) Working Group on Biospecimen Science developed a Standard PREanalytical Code (SPREC) that identifies the main preanalytical factors of clinical fluid and solid biospecimens and their simple derivatives (28). Each biospecimen is assigned a seven-element-long code that corresponds to seven preanalytical variables and contains a string of 11 (for fluids) or 13 (for solid tissues) letters in a defined order, separated by six hyphens. This SPREC is easy to implement and can be integrated into biobank quality management systems and databases. It is expected to have a particular value for multipartner validation and quality control and the execution of multicenter projects (e.g., involving proteomic, genomic, and Barcode of Life studies).

6.6.3 Specimen Transportation

Whether it is required for clinical analysis or clinical research, the specimen may be shipped to a different location for further analysis. Blood and bone marrow specimens sent to outside laboratories for molecular analysis can be shipped overnight at room temperature or with ice packs. Ideally a snap-frozen specimen should be transported in a –80°C CryoTainer or –150°C CryoCube. To decrease costs, a snap-frozen specimen can be transported in at least 10 lb dry ice overnight. Once it arrives, the specimen should be stored immediately in a –140°C freezer. FFPE specimens are stable and can be shipped overnight at room temperature.

6.6.4 Specimen Storage

6.6.4.1 *Tissue Specimens*

Snap-frozen tissue specimens should be stored in a –140°C freezer on an emergency power.

FFPE specimens are stable at room temperature, with minimal DNA degradation. However, paraffin tissue blocks should be stored in a cool, dark place and not exposed to high humidity. FFPE blocks for genomic testing may be stored under refrigeration.

For the storage of unstained FFPE slides, preventive measures such as low-temperature storage or coating with a thin layer of paraffin should be undertaken to avoid deterioration of nucleic acid quality (7). However, in principle, long-term storage of unstained FFPE slides for genomic testing should be avoided, and unstained FFPE slides should preferably be freshly prepared from the FFPE block, if possible.

6.6.4.2 *Specimen Derivatives*

Isolated DNA of sufficient purity can be stored at room temperature in a buffered solution, such as Tris-EDTA, for several months or at least 1 year at 4°C in a refrigerator. Purified DNA can be stored in a freezer at –20°C to –70°C in tightly sealed tubes for up to 10 years or longer. Storage in a freezer is preferred for long-term storage; however, a clean DNA preparation in frequent use is better stored in the refrigerator to avoid DNA damage caused by multiple cycles of freezing/thawing.

RNA is extremely susceptible to degradation by ribonucleases that are ubiquitous in the environment. Therefore, special precautions are needed (18). RNA collection, transport, and storage conditions can be different by genes and assays, so it must be performed by validated protocols (29). RNA suspended in water must be frozen at –70°C soon after extraction and can be stored long term as such. Freezing and thawing RNA more than three times affects its stability and recovery (1).

Proteins are an extremely heterogeneous class of biological macromolecules. Many are unstable when not in their native environments, which can vary considerably among cell compartments and extracellular fluids. If certain buffer conditions are not maintained, extracted proteins may not function properly or remain soluble. Proteins can lose structural integrity and activity as a result of proteolysis, aggregation, and suboptimal buffer conditions.

Purified proteins often need to be stored for an extended period while retaining their original structural integrity and/or activity. The extent of storage "shelf life" can vary from a few days to more than a year and is dependent on the nature of the protein and the storage conditions used. Optimal conditions for storage are distinctive to each protein; nevertheless, it is possible to suggest some general guidelines for protein storage and stability.

Common conditions for protein storage are summarized and compared in Table 6.6. Generally, there are tradeoffs associated with each method. For example, proteins stored in solution at 4°C can be dispensed conveniently as needed but require more diligence to prevent microbial or proteolytic degradation; such proteins may not be stable for more than a few days or weeks. By contrast, lyophilization allows for long-term storage of protein with very little threat of degradation, but the protein must be reconstituted before use and may be damaged by the lyophilization process (30).

6.6.5 Data Storage and Information Security

Biospecimen resource informatics systems should provide role- and project-based access control to system functionality and data (31). Role-based access control (RBAC) should support at least the flat National Institute of Standards and Technology (NIST) level and preferably the hierarchical level as well. Project-based security should implement a separate RBAC for access to data based on project/study/protocol privileges. Biospecimen resource informatics systems that store protected health information

TABLE 6.6

Comparison of Protein Storage Conditions

Storage conditions	Solution at 4°C	Solution in 25–50% glycerol or ethylene glycol at –20°C	Frozen at –20° to –80° or in liquid nitrogen	Lyophilized (usually also frozen)
Typical shelf life	1 month	1 year	Years	Years
Requires sterile conditions or addition of antibacterial agent	Yes	Usually	No	No
Number of times a sample may be remove for use	Many	Many	Once (repeated freeze-thaw cycles degrade proteins)	Once (it is impractical to lyophilize repeatedly)

(PHI)/personally identifiable information (PII) should adhere to all security regulations for such data (e.g. HIPAA, HITECH). These systems should also meet the criteria for NIST data stored and accessed at the Federal Information Security Management Act (FISMA) moderate level.

Secure data storage collectively refers to the manual and automated computing processes and technologies used to ensure stored data security and integrity. This can include physical protection of the hardware on which the data is stored, as well as security software. Physical protection applies to data at rest stored in computer/server hard disks, portable devices—like external hard drives or USB drives—as well as online/cloud, network-based storage area network (SAN) or network attached storage (NAS) systems. It involves protecting both storage resources and the data stored on them—both on premises and in external data centers and the cloud—from accidental or deliberate damage or destruction and from unauthorized users and uses. It's an area that is of critical importance to enterprises because most data breaches are ultimately caused by a failure in data storage security.

Security (user) codes should be established to permit only specifically authorized individuals to access patient data or alter programs. A system that allows different levels of user access to the system based on the user's authorization is desirable and usually provides effective security. Examples of best practices include these requirements: periodic alteration of passwords by users, minimum character length for passwords, password complexity requirements (e.g. a combination of alphanumeric characters), and recording of failed log-on attempts with user lock-out after a defined number of unsuccessful log-on attempts.

Biorepository computers often serve multiple functions. Many of these computers are connected in a network. The security of the system should be enough to prevent the casual user from installing software. Such unauthorized installation may cause instability of the operating system or introduce other unwanted consequences. Many operating systems allow procedures to restrict certain users from installing software.

Information sent over a public domain such as the Internet is considered in the public domain. Thus, it is potentially accessible to all parties on that network. Systems must be in place to protect network traffic, such as firewalls and data encryption schemes.

In order to respond to these technology trends and deal with the inherent security vulnerabilities in their storage systems, experts recommend that organizations implement the following data security best practices (32):

1. Data storage security policies—Biorepositories should have written policies specifying the appropriate levels of security for the different types of data that they have. Obviously, public data needs far less security than restricted or confidential data, and the organization needs to have security models, procedures, and tools in place to apply appropriate protections. The policies should also include details on the security measures that should be deployed on the storage devices used by the organization.
2. Access control—Role-based access control is a must-have for a secure data storage system, and in some cases, multi-factor authentication may be appropriate. Administrators should also be sure to change any default passwords on their storage devices and to enforce the use of strong passwords by users.
3. Encryption—Data should be encrypted both while in transit and at rest in the storage systems. Storage administrators also need to have a secure key management system for tracking their encryption keys.
4. Data loss prevention—Many experts say that encryption alone is not enough to provide full data security. They recommend that organizations also deploy data loss prevention (DLP) solutions that can help find and stop any attacks in progress.
5. Strong network security—Storage systems don't exist in a vacuum; they should be surrounded by strong network security systems, such as firewalls, anti-malware protection, security gateways, intrusion detection systems, and possibly advanced analytics and machine learning-based security solutions. These measures should prevent most cyber attackers from ever gaining access to the storage devices.
6. Strong endpoint security—Similarly, organizations also need to make sure that they have appropriate security measures in place on the computers, smartphones, and other devices that will be accessing the stored data. These endpoints, particularly mobile devices, can otherwise be a weak point in an organization's cyber defenses.
7. Redundancy—Redundant storage, including RAID technology, not only helps to improve availability and performance; in some cases, it can also help organizations mitigate security incidents.
8. Backup and recovery—Some successful malware or ransomware attacks compromise corporate networks so completely that the only way to recover is to restore from backups. Storage managers need to make sure that their backup systems and processes are adequate for these types of events, as well as for disaster recovery purposes. In addition, they need to make sure that backup systems have the same level of data security in place as primary systems.

6.7 Summary

Specimen acquisition is the starting point and the most critical step in precision pathology. An error in molecular pathology may not always change the final diagnosis, but an error in precision pathology will miss an opportunity for the patient to get effective treatment and live a longer life. If an accurate and high-quality patient specimen is not obtained, all the following steps will be in vain, regardless of the cutting-edge technology and other fancy tools being used; this is the so-called "garbage in, garbage out" principle, not to mention all the resources that might have been wasted by the error. Therefore, precautions should be taken at every step in specimen acquisition, from test ordering to accurate patient identification, correct specimen collection, specimen preservation, specimen preparation for testing, proper assays used in analysis, data analysis, and patient data security. Next, we will examine the precision pathology of each unique organ and system.

REFERENCES

1. Coleman WB, Tsongalis GJ, eds. Molecular Diagnostics: For the Clinical Laboratorian, 2nd ed. Humana Press, 2005.
2. Kotikalapudi R, Patel RK. Comparative study of the influence of EDTA and sodium heparin on long term storage of cattle DNA. Cell J. 2015;17(1):181–6.
3. Del Monte U. Does the cell number 10(9) still really fit one gram of tumor tissue? Cell Cycle (Georgetown, Tex.). 2009;8(3):505–6.
4. Hsu LH, Ko JS, Liu CC, et al. Conventional transbronchial needle aspiration is promising for identifying EGFR mutations in lung adenocarcinoma. Thorac Cancer. 2019;10(4):856–63.
5. Gleeson FC, Levy MJ, Roden AC, et al. EUS fine-needle pancreatic core biopsy can determine eligibility for tumor-agnostic immunotherapy. Endosc Int Open. 2018;6(10):E1278–82.
6. Ludgate JL, Wright J, Stockwell PA, et al. A streamlined method for analysing genome-wide DNA methylation patterns from low amounts of FFPE DNA. BMC Med Genomics. 2017;10(1):54.
7. Hatanaka Y, Kuwata T, Morii E, et al. The Japanese Society of Pathology Practical Guidelines on the handling of pathological tissue samples for cancer genomic medicine. Pathol Int. 2021;71(11):725–40.
8. Naito Y, Aburatani H, Amano T, et al. Clinical practice guidance for next-generation sequencing in cancer diagnosis and treatment (edition 2.1). Int J Clin Oncol. 2021;26(2):233–83.
9. Cheng DT, Mitchell TN, Zehir A, et al. Memorial Sloan Kettering-Integrated Mutation Profiling of Actionable Cancer Targets (MSK-IMPACT): A hybridization capture-based next-generation sequencing clinical assay for solid tumor molecular oncology. J Mol Diagn. 2015;17(3):251–64.
10. Carson KR, Salahudeen A, Kaneva K, et al. Paired tumor/normal sequencing reduces apparent racial differences in tumor mutational burden (TMB). J Clin Oncol. 2022;40(suppl 16):abstr 3138.
11. Definition of Variant. NCI Dictionary of Genetics Terms. NCI. Retrieved December 1, 2022. www.cancer.gov/publications/dictionaries/genetics-dictionary/def/variant.
12. Human genome reference sequence. National Human Genome Research Institute. May 10, 2022. Retrieved December 1, 2022. www.genome.gov/genetics-glossary/Human-Genome-Reference-Sequence.
13. Barbosa A, Pinto P, Peixoto A, et al. Next generation sequencing of tumor and matched plasma samples: Identification of somatic variants in ctDNA from ovarian cancer patients. Front Oncol. 2021;11:754094.
14. Solit D. Next-generation sequencing "not overhyped": MSK-IMPACT hits 65,000 samples and counting. 24 February 2021. Retrieved 21 December 2022. www.mskcc.org/clinical-updates/next-generation-sequencing-not-overhyped-msk-impact-hits-65000-samples-and-counting.
15. Ptashkin RN, Ewalt MD, Jayakumaran G, et al. Enhanced clinical assessment of hematologic malignancies through routine paired tumor:normal sequencing. Nat Commun. 2023;14(1):6895.
16. Mitchell M. Biobanking and reference materials: How new samples and biospecimen types raise the standard. AMP Reference Material Forum. 2022 Annual Meeting of Association of Molecular Pathology, Phoenix, AZ, 1–5 November 2022.
17. Plebani M. Quality indicators to detect pre-analytical errors in laboratory testing. Clin Biochem Rev. 2012;33(3):85–88.
18. College of American Pathologists (CAP) Molecular Pathology Checklist. 22 September 2021. www.cap.org/laboratory-improvement/accreditation/accreditation-checklists.
19. Shen CH, ed. Diagnostic Molecular Biology. Elsevier, 2019.
20. College of American Pathologists (CAP) Biorepository Checklist. 24 October 2022. www.cap.org/laboratory-improvement/accreditation/accreditation-checklists
21. Jennings LJ, Arcila ME, Corless C, et al. Guidelines for validation of next-generation sequencing-based oncology panels: A joint consensus recommendation of the Association for Molecular Pathology and College of American Pathologists. J Mol Diagn. 2017;19(3):341–65.
22. Buckingham L, ed. Molecular Diagnostics: Fundamentals, Methods and Clinical Applications. 3rd edition. F.A. Davis Company, 2019.
23. Krohn RI. The colorimetric detection and quantitation of total protein. Curr Protoc Cell Biol. 2011; Appendix 3:3H.
24. Overview of protein assays methods. ThermoFisher Scientific. Retrieved 21 December 2022. www.thermofisher.com/us/en/home/life-science/protein-biology/protein-biology-learning-center/protein-biology-resource-library/pierce-protein-methods/overview-protein-assays.html.
25. Engel KB, Vaught J, Moore HM. National cancer institute biospecimen evidence-based practices: A novel approach to pre-analytical standardization. Biopreserv Biobank. 2014; 12(2):148–50.
26. Standardization of biospecimen collection kits is an effective way to ensure greater consistency in biospecimen collection. CAP Today, December 2014. Retrieved 21 December 2022. www.captodayonline.com/standardization-biospecimen-collection-using-biospecimen-kits/.
27. Biorepository Accreditation Program. College of American Pathologists. Retrieved 21 December 2022. www.cap.org/laboratory-improvement/accreditation/biorepository-accreditation-program.
28. Betsou F, Lehmann S, Ashton G, et al. Standard pre-analytical coding for biospecimens: Defining the sample PREanalytical code. Cancer Epidemiol Biomarkers Prev. 2010;19(4):1004–11.
29. ACMG Technical Standards for Clinical Genetics Laboratories (2021 Revision), Section G: Clinical Molecular Genetics Technical Laboratory Standards. Retrieved 21 December 2022. www.acmg.net/PDFLibrary/ACMG%20Technical%20Lab%20Standards%20Section%20G.pdf.
30. Protein stability and storage. ThermoFisher. Tech Tip#43. Retrieved 21 December 2022. https://tools.thermofisher.com/content/sfs/brochures/TR0043-Protein-storage.pdf.
31. Biospecimen resource informatics: Data management and inventory control and tracking. National Cancer Institute, Division of Cancer Treatment & Diagnosis, Cancer Diagnosis Program, Biorepositories and Biospecimen Research Brach. 29 March 2016. Retrieved 21 December 2022. https://biospecimens.cancer.gov/bestpractices/to/bri.asp.
32. Data storage security. HypertechDirect 2021. Retrieved 21 December 2022. https://hypertecdirect.com/knowledge-base/data-storage-security/.

7

Skin Cancers

Benjamin K. Stoff, Zachary Wolner, and Rebecca Leibowitz

7.1 Introduction

Skin cancer is the most common malignancy in the United States, representing one out of every three newly diagnosed cancers (1). Although many types of skin cancer exist, they can be divided into two major groups—melanoma and keratinocyte carcinoma (often referred to as "non-melanoma skin cancer" (NMSC)). Basal cell carcinoma (BCC) and cutaneous squamous cell carcinoma (cSCC) are keratinocyte carcinomas and represent the majority of skin cancers. Although melanoma only accounts for approximately 2% of skin cancer, it is responsible for more than 80% of skin cancer mortality (1). The gold standard for diagnosing cutaneous malignancies is biopsy with histopathological examination, albeit with variability in the interpretation of melanocytic lesions across pathologists (2). Once diagnosed, the mainstay of treatment for early-stage melanoma is wide local excision with surgical margins determined by microscopic tumor stage (3). Although the incidence of melanoma has continued to increase over time, mortality rates have declined due to the advent of novel systemic therapies for advanced disease (4). While surgery remains the optimal therapy for localized melanoma and keratinocyte carcinoma, first-line therapies for locally advanced, unresectable, or metastatic disease include systemic treatments and radiation (5, 6). Precision pathology holds promise for current diagnostic challenges and may contribute to staging and directing treatment of cutaneous malignancies.

7.2 Melanoma

The malignant transformation of melanocytes into melanoma is strongly linked to ultraviolet (UV) exposure (7). Histologically, there are several growth patterns of melanoma determined by the intraepidermal pattern of involvement, with superficial spreading melanoma and nodular melanoma accounting for 65% and 20% of cases, respectively (8). Superficial spreading melanoma is characterized histologically by horizontal proliferation of malignant melanocytes within the epidermis. Typical histologic features include epithelioid cytomorphology, irregular melanocytic nests, poor circumscription, asymmetry, and extension of melanocytes superior to the basal layer of the epidermis, otherwise known as pagetoid scatter or spread. On the other hand, nodular melanoma is believed to lack a horizontal growth phase and immediately progresses into vertical growth with limited epidermal involvement (Figure 7.1). As such, this subtype tends to present at a later stage and has a worse prognosis (9). Despite ongoing advances in genetics, the depth of invasion, also known as Breslow thickness, and ulceration have remained the most important prognostic factors of the primary tumor.

7.2.1 Genetic Aberrations

Melanocytic neoplasms can be viewed on a spectrum of accumulated genetic alterations (Figure 7.2). The majority of melanocytic neoplasms harbor a mutation that activates the mitogen-activated protein kinase (MAPK) signaling pathway, with *BRAF* and *NRAS* being the most common initiating oncogenes. BRAF is a serine/threonine kinase that promotes melanomagenesis via deregulated activation of downstream effectors of the MAPK pathway (Figure 7.3). *BRAF* V600E mutation is present in over 90% of nevi, and *BRAF* V600 mutations are present in 50% of melanomas (10).

Shain et al. sequenced hundreds of cancer genes in 37 primary melanomas and their adjacent precursor lesions to further characterize their genetic evolution. Seventy-seven percent of atypical melanocytic precursor neoplasms (such as dysplastic nevi) and in-situ melanomas possess mutations to the telomerase reverse transcriptase (TERT) promoter, while further evolution to invasive melanoma and subsequent metastatic disease is marked by mutations in cyclin-dependent kinase inhibitor 2A (*CDKN2A*) and *TP53*/*PTEN*, respectively (11).

The Cancer Genome Atlas network cataloged somatic alterations of 333 melanomas to create a framework for genomic classification. The largest genomic subtype is *BRAF* mutations (52%), followed by *RAS* mutations (28%) including *NRAS*, *KRAS*, and *HRAS*, and *NF1* (14%). These three aberrations serve to constitutively activate the MAPK pathway. The least common was called Triple-wild type (6%), as it lacked the formerly mentioned mutations (12). Additional aberrations in *CDKN2A* or *CDK4* of the p16-retinoblastoma (Rb) pathway are needed to escape senescence and continue tumor progression (13).

In addition to genetic aberrations in acquired nevi, there are inherited genetic mutations that can predispose patients to melanoma. Familial atypical multiple mole melanoma (FAMMM) syndrome is an autosomal dominant condition characterized by a family history of melanoma and multiple melanocytic lesions. Patients with FAMMM have about a 58% to 92% lifetime risk of developing melanoma, which is 25 to 45 times the risk of the average population (14, 15). Approximately 40% of cases of FAMMM are associated with mutations in *CDKN2A* (14).

DOI: 10.1201/9781003513469-7

Tumor	Subtype	H&E Characteristics	Stains	Representative Example
Melanoma	Superficial Spreading	• Horizontal proliferation within epidermis • Irregular melanocytic nests • Pagetoid scatter	• SOX10 • Melan-A • PRAME • Loss of p16	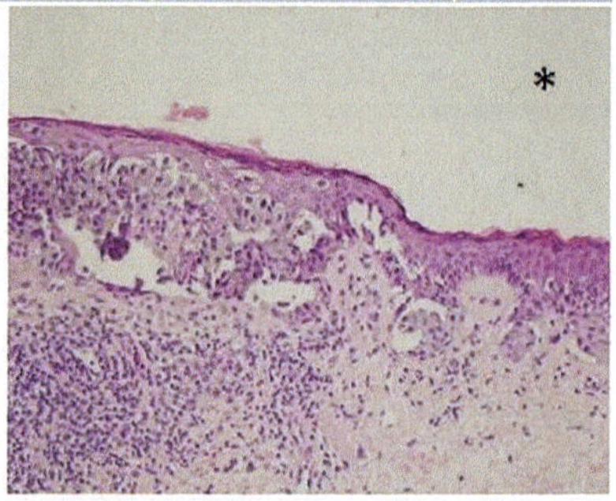
	Nodular	• Vertical growth with limited epidermal involvement		
Basal Cell Carcinoma	Superficial	• Clusters of basaloid cells extending from the epidermis • No reticular dermal invasion	• BerEP4	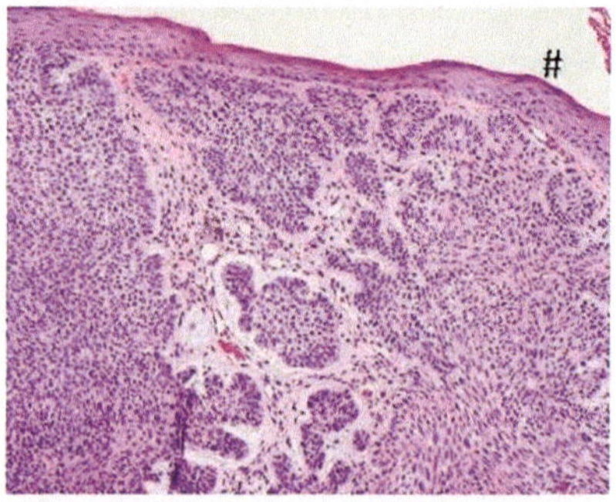
	Nodular	• Islands of basophilic cells • Peripheral palisading • Retraction artifact • Mucinous stroma		
	Morpheaform	• Thin strands of cells invading the dermis • Surrounded by fibrous stroma		
	Micronodular	• Similar to nodular subtype; organized into small nodules		
Squamous Cell Carcinoma	Acantholytic	• Pseudoglandular with acantholysis	• E-cadherin • Podoplanin • p63 • p40	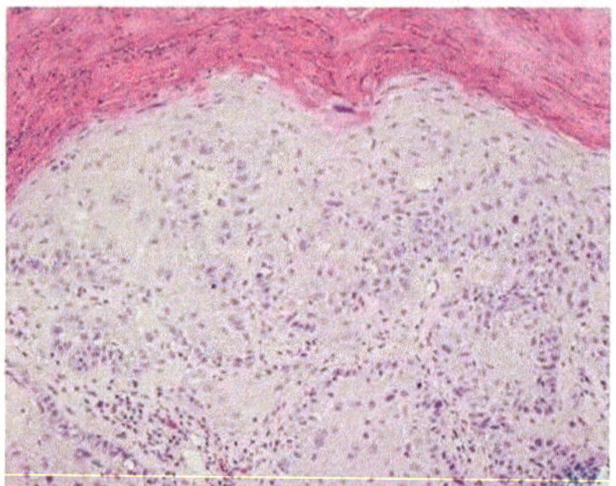
	Spindle Cell	• Atypical spindled squamous cells with collagen fibers and abundant stroma		
Merkel Cell Carcinoma	-	• Sheets of basaloid cells with a "salt and pepper" chromatin pattern • Minimal cytoplasm	• CK-20 • Pancytokeratin AE1/AE3 • CAM 5.2 • Neurofilament	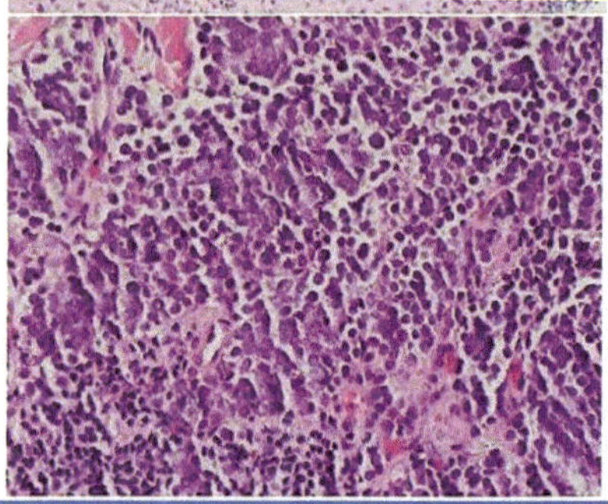

*) melanoma, superficial spreading growth pattern #) basal cell carcinoma, nodular growth pattern

FIGURE 7.1 Key features and examples of cutaneous malignancies.

This syndrome also has a strong association with pancreatic cancer, with FAMMM patients at a 13–22 times greater risk of developing pancreatic cancer as compared to the general population. This risk increases to 38-fold in FAMMM patients with mutations in *CDKN2A* (16). Because a strong correlation exists between FAMMM, mutant *CDKN2A*, and pancreatic cancer, it is recommended by the National Comprehensive Cancer Network (NCCN) that patients suspected of having FAMMM syndrome should undergo genetic screening for *CDKN2A* mutant (17).

Despite this taxonomy of genetic mutations, diagnosis of melanocytic lesions is challenging and, in some cases, not entirely reproducible. Multiple studies have revealed substantial inter- and intra-observer variability in melanoma diagnosis by pathologists (18). In one study, US pathologists were randomized to interpret skin biopsies to determine diagnostic concordance with a consensus diagnosis by experienced pathologists. Diagnoses ranging from moderately dysplastic nevi (class II) to early-stage invasive melanoma (class IV) were neither accurate nor reproducible, while lesions that belonged to classes I (benign nevi)

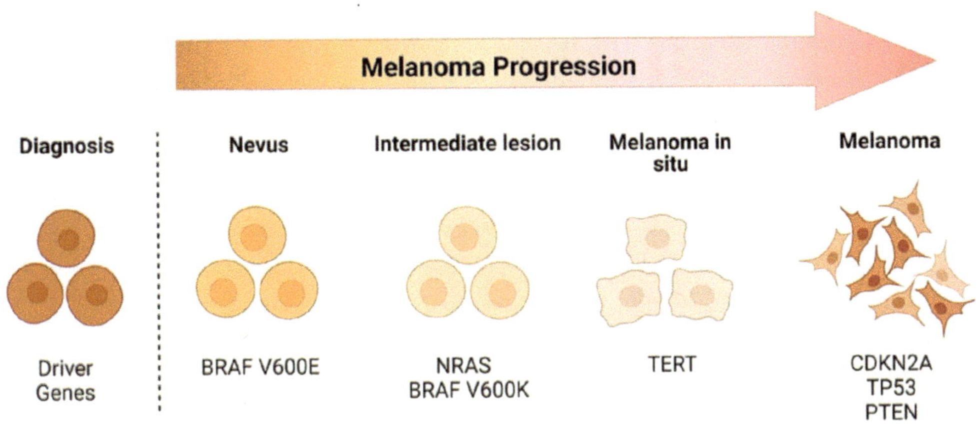

FIGURE 7.2 Progression of genetic abnormalities of melanoma. The proposed stereotypical pattern of melanoma evolution and associated mutations. This schematic is modeled after Shain et al. (11; adapted from Growth Factors Involved in Cardiomyocyte Differentiation by BioRender.com).

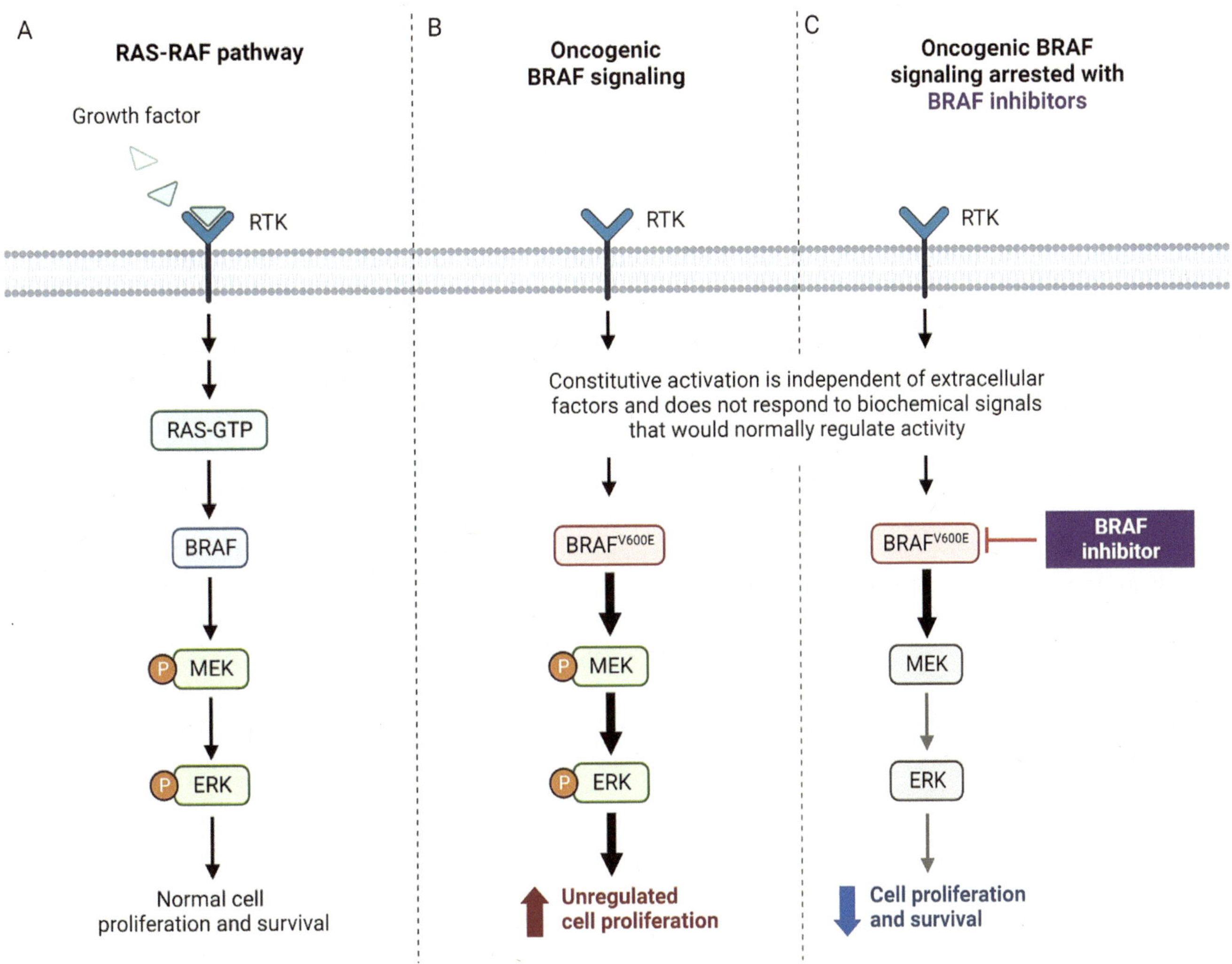

FIGURE 7.3 BRAF signaling pathways (adapted from Vemurafenib in Oncogenic BRAF Signaling Pathway in Melanoma by BioRender.com). Panel A represents the normal activation of RAS-GTP via extracellular growth factors interacting with receptor tyrosine kinase (RTK) and subsequent downstream signaling. Panel B represents the oncogenic BRAF signaling pathway in which constitutive activation is independent of extracellular growth factors. Panel C represents the oncogenic BRAF signaling pathway arrested with BRAF inhibitors, thus blocking the constitutive activation of MEK by mutant *BRAF* V600E.

and V (high-stage invasive melanoma) had much higher rates of inter-observer agreement (2). Supplementing histologic assessment with immunohistochemical staining and other ancillary techniques (see subsequently) may help improve upon diagnostic discrepancies of melanocytic lesions.

7.2.2 Immunohistochemistry

Melanoma can be a challenging diagnosis to make using histopathology alone. Immunohistochemistry (IHC) is frequently employed to establish melanocytic lineage, reveal the full extent of the melanocytic proliferation, and more recently to support malignancy in the setting of borderline histologic features and determine *BRAF* V600E mutation status. One such stain is SOX10, a nuclear transcription factor involved in the differentiation of neural crest progenitor cells to melanocytes. SOX10 has been shown to be an extremely sensitive marker for melanocytes but can stain other cells, such as myoepithelial cells and some nerve sheath neoplasms (19). As a result of nuclear expression and greater specificity, SOX10 has gained favor over S100 protein by many dermatopathologists. Melan-A is a more specific marker for melanocytic lesions, but it is not expressed in desmoplastic melanoma, a relatively uncommon variant of melanoma characterized by spindle cell morphology that can be difficult to diagnose due to significant variability in epidermal involvement, perineural invasion, tumor cellularity, and degree of fibrosis (20, 21). Another marker that may be helpful in differentiating nevi from melanoma is p16, the product of a tumor suppressor gene involved in G1 to S checkpoint regulation. This protein marker is present in most benign nevi, while its absence may represent progression to melanoma in up to 50 to 98% of cases (20). A newer IHC stain, preferentially expressed antigen in melanoma (PRAME), can potentially aid in differentiating melanoma from benign lesions. Lezcano et al. recently evaluated 400 melanocytic tumors by IHC for PRAME. They found >75% of melanocytes exhibited strong expression in 87% of metastatic melanoma, 83.2% of primary melanoma, and only 13.6% of melanocytic nevi (22).

7.2.3 Fluorescence *In Situ* Hybridization and Comparative Genomic Hybridization

For ambiguous melanocytic lesions, fluorescence *in situ* hybridization (FISH) and comparative genomic hybridization (CGH) have shown promise as diagnostic aids. Conventional melanoma FISH targets sequences on chromosomes 6, 8, 9, and 11 and demonstrates a reported sensitivity of 75–100% and specificity of about 95% in unequivocal cases; however, its utility in the diagnosis of histologically ambiguous cases remains uncertain. Positivity is determined by absolute or relative gain of 6p25, loss of 6q23, gain of 11q13, loss of 9p21, or gain of 8q24. More specifically, homozygous deletion of 9p21 has been correlated with clinically aggressive behavior in histologically ambiguous melanomas. CGH is similar to FISH in that it also assesses for chromosomal gains and losses, although it is not restricted to those assessed by FISH. The clinical utility of CGH is limited by its requirement for greater tumor tissue, lower resolution, limited availability, and expense. Nevertheless, one study demonstrated that CGH results were in agreement with expert consensus diagnosis 71% of the time (23). Although an extensive review of FISH and CGH is beyond the scope of this chapter, interested readers may review cited references for further details (24, 25).

7.2.4 Genomic Expression Profiling

Genomic expression profiling (GEP) is one of the newest technologies to aid in diagnosis and prognosis of melanocytic lesions (Table 7.1). GEP is a neural network-based model that uses select gene expression levels to predict diagnosis and risk of a clinical outcome (26). Two tests, MyPath and DiffDx, are 23 and 35 GEPs, respectively, that have been marketed as an adjunct to conventional histology for diagnosis of ambiguous melanocytic lesions. These tests were developed and validated on unequivocal melanocytic nevi and melanomas, and equivocal lesions or those with an indeterminate score on the test were excluded (27). They utilize quantitative RT-PCR to analyze the expression of selected genes involved in melanoma pathogenesis and subsequently generate a score that classifies a lesion as benign, indeterminate, or malignant. In an analysis of 70 histopathologically challenging melanoma cases, FISH demonstrated 84% agreement with final interpretation, while myPath showed 74% overall agreement (23). Despite limited evidence, over 2,600 tests were ordered in 2021 (28). While diagnostic aids are needed in classifying diagnostically challenging melanocytic neoplasms, high-quality prospective studies are essential in determining the value of GEP in the diagnosis of melanocytic lesions. Table 7.1 provides a summary of the studies assessing the utility of GEP.

While these modalities may be useful in establishing a diagnosis of melanoma, GEPs are also being used for prognosis, including to triage sentinel lymph node biopsies (SLNB) and to assess risk of clinical outcomes. SLNB plays a vital role in staging and prognostication of melanoma, but it carries a risk of hemorrhage, infection, and lymphedema (29). To avoid unnecessary SLNB in patients who may not need them and identify patients at higher risk for lymph node metastasis, GEPs have been developed to predict SLNB positivity.

In this vein, in 2021, Whitman et al. incorporated clinicopathologic information into a GEP assay to create the integrating 31-gene expression profiling (i31-GEP) neural network algorithm to predict SLNB positivity (Table 7.1). While the clinical utility of GEP in prior studies was uncertain, use of the i31-GEP-SLNB model had greater net benefit for patients with T1b, T2a, and T2b melanoma as compared to those with T1a. Among patients with T1b disease, the i31-GEP conferred a 23% decrease in negative SLNB (without SLN metastasis) and no increase in the number of patients with a missed diagnosis of SLN metastasis compared to SLNB alone. Given these results, this test has the potential to decrease morbidity and improve yield associated with SLNB (30). Current evidence for GEP evaluates performance for small groups of patients, often without consideration of all staging-relevant clinicopathologic features. Furthermore, analyses often lack survival outcomes as compared with data from the American Joint Committee on Cancer 8th (AJCC8) edition melanoma staging system international database (26). While there is a need and promise for GEP in melanoma prognosis, more rigorous and higher-quality studies are needed.

TABLE 7.1

Comparison of Gene Expression Profiling Studies for Melanoma and Cutaneous Squamous Cell Carcinoma

Test	Publication	Type	Methods	Findings
31-GEP: Melanoma	Hsueh et al. [77, 78]	Prospective	• 342 patients • 67% Stage I • 22% Stage II • 11% Stage III • Metastatic event/median event-free f/u: 3.5 y	• Class 1A: 3-y 96% RFS; 97% DMFS • Class 1B: 3-y 91% RFS; 93% DMFS • Class 2A: 3-y 80% RFS; 84% DMFS • Class 2B: 3-y 62% RFS; 80% DMFS • Recurrences correctly classified stages I-III: 60% (26/43)
31-GEP: Melanoma	Vetto et al. [79]	Prospective	• 838 patients • T1/T2 patient with SLNB (or eligible) divided into two cohorts	*Cohort 1* • Class 1A: 6.2% SLNB+ • Class 2B: 8.3% SLNB+ *Cohort 2* • Class 1A: 6.3% SLNB+ • Class 2A 24.5% SLNB+
i31-GEP: Melanoma	Whitman et al. [30]	Retrospective	• 1,674 patients • 42% T1 • 32% T2 • 18% T3 • 8% T4	*PPV and NPV for +SLNB* • T1a-HR: 4% PPV; 98% NPV • T1b: 8% PPV; 98% NPV • T2a: 13% PPV; 96% NPV • T2b: 13% PPV; 100% NPV • T3–4: N/A [80]
GEP: Melanocytic Lesions	Reimann et al. [23]	Prospective	• 268 cases • 74% morphologically unequivocal • 26% morphologically ambiguous	• Sensitivity morphologic diagnosis: 67% • Specificity morphologic diagnosis: 81%
40-GEP: cSCC	Wysong et al. [63]	Retrospective	• 321 cases • 58% T1 (BWH) • 31% T2a (BWH) • 9% T2b (BWH) • 2% T3 (BWH)	*Metastatic risk* • Class 2B v. 1/2A: 60% PPV; 88% NPV • Class 2 v. 1: 29% PPV; 91% NPV

Source: (see further ref. 26)

Abbreviations: BWH, Brigham and Women's Hospital; f/u, follow-up; GEP, gene expression profile; i31-GEP, integrating 31-gene expression profile; HR, high risk; NPV, negative predictive value; PPV, positive predictive value; RFS, recurrence-free survival; cSCC, cutaneous squamous cell carcinoma; SLNB, sentinel lymph node biopsy.

7.2.5 Next-Generation Sequencing

Next-generation sequencing (NGS) has emerged as another adjunct to melanoma diagnostics. A recent study utilized NGS to differentiate between melanoma and all other lesions, as well as malignant vs. benign lesions. One analysis assessed the number of small nucleotide variants per tumor and demonstrated that melanocytic lesions had a median of 18 variants per tumor, while all other lesions had a median of just 8 variants per tumor. A similar trend was observed when comparing benign and malignant tumors, with a median of 16 variants per tumor in malignant lesions and a median of 7 variants for those classified as benign. NGS also appears to yield greater diagnostic accuracy as it was found to have 100% concordance with consensus diagnoses, while FISH, for example, yielded 83% concordance (31).

7.2.6 Staging

Melanoma treatment is ultimately guided by staging as defined by the AJCC8. In this staging system, the tumor (T) category of staging is stratified based on tumor thickness, with T1 as less than 1 mm, T2 between 1 and 2 mm, T3 between 2 and 4 mm, and T4 greater than 4 mm. Additionally, the T category is further subdivided into "a" and "b" substrata based on the presence of ulceration, with "a" denoting absence of ulceration and "b" presence of ulceration. Furthermore, the 8th edition of this staging system has eliminated mitotic rate as a T-category criterion; however, mitotic rate remains a major prognostic determinant in melanoma. The nodal (N) category is defined by the number and extent of involved lymph nodes and presence of regional nodal metastasis found at SLNB. The third and final component of the AJCC8 melanoma staging system is the metastasis (M) category, as determined by the site of distant metastasis and serum lactate dehydrogenase level (32).

7.2.7 Immunotherapy and Targeted Treatment

In situ or stage I melanoma is typically treated with excision, with SLNB also typically performed for stage T1b and above. If SLNB is positive, adjuvant therapy may include lymph node dissection and, in some cases, systemic therapy with immune checkpoint inhibition or targeted therapy such as BRAF inhibition. Treatment of stage II is the same as previously: primary tumors are removed via wide excision, a sentinel lymph node biopsy is performed, and adjuvant therapy is considered for patients with advanced primary tumors or positive SLNB (33). To further guide treatment, tumor stage III or higher are often genetically profiled to assess for specific mutations, such as *BRAF* V600. If positive, a BRAF inhibitor can be added as adjuvant therapy. Half of patients treated with a BRAF inhibitor develop disease progression 6 months after treatment initiation (34). This failure of treatment has largely been attributed to acquired resistance mechanisms, such as mutant *BRAF* and activating mutations in *MEK1*. To circumvent this, a MEK inhibitor, such as trametinib, should be initiated at the same time as BRAF inhibition. MEK is a downstream target of BRAF, and its inhibition has proven to be an effective method of overcoming resistance to BRAF inhibitors (3). Systemic treatments for stage IV melanoma have rapidly evolved in recent years. Immunotherapy has become the first-line treatment for widespread metastatic disease and has drastically improved progression-free and overall survival. While there are no specific mutational targets associated with immunotherapy, current evidence does not support testing the tumor for PD-L1 to guide therapy (5). One option specific to advanced-stage melanoma targets c-*KIT*, a proto-oncogene encoding a tyrosine kinase that is often mutated in unresectable stage III and IV melanoma (33). It has been shown that KIT inhibition with imatinib results in durable clinical responses in 16% of patients harboring c-*KIT* mutations; however, response to this therapy is unpredictable (35).

7.2.8 Summary

The diagnosis and prognosis of melanocytic lesions remain challenges. While genetic profiling, through FISH/CGH and GEPs, offers potential benefit, further evaluation is needed to better incorporate these modalities into established guidelines. Time-tested histologic parameters, such as Breslow thickness, continue to carry significant prognostic value. Genetic profiling currently aids in selection of patients eligible for BRAF inhibition, and further investigation may lead to development of new treatments and identification of candidates for adjuvant immunotherapy.

7.3 Basal Cell Carcinoma

Basal cell carcinoma (BCC) is the most common malignancy in the United States and accounts for over 90% of skin cancers (36, 37). Similar to melanoma, BCC can manifest with one of several different growth patterns, such as nodular, superficial, morpheaform, infiltrative, and micronodular variants. Superficial BCC may demonstrate multiple clusters of basaloid cells extending from the epidermis without reticular dermal invasion (38). Nodular BCCs are the most common variant and, like superficial BCC, are known to have lower risk of recurrence than other subtypes (36). Histologically, this variant may present with islands of basophilic cells with peripheral palisading, retraction artifact from adjacent stroma and mucinous stroma (38). Micronodular BCCs are histologically similar to the nodular subtype, except that they are composed of multiple smaller nodules. Furthermore, they have a higher risk of recurrence than nodular BCC (36, 38). Morpheaform BCC displays thin strands of tumor cells invading the reticular dermis, surrounded by fibrous stroma (Figure 7.1). This is another subtype with a higher rate of recurrence and perineural invasion (36, 38).

7.3.1 Genetic Aberrations

Like melanoma, BCC results from mutations in both oncogenes and tumor suppressor genes. Eighty-five percent of BCCs contain mutations in the Sonic hedgehog (Hh) pathway (Figure 7.4), with patched (*PTCH1*) and smoothened (*SMO*) accounting for 93% of the observed genetic aberrations (39). In one study, single-strand conformational polymorphism screening was used to demonstrate that the inactivation of *PTCH1* is a necessary step in the development of BCC. Furthermore, *PTCH1* was found to be expressed at much higher levels in tumor cells as compared to normal skin cells, which suggests that the wild-type gene's inactivation generates overexpression of the mutant transcript (40). Although mutations in the Hh pathway are almost uniformly involved in BCC tumorigenesis, the mutational profile differs across BCCs, with varying levels of risk of recurrence. BCCs with high risk of recurrence, such as morpheaphorm BCCs, are more likely to have mutations in *MYCN*, protein phosphatase 6 catalytic subunit (*PPP6C*) and protein tyrosine phosphatase non-receptor type 14 (*PTPN14*) than BCCs with low risk of recurrence, like superficial BCCs. Additionally, BCC mutational profiles can be used to predict tumor responsiveness to treatment with an SMO inhibitor, such as vismodegib. Patients with a BCC on vismodegib who develop resistance have at least a 2.2-fold greater frequency of *SMO* mutations than vismodegib-naïve BCCs (39).

7.3.2 Immunohistochemistry

Although BCC can usually be distinguished from other lesions on H&E stain, the distinction may be more complicated and require IHC in some cases. Ensuring an accurate diagnosis of BCC vs. cutaneous squamous cell carcinoma (cSCC), for example, is important, as the two diagnoses can have different prognoses. BerEP4 is a monoclonal antibody directed against a protein moiety of two glycopeptides on human epithelial cells (41). Beer et al. compared BerEP4 and epithelial membrane antigen (EMA) staining in 39 BCCs and 23 cSCCs. All BCCs tested were positive for BerEP4 and negative for EMA, while all cSCCs were negative for BerEP4, and 96% were positive for EMA (42). BerEP4 and EMA appear to be useful in distinguishing between the two. There are other tumors that mimic the clinical and histological characteristics of BCC; thus, IHC can be critical in the distinction between BCC and other similar neoplasms. Trichoepithelioma, for example, is a benign neoplasm that shares many of the same histologic features as BCC; however, stromal CD10 staining and tumor expression of BCL2, cytokeratin 15 (CK15), and D2–40 in the outermost layer of basaloid nests have been shown to be reliable markers for distinguishing trichoepithelioma from BCC (43). Further, colonization of trichoepitheliomas by Merkel cells (showing cytokeratin 20 (CK20) expression) may also confer diagnostic benefit (44).

7.3.3 Staging

The vast majority of BCCs are managed locally with surgical or destructive interventions. Certain tumors present a higher risk for recurrence and even rare metastasis. Two staging systems, AJCC8 and Brigham and Women's Hospital (BWH), have been developed to help identify tumors at higher risk for poorer outcomes. In the

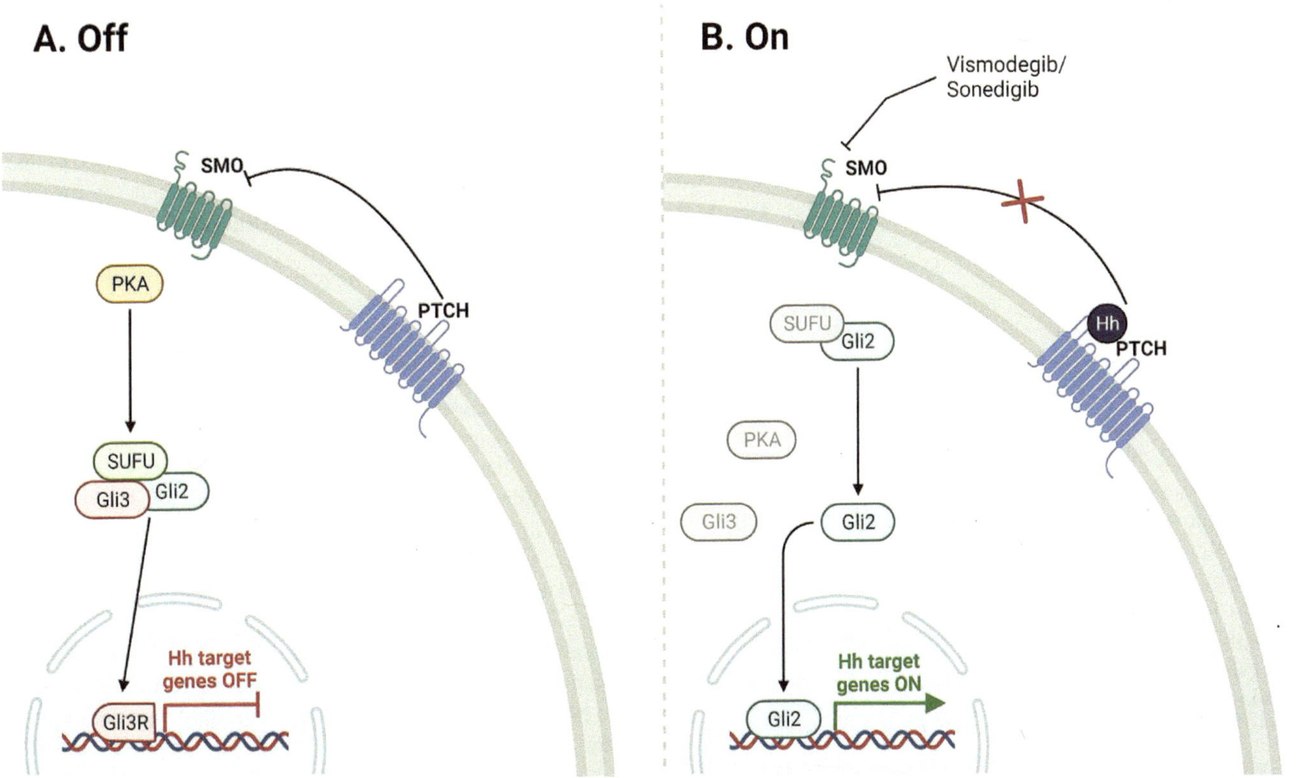

FIGURE 7.4 Sonic hedgehog signaling pathways (adapted from Hedgehog Signaling Pathway by BioRender.com). Panel A represents the patched PTCH1 signaling pathway in the absence of Sonic hedgehog (Hh) ligand. In this pathway, PTCH1 represses smoothened (SMO), ultimately resulting in transcriptional repression of Hh target genes. Panel B represents the SHH pathway in the presence of Hh ligand. In this pathway, Hh binds to PTCH1, releasing the inhibition of SMO and allowing SMO to activate the GLI-family transcription factors. These transcription factors ultimately result in the transcriptional activation of Hh target genes. In the presence of SMO inhibitors, such as vismodegib and sonedigib, SMO is prevented from activating the GLI-family transcription factors and thus represses uncontrolled cell growth and proliferation.

AJCC8, the tumor (T) category of staging is stratified based on maximum clinical tumor dimension, with T1 as less than 20 mm, T2 between 20 and 40 mm, and T3 greater than 40 mm. Additionally, T1 and T2 tumors can be upstaged to T3 if deep invasion (>6 mm thickness and/or beyond subcutaneous fat) or specified perineural invasion (diameter ≥0.1 mm) exists. T4 stage is defined by gross bone cortical or marrow invasion (45).

A novel tumor staging system for BCC was developed by BWH to better predict risk of metastasis and death. When compared with the AJCC8, the BWH staging system demonstrated higher specificity and positive predictive value for the identification of cases at risk of metastasis and/or death. Ultimately, the BWH system minimizes inappropriate upstaging more likely to be observed with the AJCC8 staging system (46).

7.3.4 Treatment

While most BCCs can be treated with local destruction, wide local excision, or Mohs micrographic surgery, higher-risk BCCs, such as metastatic or unresectable tumors, may require targeted therapy or immunotherapy. Almost all BCCs harbor genetic aberrations that cause a loss of function of PTCH1, resulting in SMO hyperactivity. As a first-line therapy for locally advanced or metastatic BCC, SMO-inhibitors, vismodegib and sonedigib, work to counteract this aberrant pathway activation and subsequent over-proliferation of basal cells (Figure 7.3) (47). In a meta-analysis that reviewed the efficacy of these treatments, the weighted average therapeutic response, either partial or complete, to vismodegib was 62.1%. The weighted average response rate in locally advanced disease was 64.7%, while that of metastatic BCC was 33.6% (48).

Vismodegib has also been studied in the context of basal cell nevus syndrome, a rare, heritable disease that can cause thousands of BCCs in an affected patient. This syndrome is marked by the presence of one defective copy of *PTCH1*. In a phase II trial that tested the efficacy and safety of vismodegib in patients with basal cell nevus syndrome, it was found that the per-patient rate of new surgically eligible BCCs was only 2 for those treated with the drug, as compared to 34 in the placebo group. Furthermore, the percent change in tumor size was greater in those treated than in those who received the placebo (−56% vs. −13%) (49).

For those patients who do not respond or experience recurrence on hedgehog inhibitor therapy, there exist alternative immunotherapies. Cemiplimab is a PD-1 antibody approved for the treatment of advanced cSCC and non-small cell lung cancer. In a more recent phase II trial, it was shown to also have antitumor activity against BCCs. In this study, 31% of patients had an objective response to cemiplimab therapy, with 6% exhibiting a complete response and 25% a partial response (50).

7.4 Squamous Cell Carcinoma

cSCC accounts for up to 20% of NMSCs (51). Risk factors for the development of cSCC are similar to those of BCC and include excess UV exposure, immunocompromised state, chronic wounds, and tanning bed use (52). cSCC, however, is responsible for the majority of NMSC-related metastasis and death (53). The most common subtype carries the greatest risk of metastasis. On histology, this subtype demonstrates atypically enlarged, hyperchromatic keratinocytes that invade into the dermis with associated keratin formation. There are several histologic subtypes of cSCC, all of which carry varying prognoses. Acantholytic cSCC is the subtype that carries the second greatest risk for metastasis. This subtype produces a pseudoglandular appearance on histology secondary to acantholysis. Spindle cell cSCC, otherwise known as pleomorphic or sarcomatoid cSCC, is a rare subtype associated with trauma, radiation and UV exposure. On histology, this subtype may display atypical, spindled squamous cells intertwined with collagen fibers and surrounded by abundant stroma (Figure 7.1). Verrucous cSCCs have the most favorable prognosis and, as such, appear well differentiated with minimal atypia on histology (54).

7.4.1 Genetic Aberrations

UV radiation exposure is the most common environmental carcinogen responsible for initiating mutations in cSCC (55). *TP53*, a tumor suppressor gene involved in the response to UV damage, has been shown to be mutated in 100% of high-risk primary head and neck cutaneous cSCCs (56). Similarly, *CDKN2A*, a gene integral to cell cycle progression through TP53, is mutated in 21 to 62% of cSCCs (57). Moreover, 60% of cSCC cases exhibited mutations in other major tumor suppressor genes, such as *APC*, *ATM*, and *RB1*. Other genes implicated in cSCC include those that encode receptor tyrosine kinases, such as *ERBB4*, *KIT*, and *ABL1*. In a study by Zilberg et al., targeted sequencing of 48 genes was performed on DNA from 24 primary head and neck cSCCs. They found that *FGFR2* mutations were only observed in cases with perineural invasion, while changes in the DNA repair gene *MLH1* were only seen in patients under 45 years of age (56).

Immunocompromised patients are at higher risk for developing skin cancer, particularly squamous cell carcinoma. In solid organ transplant patients, the risk of cSCC is 60 to 250 times that of the general population (58). This has been attributed to decreased immuno-surveillance and exposure to oncogenic human papilloma virus (HPV), particularly in the lower anogenital tract. This is due to regulation of TP53 and Rb (58). HPV-associated squamous intraepithelial lesions and invasive SCC fall outside the scope of this chapter, but helpful resources are cited here (59).

7.4.2 Immunohistochemistry

IHC markers can aid in diagnosis, prognosis, and therapeutic decisions for cSCC. Markers of mesenchymal epithelial transition, such as cytoplasmic E-cadherin and podoplanin, have been used to identify tumors with increased risk of recurrence, lymphatic invasion, and metastasis. Neural markers, such as S-100, can aid in H&E examination for perineural invasion (60). P63 has been shown to have high sensitivity but variable specificity in distinguishing spindle cell SCC (SpSCC) from other spindle cell malignancies like atypical fibroxanthoma (AFX). In an investigation by Buonaccorsi and Plaza, 7/10 SpSCCs stained positive for p63, while only 1/42 AFX tumors demonstrated positive staining (61). P40 has been shown to have similar sensitivity to p63 in detecting SpSCC; however, p40 exhibits significantly superior specificity compared to p63 in the distinction between SpSCC and AFX (48). In the section on BCC, we highlight how IHC can help distinguish cSCC from BCC.

7.4.3 Staging

AJCC8 defines tumor stage based on clinical size, depth of invasion, and perineural invasion. Another staging system developed by BWH has been shown to better predict outcomes of high-risk cSCCs, similar to BCC (Figure 7.5). In a cohort study of 459 patients with head and neck cSCC, twice as many tumors were categorized as high-grade cSCC (T3/T4) using AJCC8 compared to BWH criteria; thus, BWH minimizes inappropriate upstaging of low-risk cSCC. Yet the BWH tumor classification system exhibited higher specificity and positive predictive value for recognizing patients at risk for metastasis and death (62).

To better identify patients at higher risk for metastasis, a prognostic 40-GEP was developed. Wysong et al. aimed at validating this test, comparing risk prediction performance of the 40-GEP, AJCC8, and BWH in 321 patients with cSCC, 52 of which had developed metastases (Table 7.1). The 40-GEP highest risk group (Class 2B) had a positive predictive value (PPV) of 60% for metastasis, more than double what was observed using the BWH staging system (58, 59). Yet when the higher risk group (Class 2A) was added to the comparison, the PPV fell to 28.8%. All three tests have high negative predictive values, ranging from 86.3 to 91.1% (64). While GEP offers promise in aiding risk stratification, more studies are needed to validate clinical utility.

7.4.4 Treatment

Like other NMSCs, cSCC can be treated with surgical excision, radiotherapy, and systemic therapies depending on patient factors and tumor stage. The advent of immunotherapies has improved outcomes for patients with cSCC refractory to traditional treatments. Cemiplimab, a PD1 antibody also used in the setting of treatment-resistant BCC, is the only FDA-approved therapy for patients with locally advanced or metastatic cSCC who are ineligible for surgery or radiation therapy. This monoclonal antibody has demonstrated a disease control rate (percentage of patients with advanced or metastatic cSCC who have achieved complete or partial response or stable disease) of 72.5%. In a phase II trial to assess efficacy of cemiplimab in the treatment of advanced cSCC, the overall complete response rate (percentage of patients who achieved disappearance of all target lesions) was found to be 16.1% (65).

7.5 Merkel Cell Carcinoma

Merkel cell carcinoma (MCC) is a rare primary cutaneous tumor classically described as neuroendocrine but with new evidence suggesting a possible origin from dermal pre-/pro-B cells (66).

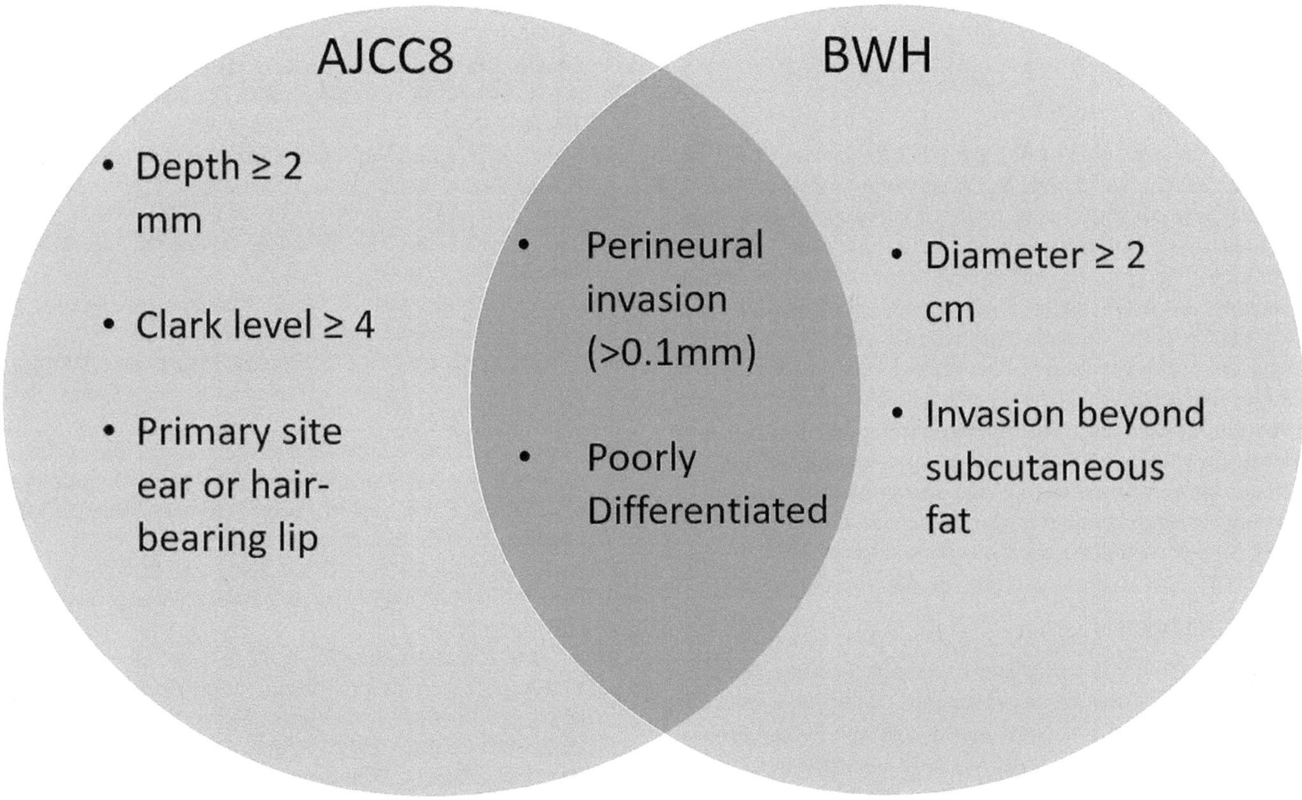

FIGURE 7.5 Comparison of high-risk features as defined by AJCC8 and BWH staging systems for cSCC. The far-left section represents high-risk features for cSCC defined by AJCC8. The far-right section represents high-risk features for cSCC defined by the BWH staging system. The center section represents high-risk features that are shared by both staging systems ref.(63).

These tumors can be particularly aggressive, with an average 5-year survival of 51% for local disease and 14% for distant disease (67). MCC typically occurs in sun-exposed areas, such as the head, neck, and extremities, and its incidence is skewed toward the elderly population, with a median age at presentation between 67 and 76 years (68). MCC has two pathways of pathogenesis: virus-associated pathway with clonal integration of the Merkel cell polyomavirus (MCV) and virus-independent pathway with UV radiation as the primary driver. In one study, MCV sequences were integrated into the genome of 80% of MCC tumors. Immunocompromised patients are at higher risk for MCC (69). As such, host immune system integrity has emerged as the most important prognostic biomarker in MCC, with higher densities of MCC-associated CD8+ T-cells correlated with improved survival (70).

7.5.1 Genetic Aberrations

The two distinct pathways, MCV-positive and MCV-negative, for MCC result in two genetic landscapes. Harms et al. utilized whole-exome sequencing on 49 MCCs and demonstrated a dichotomy of mutational burden between MCV-positive and MCV-negative MCCs. MCV-negative tumors exhibited an average of 1121 singe nucleotide variants per exome, while MCV-positive tumors maintained an average of 12.5 variants (71). Moreover, both subgroups demonstrated mutations that activate the PI3K pathway and inactivate the Notch pathway. Mutations in *Rb* and *TP53* were frequently observed in MCV-negative tumors; however, MCV-positive tumors never displayed mutations in these oncogenes (71). Further research into the genetic makeup may help explain why MCV-positive MCC generally confers a more favorable prognosis than MCV-negative MCC (67).

7.5.2 Immunohistochemistry

MCC appears as sheets of basaloid cells within the dermis with a "salt and pepper" chromatin pattern and minimal cytoplasm (Figure 7.1). Often, a diagnosis of MCC cannot be made with standard histology alone, and IHC must be utilized as an adjunct. MCC classically stains with CK20, a low molecular weight keratin, in a paranuclear dot-like pattern. However, CK20 only has a 75% sensitivity in MCC. Neurofilament can also be a useful adjunct in CK20-negative MCC. Additionally, MCC commonly stains positive for neuroendocrine markers, such as chromogranin, synaptophysin, and insulinoma-associated protein 1 (INSM-1); however, these markers lack specificity for MCC (67). Furthermore, certain immunohistochemical features are inversely correlated with survival, with p63 immunopositivity demonstrating the strongest prognostic value (67). Stetsenko et al. showed that p63 expression was associated with significantly higher MCC-specific mortality, with 63% cumulative mortality at 5 years among patients with p63-positive tumors and 31% among those with p63-negative tumors (72).

7.5.3 Staging

MCC tumors are staged using the AJCC8 system. Unlike the other cancers discussed here, SLNB should be considered for all new diagnoses of MCC, as up to 1/3 of patients can have occult nodal disease (73). Other prognostic indicators, such as the concentration of specific viral oncoprotein antibodies, can be used as an adjunct to AJCC8 staging. Paulson et al. examined MCV antibody titer levels in 219 patients with newly diagnosed MCC and found 114 (52%) were seropositive. Titer levels were followed in seropositive patients, and they found that an increasing oncoprotein antibody titer had a positive predictive value of 66%, and a decreasing MCV antibody titer had a negative predictive value of 97% for MCC recurrence (74). Viral oncoprotein antibodies may not only be useful in initial prognosis but also as a tool for monitoring for recurrent disease and treatment response.

7.5.4 Treatment

Surgical excision and radiotherapy represent first-line therapies for MCC, with postoperative radiotherapy conferring a reduction in risk of local recurrence and improvement in 3-year survival from 48% to 76% (75). For patients with advanced or unresectable MCC, alternative treatments such as systemic immunotherapy can be employed. One such option is pembrolizumab, a PD-L1 pathway inhibitor. In a phase II trial that assessed safety and efficacy of pembrolizumab in the treatment of advanced MCC, the objective response to treatment among 50 patients naïve to systemic treatment was 56%. Although there was no significant difference in treatment response between patients with MCV-positive vs. MCV-negative tumors, progression-free survival and overall survival were improved in patients with PD-L1-positive tumors (76).

REFERENCES

1. American Cancer Society. Cancer Facts & Figures 2017. Available from: www.cancer.org/research/cancer-facts-statistics/all-cancer-facts-figures/cancer-facts-figures-2017.html.
2. Elmore JG, Barnhill RL, Elder DE, et al. Pathologists' diagnosis of invasive melanoma and melanocytic proliferations: Observer accuracy and reproducibility study. BMJ. 2017;357:j2813.
3. Domingues B, Lopes JM, Soares P, et al. Melanoma treatment in review. Immunotargets Ther. 2018;7:35–49.
4. Siegel RL, Miller KD, Jemal A. Cancer statistics, 2020. CA Cancer J Clin. 2020;70(1):7–30.
5. Coit DG. NCCN guidelines and quality cancer care: Where have we come from, and where should we be going? J Natl Compr Canc Netw. 2016;14(4):373–7.
6. Olencki T. Optimal treatment of unresectable nonmelanoma skin cancers. J Natl Compr Canc Netw. 2014;12(5 Suppl):789–92.
7. Gandini S, Sera F, Cattaruzza MS, et al. Meta-analysis of risk factors for cutaneous melanoma: II. Sun exposure. Eur J Cancer. 2005;41(1):45–60.
8. Greenwald HS, Friedman EB, Osman I. Superficial spreading and nodular melanoma are distinct biological entities: A challenge to the linear progression model. Melanoma Res. 2012;22(1):1–8.
9. Smoller BR. Histologic criteria for diagnosing primary cutaneous malignant melanoma. Mod Pathol. 2006;19(Suppl 2):S34–40.
10. Ascierto PA, Kirkwood JM, Grob JJ, et al. The role of BRAF V600 mutation in melanoma. J Transl Med. 2012;10:85.
11. Shain AH, Yeh I, Kovalyshyn I, et al. The genetic evolution of melanoma from precursor lesions. N Engl J Med. 2015;373(20):1926–36.
12. Cancer Genome Atlas Network. Genomic classification of cutaneous melanoma. Cell. 2015;161(7):1681–96.
13. Castellano M, Pollock PM, Walters MK, et al. CDKN2A/p16 is inactivated in most melanoma cell lines. Cancer Res. 1997;57(21):4868–75.
14. Eckerle Mize D, Bishop M, Resse E, et al. Familial atypical multiple mole melanoma syndrome. In: Riegert-Johnson DL, Boardman LA, Hefferon T, et al., editors. Cancer Syndromes. Bethesda, MD: National Center for Biotechnology Information; 2009.
15. National Cancer Institute. Cancer Stat Facts: Melanoma of the Skin 2022. Available from: https://seer.cancer.gov/statfacts/html/melan.html
16. Soura E, Eliades PJ, Shannon K, et al. Hereditary melanoma: Update on syndromes and management: Genetics of familial atypical multiple mole melanoma syndrome. J Am Acad Dermatol. 2016;74(3):395–407; quiz 8–10.
17. Pauley K, Khan A, Kohlmann W, et al. Considerations for germline testing in melanoma: Updates in behavioral change and pancreatic surveillance for carriers of CDKN2A pathogenic variants. Front Oncol. 2022;12:837057.
18. Davis LE, Shalin SC, Tackett AJ. Current state of melanoma diagnosis and treatment. Cancer Biol Ther. 2019;20(11):1366–79.
19. Willis BC, Johnson G, Wang J, et al. SOX10: A useful marker for identifying metastatic melanoma in sentinel lymph nodes. Appl Immunohistochem Mol Morphol. 2015; 23(2):109–12.
20. Ohsie SJ, Sarantopoulos GP, Cochran AJ, et al. Immunohistochemical characteristics of melanoma. J Cutan Pathol. 2008;35(5):433–44.
21. Chen LL, Jaimes N, Barker CA, et al. Desmoplastic melanoma: A review. J Am Acad Dermatol. 2013;68(5):825–33.
22. Lezcano C, Jungbluth AA, Nehal KS, et al. PRAME expression in melanocytic tumors. Am J Surg Pathol. 2018;42(11):1456–65.
23. Reimann JDR, Salim S, Velazquez EF, et al. Comparison of melanoma gene expression score with histopathology, fluorescence in situ hybridization, and SNP array for the classification of melanocytic neoplasms. Mod Pathol. 2018;31(11):1733–43.
24. Miedema J, Andea AA. Through the looking glass and what you find there: Making sense of comparative genomic hybridization and fluorescence in situ hybridization for melanoma diagnosis. Mod Pathol. 2020;33(7):1318–30.
25. Gerami P, Jewell SS, Morrison LE, et al. Fluorescence in situ hybridization (FISH) as an ancillary diagnostic tool in the diagnosis of melanoma. Am J Surg Pathol. 2009;33(8):1146–56.
26. Grossman D, Okwundu N, Bartlett EK, et al. Prognostic gene expression profiling in cutaneous melanoma: Identifying the knowledge gaps and assessing the clinical benefit. JAMA Dermatol. 2020;156(9):1004–11.
27. Clarke LE, Flake DD, Busam K, et al. An independent validation of a gene expression signature to differentiate

malignant melanoma from benign melanocytic nevi. Cancer. 2017;123(4):617–28.
28. Castle Biosciences. Castle Biosciences Announces Preliminary Fourth Quarter and Full-Year 2021 Results 2022. Available from: https://ir.castlebiosciences.com/news/news-details/2022/Castle-Biosciences-Announces-Preliminary-Fourth-Quarter-and-Full-Year-2021-Results/default.aspx
29. Moody JA, Ali RF, Carbone AC, et al. Complications of sentinel lymph node biopsy for melanoma—A systematic review of the literature. Eur J Surg Oncol. 2017;43(2):270–7.
30. Whitman ED, Koshenkov VP, Gastman BR, et al. Integrating 31-gene expression profiling with clinicopathologic features to optimize cutaneous melanoma sentinel lymph node metastasis prediction. JCO Precis Oncol. 2021;5.
31. Zarabi SK, Azzato EM, Tu ZJ, et al. Targeted next generation sequencing (NGS) to classify melanocytic neoplasms. J Cutan Pathol. 2020;47(8):691–704.
32. Keung EZ, Gershenwald JE. The eighth edition American Joint Committee on Cancer (AJCC) melanoma staging system: Implications for melanoma treatment and care. Expert Rev Anticancer Ther. 2018;18(8):775–84.
33. American Cancer Society. Treatment of Melanoma Skin Cancer, by Stage 2022. Available from: www.cancer.org/cancer/melanoma-skin-cancer/treating/by-stage.html
34. Rizos H, Menzies AM, Pupo GM, et al. BRAF inhibitor resistance mechanisms in metastatic melanoma: Spectrum and clinical impact. Clin Cancer Res. 2014;20(7):1965–77.
35. Carvajal RD, Antonescu CR, Wolchok JD, et al. KIT as a therapeutic target in metastatic melanoma. JAMA. 2011;305(22):2327–34.
36. Kim DP, Kus KJB, Ruiz E. Basal cell carcinoma review. Hematol Oncol Clin North Am. 2019;33(1):13–24.
37. UCSF Health. Basal Cell and Squamous Cell Carcinoma 2022. Available from: www.ucsfhealth.org/conditions/basal-cell-and-squamous-cell-carcinoma
38. McDaniel B, Badri T, Steele RB. Basal Cell Carcinoma. 2022. In: StatPearls [Internet]. Treasure Island, FL: StatPearls Publishing. Available from: www.ncbi.nlm.nih.gov/books/NBK482439/.
39. Bonilla X, Parmentier L, King B, et al. Genomic analysis identifies new drivers and progression pathways in skin basal cell carcinoma. Nat Genet. 2016;48(4):398–406.
40. Gailani MR, Stahle-Backdahl M, Leffell DJ, et al. The role of the human homologue of Drosophila patched in sporadic basal cell carcinomas. Nat Genet. 1996;14(1):78–81.
41. Latza U, Niedobitek G, Schwarting R, et al. Ber-EP4: New monoclonal antibody which distinguishes epithelia from mesothelial. J Clin Pathol. 1990;43(3):213–9.
42. Beer TW, Shepherd P, Theaker JM. Ber EP4 and epithelial membrane antigen aid distinction of basal cell, squamous cell and basosquamous carcinomas of the skin. Histopathology. 2000;37(3):218–23.
43. Tebcherani AJ, de Andrade HF, Jr., Sotto MN. Diagnostic utility of immunohistochemistry in distinguishing trichoepithelioma and basal cell carcinoma: Evaluation using tissue microarray samples. Mod Pathol. 2012;25(10):1345–53.
44. Katona TM, Perkins SM, Billings SD. Does the panel of cytokeratin 20 and androgen receptor antibodies differentiate desmoplastic trichoepithelioma from morpheaform/infiltrative basal cell carcinoma? J Cutan Pathol. 2008;35(2):174–9.
45. Keohane SG, Proby CM, Newlands C, et al. The new 8th edition of TNM staging and its implications for skin cancer: A review by the British Association of Dermatologists and the Royal College of Pathologists, U.K. Br J Dermatol. 2018;179(4):824–8.
46. Morgan FC, Ruiz ES, Karia PS, et al. Brigham and Women's Hospital tumor classification system for basal cell carcinoma identifies patients with risk of metastasis and death. J Am Acad Dermatol. 2021;85(3):582–7.
47. Sekulic A, Migden MR, Oro AE, et al. Efficacy and safety of vismodegib in advanced basal-cell carcinoma. N Engl J Med. 2012;366(23):2171–9.
48. Henderson SA, Torres-Cabala CA, Curry JL, et al. p40 is more specific than p63 for the distinction of atypical fibroxanthoma from other cutaneous spindle cell malignancies. Am J Surg Pathol. 2014;38(8):1102–10.
49. Tang JY, Ally MS, Chanana AM, et al. Inhibition of the hedgehog pathway in patients with basal-cell nevus syndrome: Final results from the multicentre, randomised, double-blind, placebo-controlled, phase 2 trial. Lancet Oncol. 2016;17(12):1720–31.
50. Stratigos AJ, Sekulic A, Peris K, et al. Cemiplimab in locally advanced basal cell carcinoma after hedgehog inhibitor therapy: An open-label, multi-centre, single-arm, phase 2 trial. Lancet Oncol. 2021;22(6):848–57.
51. Burton KA, Ashack KA, Khachemoune A. Cutaneous squamous cell carcinoma: A review of high-risk and metastatic disease. Am J Clin Dermatol. 2016;17(5):491–508.
52. Green AC, Olsen CM. Cutaneous squamous cell carcinoma: An epidemiological review. Br J Dermatol. 2017;177(2):373–81.
53. Yanofsky VR, Mercer SE, Phelps RG. Histopathological variants of cutaneous squamous cell carcinoma: A review. J Skin Cancer. 2011;2011:210813.
54. Lohmann CM, Solomon AR. Clinicopathologic variants of cutaneous squamous cell carcinoma. Adv Anat Pathol. 2001;8(1):27–36.
55. Nagarajan P, Asgari MM, Green AC, et al. Keratinocyte carcinomas: Current concepts and future research priorities. Clin Cancer Res. 2019;25(8):2379–91.
56. Zilberg C, Lee MW, Yu B, et al. Analysis of clinically relevant somatic mutations in high-risk head and neck cutaneous squamous cell carcinoma. Mod Pathol. 2018;31(2):275–87.
57. Di Nardo L, Pellegrini C, Di Stefani A, et al. Molecular genetics of cutaneous squamous cell carcinoma: Perspective for treatment strategies. J Eur Acad Dermatol Venereol. 2020;34(5):932–41.
58. Que SKT, Zwald FO, Schmults CD. Cutaneous squamous cell carcinoma: Incidence, risk factors, diagnosis, and staging. J Am Acad Dermatol. 2018;78(2):237–47.
59. Darragh TM, Colgan TJ, Cox JT, et al. The lower anogenital squamous terminology standardization project for HPV-Associated Lesions: Background and consensus recommendations from the College of American Pathologists and the American Society for Colposcopy and Cervical Pathology. Arch Pathol Lab Med. 2012;136(10):1266–97.
60. Balasescu E, Gheorghe AC, Moroianu A, et al. Role of immunohistochemistry in the diagnosis and staging of cutaneous squamous-cell carcinomas (Review). Exp Ther Med. 2022;23(6):383.
61. Buonaccorsi JN, Plaza JA. Role of CD10, wide-spectrum keratin, p63, and podoplanin in the distinction of epithelioid and spindle cell tumors of the skin: An immunohistochemical study of 81 cases. Am J Dermatopathol. 2012;34(4):404–11.

62. Ruiz ES, Karia PS, Besaw R, et al. Performance of the American Joint Committee on Cancer Staging Manual, 8th Edition vs the Brigham and Women's Hospital tumor classification system for cutaneous squamous cell carcinoma. JAMA Dermatol. 2019;155(7):819–25.
63. Chu MB, Slutsky JB, Dhandha MM, et al. Evaluation of the definitions of "high-risk" cutaneous squamous cell carcinoma using the American joint committee on cancer staging criteria and national comprehensive cancer network guidelines. J Skin Cancer. 2014;2014:154340.
64. Wysong A, Newman JG, Covington KR, et al. Validation of a 40-gene expression profile test to predict metastatic risk in localized high-risk cutaneous squamous cell carcinoma. J Am Acad Dermatol. 2021;84(2):361–9.
65. Garcia-Foncillas J, Tejera-Vaquerizo A, Sanmartin O, et al. Update on management recommendations for advanced cutaneous squamous cell carcinoma. Cancers (Basel). 2022;14(3).
66. Zur Hausen A, Rennspiess D, Winnepenninckx V, et al. Early B-cell differentiation in Merkel cell carcinomas: Clues to cellular ancestry. Cancer Res. 2013;73(16):4982–7.
67. Coggshall K, Tello TL, North JP, et al. Merkel cell carcinoma: An update and review: Pathogenesis, diagnosis, and staging. J Am Acad Dermatol. 2018;78(3):433–42.
68. Andea AA, Coit DG, Amin B, et al. Merkel cell carcinoma: Histologic features and prognosis. Cancer. 2008;113(9):2549–58.
69. Feng H, Shuda M, Chang Y, et al. Clonal integration of a polyomavirus in human Merkel cell carcinoma. Science. 2008; 319(5866):1096–100.
70. Farah M, Reuben A, Spassova I, et al. T-cell repertoire in combination with T-cell density predicts clinical outcomes in patients with Merkel cell carcinoma. J Invest Dermatol. 2020;140(11):2146–56e4.
71. Goh G, Walradt T, Markarov V, et al. Mutational landscape of MCPyV-positive and MCPyV-negative Merkel cell carcinomas with implications for immunotherapy. Oncotarget. 2016;7(3):3403–15.
72. Stetsenko GY, Malekirad J, Paulson KG, et al. p63 expression in Merkel cell carcinoma predicts poorer survival yet may have limited clinical utility. Am J Clin Pathol. 2013;140(6):838–44.
73. Iyer JG, Storer BE, Paulson KG, et al. Relationships among primary tumor size, number of involved nodes, and survival for 8044 cases of Merkel cell carcinoma. J Am Acad Dermatol. 2014;70(4):637–43.
74. Paulson KG, Lewis CW, Redman MW, et al. Viral oncoprotein antibodies as a marker for recurrence of Merkel cell carcinoma: A prospective validation study. Cancer. 2017;123(8):1464–74.
75. Zwijnenburg EM, Lubeek SFK, Werner JEM, et al. Merkel cell carcinoma: New trends. Cancers (Basel). 2021;13(7).
76. Nghiem P, Bhatia S, Lipson EJ, et al. Durable tumor regression and overall survival in patients with advanced Merkel cell carcinoma receiving pembrolizumab as first-line therapy. J Clin Oncol. 2019;37(9):693–702.

8

Bone and Soft Tissue Tumors

Armita Bahrami

8.1 Introduction

Connective tissue, the most abundant and diverse tissue type in the body, gives rise to a variety of mesenchymal neoplasms, forming the basis for the classification of bone and soft tissue tumors. The World Health Organization categorizes these tumors into several major groups, such as adipocytic, fibroblastic, myofibroblastic, and chondrogenic, and others, each comprising distinct subcategories with unique clinical, histologic, and genetic characteristics. Moreover, tumors originating from other cellular lineages add to the diverse spectrum of bone and soft tissue neoplasms. The rarity and diversity of these tumor subtypes present considerable challenges in their diagnosis and management.

Over the past two decades, advancements in molecular genetics have significantly enhanced our understanding of the molecular mechanisms underlying mesenchymal neoplasms. A considerable subset of these tumors is driven by chromosomal translocations, while others display complex genomic profiles involving multiple oncogenes and tumor suppressor genes. In sarcomas with simpler genomic profiles resulting from translocations, single gene mutations, or amplifications, specific driver genes have been identified. Certain genetic alterations serve as unique identifiers for specific tumor types, while others are common across different neoplasms.

Recent advancements in next-generation sequencing technology have enabled its clinical application using formalin-fixed paraffin-embedded tissue samples. FDA–approved molecular diagnostic assays now allow the screening of a wide range of cancer-associated mutations, covering the entire spectrum of genetic alterations in a single assay. This approach is particularly valuable when conventional histology-based diagnosis is challenging.

In precision oncology, matching patients with clinical trials based on specific molecular pathways has shown notable success, particularly in sarcomas or aggressive mesenchymal tumors with translocations involving receptor tyrosine kinases or growth factors. However, these cases represent a small fraction of adult sarcomas. More commonly, translocation-driven sarcomas involve chimeric genes that encode transcription factor proteins where targeted therapies are lacking. Challenges also arise with sarcomas that harbor rare mutations or novel gene fusions, as there may be limited guidance from existing literature on their behavior. However, the increasing genetic profiling of sarcomas and the development of comprehensive databases are generating valuable research data, offering hope for the future development of targeted drugs for these rare tumors (1–3).

The subsequent sections of this chapter delve into the frequent genetic alterations observed in different histologic subtypes of mesenchymal tumors, emphasizing the opportunity for diagnostic precision and the potential for molecularly targeted therapies derived from these alterations. Table 8.1 provides a comprehensive summary of the recurrent fusion genes identified across various sarcoma subtypes. This summary highlights that certain genetic changes may occur across different tumor types, thereby underlining the necessity of a comprehensive diagnostic approach (Figure 8.1). Integrating histologic and molecular parameters is pivotal for accurate tumor classification, which is crucial for devising personalized treatment strategies.

TABLE 8.1
Recurrent Gene Rearrangements and Associated Mesenchymal Tumors

Gene Name	Associated Mesenchymal Tumors
ALK	Inflammatory myofibroblastic tumor*, benign fibrous histiocytoma, leiomyosarcoma
BCOR	Undifferentiated small round cell sarcoma*
CAMTA1	Epithelioid hemangioendothelioma*
CCNB3	Undifferentiated small round cell sarcoma*
CIC	Undifferentiated small round cell sarcoma*
CSF1	Tenosynovial giant cell tumor*
ETV6	Infantile fibrosarcoma*
EWSR1	Ewing sarcoma*, angiomatoid fibrous histiocytoma*, extraskeletal myxoid chondrosarcoma*, clear cell sarcoma*, desmoplastic small round cell tumor*, sclerosing epithelioid fibrosarcoma*, myoepithelioma/myoepithelial carcinoma*, round cell sarcoma with EWSR1-non-ETS fusions*, myxoid liposarcoma, low-grade fibromyxoid sarcoma,

(Continued)

DOI: 10.1201/9781003513469-8

TABLE 8.1 (Continued)

Gene Name	Associated Mesenchymal Tumors
FOS	Osteoid osteoma*, osteoblastoma*, epithelioid hemangioma*, proliferative fasciitis*
FOSB	Osteoblastoma*, pseudomyogenic hemangioendothelioma*, epithelioid hemangioma
FOXO1	Alveolar rhabdomyosarcoma*
FUS	Myxoid liposarcoma*, low-grade fibromyxoid sarcoma*, Ewing sarcoma, angiomatoid fibrous histiocytoma, myoepithelioma/myoepithelial carcinoma, undifferentiated round cell sarcoma
HMGA2	Lipoma*, lipoblastoma
NCOA2	Angiofibroma of soft tissue*, mesenchymal chondrosarcoma*, congenital/infantile spindle cell rhabdomyosarcoma*
NOTCH1/2/3	Glomus tumor*
NR4A3	Extraskeletal myxoid chondrosarcoma*
NTRK1/2/3	Infantile fibrosarcoma*, *NTRK*-rearranged spindle cell neoplasm*, inflammatory myofibroblastic tumor
PDGFB	Dermatofibrosarcoma protuberans*, giant cell fibroblastoma*
PDGFD	Dermatofibrosarcoma protuberans
PHF1	Ossifying fibromyxoid tumor*
PLAG1	Lipoblastoma*, mixed tumor of soft tissue*
PRDM10	Superficial CD34-positive fibroblastic tumor*
RELA	Cellular myopericytoma (perivascular myoid tumor)*
RET	Lipofibromatosis, inflammatory myofibroblastic tumor
ROS1	Lipofibromatosis, inflammatory myofibroblastic tumor
SRF	Cellular myopericytoma (perivascular myoid tumor)*, congenital/infantile spindle cell rhabdomyosarcoma
SS18	Synovial sarcoma*
STAT6	Solitary fibrous tumor*
TAF15	Extraskeletal myxoid chondrosarcoma*
TCF12	Extraskeletal myxoid chondrosarcoma, spindle cell/sclerosing rhabdomyosarcoma
TFE3	Alveolar soft part sarcoma*, epithelioid hemangioendothelioma*, ossifying fibromyxoid tumor, PEComa
USP6	Aneurysmal bone cyst*, fibroma of tendon sheath*, myositis ossificans*, nodular fasciitis*, fibro-osseous pseudotumor of digits*
WWTR1	Epithelioid hemangioendothelioma*
YWHAE	Undifferentiated round cell sarcoma of infancy*

An asterisk (*) next to a tumor type indicates that it is a commonly associated mesenchymal tumor for the corresponding gene.

8.2 Fibroblastic and Myofibroblastic Tumors

Fibroblastic and myofibroblastic tumors span a spectrum of entities, ranging from nodular fasciitis to fibromatosis to variants of fibrosarcoma. This diverse category presents unique diagnostic challenges due to their morphologic heterogeneity and overlapping features (Figure 8.2). Molecular diagnostic testing plays a valuable role in identifying unique alterations, aiding in accurate classification, especially in small biopsies.

8.2.1 Benign Fibroblastic and Myofibroblastic Tumors

Several benign fibroblastic and myofibroblastic tumors, such as aneurysmal bone cyst, nodular fasciitis, myositis ossificans, fibro-osseous pseudotumor of digits, and fibroma of tendon sheath, commonly exhibit fusions involving the *USP6* gene (4). These fusions include the entire coding sequence of *USP6* and the promoter of one of several potential partner genes. In proliferative fasciitis/proliferative myositis, fusions involving the *FOS* gene have been identified (5). The detection of these fusions through genetic testing provides valuable support for a benign diagnosis.

Other benign mesenchymal tumors are also associated with specific genetic markers (Figure 8.3). For instance, fibrous hamartoma of infancy is linked to *EGFR* exon 20 insertion/duplication (6), while calcifying aponeurotic fibroma is characterized by recurrent *FN1::EGF* fusions (7). Myofibroblastoma, cellular angiofibroma, and superficial acral fibromyxoma are related tumors that exhibit loss of 13q14, including *RB1* (8). For angiofibroma of soft tissue, a benign fibroblastic tumor, chromosomal translocations resulting in the *AHRR::NCOA2* fusion are frequently observed (9). Recent findings have unveiled a newly described mesenchymal tumor associated with the *EWSR1::SMAD3* fusion (10). This tumor type typically originates in the acral region and demonstrates a potential for local recurrence.

8.2.2 Intermediate Fibroblastic and Myofibroblastic Tumors

Intermediate fibroblastic and myofibroblastic tumors encompass a diverse group of neoplasms exhibiting varying levels of local aggressiveness and rare metastasis. The prototypical example is desmoid-type fibromatosis, in which most cases can be attributed to a mutation in the *CTNNB1* gene. This mutation leads to the accumulation of β-catenin in the nucleus and subsequent

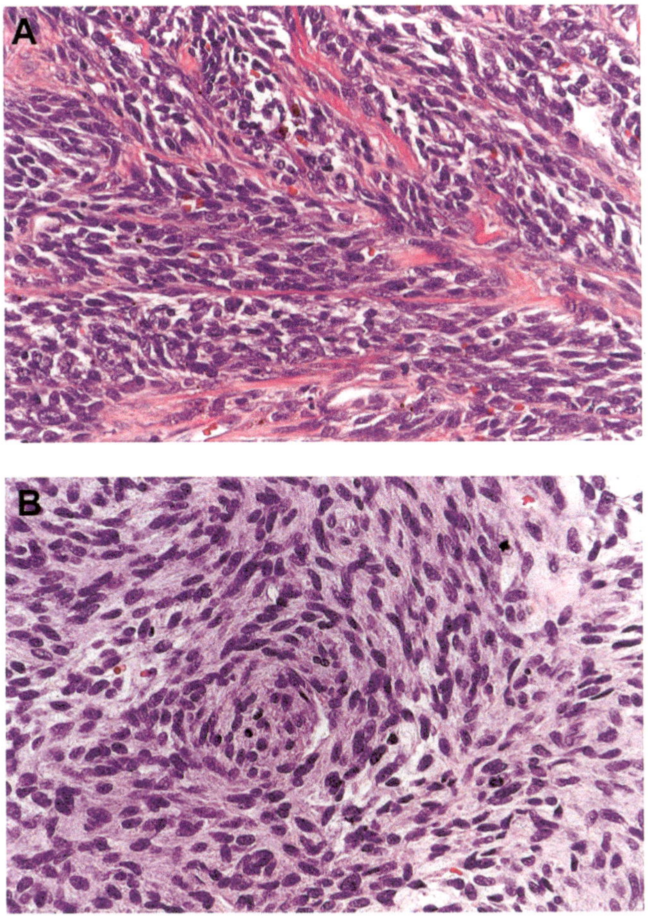

FIGURE 8.1 Photomicrographs illustrating the histologic diversity of tumors associated with the *EWSR1::ATF1* gene fusion (H&E). (A) Clear cell sarcoma of soft tissue, a malignant tumor characterized by a significant risk of distant metastasis, harboring the *EWSR1::ATF1* fusion. (B) Angiomatoid fibrous histiocytoma, an intermediate neoplasm with an extremely rare metastatic potential, also carrying the *EWSR1::ATF1* fusion.

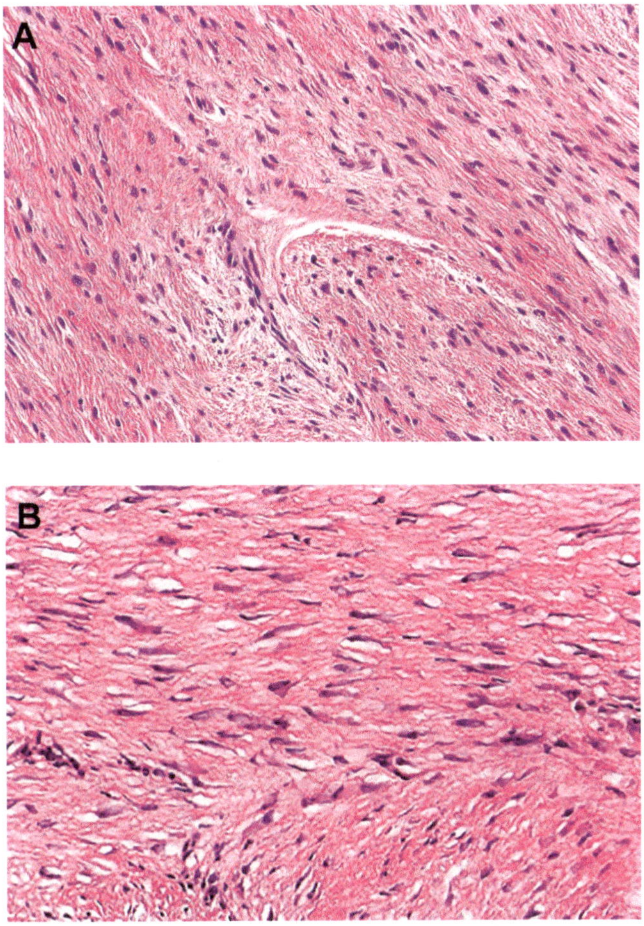

FIGURE 8.2 Photomicrographs illustrating the deceptively bland and uniform apperance of tumor cells in low-grade fibromyxoid sarcoma (A, H&E), closely simulating the cells in fibromatosis (B, H&E).

activation of the Wnt signaling pathway. In some cases, inactivating *APC* mutations are present, associated with Gardner syndrome (11, 12). The identification of *APC* mutations in desmoid tumors may prompt physicians to recommend genetic counseling and germline genetic testing.

Lipofibromatosis, also known as infantile fibromatosis, primarily affects young children and is characterized by a high rate of local recurrence. Various fusions involving genes encoding EGF family ligands (EGF, HBEGF, TGF-α), receptor tyrosine kinases (PDGFRB, RET, ROS1, EGFR), or the serine/threonine kinase BRAF have been observed (13). Detection of kinase fusions may lead to the consideration of tyrosine kinase inhibitors (TKIs) in patients with unresectable tumors.

Dermatofibrosarcoma protuberans (DFSP) and giant cell fibroblastoma are closely related tumors, primarily characterized by the *COL1A1::PDGFB* gene fusion. This fusion, arising from a translocation between chromosomes 17 and 22 at loci 17q22 and 22q13, occurs in over 90% of DFSP cases. Additionally, some cases exhibit supernumerary ring chromosomes composed of fragments from these loci (14). However, approximately 8% of DFSP cases present a deviation from this common fusion pattern, displaying alternative fusions often involving the *PDGFD* gene with partners like *COL6A3*, *EMILIN2*, and *TNC* (15). For adults with recurrent or metastatic DFSP, TKIs such as imatinib mesylate have been approved by the FDA as a treatment option (16). Given the various morphologic variants of DFSP, molecular testing to detect *PDGFB* or *PDGFD* alterations is essential for accurate diagnosis in cases with unusual morphology (Figure 8.4). The genetic or molecular drivers behind more aggressive DFSP phenotypes, including fibrosarcomatous change and metastasis, remain to be fully elucidated.

Solitary fibrous tumor (SFT) is a distinct mesenchymal tumor that exhibits a spectrum of behavior, from benign to low-malignant potential to fully malignant, which is characterized by the presence of the *NAB2::STAT6* gene fusion, resulting from a paracentric inversion of chromosome 12q. This fusion leads to STAT6 overexpression, which can be assessed immunohistochemically (17, 18). The *NAB2::STAT6* gene fusion is highly specific to SFT, and its presence, even in sarcomas without histologic resemblance to SFT, is diagnostic for SFT, including dedifferentiated or poorly differentiated cases. Predicting the behavior of SFT solely based on histologic features can be challenging. At the molecular level, the presence of *TERT* promoter mutations or *TP53* mutations has been associated with an increased risk of malignant behavior (19).

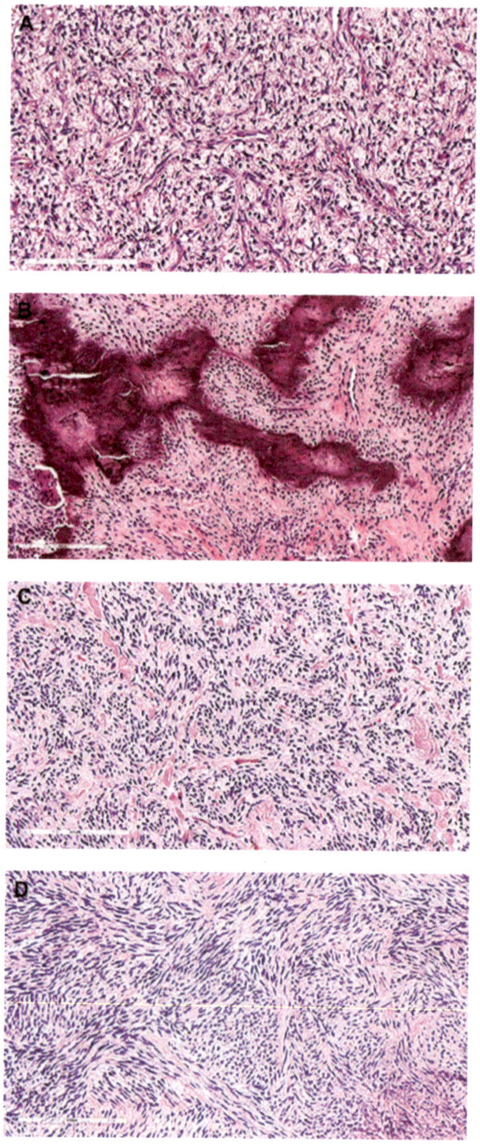

FIGURE 8.3 Photomicrographs of benign fibroblastic tumors demonstrating their histologic overlap but distinct genetic profiles (H&E). (A) Angiofibroma of soft tissue, harboring *AHRR::NCOA2* fusion. (B) Calcifying aponeurotic fibroma, characterized by the recurrent *FN1::EGF* fusion. (C) Cellular spindle cell lipoma, an *RB1*-deleted tumor. (D) An emerging distinct fibroblastic tumor with the *EWSR1::SMAD3* fusion.

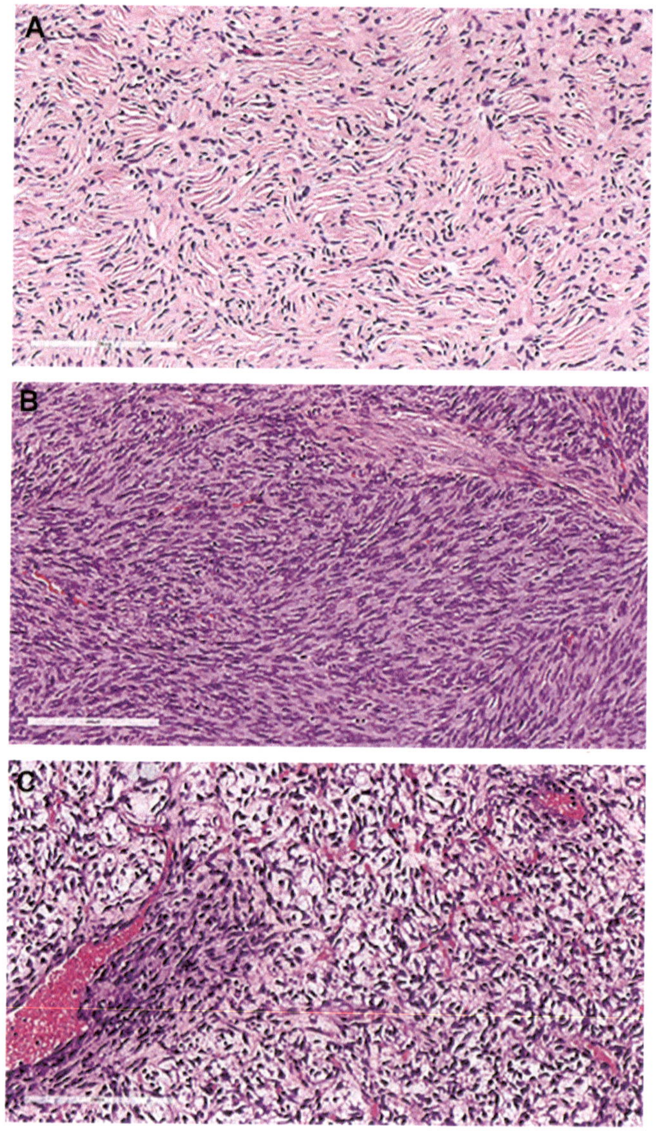

FIGURE 8.4 Photomicrographs of dermatofibrosarcoma protuberans (DFSP) and its variants (H&E), characterized by the *COL1A1::PDGFB* fusion. (A) Conventional DFSP, displaying the classic histologic features. (B) Fibrosarcomatous DFSP, showing the transition to a more aggressive fibrosarcomatous phenotype. (C) Myxoid fibrosarcomatous DFSP, illustrating the myxoid variation within fibrosarcomatous DFSP.

Inflammatory myofibroblastic tumor (IMT) is characterized by a proliferation of neoplastic myofibroblasts intermingled with chronic inflammatory cells. The genetic makeup of IMT is diverse. Approximately 50–60% of children and adults with IMT exhibit gene fusions involving *ALK* with various partner genes. These fusions result in a chimeric protein with a constitutively active ALK kinase domain and can be detected through ALK overexpression using immunohistochemistry. *ROS1* and *NTRK3* gene rearrangements are present in 5–10% of cases each. Notably, *RANBP2::ALK* or *RRBP1::ALK* fusions are frequently associated with the more aggressive epithelioid subtype of IMT (20). Fusions involving other kinases, such as *RET*, *ROS1*, and *PDGFRB*, are rarely observed (21). IMTs generally have a low potential for malignancy, with metastatic disease occurring in rare cases (approximately 5%). The genetic alterations driving aggressive behavior in IMTs are not yet fully understood. In July 2022, crizotinib, an ALK inhibitor, was granted an FDA approval for the treatment of ALK-positive IMT in patients with relapsed, refractory, or inoperable tumors. Other TKIs are also being evaluated in clinical trials for *ALK* and other kinase gene fusion-positive tumors (22, 23).

Superficial CD34-positive fibroblastic tumor arises in the dermis or subcutis and is characterized by the presence of cells with granular to glassy cytoplasm, pleomorphic nuclei, low mitotic activity, diffuse CD34 expression, and a favorable prognosis (Figure 8.5). *PRDM10* rearrangements are frequently found in this tumor and serve as a distinguishing feature from pleomorphic sarcoma (24, 25).

Infantile fibrosarcoma (IFS) primarily affects infants and rarely metastasizes. The *ETV6::NRTK3* gene fusion is a key

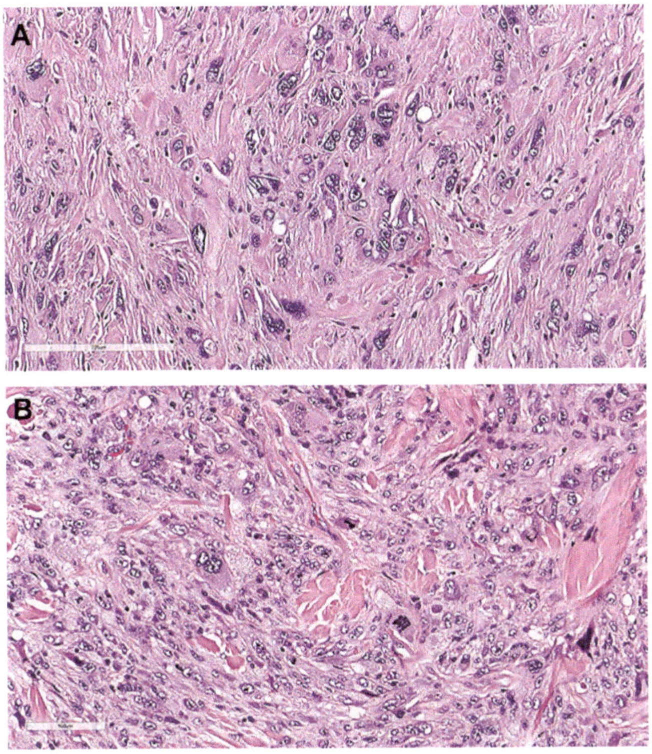

FIGURE 8.5 Comparison between superficial CD34-positive fibroblastic tumor (A) and pleomorphic dermal sarcoma (B) (H&E).

genetic marker of these tumors. Less frequently, IFS and its variants, known as IFS-like tumors, are associated with fusions involving other receptor tyrosine kinase family genes (e.g., *NTRK1*, *NTRK2*, *RET*, *MET*, or *RAF1*) or *BRAF* (26). Targeted therapies using tropomycin receptor kinase (TRK) inhibitors, such as larotrectinib and entrectinib, have proven effective for the treatment of patients with unresectable or metastatic *NTRK*-fusion IFS (27). Larotrectinib is a selective pan-TRK inhibitor used for sarcomas harboring *NTRK* fusions, while entrectinib inhibits ROS1 and ALK in addition to pan-TRK, making it suitable for tumors harboring *NTRK*, *ROS1*, or *ALK* fusions (28).

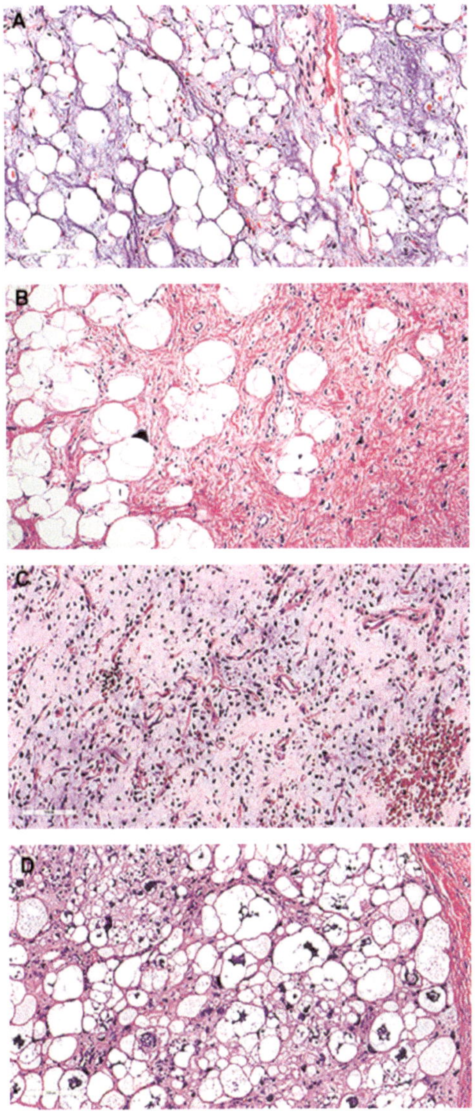

FIGURE 8.6 Photomicrographs of lipomatous tumors, each tumors with distinct histologic and molecular characteristics (H&E). (A) Lipoblastoma, a benign tumor displaying *PLAG1* fusion. (B) Atypical lipomatous tumor, a locally aggressive, non-metastasizing tumor with *MDM2* amplification. (C) Low-grade myxoid liposarcoma, characterized by *DDIT3* fusion. (D) Pleomorphic liposarcoma, a high-grade sarcoma lacking tumor-specific gene fusion or mutation.

8.2.3 Malignant Fibroblastic Tumors

Malignant fibroblastic tumors encompass various subtypes with distinct clinical and genetic characteristics.

Myxofibrosarcoma (MFS) is a malignant fibroblastic tumor typically found in the superficial soft tissues, predominantly in the extremities of older adults. It exhibits infiltrative growth patterns, making complete excision challenging and leading to frequent recurrences. Compared to conventional MFS, the epithelioid subtype demonstrates a more aggressive clinical course. Myxofibrosarcomas have a complex karyotype, and commonly mutated genes include *TP53*, *CDKN2A*, *CDKN2B*, *ATRX*, *RB1*, and *NF1* (2, 3). Clinical trials are currently evaluating the effectiveness of immune checkpoint inhibitors in patients with locally advanced, unresectable, or metastatic MFS (29).

Low-grade fibromyxoid sarcoma (LGFMS) is a variant of fibrosarcoma that predominantly arises in deep soft tissues, featuring alternating collagenous and myxoid areas with uniform, deceptively bland-appearing spindle cells, with low mitotic rate. LGFMS is notable for its tendency to metastasize later in the disease course. These tumors are characterized by the presence of the *FUS*::*CREB3L2* gene fusion, which results from a t(7;16) translocation observed in the majority of cases. This gene fusion serves as a useful diagnostic marker, especially in small biopsy samples (Figure 8.2). Rare cases may exhibit *FUS/EWSR1::CREB3L1* fusions (30).

Sclerosing epithelioid fibrosarcoma (SEF) is a rare variant of fibrosarcoma that shares some histologic features with LGFMS but tends to have a more aggressive clinical course. The most common genetic alteration in SEF is the *EWSR1::CREB3L1* gene fusion (31). In some cases, SEF may exhibit gene fusions involving another CREB-TF encoding gene (*CREB3L2* or *CREB3L3*) joined with *EWSR1*, and less commonly, with *FUS* (32).

8.3 Fibrohistiocytic Tumors

Tenosynovial giant cell tumor is a fibrohistiocytic neoplasm that originates in the synovium and tendon sheaths. It encompasses three subtypes: the localized type, the diffuse type (also known as pigmented villonodular synovitis), and the malignant variant, characterized by sarcomatous dedifferentiation. The pathogenesis involves a *CSF1* gene rearrangement present in a small subset of cells within the tumor, resulting in excessive production of CSF1 protein (33). Targeted therapy with CSF1R inhibitors, such as pexidartinib hydrochloride, offers a viable option for managing metastatic or unresectable tumors through reducing CSF1 protein production (34).

8.4 Adipocytic Tumors

Adipocytic tumors encompass a diverse group of neoplasms, ranging from benign to locally aggressive to malignant (Figure 8.6). These tumors can often be identified by specific chromosomal translocations or gene amplifications. Molecular diagnostic testing plays a crucial role, particularly in challenging cases or when dealing with small biopsy specimens.

Ordinary lipomas, the most common benign lipomatous tumors, frequently exhibit fusions involving the *HMGA2* gene, typically with *LPP* (lipoma preferred partner) (35) or occasionally with other fusion partners. Lipoblastoma, which primarily affects infants and children, is associated with chromosomal translocations that activate the *PLAG1* gene (8q12) (36). Detection of *PLAG1* gene rearrangements helps differentiate lipoblastoma from histologic mimics, such as myxoid liposarcoma (Figure 8.6).

Atypical lipomatous tumor/well-differentiated liposarcoma (ALT/WDL) is a locally aggressive adipocytic neoplasm characterized by *MDM2* gene amplification. ALT/WDL contains supernumerary ring or giant marker chromosomes created by amplified sequences of the 12q14-q15 region containing *MDM2* (12q15) and *CDK4* (12q14.1), along with other nearby genes. The detection of *MDM2* gene amplification is a valuable diagnostic tool, especially when diagnostic areas are not easily discernible on traditional H&E-stained sections. If *MDM2* and/or *CDK4* amplification is detected in non-lipomatous tumors, it may suggest a diagnosis of dedifferentiated liposarcoma, a fully malignant non-lipomatous tumor progressing from ALT/WDL. Amplification of *MDM2* and/or *CDK4* can also help select patients for clinical trials evaluating the efficacy of therapies targeting dedifferentiated liposarcoma, such as MDM2 inhibitors (e.g., siremadlin) or CDK4/6 inhibitors (e.g., palbociclib) (37, 38).

Myxoid liposarcoma is characterized by a specific chromosomal translocation resulting in the *FUS::DDIT3* or *EWSR1::DDIT3* gene fusion (Table 8.1) (39). The presence of these gene fusions is valuable in distinguishing pure round cell, high-grade myxoid liposarcoma from other round cell sarcomas, as their prognosis and treatment strategies vary (40).

Pleomorphic liposarcoma is characterized by pleomorphic lipoblasts set within a background akin to that of pleomorphic sarcoma. Unlike other subtypes of liposarcoma, it exhibits a complex genomic profile with alterations in multiple genes, including *RB1*, *TP53*, *ATRX*, and *NF1*, but no tumor-specific gene mutation (2). Clinical trials are currently investigating the efficacy of immune checkpoint inhibitors combined with other treatments, such as chemotherapy, for advanced/metastatic tumors (41).

Myxoid pleomorphic liposarcoma is an extremely rare and aggressive liposarcoma that primarily affects children and adolescents. It exhibits a combination of histologic features seen in myxoid and pleomorphic liposarcomas. This subtype, characterized by widespread loss of heterozygosity (42), is differentiated from myxoid liposarcoma and dedifferentiated liposarcoma by the absence of the *DDIT3* gene fusion and *MDM2* gene amplification, respectively.

8.5 Vascular Tumors

Vascular neoplasms represent a biologically diverse spectrum, encompassing benign lesions such as hemangiomas, locally aggressive tumors like epithelioid hemangioma, intermediate forms such as pseudomyogenic hemangioendothelioma, and malignant varieties including epithelioid hemangioendothelioma and angiosarcoma. Distinguishing between these entities can be challenging, particularly in small biopsies. Therefore, detecting specific genetic alterations associated with each tumor type can be helpful in achieving an accurate diagnosis.

For example, anastomosing hemangioma may resemble a well-differentiated angiosarcoma, but it carries distinctive *GNAQ*, *GNA14*, and *GNA11* mutations (43). Spindle cell hemangioma, often associated with Maffucci syndrome, exhibits *IDH1* or *IDH2* hotspot mutations (44, 45). Epithelioid hemangioma, with its potential for solid growth or atypical features, often presents a diagnostic challenge, as it can be confused with malignant vascular tumors. This confusion is alleviated by the identification of recurrent gene fusions involving *FOS* fused with various partner genes (*VIM*, *LMNA*, *MBNL1*), or *FOSB* fused with several other partner genes (*ZFP36*, *SETD1B*, *WWTR1*), which are distinctive for epithelioid hemangioma (46).

Pseudomyogenic hemangioendothelioma, a rarely metastasizing neoplasm, is characterized by *FOSB* rearrangements, frequently involving *SERPINE1* or *ACTB*, and less commonly with other partner genes (e.g., *CLTC* or *POTE1*) (47). Epithelioid hemangioendothelioma is a low-grade malignant vascular tumor displaying epithelioid endothelial cells, chondromyxoid matrix, and a cord-like arrangement of cells. Epithelioid hemangioendothelioma typically arises from the translocation t(1;3)(p36;q23-q25), leading to the *WWTR1::CAMTA1* fusion (48). A subset, however, exhibits the *YAP1::TFE3* fusion, distinguished by unique morphology and clinical characteristics (49).

Angiosarcomas have a complex karyotype and harbor recurrent mutations in angiogenic signaling pathway genes, including *PLCG1*, *PTPRB* and *KDR* (*VEGFR2*) (50, 51). Less common recurrent gene alterations involve *PIK3CA* (10%), *TP53* (25%), or *FLT4* (*VEGFR3*). Post-radiation and chronic lymphedema-associated angiosarcomas are characterized by high-level *MYC* amplification and, in 25% of cases, *FLT4* (*VEGFR3*) coamplification, which is associated with worse prognosis. *MYC* amplification is particularly useful in distinguishing post-irradiation atypical vascular lesions from angiosarcomas (51, 52).

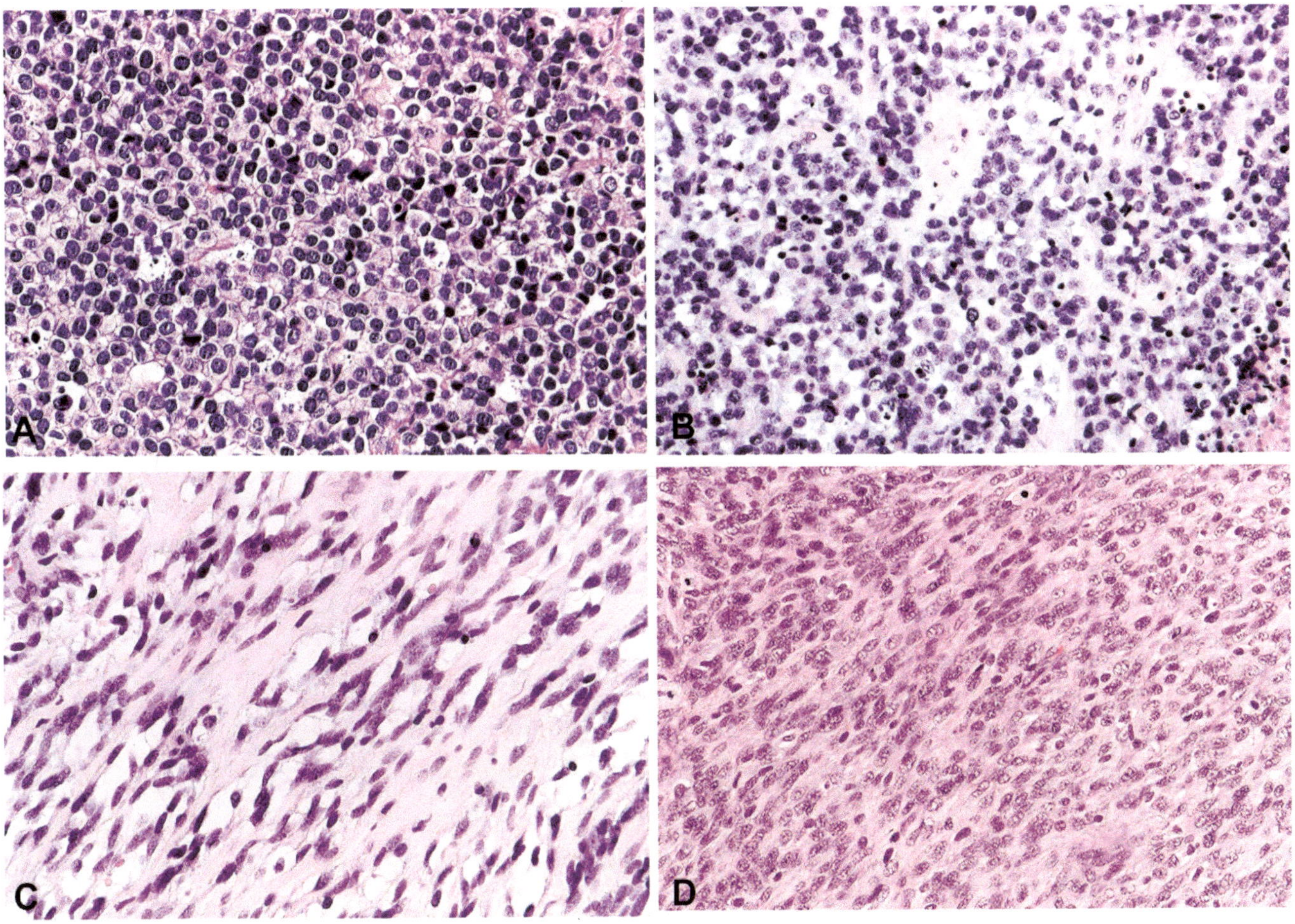

FIGURE 8.7 Histologic subtypes of rhabdomyosarcoma with distinct molecular and prognostic characteristics (H&E). (A) Solid variant of alveolar rhabdomyosarcoma, carrying *FOXO1* fusion. (B) Embryonal rhabdomyosarcoma with round cell features, lacking *FOXO1* fusion. (C) Sclerosing rhabdomyosarcoma, with *MYOD1* mutation. (D) Congenital/infantile spindle cell rhabdomyosarcoma, with *VGLL2* fusion.

8.6 Pericytic (Perivascular) Tumors

Pericytic (perivascular) tumors encompass a group of lesions derived from perivascular modified smooth muscle cells. This category includes glomus tumors, myopericytoma (including myofibroma), and angioleiomyoma. Approximately half of benign or malignant glomus tumors exhibit rearrangements in *NOTCH* family genes (*NOTCH1/2/3*), most commonly *NOTCH2* fused to *MIR143* (53). A small subset of cases with malignant features may harbor *BRAF* p.V600E mutations, providing potential targeted therapy options for patients with progressive disease (54). Myopericytoma/myofibroma and myopericytomatosis are associated with mutations in *PDGFRB*, while germline *PDGFRB* mutations underlie familial infantile myofibromatosis (55). Cellular/atypical myofibromas are linked to *SRF::RELA* gene fusions (56).

8.7 Smooth Muscle Tumors

Leiomyosarcomas are characterized by a high level of genomic instability, including chromothripsis, and a moderate mutation burden. The most frequently observed gene alterations in leiomyosarcomas are *TP53*, *RB1*, *ATRX*, and *PTEN* (2, 57). Although rare, some leiomyosarcomas harbor *ALK* gene rearrangement, presenting opportunities for targeted therapy (58).

8.8 Skeletal Muscle Tumors

Rhabdomyosarcomas (RMSs) are classified into four main histologic subtypes: embryonal, alveolar, spindle cell/sclerosing, and pleomorphic (Figure 8.7). The spindle cell/sclerosing subtype include at least two distinct molecular and biological categories.

Embryonal RMS is characterized by aneuploidy and loss of heterozygosity at 11p15.5 including the *IGF2* gene. Common driver mutations in the RAS pathway (*NRAS*, *KRAS*, *HRAS*, *NF1*, *FGFR4*), occur in a mutually exclusive pattern. Other recurrent mutations involve *PTEN*, *PIK3CA*, *FBXW7*, and *CTNNB1* (59). *TP53* mutations are linked to the anaplastic variant.

Alveolar RMS is distinguished by *PAX3::FOXO1 PAX7::FOXO1* gene fusions. Differentiating embryonal rhabdomyosarcoma with a round cell phenotype from the solid variant of alveolar RMS is challenging due to overlapping features. Detecting these gene fusions is crucial for therapeutic and risk group classification, offering more precision than histologic differentiation (60). Prognoses are generally poorer with *PAX3* fusions compared to *PAX7* fusions (61). Other rare fusion variants include *PAX3* with *FOXO4*, *NCOA1*, or *FGFR1*.

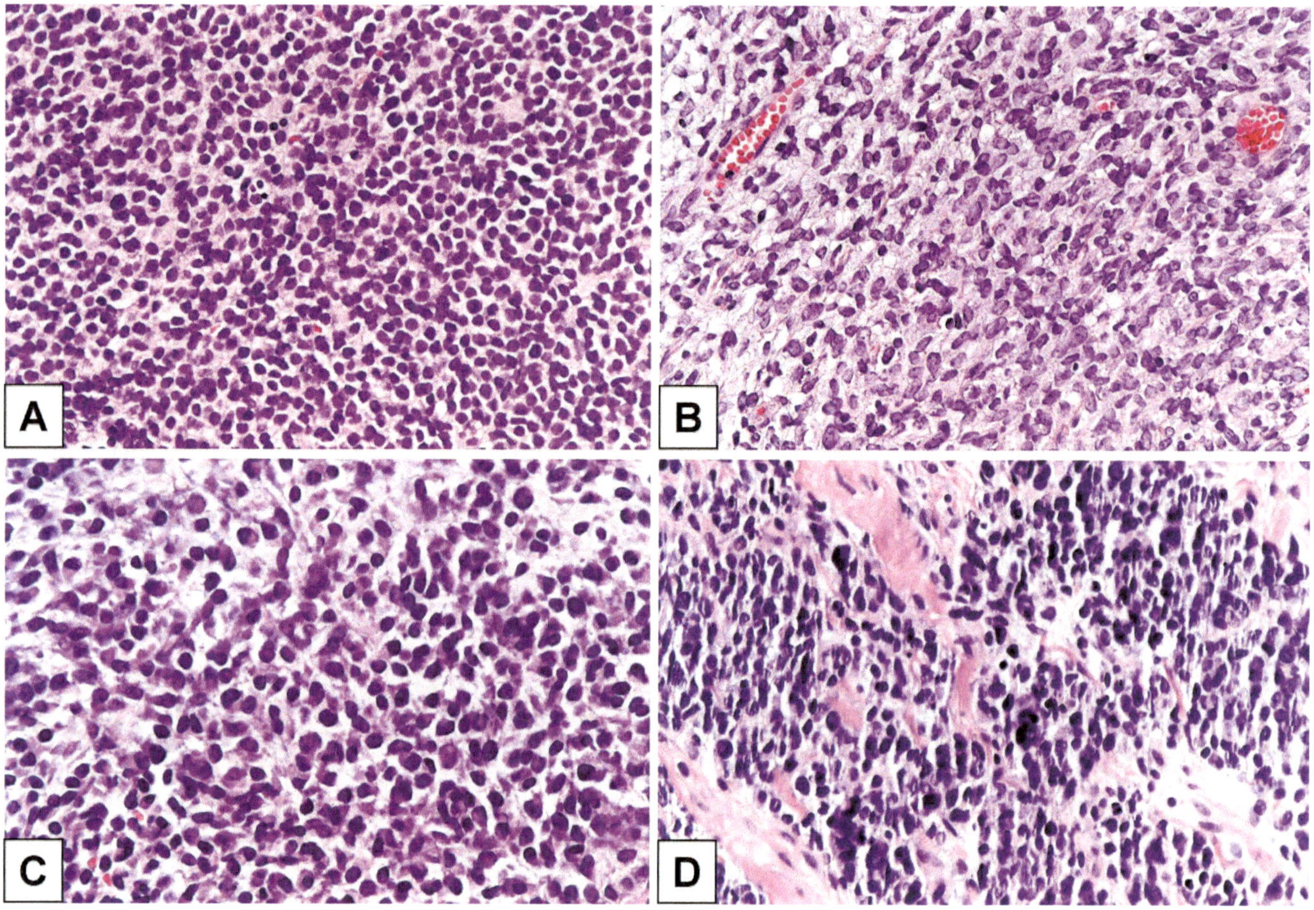

FIGURE 8.8 Photomicrographs of undifferentiated small round cell sarcoma subtypes, each exhibiting a pathognomonic genetic alteration (H&E). (A) Classic Ewing sarcoma, characterized by *EWSR1::FLI1* fusion. (B) *BCOR*-rearranged sarcoma, exhibiting *BCOR* gene rearrangement. (C) *CIC*-rearranged sarcoma, identified by *CIC*-related gene fusions. (D) Desmoplastic small round cell tumor, defined by the *EWSR1::WT1* fusion.

Spindle cell/sclerosing RMS is a diverse group both genetically and biologically. One subgroup includes the *MYOD1* (p.L122R) mutant sclerosing subtype, with about a third of cases also showing *PIK3CA* mutations (62). The infantile/congenital spindle cell variant, often fusion-positive, involves fusions like *NCOA2*, *VGLL2*, *SRF*, *TEAD1*, and *CITED2* (63, 64). A new variant, characterized by *ALK* and cytokeratin expression favors intraosseous locations, and harbors fusions like *TFCP2* with *EWSR1* or *FUS*, or *MEIS1*::*NCOA2* (65).

Ectomesenchymomas, displaying a mixture of RMS and neuronal/neuroblastic components, frequently have *HRAS* mutations (66). Lastly, pleomorphic RMS exhibits a genomic profile similar to undifferentiated pleomorphic sarcomas.

8.9 Peripheral Nerve Sheath Tumors

Genetic alterations in neurbromas primarily occur through biallelic inactivation of the tumor suppressor gene. Atypical neurofibromas/atypical neurofibromatous neoplasms with uncertain biological potential are distinguished by the acquisition of additional deletions in the *CDKN2A*/*CDKN2B* genes, which encode the cell-cycle regulatory proteins p16 and p15 (67). As these tumors progress towards malignant degeneration, they undergo further chromosomal copy number alterations. Malignant peripheral nerve sheath tumors (MPNSTs) exhibit a complex karyotype characterized by recurrent mutations involving not only *NF1* and *CDKN2A*/*B* but also the core components (*EED* or *SUZ12*) of the PRC2 complex (68, 69). In high-grade MPNSTs, approximately 80% of cases show a loss of PRC2 activity, resulting in the complete absence of H3K27me3 expression, which can be assessed immunohistochemically (70).

8.10 Tumors of Uncertain Differentiation

A significant portion of mesenchymal tumors have an uncertain cell of origin, as they do not fit into any specific cell type. This category encompasses various subtypes, each characterized by unique morphology, molecular genetics, and biological behavior. Diagnosis typically requires a comprehensive approach, integrating morphologic, immunohistochemical, and molecular genetic analyses.

8.10.1 Small Round Cell Sarcomas

Small round cell sarcomas are a heterogeneous group characterized by cells with small, round shapes and dense chromatin (Figure 8.8). They comprise different histologic subtypes, each with varying treatment options and prognoses. Detecting genetic alterations associated with specific types of round cell sarcomas can aid in diagnosis when morphologic and immunohistochemical techniques alone are inconclusive.

Desmoplastic small round cell tumor is characterized by a unique chromosomal translocation, t(11;22)(p13;q12), resulting in the *EWSR1::WT1* gene fusion. Ewing sarcoma is commonly linked to chromosomal translocations that fuse the *EWSR1* gene with an ETS family gene, predominantly *FLI1* (in 85% of cases) and *ERG* (5%). The co-occurrence of *STAG2* and *TP53* genetic alterations is typically associated with a poorer prognosis (71). Other high-grade undifferentiated round cell sarcomas include sarcoma with *CIC* rearrangement, which involves the *CIC::DUX4* fusion (95%) or the *CIC*-non-*DUX4* fusion (5%) (72); sarcoma with *BCOR* alterations (*BCOR* fusion or *BCOR* internal tandem duplication) (73, 74); and round cell sarcoma with *EWSR1*::non-ETS (*EWSR1/FUS::NFATC2*, and *EWSR1::PATZ1*) (75). Each of these tumors presents with varying prognoses and responses to conventional systemic therapies. The lack of targeted therapies or specific cancer treatment strategies for these subtypes of round cell sarcomas remains a significant challenge in oncology.

8.10.2 Tumors of Uncertain Differentiation—Spindle Cell Phenotype

Mesenchymal tumors with a spindle cell phenotype of uncertain differentiation represent a diverse group, exhibiting behaviors ranging from benign to malignant.

Intramuscular myxoma is a benign mesenchymal tumor characterized by a hypovascular myxoid stroma. Its genetic hallmark is an activating point mutation in the *GNAS* gene (76), which helps differentiate it from its morphologic mimics like low-grade myxoid sarcoma. Intramuscular myxoma may occur in the setting of Mazabraud syndrome, a rare condition characterized by the presence of fibrous dysplasia of bone and multiple intramuscular myxomas (77).

Angiomatoid fibrous histiocytoma (AFH), a mesenchymal neoplasm of uncertain differentiation, shows low malignant potential. It is characterized by monotonous, histiocyte-like cells and cystic hemorrhage. Over 90% of AFH cases exhibit an *EWSR1::CREB1* gene fusion. Other variants include *EWSR1/FUS::ATF1* fusions (78).

NTRK-rearranged spindle cell neoplasms are currently classified as tumors of uncertain differentiation, but recent evidence suggests a possible myofibroblastic lineage (79). They exhibit CD34 and S100 expression, and *NTRK* gene fusion, which activates the TRK signaling pathway. This fusion renders patients eligible for TRK inhibitors like entrectinib and larotrectinib, which are effective in treating metastatic or unresectable cases (27).

Synovial sarcoma, a malignant neoplasm with variable epithelial differentiation, is distinguished by a unique chromosomal translocation that results in *SS18::SSX* gene fusions. Two-thirds of cases involve *SSX1*, one-third involve *SSX2*, and rare cases involve *SSX4* (80, 81). This genetic hallmark is especially useful in diagnosing poorly differentiated synovial sarcomas with a round cell phenotype.

Clear cell sarcoma, a malignant mesenchymal tumor showing melanocytic differentiation, is characterized primarily by the *EWSR1::ATF1* gene fusion, and less commonly by the *EWSR1::CREB1* or *EWSR1::CREM* gene fusions (82). These genetic markers are invaluable for differentiating clear cell sarcoma from melanoma.

Undifferentiated pleomorphic sarcomas (UPSs) are noted for their genomic complexity, exhibiting complex karyotypes and extensive structural rearrangements. Although they lack tumor-specific amplifications or mutations, genes such as *TP53*, *ATRX*, *RB1*, *CDKN2A*, and *CDKN2B* are frequently altered (2). Genomic profiling is crucial in distinguishing UPS from dedifferentiated tumors that lack morphologic and immunohistochemical differentiation features. Examples of such dedifferentiated tumors include melanomas, liposarcomas, chondrosarcomas, and dedifferentiated solitary fibrous tumors. Current clinical trials are assessing the efficacy of immune checkpoint inhibitors, like pembrolizumab, in UPS with a high tumor mutational burden, particularly for unresectable or metastasized tumors (83, 84).

8.10.3 Tumors of Uncertain Differentiation—Epithelioid Cell Phenotype

A wide range of mesenchymal tumors, including benign, borderline, and malignant types, can exhibit an epithelioid cell appearance. Epithelioid sarcoma (ES), a malignant tumor of uncertain differentiation, is characterized by epithelioid features and is divided into proximal and distal subtypes. Both subtypes demonstrate complete loss of INI-1 nuclear protein expression, a product of the *SMARCB1* gene, which is detectable through immunohistochemical analysis. This loss usually results from homozygous *SMARCB1* deletion, less commonly from heterozygous deletion, or from negative transcriptional dysregulation by microRNAs (85, 86). In rare cases, other SWI/SNF chromatin-remodeling complex members, like *SMARCA4* (BRG1), are lost (87). While pediatric malignant rhabdoid tumor also exhibits INI-1 loss, ES is distinct due to its complex copy-number alterations and high mutational burden. In January 2020, the FDA granted accelerated approval for tazemetostat hydrobromide, an EZH2 inhibitor, for treating metastatic or unresectable ES in adults and pediatric patients aged 16 and older (88).

Extraskeletal myxoid chondrosarcoma (EMC) is characterized by small eosinophilic cells within a myxoid/chondromyxoid matrix. Some EMC cases may display high-grade features and loss of INI-1 expression, leading to potential diagnostic confusion with other INI-1-deficient tumors. Over 90% of EMC cases exhibit an *NR4A3* gene rearrangement, usually fusing with *EWSR1* and less commonly with *TAF15*, which differentiates EMC from morphologic mimics (89, 90).

Myoepithelial tumors of soft tissue, encompassing myoepithelioma, myoepithelial carcinoma, and mixed tumors, resemble their salivary gland and skin counterparts. More than half of these tumors exhibit *EWSR1* gene rearrangement, fusing with various genes like *ZNF44*, *PBX1*, *PBX3*, and *POU5F1* (91). The presence of an *EWSR1* fusion, along with specific morphologic and immunohistochemical characteristics, supports the diagnosis of myoepithelial tumors. Myoepithelial tumors with a mixed tumor phenotype frequently show *PLAG1* gene rearrangements (92).

Alveolar soft part sarcoma (ASPS) is a rare malignant mesenchymal neoplasm characterized by large epithelioid cells with abundant cytoplasm. It is driven by the *ASPSCR1::TFE3* fusion resulting from the der(17)t(X;17)(p11.2;q25) chromosomal translocation. Atezolizumab, a monoclonal antibody targeting programmed cell death-ligand 1 (PD-L1), has shown promising results in ASPS (93). In December 2022, it received FDA approval for the treatment of metastatic and unresectable tumors (94).

PEComas are rare mesenchymal tumors composed of perivascular epithelioid cells, characterized by coexpression of myoid and melanocytic markers, and often associated with *TSC2* alterations leading to activation of the mTOR signaling pathway. In cases without *TSC2* mutations, *TFE3* gene fusions are observed (95). Malignant PEComas, known for their aggressive behavior and metastatic potential, are treated with the mTOR inhibitor sirolimus for unresectable or metastatic conditions (96).

8.11 Chondrogenic Tumors

Mutations in the isocitrate dehydrogenase genes (*IDH1* or *IDH2*) are prevalent in chondrogenic tumors, including enchondroma, periosteal chondroma, and grade 1–3 central chondrosarcomas, but are absent in other mesenchymal tumors (97). Enchondromatosis patients typically exhibit somatic mosaic mutations in *IDH1* or *IDH2* (44, 45). On the other hand, osteochondromas often involve biallelic inactivation of the *EXT1* or *EXT2* genes (98).

Low-grade chondrosarcomas/atypical cartilaginous tumors are distinguished from enchondromas by the presence of copy number gains and losses, predominantly affecting *CDKN2A* (99). Higher-grade tumors, like grade 2 and 3 central chondrosarcomas, are characterized by aneuploidy and complex karyotypes. In addition to *IDH* mutations, other common alterations in these tumors include *CDKN2A* and *COL2A1* (100, 101). Secondary chondrosarcomas that arise from osteochondromas show chromosomal instability and complex karyotypes similar to those in higher-grade central chondrosarcomas. However, they are distinguishable by the presence of mutant *EXT1* or *EXT2* genes. Dedifferentiated chondrosarcomas, while also harboring *IDH1*/*IDH2* mutations, exhibit additional mutations in genes such as *TP53*, the *TERT* promoter, and *CDKN2A/B* (102). Mesenchymal chondrosarcoma is characterized by the unique *HEY1::NCOA2* fusion, which is found in nearly all cases (103). This fusion is particularly helpful in diagnosing biopsies of undifferentiated round cell tumors where the cartilaginous component is not evident.

Chondroblastoma is frequently associated with *H3–3B* mutations, leading to amino acid substitutions (Lys36Met) and a subsequent reduction in global H3K36 methylation (104). Chondromyxoid fibroma is characterized by a specific upregulation of *GRM1* expression due to complex rearrangements (105). Finally, synovial chondromatosis, which includes both benign and malignant variants, typically exhibits recurrent fusions involving the *FN1* and *ACVR2A* genes (106, 107).

8.12 Osteogenic Tumors

Both osteoblastomas and osteoid osteomas are driven by rearrangement of the *FOS* gene, which fuses with various partner genes such as *ANKH*, *RUNX2*, and *CEMIP* (108). Detecting *FOS* rearrangement can help differentiate osteoblastomas with atypical features from osteosarcoma.

Amplification of 12q13-q15, involving *MDM2* and *CDK4*, is commonly observed in parosteal osteosarcoma as well as low-grade central osteosarcoma (109, 110). High-grade conventional osteosarcoma is characterized by a high number of structural variations and copy number alterations, indicating genomic instability. Around half of osteosarcomas exhibit numerous point mutations near chromosomal breaks, a phenomenon known as kataegis. *TP53* is altered in over 90% of pediatric osteosarcomas, with approximately 55% of *TP53* alterations caused by a unique mechanism of gene inactivation through *TP53* intron 1 rearrangement. Osteosarcoma shows relatively few recurrent single-nucleotide variations. Besides *TP53*, other frequently mutated genes in osteosarcoma include *ATRX* and *RB1* (111).

8.13 Giant Cell-Rich Tumors

As mentioned earlier, rearrangements of the *USP6* gene, in partnership with various other genes, underlie the molecular changes seen in aneurysmal bone cyst (112). Pathogenic *H3–3A* mutations are present in nearly all giant cell tumors of bone, with the vast majority (90%) involving amino acid substitutions such as Gly34Trp, less commonly Gly34Leu, and rarely other mutations (104). The mononuclear tumor cells express RANK-L (receptor activator of nuclear factor kappaB ligand), which plays a role in osteoclast differentiation, proliferation, and survival. Denosumab, an inhibitor of RANK ligand, has been FDA-approved for the treatment of unresectable giant cell tumors in adults and post-pubertal adolescents (113). Malignant transformation in giant cell tumors has been associated with *TERT* activation and *TP53* mutations (114, 115). In non-ossifying fibromas, over 80% of cases exhibit mutually exclusive hotspot mutations in *KRAS*, *FGFR1*, and *NF1* (116).

8.14 Notochordal Tumors

Notochordal tumors, particularly chordoma, are marked by the expression of brachyury, a transcription factor encoded by the *TBXT* gene. Common genetic mutations in chordoma include *CDKN2A/B*, *LYST*, and mutations in the PI3K signaling pathway (117). In a subset of chordomas, *EGFR* expression is noted, which is essential for determining eligibility for EGFR inhibitor therapies (118). Poorly differentiated chordoma is often characterized by the loss of the SMARCB1 protein, typically due to deletions in the *SMARCB1* gene, affecting the tumor behavior (119, 120).

8.15 Summary

In recent decades, remarkable progress has been made in unraveling the genetic landscape of various sarcoma subtypes. The discovery of genetic alterations specific to different types of sarcoma has not only improved our understanding of their pathogenesis but also directly impacted patient care. Key to this progress has been the development of comprehensive molecular assays, which have revolutionized the screening for relevant genes in patient tumor samples. Integrating molecular genetic insights with histologic assessments aids in precise tumor classification and opens doors to identifying biomarkers for clinical trials. Although the number of actionable biomarkers in sarcomas remains limited, burgeoning databases and ongoing research offer hope for the development of novel treatments for this varied and challenging group of neoplasms.

REFERENCES

1. Pestana RC, Serrano C. Analysis of histology-agnostic targets among soft tissue and bone sarcomas in the AACR GENIE database. Front Oncol. 2022;12:1079909.
2. Pugh TJ, Bell JL, Bruce JP, et al. AACR Project GENIE: 100,000 cases and beyond. Cancer Discov. 2022;12(9):2044–2057.
3. André F, Arnedos M, Baras AS, et al. AACR Project GENIE: Powering precision medicine through an international consortium. Cancer Discov. 2017;7(8):818–831.
4. Hiemcke-Jiwa LS, van Gorp JM, Fisher C, et al. USP6-Associated neoplasms: A rapidly expanding family of lesions. Int J Surg Pathol. 2020;28(8):816–825.
5. Makise N, Mori T, Motoi T, et al. Recurrent FOS rearrangement in proliferative fasciitis/proliferative myositis. Mod Pathol. 2021;34(5):942–950.
6. Park JY, Cohen C, Lopez D, et al. Exon 20 insertion/duplication mutations characterize fibrous hamartoma of infancy. Am J Surg Pathol. 2016;40(12):1713–1718.
7. Puls F, Hofvander J, Magnusson L, et al. Gene fusions are recurrent in calcifying aponeurotic fibroma. J Pathol. 2016;238(4):502–507.
8. Libbrecht S, Van Dorpe J, Creytens D. The rapidly expanding group of RB1-deleted soft tissue tumors: An updated review. Diagnostics (Basel). 2021;11(3).
9. Jin YS, Möller E, Nord KH, et al. Fusion of the AHRR and NCOA2 genes through a recurrent translocation t(5;8)(p15;q13) in soft tissue angiofibroma results in upregulation of aryl hydrocarbon receptor target genes. Gene Chromosome Cancer. 2012;51(5):510–520.
10. Kao YC, Flucke U, Eijkelenboom A, et al. Novel EWSR1-SMAD3 gene fusions in a group of acral fibroblastic spindle cell neoplasms. Am J Surg Pathol. 2018;42(4):522–528.
11. Bhattacharya B, Dilworth HP, Iacobuzio-Donahue C, et al. Nuclear beta-catenin expression distinguishes deep fibromatosis from other benign and malignant fibroblastic and myofibroblastic lesions. Am J Surg Pathol. 2005;29(5):653–659.
12. Crago AM, Chmielecki J, Rosenberg M, et al. Near universal detection of alterations in CTNNB1 and Wnt pathway regulators in desmoid-type fibromatosis by whole-exome sequencing and genomic analysis. Genes Chromosomes Cancer. 2015;54(10):606–615.
13. Al-Ibraheemi A, Folpe AL, Perez-Atayde AR, et al. Aberrant receptor tyrosine kinase signaling in lipofibromatosis: A clinicopathological and molecular genetic study of 20 cases. Modern Pathol. 2019;32(3):423–434.
14. Simon MP, Pedeutour F, Sirvent N, et al. Deregulation of the platelet-derived growth factor B-chain gene via fusion with collagen gene COL1A1 in dermatofibrosarcoma protuberans and giant-cell fibroblastoma. Nat Genet. 1997;15(1):95–98.
15. Dadone-Montaudié B, Alberti L, Duc A, et al. Alternative PDGFD rearrangements in dermatofibrosarcomas protuberans without PDGFB fusions. Mod Pathol. 2018;31(11):1683–1693.
16. Beaziz J, Battistella M, Delyon J, et al. Long-term outcome of neoadjuvant tyrosine kinase inhibitors (TKI) in locally advanced dermatofibrosarcoma protuberans (DFSP). Ann Oncol. 2019;30(suppl. 5):V698.
17. Doyle LA, Vivero M, Fletcher CDM, et al. Nuclear expression of STAT6 distinguishes solitary fibrous tumor from histologic mimics. Mod Pathol. 2014;27(3):390–395.
18. Robinson DR, Wu YM, Kalyana-Sundaram S, et al. Identification of recurrent NAB2-STAT6 gene fusions in solitary fibrous tumor by integrative sequencing. Nat Genet. 2013;45(2):180–185.
19. Bahrami A, Lee S, Schaefer IM, et al. TERT promoter mutations and prognosis in solitary fibrous tumor. Mod Pathol. 2016;29:13a–14a.
20. Lee JC, Li CF, Huang HY, et al. ALK oncoproteins in atypical inflammatory myofibroblastic tumours: Novel RRBP1-ALK fusions in epithelioid inflammatory myofibroblastic sarcoma. J Pathol. 2017;241(3):316–323.
21. Antonescu CR, Suurmeijer AJ, Zhang L, et al. Molecular characterization of inflammatory myofibroblastic tumors with frequent ALK and ROS1 gene fusions and rare novel RET rearrangement. Am J Surg Pathol. 2015;39(7):957–967.
22. Gros L, Dei Tos AP, Jones RL, et al. Inflammatory myofibroblastic tumour: State of the art. Cancers. 2022;14(15):3662.
23. Butrynski JE, D'Adamo DR, Hornick JL, et al. Crizotinib in ALK-rearranged inflammatory myofibroblastic tumor. N Engl J Med. 2010;363(18):1727–1733.
24. Puls F, Carter JM, Pillay N, et al. Overlapping morphological, immunohistochemical and genetic features of superficial CD34-positive fibroblastic tumor and PRDM10-rearranged soft tissue tumor. Mod Pathol. 2022;35(6):767–776.
25. Perret R, Michal M, Carr RA, et al. Superficial CD34-positive fibroblastic tumor and PRDM10-rearranged soft tissue tumor are overlapping entities: A comprehensive study of 20 cases. Histopathology. 2021;79(5):810–825.
26. Kao YC, Fletcher CDM, Alaggio R, et al. Recurrent BRAF gene fusions in a subset of pediatric spindle cell sarcomas: Expanding the genetic spectrum of tumors with overlapping features with infantile fibrosarcoma. Am J Surg Pathol. 2018;42(1):28–38.
27. Cocco E, Scaltriti M, Drilon A. NTRK fusion-positive cancers and TRK inhibitor therapy. Nat Rev Clin Oncol. 2018;15(12):731–747.
28. Drilon A, Siena S, Ou SI, et al. Safety and antitumor activity of the multitargeted pan-TRK, ROS1, and ALK inhibitor entrectinib: Combined results from two Phase I trials (ALKA-372–001 and STARTRK-1). Cancer Discov. 2017;7(4):400–409.
29. Yamashita A, Suehara Y, Hayashi T, et al. Molecular and clinicopathological analysis revealed an immuno-checkpoint inhibitor as a potential therapeutic target in a subset of high-grade myxofibrosarcoma. Virchows Archiv. 2022;481(4):1–17.
30. Guillou L, Benhattar J, Gengler C, et al. Translocation-positive low-grade fibromyxoid sarcoma: Clinicopathologic and molecular analysis of a series expanding the morphologic spectrum and suggesting potential relationship to sclerosing epithelioid fibrosarcoma: A study from the French Sarcoma Group. Am J Surg Pathol. 2007;31(9):1387–1402.
31. Arbajian E, Puls F, Antonescu CR, et al. In-depth genetic analysis of sclerosing epithelioid fibrosarcoma reveals recurrent genomic alterations and potential treatment targets. Clin Cancer Res. 2017;23(23):7426–7434.
32. Doyle LA, Wang WL, Dal Cin P, et al. MUC4 is a sensitive and extremely useful marker for sclerosing epithelioid fibrosarcoma. Am J Surg Pathol. 2012;36(10):1444–1451.
33. West RB, Rubin BP, Miller MA, et al. A landscape effect in tenosynovial giant-cell tumor from activation of CSF1 expression by a translocation in a minority of tumor cells. Proc Natl Acad Sci USA. 2006;103(3):690–695.

34. Cannarile MA, Weisser M, Jacob W, et al. Colony-stimulating factor 1 receptor (CSF1R) inhibitors in cancer therapy. J Immunother Cancer. 2017;5(1):53.
35. Petit MM, Mols R, Schoenmakers EF, et al. LPP, the preferred fusion partner gene of HMGIC in lipomas, is a novel member of the LIM protein gene family. Genomics. 1996;36(1):118–129.
36. Hibbard MK, Kozakewich HP, Dal Cin P, et al. PLAG1 fusion oncogenes in lipoblastoma. Cancer Res. 2000;60(17):4869–4872.
37. Dickson MA, Schwartz GK, Keohan ML, et al. Progression-free survival among patients with well-differentiated or dedifferentiated liposarcoma treated with CDK4 inhibitor palbociclib: A phase 2 clinical trial. JAMA Oncol. 2016;2(7):937–940.
38. Abdul Razak AR, Bauer S, Suarez C, et al. Co-targeting of MDM2 and CDK4/6 with siremadlin and ribociclib for the treatment of patients with well-differentiated or dedifferentiated liposarcoma: Results from a proof-of-concept, Phase Ib study. Clin Cancer Res. 2022;28(6):1087–1097.
39. Hisaoka M, Tsuji S, Morimitsu Y, et al. Detection of TLS/FUS-CHOP fusion transcripts in myxoid and round cell liposarcomas by nested reverse transcription-polymerase chain reaction using archival paraffin-embedded tissues. Diagn Mol Pathol. 1998;7(2):96–101.
40. Gronchi A, Hindi N, Cruz J, et al. Trabectedin and RAdiotherapy in Soft Tissue Sarcoma (TRASTS): Results of a phase I study in myxoid liposarcoma from Spanish (GEIS), Italian (ISG), French (FSG) Sarcoma Groups. EClinicalMedicine. 2019;9:35–43.
41. Assi T, Ngo C, Faron M, et al. Systemic therapy in advanced pleomorphic liposarcoma: A comprehensive review. Curr Treat Options Oncol. 2023;24(11):1598–1613.
42. Dermawan JK, Hwang S, Wexler L, et al. Myxoid pleomorphic liposarcoma is distinguished from other liposarcomas by widespread loss of heterozygosity and significantly worse overall survival: A genomic and clinicopathologic study. Mod Pathol. 2022;35(11):1644–1655.
43. Liau JY, Tsai JH, Lan J, et al. GNA11 joins GNAQ and GNA14 as a recurrently mutated gene in anastomosing hemangioma. Virchows Arch. 2020;476(3):475–481.
44. Amary MF, Damato S, Halai D, et al. Ollier disease and Maffucci syndrome are caused by somatic mosaic mutations of IDH1 and IDH2. Nat Genet. 2011;43(12):1262–1265.
45. Pansuriya TC, van Eijk R, d'Adamo P, et al. Somatic mosaic IDH1 and IDH2 mutations are associated with enchondroma and spindle cell hemangioma in Ollier disease and Maffucci syndrome. Nat Genet. 2011;43(12):1256–1261.
46. Huang SC, Zhang L, Sung YS, et al. Frequent FOS gene rearrangements in epithelioid hemangioma: A molecular study of 58 cases with morphologic reappraisal. Am J Surg Pathol. 2015;39(10):1313–1321.
47. Walther C, Tayebwa J, Lilljebjörn H, et al. A novel SERPINE1-FOSB fusion gene results in transcriptional up-regulation of FOSB in pseudomyogenic haemangioendothelioma. J Pathol. 2014;232(5):534–540.
48. Errani C, Zhang L, Sung YS, et al. A novel WWTR1-CAMTA1 gene fusion is a consistent abnormality in epithelioid hemangioendothelioma of different anatomic sites. Genes Chromosomes Cancer. 2011;50(8):644–653.
49. Antonescu CR, Le Loarer F, Mosquera JM, et al. Novel YAP1-TFE3 fusion defines a distinct subset of epithelioid hemangioendothelioma. Genes Chromosomes Cancer. 2013;52(8):775–784.
50. Behjati S, Tarpey PS, Sheldon H, et al. Recurrent PTPRB and PLCG1 mutations in angiosarcoma. Nat Genet. 2014;46(4):376–379.
51. Huang SC, Zhang L, Sung YS, et al. Recurrent CIC gene abnormalities in angiosarcomas: A molecular study of 120 cases with concurrent investigation of PLCG1, KDR, MYC, and FLT4 gene alterations. Am J Surg Pathol. 2016;40(5):645–655.
52. Guo T, Zhang L, Chang NE, et al. Consistent MYC and FLT4 gene amplification in radiation-induced angiosarcoma but not in other radiation-associated atypical vascular lesions. Genes Chromosomes Cancer. 2011;50(1):25–33.
53. Mosquera JM, Sboner A, Zhang L, et al. Novel MIR143-NOTCH fusions in benign and malignant glomus tumors. Genes Chromosomes Cancer. 2013;52(11):1075–1087.
54. Karamzadeh Dashti N, Bahrami A, Lee SJ, et al. BRAF V600E mutations occur in a subset of glomus tumors, and are associated with malignant histologic characteristics. Am J Surg Pathol. 2017;41(11):1532–1541.
55. Arts FA, Sciot R, Brichard B, et al. PDGFRB gain-of-function mutations in sporadic infantile myofibromatosis. Hum Mol Genet. 2017;26(10):1801–1810.
56. Antonescu CR, Sung YS, Zhang L, et al. Recurrent SRF-RELA fusions define a novel subset of cellular myofibroma/myopericytoma: A potential diagnostic pitfall with sarcomas with myogenic differentiation. Am J Surg Pathol. 2017;41(5):677–684.
57. Yang CY, Liau JY, Huang WJ, et al. Targeted next-generation sequencing of cancer genes identified frequent TP53 and ATRX mutations in leiomyosarcoma. Am J Transl Res. 2015;7(10):2072–2081.
58. Davis LE, Nusser KD, Przybyl J, et al. Discovery and characterization of recurrent, targetable ALK fusions in leiomyosarcoma. Mol Cancer Res. 2019;17(3):676–685.
59. Shern JF, Chen L, Chmielecki J, et al. Comprehensive genomic analysis of rhabdomyosarcoma reveals a landscape of alterations affecting a common genetic axis in fusion-positive and fusion-negative tumors. Cancer Discov. 2014;4(2):216–231.
60. Shern JF, Selfe J, Izquierdo E, et al. Genomic classification and clinical outcome in rhabdomyosarcoma: A report from an international consortium. J Clin Oncol. 2021;39(26):2859–2871.
61. Sorensen PH, Lynch JC, Qualman SJ, et al. PAX3-FKHR and PAX7-FKHR gene fusions are prognostic indicators in alveolar rhabdomyosarcoma: A report from the children's oncology group. J Clin Oncol. 2002;20(11):2672–2679.
62. Kohsaka S, Shukla N, Ameur N, et al. A recurrent neomorphic mutation in MYOD1 defines a clinically aggressive subset of embryonal rhabdomyosarcoma associated with PI3K-AKT pathway mutations. Nat Genet. 2014;46(6):595–600.
63. Mosquera JM, Sboner A, Zhang L, et al. Recurrent NCOA2 gene rearrangements in congenital/infantile spindle cell rhabdomyosarcoma. Genes Chromosomes Cancer. 2013;52(6):538–550.
64. Alaggio R, Zhang L, Sung YS, et al. A molecular study of pediatric spindle and sclerosing rhabdomyosarcoma: Identification of novel and recurrent VGLL2-related fusions in infantile cases. Am J Surg Pathol. 2016;40(2):224–235.
65. Le Loarer F, Cleven AHG, Bouvier C, et al. A subset of epithelioid and spindle cell rhabdomyosarcomas is associated with TFCP2 fusions and common ALK upregulation. Mod Pathol. 2020;33(3):404–419.

66. Huang SC, Alaggio R, Sung YS, et al. Frequent HRAS mutations in malignant ectomesenchymoma: Overlapping genetic abnormalities with embryonal rhabdomyosarcoma. Am J Surg Pathol. 2016;40(7):876–885.
67. Miettinen MM, Antonescu CR, Fletcher CDM, et al. Histopathologic evaluation of atypical neurofibromatous tumors and their transformation into malignant peripheral nerve sheath tumor in patients with neurofibromatosis 1-a consensus overview. Hum Pathol. 2017;67:1–10.
68. Lee W, Teckie S, Wiesner T, et al. PRC2 is recurrently inactivated through EED or SUZ12 loss in malignant peripheral nerve sheath tumors. Nat Genet. 2014;46(11):1227–1232.
69. Cortes-Ciriano I, Steele CD, Piculell K, et al. Genomic patterns of malignant peripheral nerve sheath tumor (MPNST) evolution correlate with clinical outcome and are detectable in cell-free DNA. Cancer Discov. 2023;13(3):654–671.
70. Schaefer IM, Fletcher CD, Hornick JL. Loss of H3K27 trimethylation distinguishes malignant peripheral nerve sheath tumors from histologic mimics. Mod Pathol. 2016;29(1):4–13.
71. Tirode F, Surdez D, Ma X, et al. Genomic landscape of Ewing sarcoma defines an aggressive subtype with co-association of STAG2 and TP53 mutations. Cancer Discov. 2014;4(11):1342–1353.
72. Yoshimoto T, Tanaka M, Homme M, et al. CIC-DUX4 induces small round cell sarcomas distinct from Ewing sarcoma. Cancer Res. 2017;77(11):2927–2937.
73. Puls F, Niblett A, Marland G, et al. BCOR-CCNB3 (Ewing-like) sarcoma: A clinicopathologic analysis of 10 cases, in comparison with conventional Ewing sarcoma. Am J Surg Pathol. 2014;38(10):1307–1318.
74. Kao YC, Sung YS, Zhang L, et al. Recurrent BCOR internal tandem duplication and YWHAE-NUTM2B fusions in soft tissue undifferentiated round cell sarcoma of infancy: Overlapping genetic features with clear cell sarcoma of kidney. Am J Surg Pathol. 2016;40(8):1009–1020.
75. Tsuda Y, Zhang L, Meyers P, et al. The clinical heterogeneity of round cell sarcomas with EWSR1/FUS gene fusions: Impact of gene fusion type on clinical features and outcome. Genes Chromosomes Cancer. 2020;59(9):525–534.
76. Sunitsch S, Gilg MM, Kashofer K, et al. Detection of GNAS mutations in intramuscular/cellular myxomas as diagnostic tool in the classification of myxoid soft tissue tumors. Diagn Pathol. 2018;13(1):52.
77. Majoor BCJ, van de Sande MAJ, Appelman-Dijkstra NM, et al. Prevalence and clinical features of Mazabraud syndrome: A multicenter European study. J Bone Joint Surg Am. 2019;101(2):160–168.
78. Rossi S, Szuhai K, Ijszenga M, et al. EWSR1-CREB1 and EWSR1-ATF1 fusion genes in angiomatoid fibrous histiocytoma. Clin Cancer Res. 2007;13(24):7322–7328.
79. Tauziède-Espariat A, Duchesne M, Baud J, et al. NTRK-rearranged spindle cell neoplasms are ubiquitous tumours of myofibroblastic lineage with a distinct methylation class. Histopathology. 2023;82(4):596–607.
80. Amary MF, Berisha F, Bernardi Fdel C, et al. Detection of SS18-SSX fusion transcripts in formalin-fixed paraffin-embedded neoplasms: Analysis of conventional RT-PCR, qRT-PCR and dual color FISH as diagnostic tools for synovial sarcoma. Mod Pathol. 2007;20(4):482–496.
81. Skytting B, Nilsson G, Brodin B, et al. A novel fusion gene, SYT-SSX4, in synovial sarcoma. J Natl Cancer Inst. 1999;91(11):974–975.
82. Hisaoka M, Ishida T, Kuo TT, et al. Clear cell sarcoma of soft tissue: A clinicopathologic, immunohistochemical, and molecular analysis of 33 cases. Am J Surg Pathol. 2008;32(3):452–460.
83. Widemann BC, Italiano A. Biology and management of undifferentiated pleomorphic sarcoma, myxofibrosarcoma, and malignant peripheral nerve sheath tumors: State of the art and perspectives. J Clin Oncol. 2018;36(2):160–167.
84. Keung EZ, Lazar AJ, Torres KE, et al. Phase II study of neoadjuvant checkpoint blockade in patients with surgically resectable undifferentiated pleomorphic sarcoma and dedifferentiated liposarcoma. BMC Cancer. 2018;18(1):913.
85. Dermawan JK, Singer S, Tap WD, et al. The genetic landscape of SMARCB1 alterations in SMARCB1-deficient spectrum of mesenchymal neoplasms. Mod Pathol. 2022;35(12):1900–1909.
86. Kohashi K, Yamamoto H, Kumagai R, et al. Differential microRNA expression profiles between malignant rhabdoid tumor and epithelioid sarcoma: miR193a-5p is suggested to downregulate SMARCB1 mRNA expression. Mod Pathol. 2014;27(6):832–839.
87. Kohashi K, Yamamoto H, Yamada Y, et al. SWI/SNF chromatin-remodeling complex status in SMARCB1/INI1-preserved epithelioid sarcoma. Am J Surg Pathol. 2018;42(3):312–318.
88. Gounder M, Schöffski P, Jones RL, et al. Tazemetostat in advanced epithelioid sarcoma with loss of INI1/SMARCB1: An international, open-label, phase 2 basket study. Lancet Oncol. 2020;21(11):1423–1432.
89. Flucke U, Tops BB, Verdijk MA, et al. NR4A3 rearrangement reliably distinguishes between the clinicopathologically overlapping entities myoepithelial carcinoma of soft tissue and cellular extraskeletal myxoid chondrosarcoma. Virchows Arch. 2012;460(6):621–628.
90. Huang SC, Lee JC, Hsu YC, et al. Extraskeletal myxoid chondrosarcomas: The uncommon clinicopathologic manifestations and significance of TAF15::NR4A3 fusion. Mod Pathol. 2023;36(7):100161.
91. Suurmeijer AJH, Dickson BC, Swanson D, et al. A morphologic and molecular reappraisal of myoepithelial tumors of soft tissue, bone, and viscera with EWSR1 and FUS gene rearrangements. Genes Chromosomes Cancer. 2020;59(6):348–356.
92. Bahrami A, Dalton JD, Krane JF, Fletcher CD. A subset of cutaneous and soft tissue mixed tumors are genetically linked to their salivary gland counterpart. Genes Chromosomes Cancer. 2012;51(2):140–148.
93. Chen AP, Sharon E, O'Sullivan-Coyne G, et al. Atezolizumab for advanced alveolar soft part sarcoma. N Engl J Med. 2023;389(10):911–921.
94. Bergsma EJ, Elgawly M, Mancuso D, et al. Atezolizumab as the first systemic therapy approved for alveolar soft part sarcoma. Ann Pharmacother. 2023.
95. Agaram NP, Sung YS, Zhang L, et al. Dichotomy of genetic abnormalities in PEComas with therapeutic implications. Am J Surg Pathol. 2015;39(6):813–825.
96. Wagner AJ, Malinowska-Kolodziej I, Morgan JA, et al. Clinical activity of mTOR inhibition with sirolimus in malignant perivascular epithelioid cell tumors: Targeting the pathogenic activation of mTORC1 in tumors. J Clin Oncol. 2010;28(5):835–840.
97. Amary MF, Bacsi K, Maggiani F, et al. IDH1 and IDH2 mutations are frequent events in central chondrosarcoma and central and periosteal chondromas but not in other mesenchymal tumours. J Pathol. 2011;224(3):334–343.

98. Bovée JV, Cleton-Jansen AM, Wuyts W, et al. EXT-mutation analysis and loss of heterozygosity in sporadic and hereditary osteochondromas and secondary chondrosarcomas. Am J Hum Genet. 1999;65(3):689–698.
99. Joseph NM, McGill KC, Horvai AE. Genomic profiling of low-grade intramedullary cartilage tumors can distinguish enchondroma From chondrosarcoma. Am J Surg Pathol. 2021;45(6):812–819.
100. Tarpey PS, Behjati S, Cooke SL, et al. Frequent mutation of the major cartilage collagen gene COL2A1 in chondrosarcoma. Nat Genet. 2013;45(8):923–926.
101. Asp J, Inerot S, Block JA, Lindahl A. Alterations in the regulatory pathway involving p16, pRb and cdk4 in human chondrosarcoma. J Orthop Res. 2001;19(1):149–154.
102. Dermawan JKT, Nafa K, Mohanty A, et al. Distinct IDH1/2-associated methylation profile and enrichment of TP53 and TERT mutations distinguish dedifferentiated chondrosarcoma from conventional chondrosarcoma. Cancer Res Commun. 2023;3(3):431–443.
103. Wang L, Motoi T, Khanin R, et al. Identification of a novel, recurrent HEY1-NCOA2 fusion in mesenchymal chondrosarcoma based on a genome-wide screen of exon-level expression data. Genes Chromosomes Cancer. 2012;51(2):127–139.
104. Behjati S, Tarpey PS, Presneau N, et al. Distinct H3F3A and H3F3B driver mutations define chondroblastoma and giant cell tumor of bone. Nat Genet. 2013;45(12):1479–1482.
105. Nord KH, Lilljebjörn H, Vezzi F, et al. GRM1 is upregulated through gene fusion and promoter swapping in chondromyxoid fibroma. Nat Genet. 2014;46(5):474–477.
106. Amary F, Perez-Casanova L, Ye H, et al. Synovial chondromatosis and soft tissue chondroma: Extraosseous cartilaginous tumor defined by FN1 gene rearrangement. Mod Pathol. 2019;32(12):1762–1771.
107. Agaram NP, Zhang L, Dickson BC, et al. A molecular study of synovial chondromatosis. Genes Chromosomes Cancer. 2020;59(3):144–151.
108. Fittall MW, Mifsud W, Pillay N, et al. Recurrent rearrangements of FOS and FOSB define osteoblastoma. Nat Commun. 2018;9(1):2150.
109. Wunder JS, Eppert K, Burrow SR, et al. Co-amplification and overexpression of CDK4, SAS and MDM2 occurs frequently in human parosteal osteosarcomas. Oncogene. 1999; 18(3):783–788.
110. He X, Pang Z, Zhang X, et al. Consistent amplification of FRS2 and MDM2 in low-grade osteosarcoma: A genetic study of 22 cases with clinicopathologic analysis. Am J Surg Pathol. 2018;42(9):1143–1155.
111. Chen X, Bahrami A, Pappo A, et al. Recurrent somatic structural variations contribute to tumorigenesis in pediatric osteosarcoma. Cell Rep. 2014;7(1):104–112.
112. Oliveira AM, Hsi BL, Weremowicz S, et al. USP6 (Tre2) fusion oncogenes in aneurysmal bone cyst. Cancer Res. 2004;64(6):1920–1923.
113. Tsukamoto S, Mavrogenis AF, Kido A, et al. Current concepts in the treatment of giant cell tumors of bone. Cancers (Basel). 2021;13(15).
114. Fittall MW, Lyskjaer I, Ellery P, et al. Drivers underpinning the malignant transformation of giant cell tumour of bone. J Pathol. 2020;252(4):433–440.
115. Ishihara S, Yamamoto H, Iwasaki T, et al. Histological and immunohistochemical features and genetic alterations in the malignant progression of giant cell tumor of bone: A possible association with TP53 mutation and loss of H3K27 trimethylation. Mod Pathol. 2022;35(5):640–648.
116. Baumhoer D, Kovac M, Sperveslage J, et al. Activating mutations in the MAP-kinase pathway define non-ossifying fibroma of bone. J Pathol. 2019;248(1):116–122.
117. Tarpey PS, Behjati S, Young MD, et al. The driver landscape of sporadic chordoma. Nat Commun. 2017;8(1):890.
118. Scheipl S, Barnard M, Cottone L, et al. EGFR inhibitors identified as a potential treatment for chordoma in a focused compound screen. J Pathol. 2016;239(3):320–334.
119. Choy E, MacConaill LE, Cote GM, et al. Genotyping cancer-associated genes in chordoma identifies mutations in oncogenes and areas of chromosomal loss involving CDKN2A, PTEN, and SMARCB1. PLoS One. 2014;9(7):e101283.
120. Mobley BC, McKenney JK, Bangs CD, et al. Loss of SMARCB1/INI1 expression in poorly differentiated chordomas. Acta Neuropathol. 2010;120(6):745–753.

9

Primary Central Nervous System Tumors

Mustafa Motiwala, Emal Lesha, Lawrence M. Pfeffer, Richard B. Hessler, Xianfeng F. Zhao, and Andrew B. Boucher

9.1 Introduction

There are a myriad of brain, spine, and other central nervous system (CNS) tumors that vary broadly in incidence, pathology, and etiology. While malignant CNS tumors are relatively rare (1), accounting for less than a third of all CNS tumor diagnoses, they portend a high mortality rate as the leading cause of cancer death for men aged less than 40 years old and women younger than 20 (2). According to the Central Brain Tumor Registry of the United States (3), glioblastoma multiforme (GBM) remains the most prevalent primary CNS malignancy for adults in the United States, while meningiomas are the most common non-malignant tumor. However, brain metastases from other primary cancers, particularly lung, breast, and melanoma, persist as the most common type of brain tumors overall (4), as approximately 20% of all patients with cancer develop intracranial metastases at some point in their lives (5).

With recent developments in precision diagnostics and targeted therapeutics, there exists an opportunity to improve prognosis for these patients. By understanding and appreciating the molecular genomics of CNS tumors, treatment of these pathologies can be tailored for each patient based on novel tumor characterization paradigms and classification systems (6). Thus, this chapter will focus on the molecular biomarkers and therapeutic targets for precision therapy of primary CNS tumors, with an emphasis on primary CNS malignancies and additional considerations for certain benign tumors. Please refer to the corresponding chapters on the primary tumors that metastasize to CNS for details on their precision pathology.

9.2 High-Grade Glioma

Primary CNS tumors in adults most frequently originate from the supporting glial cells and fall under the category of diffuse glioma, consisting of astrocytomas, oligodendrogliomas, and mixed glioneuronal tumors. Gliomas are classified into grades 1, 2, 3, or 4, with grades 1 and 2 considered low-grade gliomas (LGGs), whereas grades 3 and 4 are high grade (7). High-grade gliomas (HGGs) include undifferentiated or anaplastic tumors (Figure 9.1), and in adults, these are often malignant and convey a poor prognosis. Within this category, there is a threefold epigenetic delineation of HGG by its constituent driver mutations: astrocytoma isocitrate dehydrogenase (*IDH*) mutant, oligodendroglioma *IDH* mutant and 1p19q co-deleted, and GBM *IDH* wild type (8). The latter of these is the most aggressive and most common in the United States, appearing in 3.23 per 100,000 people (3). As the classification of these tumors shifts towards incorporation of molecular biomarkers in addition to the histology associated with them (9), novel diagnostic and therapeutic techniques must be considered, as they contribute to this revised nomenclature. All the same, standard of care for these tumors largely involves the same established protocols of maximal safe resection followed by concurrent chemotherapy and radiation therapy, but targeted treatments and immunotherapy merit discussion, as there is ongoing research into these approaches that may carry significant potential.

The World Health Organization (WHO) released the fifth edition of its CNS tumor classification system in 2021 and featured a diagnostic decision tree based on molecular features (10). These updates were largely gleaned from the Cancer Genome Atlas (TCGA) project, which conveys a substantial amount of information regarding the molecular biomarkers relevant to HGG. GBM is the first cancer studied by the TCGA project (11), which analyzed the DNA copy number, gene expression, and DNA methylation of 206 GBM specimens and identified frequent genetic alterations in three critical signaling pathways: 1) RTK/RAS/PI3K, 2) p53, and 3) RB Figure 9.2. The activated EGFR, PI3K, MDM2, and CDK4 molecules in these pathways provide potential therapeutic targets. *EGFR* gene alterations and chromosomal abnormalities involving the *MDM2* and *CDK4* genes may play a role in GBM pathogenesis. Based on the expression patterns of 840 genes, GBM has been categorized into four distinct molecular subtypes: proneural, neural, classical, and mesenchymal (12). Chromosome 7 amplification with concomitant loss of chromosome 10 is a highly frequent event in all the GBMs and was seen in 100% of the classical subtype. The classical subtype is also characterized by the high level of *EGFR* amplification and lack of *TP53* mutation, even though *TP53* is the most frequently mutated gene in GBM. The proneural subtype is predominantly featured by the alterations of *PDGFRA* and frequent mutations in *IDH1*. The neural subtype characteristically shows the expression of neuron markers such as *GABRA1*, *NEFL*, *SLC12A5*, and *SYT1*. Focal hemizygous deletion of a region containing *NF1* is the predominant feature of the mesenchymal subtype. A novel subtype of GBM has also been identified by the TCGA study and usually affects young adults, carries a methylation signature, and has a better survival.

Under this new scheme, secondary GBM was reclassified as astrocytoma *IDH*-mutant (Grade 4), leaving only *IDH* wild type

DOI: 10.1201/9781003513469-9

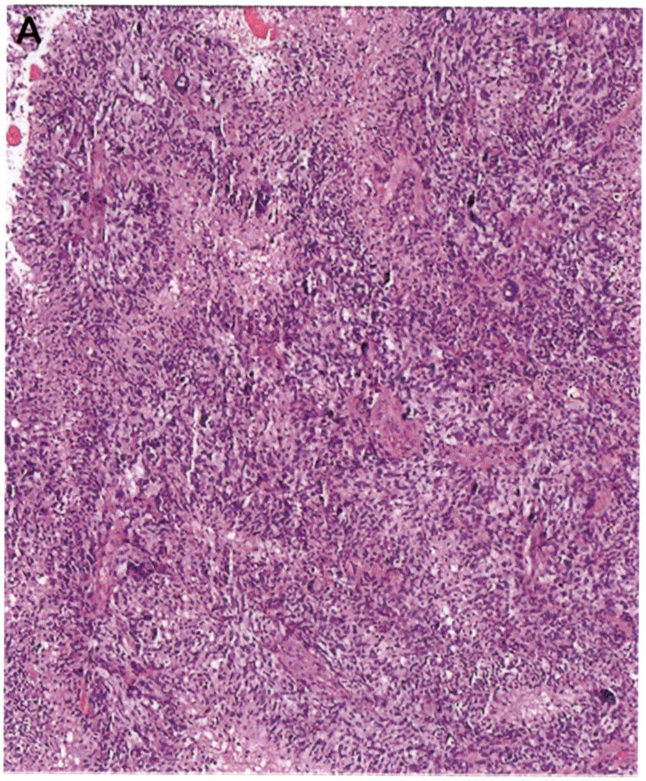

B

Results Summary

Biomarker	Biomarker Findings	Potential Therapeutic Options (in Indication)	Potential Therapeutic Options (in other Indication)	Clinical Trials
BRAF	V600E	Dabrafenib + trametinib (A)	Vemurafenib + cobimetinib (B/C), Vemurafenib (B/C), Binimetinib (C), Dabrafenib (C), Cobimetinib (C), Encorafenib + binimetinib (C)	12

Additional Biomarker Details

Microsatellite Instability (MSI)	MS-Stable	
Tumor Mutation Burden (TMB)	1.5 Muts/Mb	TMB-Low

Pertinent Negative Biomarkers Evaluated by NGS

EGFR	IDH1	IDH2	NTRK1	NTRK2	NTRK3

Biomarker Results Which May Confer Resistance To Specific Therapies

Biomarker	Biomarker Findings	Therapeutic Options Affected
None	None	None

Previously Reported Results

Biomarker	Methodology	Result
Pan-TRK	IHC	pan-TRK: Tumor cells are positive (CNS tissue) for TRK protein expression.

FIGURE 9.1 Pathology of high-grade glioma with representative NGS. (A) Aggressive neoplasm with tumor necrosis. (B) The accompanying NGS report showing the necessary information provided.

glial tumors designated as GBM, but this was not the only change based on genetic features (13). Many argue that this new "molecular marker-based diagnosis provides a more objective determination of glioma type" and complements our previous knowledge of glioma epigenetics (10, 14).

One of the most notable epigenetic alterations influencing response to treatment involves methylation of key genes. In particular, telomerase reverse transcriptase (TERT) expression is upregulated via mutations to decreased methylation of the CpG islands of *TERT* promoters (12), whereas methylation of the *MGMT* promoter in GBM leading to silencing of this DNA repair gene is well established as predictive in disease response to the alkylating agent temozolomide in the classical subtype of GBM (12, 15). Since initial reports, several clinical trials have endorsed this finding and confirmed the methylation status of *MGMT* promoter as the first predictive biomarker in neuro-oncology (16, 17). Using methylation status to predict chemosensitivity has undoubtedly changed the management of GBM, but acquired resistance to temozolomide in *MGMT*-deficient tumors has since been identified via the loss of the mismatch repair (MMR) pathway from genetic instability (18). Thus, there remains a need for the development of agents to overcome drug-resistant GBM. Currently, there are still no targeted therapies for glioma as standard of care, but our improved molecular understanding of the disease has revealed several molecules that can serve as therapeutic targets (19) (Table 9.1). Recent studies have shown that the SMARCA4/BRG1 subunit of the catalytic subunit of the SWI/SNF chromatin remodeling complex is overexpressed in GBM (20). Moreover, targeting the bromodomain of the BRG1 subunit with a small molecule inhibitor increases the chemosensitivity of GBM *in vitro* and in animal models of GBM (21, 22).

9.3 Information Classification: General

In the same vein, immunotherapies have also largely failed to improve outcomes significantly for high-grade glioma patients (23, 24). Some have credited the lack of available antigens, impaired T cell recruitment, and an immunosuppressive microenvironment for making HGG "immunologically cold tumors" (25). There are several immunotherapy strategies for the treatment of HGG with vaccines, chimeric antigen receptor T cells, and strategies to reverse immunosuppression, but regardless, there have been few advancements in targeting glioma immunologically (13).

9.4 Low-Grade Gliomas

Histologically, low-grade gliomas (LGGs) are usually composed of well-differentiated and hypercellular glia with nuclear atypia and rare mitotic activity (Figure 9.3). As compared with grade 4 glioblastoma, grade 3 was considered lower-grade glioma and analyzed together with grade 2 by TCGA, and three subtypes have been defined with distinct clinical outcomes (Figure 9.4) (26): The most favorable is the LGG with *IDH* mutant and 1p/19q co-deletion, now classified as oligodendroglioma. It carries mutations in *IDH1* or *IDH2*, which lead to abnormalities in isocitrate dehydrogenase enzyme activities, hypermethylation, and deviant gene expression (27). Simultaneous deletion of the short arm of chromosome 1 (1p) and long arm of chromosome 19 (19q) is another feature of this tumor. When the tumor harbors the *IDH1* or *IDH2* mutations without the simultaneous deletion of 1p and 19q, it is named *IDH* mutant without 1p/19q co-deletion and associated with an intermediate prognosis (28).

Unlike HGG, LGGs are well differentiated and often carry the potential for a better prognosis for patients (29). As with HGG, molecular features of LGG contribute to the revised grading by the WHO as well as survival (30). Specifically, the discovery of *IDH* mutations in LGG, either

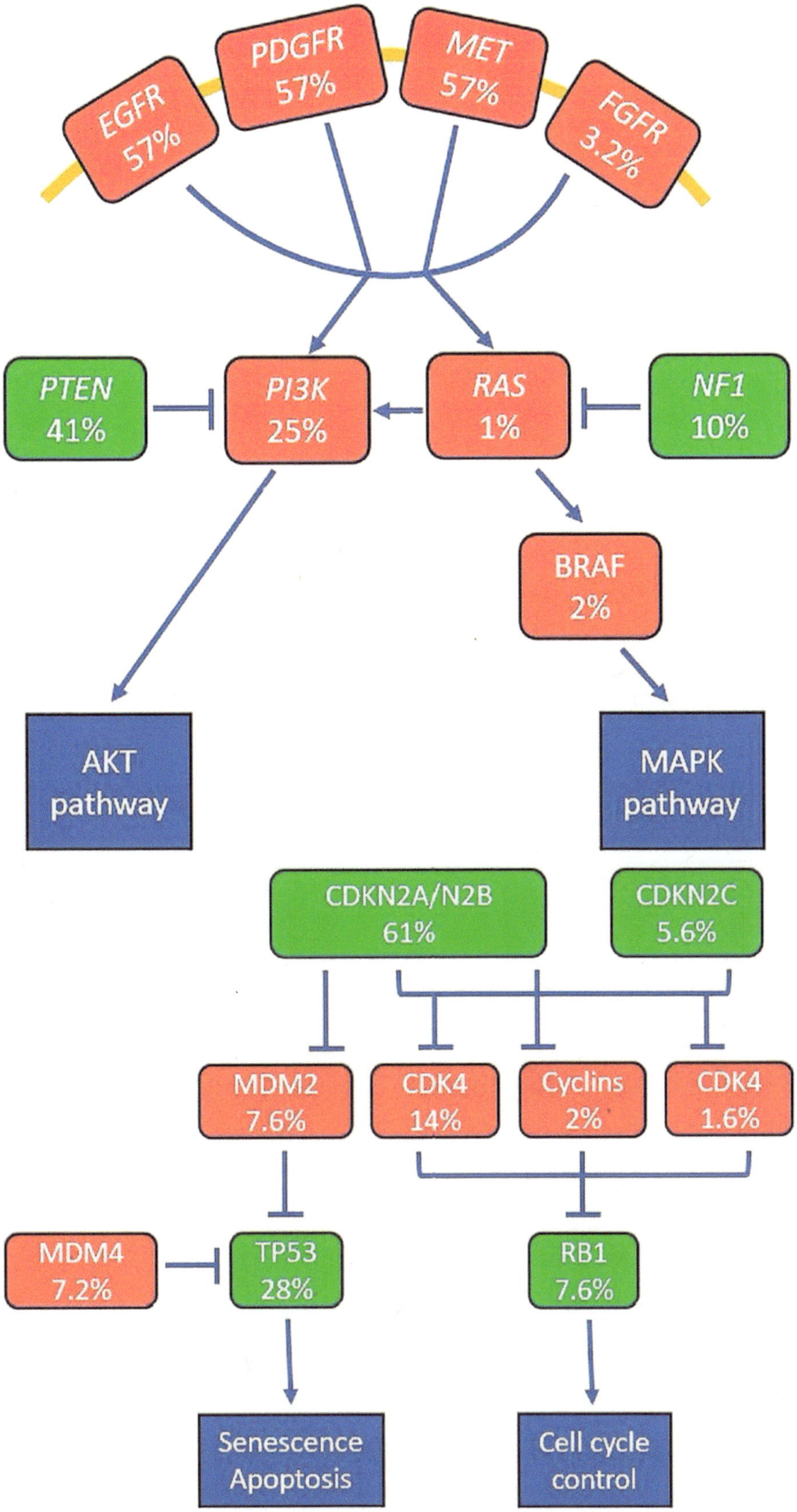

FIGURE 9.2 Critical signal transduction pathways activated in GBM (modified from reference 12). The activated oncogenes are in red, whereas the inactivated tumor suppressor genes are in green. The mutation rates in GBM are indicated as percentages. (A) Overall 90% genetic alterations are involved in activation of PI3K/AKT pathway and MAPK pathways. (B) Overall 86% genetic alterations are involved in the inactivation of senescence and apoptosis pathway, while overall 79% genetic alterations are involved in the inhibition of cell cycle control mechanism.

TABLE 9.1

Novel Therapeutic Targets for Glioblastoma

Therapy	Targets	Candidate Drugs	Current Status
Precision therapy	EGFR amplification	Depatuxizumab mafodotin	Phase 3 trial
	PI3K/AKT/mTOR pathway	Buparlisib, everolimus	Phase 2 trial
	• PTEN deletion		
	• PIK3CA mutations		
	• PIK3R1 mutations		
	VEGF	Regorafenib	Phase 2 trial
	BRAF V600E (6%)	Vemurafenib	Modest activity
	Gene fusions (50%)		
	• FGFR	Erdafitinib	
	• MET		
	• NTRK	Larotrectinib, entrectinib	
	• EGFR		
	• ROS1		
	• PDGFRA		
Immunotherapy			
Vaccine	EGFR variant III (20%)	Rindopepimut/bevacizumab	Phase 2 trial
PVSRIPO	None	N/A	21% OS rate (2 yrs)
Checkpoint	PD-1/PD-L1 and/or CTLA-4	Pembrolizumab, atezolizumab	Phase 1 trial
CAR T-cell	Variable	N/A	Preclinical trials

Source: see further ref. 19

Abbreviation: CAR, chimeric antigen receptor; OS, overall survival; PD-1, programmed death-1, PD-L1, PD1 ligand.

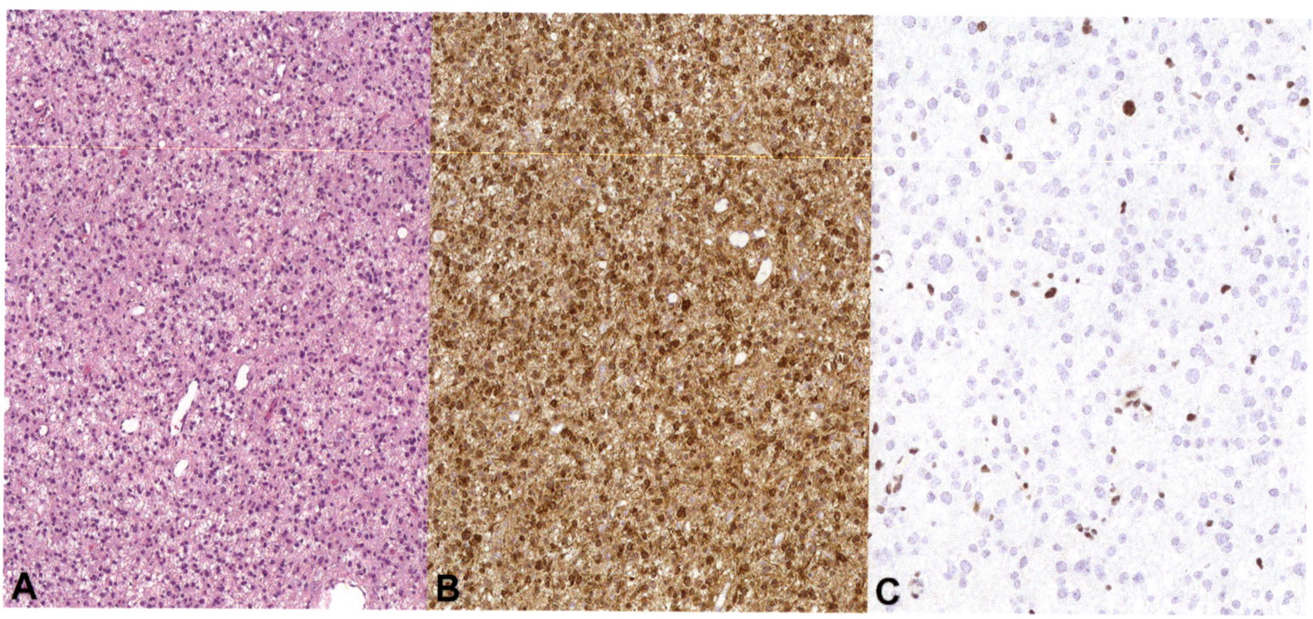

FIGURE 9.3 Pathology of low-grade glioma with *IDH* mutation. (A) Dense neurofibrils with rare mitotic figures (H&E, ×100); (B) Positive for IDH1/2 (IHC, ×100); (C) Low proliferation index (Ki67) (IHC, ×100).

in *IDH1* or *IDH2*, confers favorable survival potential compared to glioma with the wild-type *IDH1* or *IDH2* gene (31, 32). Recently, there have been advances in targeted therapies for these *IDH*-mutant tumors. Results from a Phase 3 trial with the drug vorasidenib suggest that there may be significant survival benefit with this agent that targets *IDH1* and *IDH2* mutant gliomas (33). Crucially, if this drug obtains FDA approval, it will represent the first new agent in glioma therapy in decades and carries the potential to improve treatment options when the previous mainstay of treatment has been surgical resection with the addition of non-targeted chemotherapies.

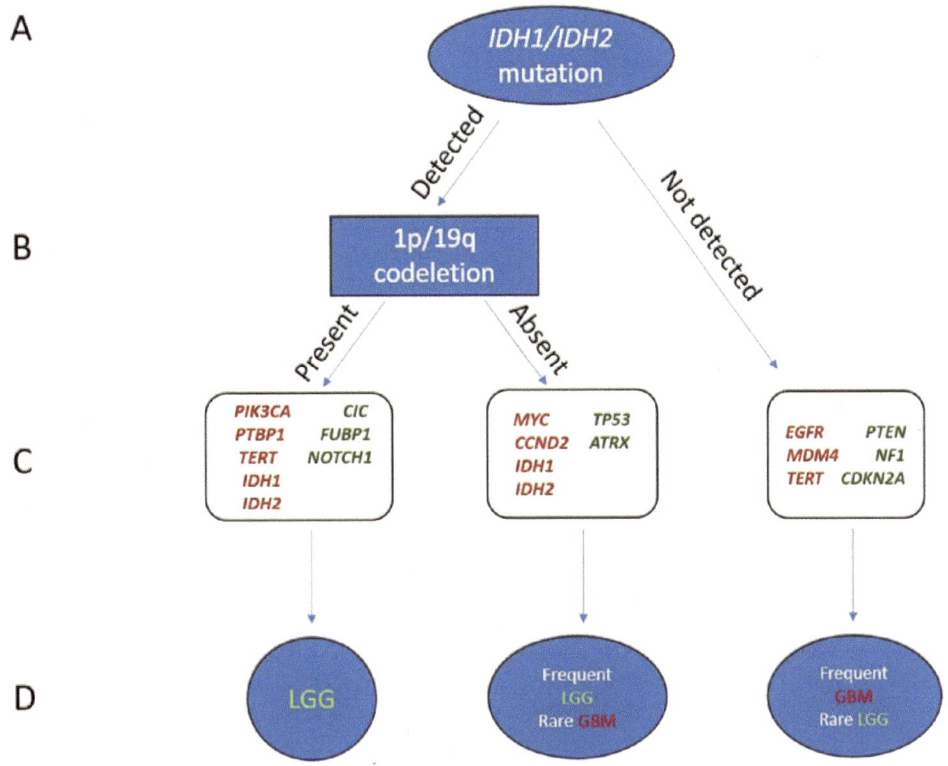

FIGURE 9.4 Defining algorithm for molecular subtypes of low-grade gliomas. (A) Identification of IDH mutation(s); (B) Identification of the 1p/19q codeletion; (C) Additional genetic alterations: activation mutations in red and inactivation mutations in green; (D) Corresponding clinical identities of LGG.

9.5 Benign CNS Tumors

9.5.1 Meningioma

Meningiomas are the most common primary CNS tumors in adults. While the majority of meningiomas are grade 1 and managed primarily with surgical resection with excellent tumor control, 15–20% of meningiomas are higher grade (grade 2 or 3) (Figure 9.5) and are associated with a poor prognosis. Surgical resection and often radiotherapy remain the first-line treatment for these higher-grade meningiomas, with pharmacotherapy used for refractory cases. In the era of precision medicine, multiple biomarkers have been identified with targeted therapies under investigation (34). Hormone-directed therapies such as somatostatin analogs octreotide and more recently pasireotide have been studied with good results in high-grade meningiomas (35, 36). Non-hormonal targeted therapies have also been studied, especially those targeting vascular endothelial growth factor (VEGF) and platelet-derived growth factor (PDGF). Bevacizumab, a VEGF monoclonal antibody, has been proven efficacious in disease control in multiple trials of patients with refractory disease (37, 38). Patients with PDGF-positive immunohistochemistry have been managed with sunitinib and vatalanib, TKIs with affinity to PDGF (39, 40).

Recent developments in genomic analyses have identified several targetable pathways in meningiomas, including the mTOR pathway, *SMO* mutations, and BAP1 tumor suppressors. For instance, mutations of *AKT1*, which are part of the mTOR pathway, are detected in 9% of meningiomas, and these tumors have a tendency for the anterior skull base. AKT inhibitor therapy has been used in case studies and recent clinical trials (34). Meningiomas harboring *BAP1* mutations are clinically aggressive. Tazemetostat, an EZH2 inhibitor that has shown inhibition for BAP1, is under investigation for high-grade meningiomas. Finally, DNA methylation pattern is another form of bioanalysis that can help further characterize meningiomas and is being

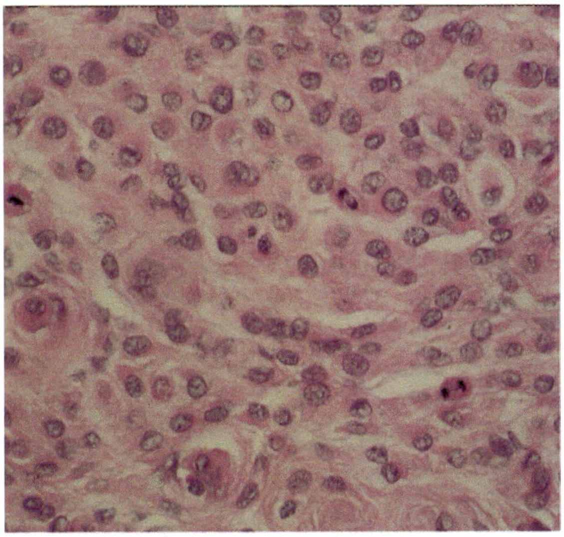

FIGURE 9.5 Pathology of atypical meningioma. High power showing the atypical neoplastic cells with vesicular nuclei and inconspicuous nucleoli. Mitotic figures are readily identified.

considered for clinical decision making. In recent years, studies of DNA methylation patterns have identified multiple genes and promoters associated with meningioma development, with subsequent targeted therapies addressing these epigenetic aberrations (41). In this regard, FAK inhibitor GSK2256098 and BRAF inhibitor dabrafenib have been utilized in clinical trials for patients with recurrent meningiomas (42, 43).

9.5.2 Craniopharyngioma

Papillary craniopharyngioma is a rare benign primary CNS tumor that occurs in children 5 to 14 years of age or adults older than 50 years within the sella and suprasellar region of the brain. The first line of treatment is maximal safe surgical resection, but these tumors tend to encase important cranial structures, so adjuvant radiation therapy is often necessary. While benign by histologic and oncologic criteria, these lesions have a high tendency to recur, with limited additional treatment options, and can cause significant morbidity due to local mass effect. Precision medicine has expanded treatment options for these tumors, as the majority of papillary craniopharyngiomas carry *BRAF* V600E mutations, making it an intriguing target for BRAF targeted therapy (44). Recently, a phase 2 clinical trial showed a 94% response using a combination BRAF inhibitor vemuraufenib and MEK inhibitor cobimetinib in patients with untreated *BRAF*-mutated papillary craniopharyngioma (45).

9.5.3 Vestibular Schwannoma

Vestibular schwannoma is a benign tumor that can present as sporadic or in association with neurofibromatosis type 2 (NF2). While the mainstay of treatment is often surgical resection, radiotherapy, or both, novel understanding of disease pathophysiology has led to the identification of several biomarkers that can be targeted via pharmacotherapy, including but not limited to VEGF, ErbB, and mTOR pathways. Bevacizumab, for instance, has been shown to have efficacy in multiple trials in patients with NF2-type vestibular schwannoma and is being considered as a first-line therapy in these patient populations (46). Lapatinib and erlotinib, TKI inhibitors with affinity for ErbB2, have also been investigated in retrospective and clinical trials (47, 48).

9.6 Testing Strategy

All brain tumors should be subjected to a frozen section evaluation at the time of surgical resection. Once suspected of diffuse glioma or glioblastoma, a portion of fresh tissue should be sent for FISH analysis for 1p/19q and molecular studies for the *IDH* mutations. A neuronal NGS panel analysis should also be carried out to identify mutations in the oncogenes and tumor suppressor genes for potential clinical trials. These results should be reported in an addendum/addenda to the original pathology report.

9.7 Conclusion

Precision pathology is revolutionizing the diagnosis and management of primary CNS tumors, addressing diagnostic and treatment challenges for the clinician and the patient. Detailed laboratory, tissue, and genomic analysis are becoming increasingly important, as they can guide clinical decision making and determine treatment options. For primary CNS tumors, we have seen molecular diagnostics change the landscape of classification and diagnoses with significant impact on prognostication and patient education. As expected, the therapeutics have lagged behind diagnostic efficacy, but there have been recent breakthroughs that support the notion that novel therapeutics and targeted therapies will alter treatment paradigms and improve outcomes for a variety of primary CNS tumors. Research trials are ongoing that suggest optimism for the future in this exciting and dynamic field of precision pathology for primary CNS tumors.

REFERENCES

1. Siegel RL, Miller KD, Fuchs HE, et al. Cancer statistics, 2021. CA Cancer J Clin. 2021;71(1):7–33.
2. Miller KD, Ostrom QT, Kruchko C, et al. Brain and other central nervous system tumor statistics, 2021. CA Cancer J Clin. 2021;71(5):381–406.
3. Ostrom QT, Cioffi G, Gittleman H, et al. CBTRUS statistical report: Primary brain and other central nervous system tumors diagnosed in the United States in 2012–2016. Neuro Oncol. 2019;21(Suppl 5):v1–v100.
4. Amsbaugh MJ, Kim C. Brain Metastasis. In: StatPearls. Treasure Island, FL: StatPearls Publishing; 2023.
5. Achrol AS, Rennert RC, Anders C, et al. Brain metastases. Nat Rev Dis Primers. 2019;5(1):5.
6. Balestrino R, Ruda R, Soffietti R. Brain metastasis from unknown primary tumour: Moving from old retrospective studies to clinical trials on targeted agents. Cancers (Basel). 2020;12(11).
7. Perry A, Wesseling P. Histologic classification of gliomas. Handb Clin Neurol. 2016;134:71–95.
8. van den Bent MJ, Geurts M, French PJ, et al. Primary brain tumours in adults. Lancet. 2023;402(10412):1564–1579.
9. Louis DN, Perry A, Wesseling P, et al. The 2021 WHO classification of tumors of the central nervous system: A summary. Neuro Oncol. 2021;23(8):1231–1251.
10. Zakharova G, Efimov V, Raevskiy M, et al. Reclassification of TCGA diffuse glioma profiles linked to transcriptomic, epigenetic, genomic and clinical data, according to the 2021 WHO CNS tumor classification. Int J Mol Sci. 2022;24(1):157.
11. Verhaak RG, Hoadley KA, Purdom E, et al. Integrated genomic analysis identifies clinically relevant subtypes of glioblastoma characterized by abnormalities in PDGFRA, IDH1, EGFR, and NF1. Cancer Cell. 2010;17(1):98–110.
12. Brennan CW, Verhaak RG, McKenna A, et al. The somatic genomic landscape of glioblastoma. Cell. 2013;155(2):462–477.
13. Nayak L, Reardon DA. High-grade gliomas. Continuum (Minneap Minn). 2017;23(6, Neuro-oncology):1548–1563.
14. Muench A, Teichmann D, Spille D, et al. A novel type of IDH wild-type glioma characterized by gliomatosis cerebri-like growth pattern, TERT promoter mutation, and distinct epigenetic profile. Am J Surg Pathol. 2023;47(12):1364–1375.
15. Hegi ME, Diserens AC, Gorlia T, et al. MGMT gene silencing and benefit from temozolomide in glioblastoma. N Engl J Med. 2005;352(10):997–1003.

16. Gusyatiner O, Hegi ME. Glioma epigenetics: From subclassification to novel treatment options. Semin Cancer Biol. 2018;51:50–58.
17. Wick W, Weller M, van den Bent M, et al. MGMT testing--the challenges for biomarker-based glioma treatment. Nat Rev Neurol. 2014;10(7):372–385.
18. Lin K, Gueble SE, Sundaram RK, et al. Mechanism-based design of agents that selectively target drug-resistant glioma. Science. 2022;377(6605):502–511.
19. Tan AC, Ashley DM, Lopez GY, et al. Management of glioblastoma: State of the art and future directions. CA Cancer J Clin. 2020;70(4):299–312.
20. Wang Y, Yang CH, Schultz AP, et al. Brahma-Related Gene-1 (BRG1) promotes the malignant phenotype of glioblastoma cells. J Cell Mol Med. 2021;25(6):2956–2966.
21. Yang C, He Y, Wang Y, et al. Next-generation bromodomain inhibitors of the SWI/SNF complex enhance DNA damage and cell death in glioblastoma. J Cell Mol Med. 2023;27(18):2770–2781.
22. Yang C, Wang Y, Sims MM, et al. Targeting the bromodomain of BRG-1/BRM subunit of the SWI/SNF complex increases the anticancer activity of temozolomide in glioblastoma. Pharmaceuticals (Basel). 2021;14(9): 904.
23. Reardon DA, Brandes AA, Omuro A, et al. Effect of nivolumab vs bevacizumab in patients with recurrent glioblastoma: The CheckMate 143 phase 3 randomized clinical trial. JAMA Oncol. 2020;6(7):1003–1010.
24. Maxwell R, Jackson CM, Lim M. Clinical trials investigating immune checkpoint blockade in glioblastoma. Curr Treat Options Oncol. 2017;18(8):51.
25. Bunse L, Bunse T, Kramer C, et al. Clinical and translational advances in glioma immunotherapy. Neurotherapeutics. 2022;19(6):1799–1817.
26. Cancer Genome Atlas Research Network; Brat DJ, Verhaak RG, et al. Comprehensive, integrative genomic analysis of diffuse lower-grade gliomas. N Engl J Med. 2015;372(26):2481–2498.
27. Yan H, Parsons DW, Jin G, et al. IDH1 and IDH2 mutations in gliomas. N Engl J Med. 2009;360(8):765–773.
28. Yip S, Butterfield YS, Morozova O, et al. Concurrent CIC mutations, IDH mutations, and 1p/19q loss distinguish oligodendrogliomas from other cancers. J Pathol. 2012;226(1):7–16.
29. Aiman WGD, Rayi A. Low-grade gliomas. In: StatPearls. Treasure Island, FL: StatPearls Publishing; 2023.
30. Bourne TD, Schiff D. Update on molecular findings, management and outcome in low-grade gliomas. Nat Rev Neurol. 2010;6(12):695–701.
31. Molenaar RJ, Radivoyevitch T, Maciejewski JP, et al. The driver and passenger effects of isocitrate dehydrogenase 1 and 2 mutations in oncogenesis and survival prolongation. Biochim Biophys Acta. 2014;1846(2):326–341.
32. Molenaar RJ, Verbaan D, Lamba S, et al. The combination of IDH1 mutations and MGMT methylation status predicts survival in glioblastoma better than either IDH1 or MGMT alone. Neuro Oncol. 2014;16(9):1263–1273.
33. Mellinghoff IK, van den Bent MJ, Blumenthal DT, et al. Vorasidenib in IDH1- or IDH2-mutant low-grade glioma. N Engl J Med. 2023;389(7):589–601.
34. Gupta S, Bi WL, Dunn IF. Medical management of meningioma in the era of precision medicine. Neurosurg Focus. 2018;44(4):E3.
35. Schulz C, Mathieu R, Kunz U, Mauer UM. Treatment of unresectable skull base meningiomas with somatostatin analogs. Neurosurg Focus. 2011;30(5):E11.
36. Norden AD, Ligon KL, Hammond SN, et al. Phase II study of monthly pasireotide LAR (SOM230C) for recurrent or progressive meningioma. Neurology. 2015;84(3):280–286.
37. Lou E, Sumrall AL, Turner S, et al. Bevacizumab therapy for adults with recurrent/progressive meningioma: A retrospective series. J Neurooncol. 2012;109(1):63–70.
38. Nayak L, Iwamoto FM, Rudnick JD, et al. Atypical and anaplastic meningiomas treated with bevacizumab. J Neurooncol. 2012;109(1):187–193.
39. Kaley TJ, Wen P, Schiff D, et al. Phase II trial of sunitinib for recurrent and progressive atypical and anaplastic meningioma. Neuro Oncol. 2015;17(1):116–121.
40. Raizer JJ, Grimm SA, Rademaker A, et al. A phase II trial of PTK787/ZK 222584 in recurrent or progressive radiation and surgery refractory meningiomas. J Neurooncol. 2014;117(1):93–101.
41. Li Z, Gao Y, Zhang J, et al. DNA methylation meningioma biomarkers: Attributes and limitations. Front Mol Neurosci. 2023;16:1182759.
42. Brastianos PK, Twohy EL, Gerstner ER, et al. Alliance A071401: Phase II trial of focal adhesion kinase inhibition in meningiomas with somatic NF2 mutations. J Clin Oncol. 2023;41(3):618–628.
43. Lee YS, Lee YS. Molecular characteristics of meningiomas. J Pathol Transl Med. 2020;54(1):45–63.
44. Brastianos PK, Taylor-Weiner A, Manley PE, et al. Exome sequencing identifies BRAF mutations in papillary craniopharyngiomas. Nat Genet. 2014;46(2):161–165.
45. Brastianos PK, Twohy E, Geyer S, et al. BRAF-MEK Inhibition in newly diagnosed papillary craniopharyngiomas. N Engl J Med. 2023;389(2):118–126.
46. Chiranth S, Langer SW, Poulsen HS, et al. A systematic review of targeted therapy for vestibular schwannoma in patients with NF2-related schwannomatosis. Neurooncol Adv. 2023;5(1):vdad099.
47. Plotkin SR, Halpin C, McKenna MJ, et al. Erlotinib for progressive vestibular schwannoma in neurofibromatosis 2 patients. Otol Neurotol. 2010;31(7):1135–1143.
48. Karajannis MA, Legault G, Hagiwara M, et al. Phase II trial of lapatinib in adult and pediatric patients with neurofibromatosis type 2 and progressive vestibular schwannomas. Neuro Oncol. 2012;14(9):1163–1170.

10

Head and Neck Cancers

Doreen N. Palsgrove and Xianfeng F. Zhao

10.1 Introduction

Head and neck cancers are a heterogeneous group of neoplasms that can be broadly grouped by site of origin: skin, oral cavity, pharynx (oropharynx, nasopharynx, hypopharynx), larynx, sinonasal tract, and salivary glands (major and minor). Excluding skin and thyroid cancers (see Chapters 7 and 18, respectively), squamous cell carcinoma (SCC) is by far the most common (>90%) tumor type among head and neck cancers, with most non-cutaneous squamous cell carcinomas SCCs arising from the mucosal epithelium in the oral cavity, pharynx, and larynx, which are known collectively as head and neck squamous cell carcinoma (HNSCC) (1).

10.2 HNSCC

The burden of HNSCC is most frequently associated with exposure to tobacco-derived carcinogens, excessive alcohol consumption, or both (2). However, the vast majority of SCCs that arise in the oropharynx—palatine tonsils, lingual tonsils (base of tongue), soft palate, uvula, and posterior pharyngeal wall (Figure 10.1)—are uniquely caused by infection with oncogenic strains of human papillomavirus (HPV), primarily HPV-16, and, to a lesser extent, HPV-18 and other strains (3). Morphologically, they are composed of atypical dysplastic squamous epithelial cells with moderate differentiation and are usually positive for CK5/6, p40, and p63.

10.2.1 Oral Cavity and Tongue

The oral cavity generally includes the following subsites: anterior tongue, gingiva (upper and lower gums), floor of mouth, buccal mucosa (inner cheeks), retromolar trigone, hard palate (roof of mouth), and mucosal lip. The vast majority of tumors that involve the oral cavity are conventional SCCs.

Known risk factors of oral SCC include any form of tobacco use and alcohol consumption, with a 30-fold increased risk for individuals who both smoke and drink heavily (4). Additional risk factors include poor oral and dental hygiene, poor nutrition, and hereditary cancer syndromes (5, 6).

Multiple studies (7, 8) have also demonstrated that the incidence and progression of HNSCC are closely associated with mutations and gene expression variations, including variation in *CTTN*, *D2HGDH*, *NLRP2*, *PEX11A*, *UPK*, and *SERPINE1* and mutations in *CCR7*, *KL*, *LGR5*, and *RORB*, which are associated with HNSCC prognosis. Frequent mutations in several genes, such as *TP53*, *CDKN2A*, and *PIK3CA*, as well as in members of the NOTCH pathway, have been reported in HPV-negative HNSCC via genomic and transcriptomic approaches (9). Mutations in oncogenic *HRAS* are rare (3%), with *HRAS* G12S being the most common alteration (10).

10.2.2 Oropharynx

Oropharyngeal squamous cell carcinoma (OPSCC) dominates the oropharyngeal tumors and arises from the base of the tongue, palatine tonsillar fossa and pillars, and lateral and posterior pharyngeal wall. Carcinogenic HPV infection is an important risk factor that accounts for ~70% and ~50% of all OPSCCs in the USA and UK, respectively (11). When only considering tonsillar subsites (lingual and palatine tonsils), high-risk HPV-driven tumorigenesis is responsible for 92% of all OPSCCs (12).

HPV infection of the mouth and throat, which is primarily transmitted through sexual contact, causes >95% of OPSCC (13) (Figure 10.2). HPV16, one of the most common high-risk HPV subtypes, is responsible for >90% of all HPV-related HNSCCs (14). In addition to HPV exposure, concomitant tobacco use may also play a part in the development of HPV-related OPSCC (15).

Owing to its improved prognosis and greater prevalence in younger individuals, numerous ongoing trials are examining the potential for treatment de-intensification as a means to improve

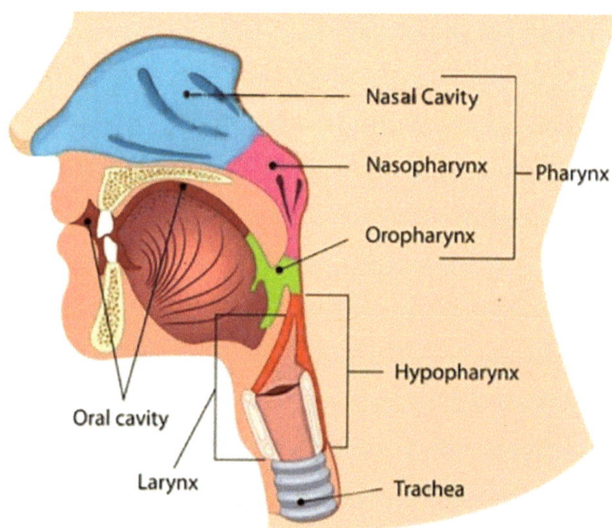

FIGURE 10.1 Anatomical locations of head and neck cancers.

DOI: 10.1201/9781003513469-10

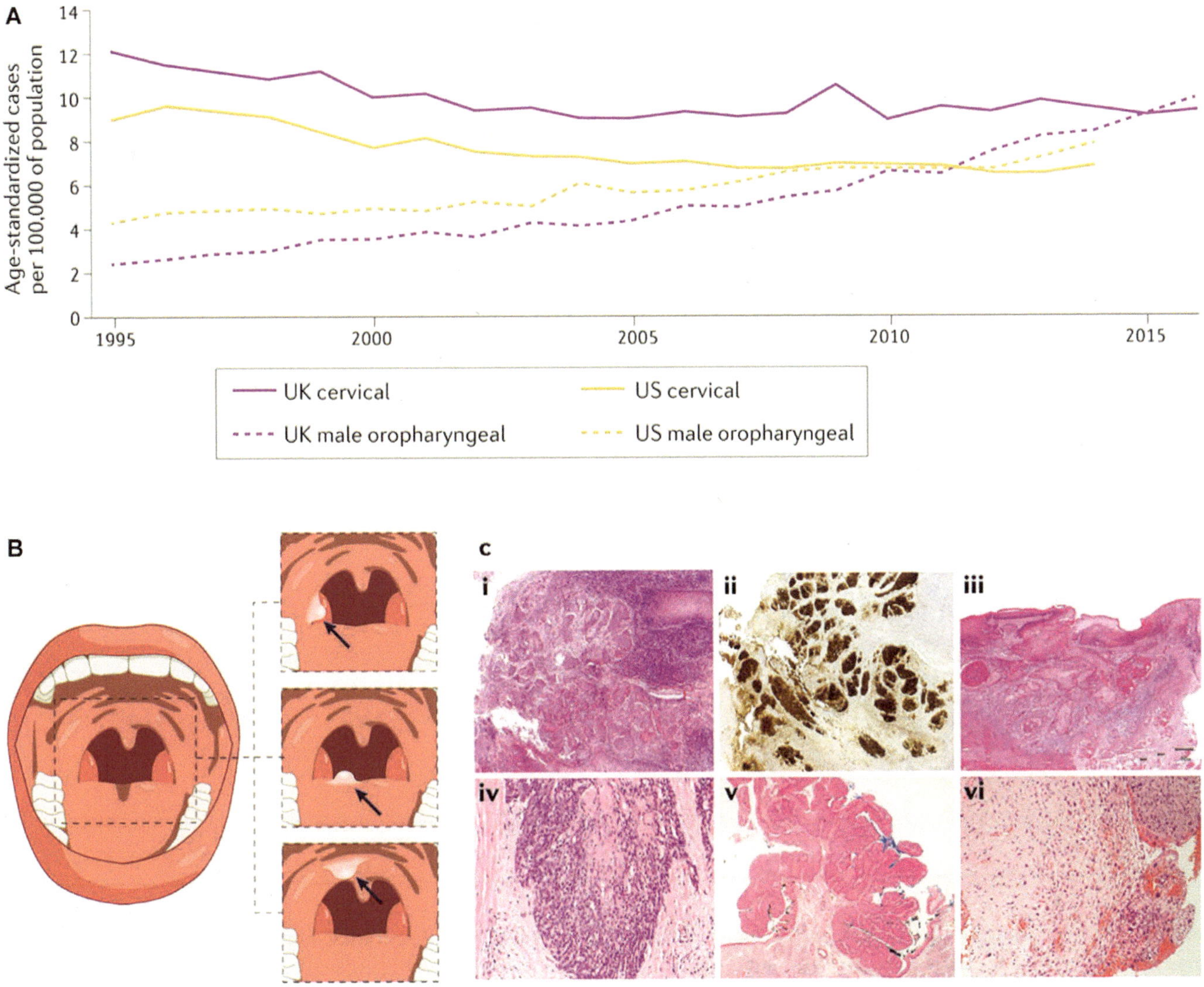

FIGURE 10.2 Incidence (A), anatomical locations (B) and histological appearance (C) of HPV+ oropharyngeal cancers (from ref 14. with permission).

quality of life while maintaining acceptable survival outcomes. In addition, owing to the distinct biology of HPV+ OPSCCs, targeted therapies and immunotherapies have become an area of particular interest. Unfortunately, the incidence of HPV+ OPSCC is expected to continue to rise over the coming decades until the benefits of gender-neutral prophylactic HPV vaccination begin to become manifest.

Oropharyngeal cancers linked to HPV infection tend to have better outcomes (prognoses) than non-HPV-driven counterparts because chemotherapy and radiation treatments work better for these cancers. This improvement in outcome, however, is not seen in people with HPV-related oropharyngeal cancers who also smoke tobacco or marijuana.

Human papillomaviruses are epitheliotropic, circular, double-stranded DNA viruses (Figure 10.3). The virus generates two oncoproteins, encoded by E6 and E7 genes, which mediate degradation of p53 and Rb proteins, respectively. This leads to the initiation of the cell cycle and DNA synthesis which is required for viral replication. Overall, HPV-associated OPSCC shows relatively fewer genetic alterations in cancer drivers than HPV-negative tumors at the exome level (16). E6 and E7 also regulate the expression of several micro-RNAs and the expression and activity of a large number of epigenetic factors. For example, E6 and E7 induce *DNMT1*, *DNMT3a*, and *DNMT3b* overexpression resulting in global DNA hypermethylation.

10.2.3 Hypopharyngeal, Laryngeal, Tracheal, and Parapharyngeal Malignancies

TP53, *FAT1*, *NOTCH1*, *KMT2C*, and *CDKN2A* were found to be most frequently mutated in HPV-negative squamous cell carcinoma originating from the hypopharynx and larynx (18).

10.3 Genomic Landscape of HNSCC

The Cancer Genome Atlas (TGCA) profiled 279 patient samples (172 from oral cavity, 33 from oropharynx, and 72 from laryngeal sites) and provided a comprehensive genomic landscape for HNSCCs (19). This study separated the specimens

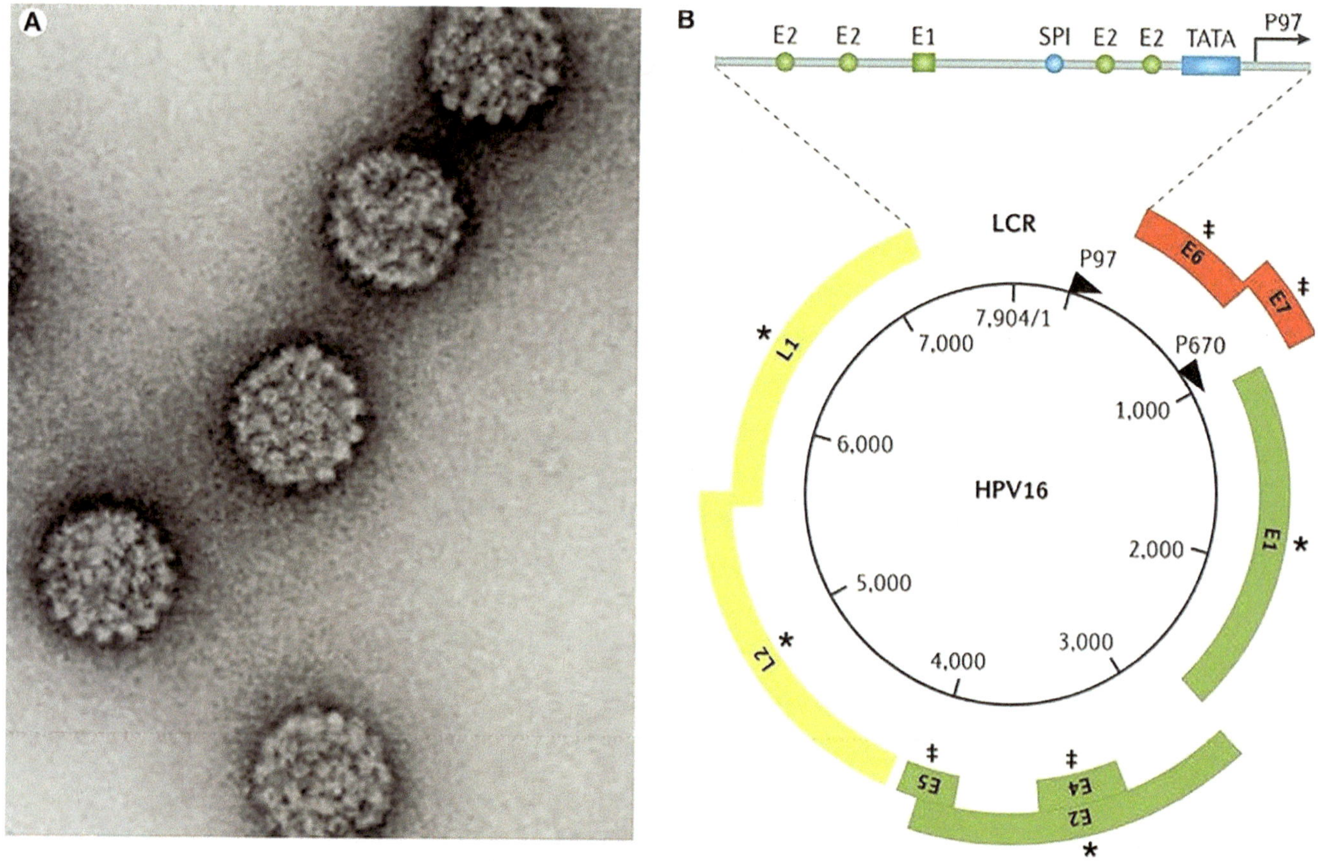

FIGURE 10.3 Viral particles (A) and genome structure (B) of a human papilloma virus (from ref. 17 with permission).

into two (36 HPV+ and 243 HPV-) groups. The most common genetic abnormalities are chromosomal copy number alterations (CNAs), which include losses of 3p and 8p and gains of 3q, 5p, and 8q. HPV+ tumors demonstrate helical domain mutations of *PIK3CA* in addition to alterations involving loss of *TRAF3* and amplification of the cell cycle gene *E2F1*, whereas HPV- tumors are featured with frequent *TP53* (83%) and *CDKN2A* (58%) mutations in addition to co-amplifications of 11q13 (*CCND1*, *FADD*, and *CTTN*) and 11q22 (*BIRC2* and *YAP1*), recurrent focal amplifications of receptor tyrosine kinase genes, and focal deletions in the nuclear set domain gene (*NSD1*) and tumor suppressor genes (for example, *FAT1*, *NOTCH1*, *SMAD4*, and *CDKN2A*). The smoking-related HNSCCs show near universal loss-of-function *TP53* mutations and *CDKN2A* inactivation, with frequent copy number alterations, including amplification of 3q26/28 and 11q13/22. Infrequent copy number alterations in conjunction with activating mutations of *HRAS* or *PIK3CA*, coupled with inactivating mutations of *CASP8*, *NOTCH1*, and *TP53* seem to be associated with a favorable prognosis. Alterations in 18 candidate genes were considered oncogenic drivers and/or therapeutic targets (Figure 10.4).

Study of the HNSCC genomic landscape led to the recognition of several pathways that are implied in the pathogenesis of HNSCC and potential targeted therapy (7). 1) Cell cycle deregulation. *CDKN2A* and *TP53* are frequently inactivated in HNSCC, while cyclin D1 expression is increased. Targeting cyclin D1 is a potential therapeutic strategy. 2) WNT signaling. It is quite remarkable that inactivating mutations in *FAT1* and *AJUBA* genes, though mutually exclusive, are identified in HNSCC (19). Furthermore, inactivation of *FAT1* frequently co-occurs with the alteration of *NOTCH1*, which together increase the beta-catenin levels. 3) Epigenetic regulations. It was observed that nuclear receptor-binding SET domain-containing protein 1 (*NSD1*) and histone-lysine N-methyltransferase 2D (*KMT2D*, also known as *MLL2*), both encoding histone-lysine N-methyltransferases, were frequently mutated in HNSCC (19). So far, the significance of these mutations remains elusive. 4) PI3K signaling. Activating mutations and amplifications of *PIK3CA* are frequently identified in HPV+ as well as HPV- HNSCC, suggesting its role as the oncogenic driver and potential therapeutic target.

10.4 Salivary Gland Tumors

Most tumors of the parotid gland are benign, and they are mainly pleomorphic adenomas (PAs). Malignant transformation into salivary ductal carcinoma (SDC) often occurs later if left untreated, which justifies complete PA removal by surgery (20). Mucoepidermoid carcinoma (MEC) is the most common malignancy that resides mainly in the minor salivary gland. Recent molecular studies shed more light on the genetic abnormalities in the salivary gland cancers and provide some novel targets for precision therapy (Table 10.1) (21). These include overexpressed androgen receptor (AR) and HER2 in advanced SDC.

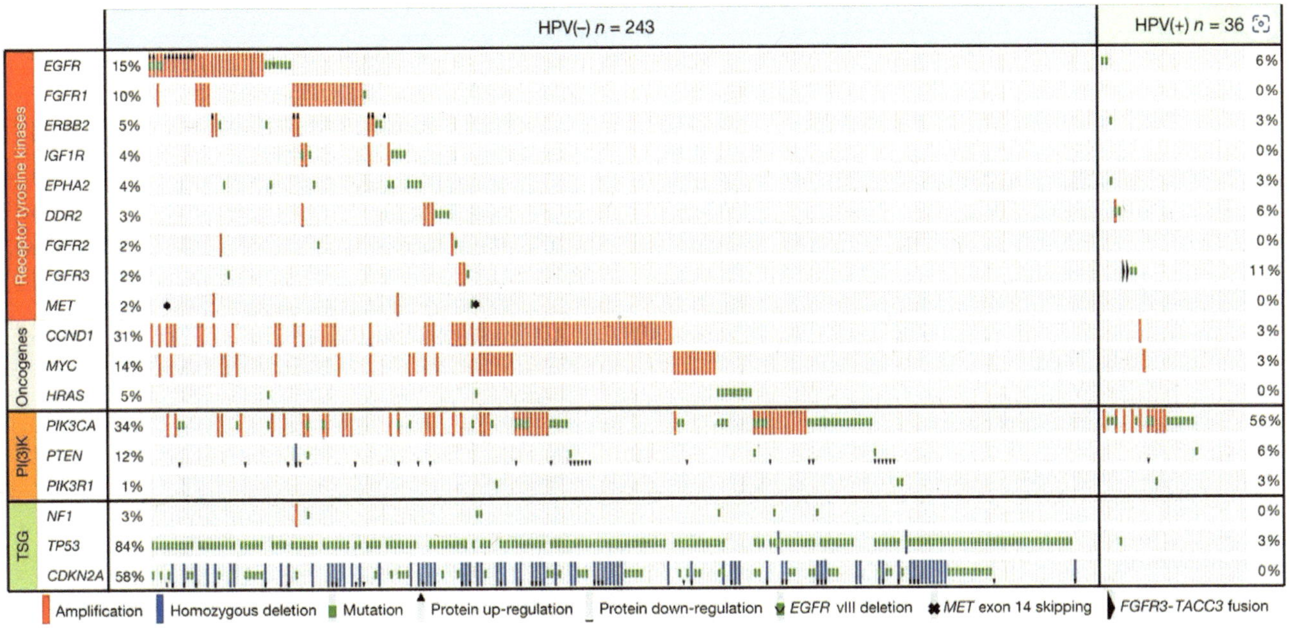

FIGURE 10.4 Eighteen candidate driver oncogenes as therapeutic targets (from ref. 18 with permission). Gene alterations for key genes are displayed by sample ($n = 279$). TSG, tumor suppressor gene.

TABLE 10.1

Genetic Alterations in Salivary Gland Tumors

Tumor Type	Chromosomal Region	Gene and Mechanism	Prevalence
Pleomorphic adenoma	8q12	*PLAG1* fusions/amplification	>50%
	12q13–15	*HMGA2* fusions/amplification	~15%
Carcinoma ex pleomorphic adenoma	8q12	*PLAG1* fusions/amplification	72.7%
	12q13–15	*HMGA2* fusions/amplification	13.6%
	17p13.1	*TP53* mutation	25–50%
Myoepithelial carcinoma	8q12	*PLAG1* fusions[a]	37.5%
	t(12,22) (q21;q12)	*EWSR1::ATF1*[a]	12.5%
Clear cell carcinoma	t(12;22) (q21;q12)	*EWSR1::ATF1*	93%
		EWSR1::CREM	<5%
Tubulotrabecular basal cell adenoma	3p22.1	*CTNNB1* hotspot mutation	37.5–80%
Membranous basal cell adenoma	16q12.1	*CYLD* mutation	36%
Basal cell adenocarcinoma	16q12.1	*CYLD* mutation	29%
Mucoepidermoid carcinoma	t(11;19) (q21;p13)	*CRTC1::MAML2*	56%
	t(11;15) (q21;q26)	*CRTC3::MAML2*	6%
	9p21.3	*CDKN2A* deletion	25%
Secretory carcinoma	t(12;15) (p13;q25)	*ETV6::NTRK3*	~95–98%
	t(12;10) (p13;q11)	*ETV6::RET*	~2–5%
	t(12;7) (p13;q31)	*ETV6::MET*	<1%
Intraductal carcinoma, intercalated duct type	10q11.21	*RET* fusions	46.7%
Intraductal carcinoma, apocrine type	3q26.32	*PIK3CA* mutations (apocrine type)	High[b]
	11p15.5	*HRAS* mutations (apocrine type)	High[b]
Epithelial-myoepithelial carcinoma	11p15.5	*HRAS* hotspot mutation[a]	77.8%
Salivary duct carcinoma	17q21.1	*HER2* amplification	31%
	8p11.23	*FGFR1* amplification	10.3%
	17p13.1	*TP53* mutation	56%
	3q26.32	*PIK3CA* mutation	33.3%
	11p15.5	*HRAS* mutation	33.3%
	Xq12	*AR* copy gain	35%
	10q23.31	*PTEN* loss	38%
		CDKN2A loss	10%

(Continued)

TABLE 10.1 (Continued)

Tumor Type	Chromosomal Region	Gene and Mechanism	Prevalence
Adenoid cystic carcinoma	6q22–23	*MYB* fusion/activation/amplification	~80%
	8q13	*MYBL1* fusion/activation/amplification	~10%
	9q34.3	*NOTCH* mutations (solid type)	13.7%
Polymorphous adenocarcinoma, classic type	14q12	*PRKD1* hotspot mutation	73%
Polymorphous adenocarcinoma, cribriform type	14q12	*PRKD1* fusions[c]	38%
	19q13.2	*PRKD2* fusions[d]	14.3%
	2p22.2	*PRKD3* fusions[d]	19%
Acinic cell carcinoma	19q31.1	*MSANTD3* fusion/amplification	4.4%
	9q31	*NR4A3* fusion/activation	86%

Source: adapted from ref. 20

Notes:

[a] Not as the malignant component of carcinoma ex pleomorphic adenoma, that is, only in de novo carcinomas.

[b] Only very few cases tested.

[c] 3/8 cases tested had ARID1A-PRKD1 fusion, 1/8 had DDX3X-PRKD1 fusion, and 4/8 had unknown fusion partners.

[d] Unknown fusion partners.

10.5 Current Treatment Challenges and Clinical Trials

Platinum-based chemotherapy (predominantly cisplatin) combined with concomitant radiation remains the mainstay for cytotoxic treatment of HNSCC (22). These cytotoxic regimens not only potentially cause secondary malignancies but also often develop drug resistance and eventually cause the treatment to fail (23).

Treatment de-intensification for HPV-related OPSCC is being pursued in clinical trials, although identifying the ~15% of patients who will have recurrent disease, and who therefore require more intensive treatment, remains a key challenge.

Prophylactic HPV vaccination, which is currently available in several countries, has been shown to decrease incidence of persistent oral infection up to 4 years after vaccination. Unfortunately, duration of protection has not been established, and the estimated population-level effect against overall oral HPV16/18/6/11 infections is only 17% because of low vaccine coverage (24).

10.5.1 Therapeutics

The molecular landscape of HNSCC has been well delineated (7, 19). The most common genetic alterations occur in tumor suppressor genes, such as *TP53* and *CDKN2A*, as inactivation mutations or deletions. Recovery of tumor suppressor functions remains more challenging than inhibiting activated oncogene products with small molecules or antibodies. Combined disruption of the PI3K/AKT/mTOR pathway and PD-1 blockade may be an effective approach in treating HNSCC (25). Guided by pharmacogenomic data, Gu et al. repurposed the JAK2 inhibitor fedratinib for low KRT18–expressing HNSCC and the topoisomerase inhibitor mitoxantrone for IL6R-activated HNSCC (26).

Immune checkpoint inhibitor (ICI) treatment with pembrolizumab and nivolumab has recently been approved in recurrent and metastatic HNSCC (27). The clinical trials leading to the approval of these agents included both HPV-related and unrelated HNSCC patients, and immunotherapy is used regardless of HPV status (28). RET inhibitor cabozantinib has gained dramatic response in the rare SDC with *NCOA4::RET* fusion (29). Androgen deprivation therapy (ADT) has shown clinical benefit in approximately 50% of AR+ SDC (30), while trastuzumab in combination with docetaxel had an objective response rate of 76% in a trial on HER2+ SDC (31).

10.5.2 Testing Strategies

Despite the lack of effective targeted therapy, as precision pathologists, we should provide as much information as possible for the optimal treatment of HNSCC. Once diagnosed histologically, the HNSCC should be analyzed for HPV positivity. Immunostains for p16 and p53 should always be performed to identify the inactivation of these tumor suppressor gene products. PI3K/AKT/mTOR pathway and cell cycle deregulation components should be analyzed to pinpoint the critical kinases that drive the development and progression of HNSCC.

10.6 Summary

As indicated by their name, head and neck cancers are any cancers arising from the head and neck region, including HNSCCs, skin cancers, thyroid cancers, adenocarcinomas, sarcomas, and lymphomas. Since HNSCC is the most common head and neck cancer, we have seen the most recent molecular advances in HNSCC. While chromosomal copy number abnormalities are common in both groups, different genetic alterations drive the development of HPV+ and HPV- HNSCC; HPV+ tumors depend on helical domain mutations of *PIK3CA*, loss of *TRAF3*, and amplification of *E2F1*, whereas HPV- tumors carry frequent *TP53* (83%) and *CDKN2A* (58%) mutations in addition to co-amplifications of 11q13 (*CCND1*, *FADD*, and *CTTN*) and 11q22 (*BIRC2* and *YAP1*), recurrent focal amplifications in receptor tyrosine kinase genes, and focal deletions in the nuclear set domain gene (*NSD1*) and tumor suppressor genes. As deletion or inactivation of tumor suppressor genes are the main drivers of HNSCC development, there remains a lack of effective targeted therapy for HNSCC. A precision pathologist should provide all the potential therapeutic targets to clinicians and be actively involved in clinical trials.

REFERENCES

1. Chow LQM. Head and neck cancer. New Eng J Med. 2020;382(1):60–72.
2. Aupérin A. Epidemiology of head and neck cancers: An update. Curr Opin Oncol. 2020;32(3):178–186.
3. Tumban E. A current update on human papillomavirus-associated head and neck cancers. Viruses. 2019;11(10):922.
4. World Cancer Day: Know the facts—tobacco and alcohol both cause cancer. 3 February 2021. World Health Organization. Retrieved on October 22, 2023. www.who.int/europe/news/item/03-02-2021-world-cancer-day-know-the-facts-tobacco-and-alcohol-both-cause-cancer#:~:text=People%20who%20use%20both%20alcohol,up%20to%2030%20times%20higher.
5. Guha N, Boffetta P, Wünsch Filho V, et al. Oral health and risk of squamous cell carcinoma of the head and neck and esophagus: Results of two multicentric case-control studies. Am J Epidemiol. 2007;166(10):1159–1173.
6. Venugopal R, Bavle RM, Konda P, Muniswamappa S, Makarla S. Familial cancers of head and neck region. J Clin Diagn Res. 2017;11(6):ZE01–ZE06.
7. Leemans C, Snijders P, Brakenhoff R. The molecular landscape of head and neck cancer. Nat Rev Cancer. 2018;18(5):269–282.
8. Ye Y, Wang J, Liang F, et al. Identification of key genes for HNSCC from public databases using bioinformatics analysis. Cancer Cell Int. 2021;21(1):549.
9. Johnson DE, Burtness B, Leemans CR, Lui VWY, Bauman JE, Grandis JR. Head and neck squamous cell carcinoma. Nat Rev Dis Primers. 2020;6(1):92.
10. Coleman N, Marcelo KL, Hopkins JF, et al. HRAS mutations define a distinct subgroup in head and neck squamous cell carcinoma. JCO Precis Oncol. 2023;7:e2200211.
11. Schache AG, Powell NG, Cuschieri KS, et al. HPV-related oropharynx cancer in the United Kingdom: An evolution in the understanding of disease etiology. Cancer Res. 2016;76(22):6598–6606.
12. Gelwan E, Malm IJ, Khararjian A, et al. Nonuniform distribution of high-risk human papillomavirus in squamous cell carcinomas of the oropharynx: Rethinking the anatomic boundaries of oral and oropharyngeal carcinoma from an oncologic HPV perspective. Am J Surg Pathol. 2017;41(12):1722–1728.
13. Pytynia KB, Dahlstrom KR, Sturgis EM. Epidemiology of HPV-associated oropharyngeal cancer. Oral Oncol. 2014;50(5):380–386.
14. Lechner M, Liu J, Masterson L, Fenton TR. HPV-associated oropharyngeal cancer: Epidemiology, molecular biology and clinical management. Nat Rev Clin Oncol. 2022;19(5):306–327.
15. Ang KK, Harris J, Wheeler R, et al. Human papillomavirus and survival of patients with oropharyngeal cancer. N Engl J Med. 2010;363(1):24–35.
16. Agrawal N, Frederick MJ, Pickering CR, et al. Exome sequencing of head and neck squamous cell carcinoma reveals inactivating mutations in NOTCH1. Science. 2011; 333(6046):1154–1157.
17. Schiffman M, Doorbar J, Wentzensen N, et al. Carcinogenic human papillomavirus infection. Nat Rev Dis Primers. 2016;2:16086.
18. Machnicki MM, Rzepakowska A, Janowska JI, et al. Analysis of mutational profile of hypopharyngeal and laryngeal head and neck squamous cell carcinomas identifies KMT2C as a potential tumor suppressor. Front Oncol. 2022;12:768954.
19. The Cancer Genome Atlas Network. Comprehensive genomic characterization of head and neck squamous cell carcinomas. Nature. 2015;517(7536):576–582.
20. Antony J, Gopalan V, Smith RA, Lam AK. Carcinoma ex pleomorphic adenoma: A comprehensive review of clinical, pathological and molecular data. Head Neck Pathol. 2012;6(1):1–9.
21. Andreasen S, Kiss K, Mikkelsen LH, et al. An update on head and neck cancer: New entities and their histopathology, molecular background, treatment, and outcome. APMIS. 2019;127(5):240–264.
22. Galluzzi L, Senovilla L, Vitale I, et al. Molecular mechanisms of cisplatin resistance. Oncogene. 2012;31(15):1869–1883.
23. Ferreira JA, Peixoto A, Neves M, et al. Mechanisms of cisplatin resistance and targeting of cancer stem cells: Adding glycosylation to the equation. Drug Resist Updat. 2016;24:34–54.
24. Diana G, Corica C. Human papilloma virus vaccine and prevention of head and neck cancer, what is the current evidence? Oral Oncol. 2021;115:105168.
25. Wang Z, Goto Y, Allevato MM, et al. Disruption of the HER3-PI3K-mTOR oncogenic signaling axis and PD-1 blockade as a multimodal precision immunotherapy in head and neck cancer. Nat Commun. 2021;12(1):2383.
26. Gu Z, Yao Y, Yang G, et al. Pharmacogenomic landscape of head and neck squamous cell carcinoma informs precision oncology therapy. Sci Transl Med. 2022;14:eabo5987.
27. Bhatia A, Burtness B. Treating head and neck cancer in the age of immunotherapy: A 2023 Update. Drugs. 2023;83(3):217–248.
28. Poulose JV, Kainickal CT. Immune checkpoint inhibitors in head and neck squamous cell carcinoma: A systematic review of phase-3 clinical trials. World J Clin Oncol. 2022;13(5):388–411.
29. Boon E, van Boxtel W, Buter J, et al. Androgen deprivation therapy for androgen receptor-positive advanced salivary duct carcinoma: A nationwide case series of 35 patients in the Netherlands. Head Neck. 2018;40(3):605–613.
30. Lee J, Park S, Jung HA, et al. A phase 2 multicenter study of docetaxel-PM and trastuzumab-pkrb combination therapy in recurrent or metastatic salivary gland carcinomas. Cancer. 2023;129(19):2966–2974.
31. Wang K, Russell JS, McDermott JD, et al. Profiling of 149 salivary duct carcinomas, carcinoma ex pleomorphic adenomas, and adenocarcinomas, not otherwise specified reveals actionable genomic alterations. Clin Cancer Res. 2016; 22(24):6061–6068.

11

Lung Cancers

Xianfeng F. Zhao, Jian Jing, and Shiyong Li

11.1 Introduction

Lung cancer remains one of the most common malignancies and the leading cause of cancer death in both men and women (1). It is classified into two major types based on morphology and clinical behaviors (2). About 80–85% of lung cancers are non-small cell lung carcinomas (NSCLCs), which consist of mainly adenocarcinoma and squamous cell carcinoma. The remaining 10–15% are small cell lung carcinomas (SCLCs). In contrast to SCLCs, which are more aggressive and sensitive to cytotoxic chemotherapy and radiotherapy, NSCLCs do not respond well to the current combined chemotherapy regimens and radiation (3). Although surgery remains the first choice for the treatment of NSCLC or even SCLC at the limited stage, approximately 70% of lung cancers present at an advanced stage and are nonresectable (3). Image-guided small biopsies and fine needle aspiration cytology specimens will be the major tissue source for pathologists in making a diagnosis and providing information for therapeutic targets (Table 11.1).

11.2 Non-Small Cell Lung Cancers

NSCLCs are subcategorized into adenocarcinoma, squamous cell carcinoma, and other rare entities based on their morphology and differentiation markers (Figure 11.1). Since most of these tumors are usually less mitotically active and thus less sensitive to radiation and cytotoxic chemotherapy, surgical resection of tumor at its limited stage remains the mainstay of treatment. Identification of various molecular targets in recent years has revolutionized therapy for NSCLCs (Table 11.2) (4). To effectively identify the precise molecular targets with limited resources, pathologists must first make the diagnosis often on small biopsies or cytology specimens.

11.2.1 Pulmonary Adenocarcinoma

Pulmonary adenocarcinoma is the most common NSCLC and characterized by tumor cells with glandular architecture and in variable growth patterns such as lepidic, acinar, papillary, micropapillary, or solid, occasionally with mucin production (2). Thyroid transcription factor (TTF) 1 and Napsin A are specific markers for adenocarcinoma of lung primary, with no expression of markers for squamous cell carcinoma, such as p40 or p63. Adenocarcinoma of the lung has seen the most advances in precision pathology as compared with other types of lung cancers. *EGFR*, *KRAS*, and *BRAF* mutations and *ALK* fusions have been identified as drivers in the development of lung adenocarcinoma. Tyrosine kinase inhibitors (TKIs) and humanized monoclonal antibodies have been developed to target EGFR, KRAS, BRAF, ALK, MET, ROS, and RET kinase activities with promising therapeutic effects (5, 6). According to the NCCN guidelines, mutational analysis of these genes is routinely required in practice (7). Recent comprehensive molecular profiling of 230 lung adenocarcinomas by the Cancer Genome Atlas (TCGA) Research Network identified 18 significantly mutated genes (Table 11.3), providing more options for specific targeted therapies. The most recent study from the Memorial

TABLE 11.1

Classification of Small Biopsy/Cytology Lung Cancers

WHO Classification	IASLC/ATS/ERS[a] Classification
Small cell carcinoma	**Small cell carcinoma**
Large cell neuroendocrine carcinoma	**Large cell neuroendocrine carcinoma**: Non-small cell carcinoma (NSCC) with neuroendocrine morphology and markers
Adenosquamous carcinoma (if both components ≥ 10%)	**NSCC, not otherwise specified (NOS)**: Morphological squamous cell carcinoma and adenocarcinoma both present
Adenocarcinoma, SCC, adeno-squamous carcinoma or large cell carcinoma with unclear immunohistochemical features	**NSCC, NOS**: Morphological squamous cell carcinoma or adenocarcinoma patterns not present, but immunohistochemical stains favor separate squamous and adenocarcinoma components
Pleomorphic, spindle cell, and/or giant cell carcinoma	**NSCC with spindle cell and/or giant cell carcinoma**

Source: modified from ref. 2

Note: [a] IASLC, International Association for the Study of Lung Cancer; ATS, American Thoracic Society; ERS, European Respiratory Society.

DOI: 10.1201/9781003513469-11

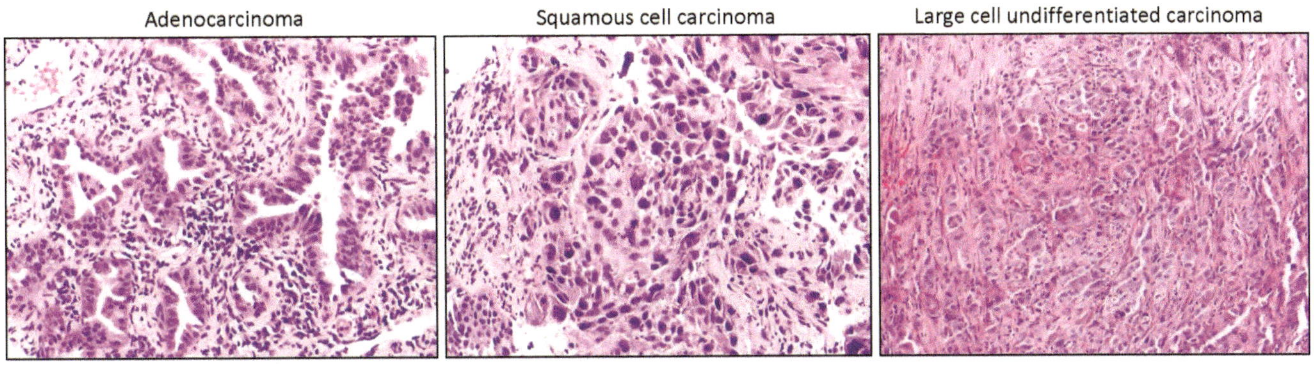

Adenocarcinoma		Squamous cell carcinoma		Large cell undifferentiated carcinoma	
CK5/6	f+	**CK5/6**	+	CK5/6	f+
CK7	+	CK7	-/+	**CK7**	+
TTF1	+	TTF1	–	TTF1	–
Napsin A	+	Napsin A	–	Napsin A	–
p40	–	**p40**	+	p40	f+
p63	f+	**p63**	+	p63	f+

FIGURE 11.1 Pathologic diagnosis of non-small cell lung cancers (NSCLCs). The typical morphology of three major NSCLCs (from left to right: lung adenocarcinoma, pulmonary squamous cell carcinoma, and large cell undifferentiated carcinoma). The immunophenotypes for differentiating these cancers are underneath the photo of each tumor.

TABLE 11.2

Biomarkers for NSCLC

Gene	Alterations	Function	Value for Targeted Therapy
ALK	C1156Y (mutation)	Gain of function	Drug resistance to crizotinib
	F1174C (predefined mutation)	Constitutive ALK phosphorylation	Drug resistance to crizotinib
	F1174L (mutation)	Transformation activity	Drug resistance to crizotinib
	F1174V (mutation)	Gain of function	Drug resistance to crizotinib
	G1202R (mutation)	Gain of function	Drug resistance to alectinib
	G1202 (deletion)	Gain of function	Drug resistance to alectinib
	G1269A (mutation)	Gain of function	Drug resistance to crizotinib
	L1152R (mutation)	Gain of function	Resistance to ceritinib and predicts response to alectinib
	L1196M (mutation)	Gain of function	Resistance to brigatinib and lorlatinib
	S1206Y (mutation)	Unknown	Drug resistance to crizotinib
	T1151 (insertion/duplication)	Unknown	Drug resistance to multiple agents
	Fusions	Activation of tyrosine kinase activity	Predictive target for ALK inhibitors
ATM	Mutation	Loss of DNA damage repair function	
	Loss	Loss of DNA damage repair function	
BRAF	V600D (predefined mutation)	Increased kinase activity	Predictive target for BRAF inhibitors
	V600E (predefined mutation)	Constitutive activation of MEK/ERK	Predictive target for BRAF inhibitors
	V600G (predefined mutation)	Increased kinase activity	Predictive target for BRAF inhibitors
	V600K (predefined mutation)	Increased kinase activity	Predictive target for BRAF inhibitors
	V600M (predefined mutation)	Increased kinase activity	Predictive target for BRAF inhibitors
	V600R (predefined mutation)	Increased kinase activity	Predictive target for BRAF inhibitors
	Y472C (missense mutation)	Impaired BRAF kinase activity, but paradoxically increases MEK and ERK Signaling through C-raf transactivation	Predictive target for BRAF inhibitors
BRCA1	Complete loss	Loss of DNA damage repair function	Predictive target for olaparib
	Mutations	Loss of DNA damage repair function	Predictive target for olaparib

(Continued)

TABLE 11.2 (Continued)

Gene	Alterations	Function	Value for Targeted Therapy
BRCA2	Complete loss	Loss of DNA damage repair function	Predictive target for olaparib
	Mutations	Loss of DNA damage repair function	Predictive target for olaparib
CDK4	Amplification	Increase of mTORC1 recruitment	Predictive target for CDK4/6 inhibitors
CHK1	Mutation	Loss of DNA damage response function	Predictive target for olaparib
EGFR	A763_Y764insFQEA (Exon 20 insertion)	Increased kinase activity	Predictive target for EGFR inhibitors
	C797S (missense substitution)	Increased kinase activity	Resistance to TKIs
	G719X (missense substitution)	Increased kinase activity	Decreased sensitivity to TKIs
	L858R (missense substitution)	Increased kinase activity	Predictive target for TKIs
	L861Q (missense substitution)	Increased kinase activity	Predictive target for TKIs
	S768I (missense substitution)	Increased kinase activity	Predictive target for TKIs
	T790M (missense substitution)	Increased ATP-binding affinity	Drug resistance
	Exon 19 insertion	Increased kinase activity	Predictive target for TKIs
	Exon 19 deletion	Increased EGFR autophosphorylation	Predictive target for TKIs
	Exon 20 insertion	Increased kinase activity	Resistance to conventional TKIs
	Expression	Increased invasive potential	Predictive target for TKIs
ERBB2	Amplification	Increased tyrosine kinase activity	Predictive target for trastuzumab
	Exon 20 insertion	Stimulates downstream PI3K-AKT and MEK-ERK pathway	May respond to motocertinib
	D769Y (missense mutation)	Increased TK receptor activity	Predictive target for neratinib and TKIs
	G776V (missense mutation)	Increased TK receptor activity	Predictive target for trastuzumab
	I767M (missense mutation)	Increased TK receptor activity	Predictive target for trastuzumab
	L755S (missense mutation)	Increased TK receptor activity	Target for tucatinib and trastuzumab
	R868W (missense mutation)	Increased TK receptor activity	Target for ado-trastuzumab emtansine and fam trastuzumab deruxtecan
	S310F (missense mutation)	Increased TK receptor activity	
	T862A (missense mutation)	Increased TK receptor activity	
	V659E (missense mutation)	Increased TK receptor activity	
	V777L (missense mutation)	Increased TK receptor activity	
	V842I (missense mutation)	Increased TK receptor activity	
FGFR2	Fusion	Activation of FGF2 pathway	May be targeted by erdafitinib
FGFR3::TACC3	Fusion	Activation of FGF3 pathway	Potential bypass resistance mechanism to TKIs
HER2	Deficient expression		Predictive biomarker for use of fulvestrant, everolimus, abemaciclib, aromatase inhibitor, etc.
	Overexpression	Increased HER2 activity	Slowed down due to negative clinical trial
IDH1	R132C (missense mutation)	Chromatin remodeling/DNA methylation	Inclusion in acute myeloid leukemia trial
KIT	Amplification	PI3K pathway activation	
KRAS	Amplification	Local aggressiveness	Inclusion criteria in clinical trials
	A11_G12dup (insertion)	Activates MAP kinase signaling	Predictive target for TKIs and immunotherapy
	G10dup	Activates MAP kinase signaling	Predictive target for TKIs and immunotherapy
	A59E (missense mutation)	Gain of function	Predictive target for TKIs and immunotherapy
	A59G (missense mutation)	Gain of function	Predictive target for TKIs and immunotherapy
	A59P (missense mutation)	Gain of function	Predictive target for TKIs and immunotherapy
	A59S (missense mutation)	Gain of function	Predictive target for TKIs and immunotherapy
	A59T (missense mutation)	Gain of function	Predictive target for TKIs and immunotherapy
	A59V (missense mutation)	Gain of function	Predictive target for TKIs and immunotherapy
	A146P (missense mutation)	Gain of function	Predictive target for TKIs and immunotherapy
	A146S (missense mutation)	Reduced response to EGFR TKIs	Predictive target for TKIs and immunotherapy
	A146T (missense mutation)	Gain of function	Predictive target for TKIs and immunotherapy
	A146V (missense mutation)	Gain of function	Predictive target for TKIs and immunotherapy
	D33E (missense mutation)	Gain of function	Predictive target for TKIs and immunotherapy
	D119N (missense mutation)	Gain of function	Predictive target for TKIs and immunotherapy
	F28L (missense mutation)	Gain of function	Predictive target for TKIs and immunotherapy
	F156L (missense mutation)	Gain of function	Predictive target for TKIs and immunotherapy
	G12A (missense mutation)	Gain of function	Predictive target for TKIs and immunotherapy
	G12C (missense mutation)	*Associated with high PD-L1 expression*	*Predictive target for TKIs and immunotherapy*

(Continued)

TABLE 11.2 (Continued)

Gene	Alterations	Function	Value for Targeted Therapy
	G12D (missense mutation)	Associated with high PD-L1 expression	Predictive target for TKIs and immunotherapy
	G12F (missense mutation)	Gain of function	Predictive target for TKIs and immunotherapy
	G12L (missense mutation)	Gain of function	Predictive target for TKIs and immunotherapy
	G12R (missense mutation)	Gain of function	Predictive target for TKIs and immunotherapy
	G12S (missense mutation)	Gain of function	Predictive target for TKIs and immunotherapy
	G12V (missense mutation)	Associated with high PD-L1 expression	Inclusion in TKI and immunotherapy trials
	G13A (missense mutation)	Gain of function	Predictive target for TKIs and immunotherapy
	G13C (missense mutation)	Gain of function	Predictive biomarker for TKIs and immunotherapy
	G13D (missense mutation)	Associated with high PD-L1 expression	
	G13E (missense mutation)	Gain of function	Predictive biomarker for TKIs and immunotherapy
	G13R (missense mutation)	Gain of function	Predictive biomarker for TKIs and immunotherapy
	G13S (missense mutation)	Gain of function	Predictive biomarker for TKIs and immunotherapy
	G13V (missense mutation)	Gain of function	Predictive biomarker for TKIs and immunotherapy
	G60R (missense mutation)	Gain of function	Predictive biomarker for TKIs and immunotherapy
	K5N (missense mutation)	Gain of function	Predictive biomarker for TKIs and immunotherapy
	K117N (missense mutation)	Gain of function	Predictive target for TKIs and immunotherapy
	K147E (missense mutation)	Gain of function	Predictive biomarker for TKIs and immunotherapy
	L19F (missense mutation)	Gain of function	Predictive biomarker for TKIs and immunotherapy
	N116S (missense mutation)	Gain of function	Predictive biomarker for TKIs and immunotherapy
	P34L (missense mutation)	Gain of function	Predictive biomarker for TKIs and immunotherapy
	P34R (missense mutation)	Gain of function	Predictive biomarker for TKIs and immunotherapy
	Q22E (missense mutation)	Gain of function	Predictive biomarker for TKIs and immunotherapy
	Q22K (missense mutation)	Gain of function	Predictive biomarker for TKIs and immunotherapy
	Q22R (missense mutation)	Gain of function	Predictive biomarker for TKIs and immunotherapy
	Q61E (missense mutation)	Gain of function	Predictive biomarker for TKIs and immunotherapy
	Q61H (missense mutation)	Gain of function	Inclusion criteria in clinical trials
	Q61K (missense mutation)	Gain of function	Inclusion criteria in clinical trials
	Q61L (missense mutation)	Gain of function	Inclusion criteria in clinical trials
	Q61P (missense mutation)	Gain of function	Inclusion criteria in clinical trials
	Q61R (missense mutation)	Gain of function	Inclusion criteria in clinical trials
	T58I (missense mutation)	Gain of function	Inclusion criteria in clinical trials
	T74P (missense mutation)	Gain of function	Predictive biomarker for TKIs and immunotherapy
	V14I (missense mutation)	Gain of function	Predictive biomarker for TKIs and immunotherapy
	V14L (missense mutation)	Gain of function	Inclusion criteria in clinical trials
	Y71H (missense mutation)	Gain of function	Inclusion criteria in clinical trials
MET	Exon 14 skipping	Poor prognosis	Predictive target for TKIs and immunotherapy
	Amplification		Immunotherapy or MET inhibitors
	MSI-High	Defect to correct DNA replication errors	
	TMB-High	Associated with TP53 mutations	
MLH1	Deficient expression	DNA damage repair	
MSH2	Deficient expression	DNA damage repair	
MSH6	Deficient expression	DNA damage repair	
NRAS	G12C (missense mutation)	Gain of function	Inclusion criteria in clinical trials
	G12D (missense mutation)	Gain of function	Inclusion criteria in clinical trials
	G12R (missense mutation)	Gain of function	Inclusion criteria in clinical trials
	G12V (missense mutation)	Gain of function	Inclusion criteria in clinical trials
	Q61H (missense mutation)	Gain of function	Inclusion criteria in clinical trials
	Q61K (missense mutation)	Gain of function	Inclusion criteria in clinical trials
	Q61L (missense mutation)	Gain of function	Inclusion criteria in clinical trials
	Q61R (missense mutation)	Gain of function	Inclusion criteria in clinical trials
NTRK1	Fusion	Constitutive TRKA activity	Predictive target for entrectinib and larotrectinib
NTRK2	Fusion	Constitutive TRKB activity	Predictive target for entrectinib and larotrectinib

(Continued)

TABLE 11.2 (Continued)

Gene	Alterations	Function	Value for Targeted Therapy
NTRK3	Fusion	Constitutive TRKC activity	Predictive target for entrectinib and larotrectinib
PDGFRA	Mutation	PI3K pathway activation	Inclusion criteria in clinical trials
	Fusion	Tyrosine kinase/growth factor	Predictive target for imatinib
PDGFRB	Fusion	Tyrosine kinase/growth factor	Predictive target for imatinib
	Mutation	PI3K pathway activation	Inclusion criteria in clinical trials
PD-L1	Expression	Promotes lung cancer invasion and metastasis	Predictive target for immunotherapy
PIK3CA	E542K (missense mutation)	Aberrant PI3K/AKT signaling	Predictive target for alpelisib
	E545K (missense mutation)	Aberrant PI3K/AKT signaling	Predictive target for alpelisib
	G118D (missense mutation)	Aberrant PI3K/AKT signaling	Predictive target for alpelisib
	H1047R (missense mutation)	Aberrant PI3K/AKT signaling	Predictive target for taselisib
PMS2	Deficient expression	DNA damage repair	
RAD51B	Mutation	DNA damage repair	
RET	Fusion	Constitutive RET kinase activity	Predictive biomarker for use of pralsetinib, selpercatinib, etc.
	Mutation	Constitutive RET kinase activity	Predictive biomarker for use of pralsetinib
ROS1	Fusion	Constitutive ROS1 kinase activity	Predictive target for crizotinib and cabozantinib
	D2033N (missense mutation)	Modification of ROS1 kinase activity	Resistance to crizotinib; may respond to cabozantinib
	G2032R (missense mutation)	Modification of ROS1 kinase activity	Resistance to crizotinib; may respond to cabozantinib
TP53	Frameshift (deletion)	Loss of tumor suppressor function	
	Nonsense mutations	Loss of tumor suppressor function	

Source: compiled from data in Mycancergenome.org

TABLE 11.3

Genetic Alterations in Lung Adenocarcinoma

Genes	Frequency	Gene Alterations	Adenosquamous Carcinoma
TP53	46%	Missense/nonsense/frame shift	
KRAS	33%	Missense	10.5%
KEAP1	17%	Missense/frame shift	
STK11	17%	Missense/nonsense/frame shift	
EGFR	14%	Missens/nonsense/in-frame indel	31.6%
NF1	11%	Missense/nonsense/frame shift	
BRAF	10%	Missense	
SETD2	9%	Missense/nonsense/frame shift	
RBM10	8%	Missense/nonsense/frame shift	
MGA	8%	Nonsense/frame shift/missense	
MET	7%	Missense	
ARID1A	7%	Nonsense/missense	
PIK3CA	7%	Missense	
SMARCA4	6%	Missense/nonsense/frame shift	
RB1	4%	Frame shift/nonsense/missense	
CDKN2A	4%	Missense/frame shift	
U2AF1	3%	Missense	
RIT1	2%	Missense/in-frame indel.	

Source: from TCGA/NCI

Sloan Kettering Cancer Center identified driver mutations in 60% (252/422, 95% CI 55 to 65%) of tumors from 830 patients (8). These mutations include: *KRAS* (107, 25%), *EGFR* (98, 23%), *ALK* rearrangements (14, 6%), *BRAF* (12, 3%), *PIK3CA* (11, 3%), *MET* amplifications (4, 2%), *HER2* (3, 1%), *MEK1* (2, 0.4%), and *NRAS* (1, 0.2%), and 95% of these alterations were mutually exclusive. Of the *EGFR* mutations (9), four types of genetic mutation are sensitive to the first-generation TKIs; they are in-frame deletion of exon 19, L858R, L861Q, and G719A/C (10). These mutations are commonly detected in adenocarcinoma of East Asian women without smoking history (11). Acquired T790M mutation (12) can be present in over 50% of the TKI-resistant cancers, which can be targeted by irreversible EGFR inhibitors (13).

11.2.2 Pulmonary Squamous Cell Carcinoma

The second most common NSCLC is pulmonary squamous cell carcinoma (pSCC), which often displays similar morphology as squamous cell carcinoma (SCC) of other origins, with three histological subclassifications: keratinizing, non-keratinizing, and basaloid SCC. It often arises from the respiratory squamous cell epithelium of the bronchus and expresses the pSCC differentiation markers, such as CK5/6, p40, and p63, which can be applied to differentiate it from other NSCLC (2) (Figure 11.1). Recent TCGA studies show that pSCC has unique genetic abnormalities (Table 11.4) (14, 15), some of which overlap with pulmonary adenocarcinoma and large cell carcinoma (6, 16). Although *EGFR* genetic abnormalities were also identified in pSCC, they are mostly amplifications, while the L861Q point mutation is rare and differs from the most common L858R mutation in pulmonary adenocarcinomas (Table 11.5) (6, 14, 17–19). Compared to adenocarcinoma, *KRAS* mutations are extremely rare in pSCC, and there is a high frequency of genetic alterations (96%) involving multiple pathways, with 64% of the alterations being potentially targetable. Activating mutations of PI3K/AKT/mTOR and EGFR tyrosine kinase pathways are mutually exclusive. A recent study from India showed that pSCC with *EGFR* genetic abnormalities benefited from TKI therapies, with targeting the exon 19 mutation being most effective (20).

11.2.3 Grey Zone Lung Cancers

Adenosquamous carcinoma (ASC) is rare and accounts for about 2–3% of all lung cancer. It is composed of both pSCC and adenocarcinoma (each component constituting at least ≥10% of the tumor) (2) and has the characteristics of both adenocarcinoma and pSCC. Since it is so rare, only limited studies have been performed (21–23). Wang et al. analyzed 76 ASCs (18) and found 24 (31.6%) with *EGFR* mutations, 8 (10.5%) with *KRAS* mutations, 2 (2.6%) with *AKT1* (2.6%) mutations, 1 (1.3%) with *ERBB2* insertion mutation, 1 (1.3%) with *PIK3CA* mutation, 4 (5.3%) with *ALK* fusions, and 3 (4%) with *KIF5B::RET* fusions. No *BRAF* mutation was found by this study (18). Mutation frequencies may vary between different studies, but all suggested that pathologists follow the guidelines for molecular test of NSCLC, and ASC with the *EGFR* mutations did respond to TKI therapies (22, 23).

Large cell lung carcinoma (LCLC) is a poorly differentiated NSCLC that lacks the morphological and immunohistochemical features of adenocarcinoma, pSCC, or SCLC. As its name implies, this tumor shows sheets or nests of large polygonal cells with moderate amount of cytoplasm, vesicular nuclei, and prominent nucleoli (Figure 11.1). If without architecture, it may resemble melanoma, large cell lymphoma, malignant mesothelioma, or hemangioendothelioma. Therefore, further stains with S100, CD45, or CD31 are recommended by WHO classification, and CD56, chromogranin, CK5/6, CK7, p40, p63, synaptophysin, and TTF1 have been used in resected specimens to differentiate LCLC from other lung cancers (Figure 11.1). CK7 is almost always positive, whereas TTF1 is always negative. The WHO 4th classification ranked it as the third most common lung cancer (~10%), but the updated WHO 5th classification suggests most of the cases can be further classified into large cell undifferentiated carcinoma (LCUC) adenocarcinomas (LCUC-AD) or squamous cell carcinomas (LCUC-SCC) (16). With limited amount of specimen for a comprehensive IHC workup, it should be diagnosed as NSCLC, not otherwise specified (Table 11.1). PD-L1 is overexpressed in the majority of the LCLC cases, and actionable genetic abnormalities have been identified and can be potential therapeutic targets (24).

11.2.4 Common Therapeutic Targets

11.2.4.1 EGFR

Although EGFR is the second most common molecule with targetable mutations, it drew the most attention owing to the FDA-approved small molecules commercially available to target its mutations. Activating mutations in the *EGFR* gene occur in 10–20% of Caucasian and at least 50% of Asian NSCLC patients (25). Although *EGFR* mutations are predominantly identified in women and non-smoker patients, a recent study from the Memorial Sloan Kettering Cancer Center and Weil Medical College showed that a significant number of men (19% vs. 25% in women) and smokers (21% vs. 52% in non-smokers) can also harbor those mutations (26).

Two mutations, deletions in exon 19 and the single amino acid substitution L858R in exon 21, often referred to as "classical" *EGFR* mutations, together account for ~85% of observed *EGFR* mutations in NSCLC and confer sensitivity to EGFR-targeting TKIs. Other mutations account for the remaining ~15% of *EGFR* mutations in NSCLC, which include point mutations, deletions, and insertions within exons 18–25 of the *EGFR* gene.

As with other oncogene products, mutated EGFR acquires constitutive activation of its tyrosine kinase activity and promotes cancer growth. Since first-generation TKIs selectively compete with ATP for binding to mutated EGFR, they are reversible inhibitors on EGFR activities. When T790M mutation occurs, the affinity of mutated EGFR for ATP is increased and thus confers resistance to inhibitors by hindering their binding to EGFR. Third-generation TKIs overcome resistance by irreversibly changing the conformation of the mutated EGFR that is no longer able to bind ATP.

11.2.4.2 Other Kinases

ALK1 is initially identified in anaplastic large cell lymphoma (ALCL), which often harbors t(2;5) and other gene rearrangements that constitutively activate ALK1 activities (27) (see Chapter 20). Instead of NPM1, the most common fusion partner of ALK1 in NSCLC is echinoderm microtubule-associated protein-like 4 (EML4) (28). Again, these *ALK* rearrangements are more common in nonsmokers with NSCLC adenocarcinomas. Because *EGFR* and *ALK* mutations are mutually exclusive, patients with *ALK* rearrangements do not usually benefit from EGFR-targeting TKIs. Instead, treatment with an ALK inhibitor is indicated (see Chapter 20, Table 20.5). *ROS1* gene alterations are present in approximately 1% of patients with NSCLC and can be targeted as well (29). Both fusion and mutations can activate rearranged during transfection (RET) kinase and lead to hyperactive RET signaling and uncontrolled cell growth. RET inhibitors are effective in targeting both wild-type and mutated RET isoforms (30).

TABLE 11.4
Somatic Gene Alterations in pSCC

Genes	Types of Alteration	Lung SCC	Head and Neck SCC
Somatic mutations			
TP53	Missense/nonsense	90%	62%
CDKN2A	Truncation/missense	15%	12%
PTEN	Truncation/missense	8%	7%
PIK3CA	Missense	15%	8%
KEAP1	Missense	12%	-
MLL2	Nonsense/missense/syn.	20%	12%
HLA-A	Truncation/splice site	3%	-
NFE2L2	Missense	15%	-
NOTCH1	Truncation	8%	11%
RB1	Missense/splice site/frame shift	7%	1%
CDKN2A/RB1 pathway		72%	
P16^{INK4A}	Homo. deletions/methylation/missense/truncation		
RB1	Down reg./truncation/missense		
CDK6	Amplification		
CCND1	Amplification		
Oxidative stress pathway		34%	
NFE2L2	Missense/amplification		
KEAP1	Missense/truncation		
CUL3	Missense/truncation/deletion		
Squamous differentiation pathway		44%	
SOX2	Amplification/overexpression		
TP63	Amplification/overexpression		
NOTCH1	Missense/truncation		
NOTCH2	Missense/truncation		
ASCL4	Missense/truncation		
FOXP1	Homozygous deletion		
PI3K/AKT/mTOR pathway		47%	
PIK3CA	Missense	16%	
AKT3	Activating	16%	
PTEN	Inactivating mutation	15%	
AKT2	Activating	4%	
TSC1	Unknown	3%	
TSC2	Unknown	3%	
STK11	Unknown	2%	
Receptor tyrosine kinase (RTK) pathway		26%	
NF1	Inactivating	11%	
EGFR	Amplification	9%	
FGFR1	Amplification/mutation	7%	
BRAF	Mutation	4%	
ERBB2	Activating	4%	
RASA1	Inactivating	4%	
FGFR2	Activating	3%	
HRAS	Activating	3%	
KRAS	Activating	3%	
ERBB3	Activating	2%	
FGFR2	Activating	2%	

TABLE 11.5

Comparison of *EGFR* Mutations between Pulmonary Adenocarcinomas and pSCC (TGCA/NCI)

	Adenocarcinoma	pSCC
Genetic alterations	Common	Rare
L858R	6.9%	2.7%
G719X	2%	0.3%
L861Q	1.5%	0.1%
Frame deletion in exon 19 (E476-A750)	16.5%	2.6%
Other mutations		0.8%
Amplification	Rare	Common

TABLE 11.6

FDA-Approved and Investigational Targeted Therapies for the Treatment of Lung Cancers with Targetable Oncogenic Drivers

Target	% NSCLC Patients	FDA-Approved Agents	FDA-Approved Agents (Off-Label Use)	Investigational Only
ALK fusions	3–7%	Crizotinib, ceritnib, brigatinib, alectinib, lorlatinib		Entrectinib, ensartinib
BRAF V600E	2–4%	Dabrafenib/trametinib	Vemurafinib	
EGFR	10–20%	Afatinib, erlotinib, dacomitinib, gefitinib, osimertinib		Poziotinib, olmutinib, nazartinib
HER2 alterations	2–4%		Afatinib, ado-trastuzumab emtansine, neratinib, dacomitinib	Poziotinib, DS-8201a
KRAS	15–30%		Trametinib	Selumetinib
MET alterations	4–6%		Crizotinib, cabozantinib	Tepotinib, capmatinib
NF1	8–10%		Trametinib	
NTRK fusions	1–4%	Larotrectinib		Entrectinib, LOXO-195
RET fusions	1–2%		Cabozantinib, vandetanib, sunitinib	LOXO-292
ROS1 fusions	1–2%	Crizotinib	Ceritinib, lorlatinib, carbozantinib	Entrectinib
SHP2	Unknown			RMC-4630

Source: from ref. 4 with permission

11.2.4.3 PD-L1

Programmed death 1 ligand (PD-L1) emerged as an effective therapeutic target when the anti-PD-L1 nivolumab was evaluated in a phase I trial of refractory solid tumors (31). Its high response rate in this study led to the use of nivolumab in treating NSCLC with PD-L1 expression. The expression level of PD-L1 in tumors is routinely assessed in a pathology laboratory with a membranous stain by immunohistochemistry. Even with a 5% cutoff for positivity, only 24–60% of patients with NSCLC showed PD-L1 expression in tumors (32). Therefore, any NSCLC or poorly differentiated lung cancer should be evaluated for PD-L1 expression in the first step of the biomarker algorithm. Potential pitfalls lie on variations from antibody to antibody, from staining method to method, and from pathologist to pathologist. More standardized procedures with designated antibodies and assistance from AI for interpretation of the results may improve the reliability and consistency of accurately reporting PD-L1 expression levels.

11.2.5 Current Targeted and Immuno-Therapeutic Agents

The eventual goal of identifying all these biomarkers is effective therapy. Up to now, several dozens of small molecules have either been approved by the FDA or are currently in clinical trials for the treatment of NSCLCs. The following drugs have proved effective in the targeted therapy of NSCLCs (Table 11.6) (4). The drugs already approved by the FDA for clinical use in NSCLCs include agents targeting *EGFR* mutations, *ALK* fusions, *BRAF* V600E mutation, *NTRK* fusions, *KRAS* G12C, and *ROS1* fusions. Several drugs approved by the FDA for treatment of other solid tumors also showed efficacy for NSCLCs. These include drugs targeting the *BRAF* V600E in melanoma; drugs targeting HER2 for breast cancers; a drug inhibiting MEK for pancreatic cancers with *KRAS* mutations and neurofibromatosis with *NF1* mutations; and drugs targeting MET alterations, RET fusions, and ROS1 fusions in other solid tumors (4). Numerous small molecules targeting various activated kinases are being investigated for effectiveness in targeted therapy for NSCLC. At the time of this publication, more small molecules might have been approved by the FDA for the treatment of NSCLC; the most updated list of drugs can be found on the American Cancer Society website (www.cancer.org/cancer/lung-cancer/treating-non-small-cell/targeted-therapies.html) with the following links:

- Drugs that target tumor blood vessel growth (angiogenesis)
- Drugs that target cells with KRAS gene changes
- Drugs that target cells with EGFR gene changes
- Drugs that target cells with ALK gene changes
- Drugs that target cells with ROS1 gene changes

- Drugs that target cells with BRAF gene changes
- Drugs that target cells with RET gene changes
- Drugs that target cells with MET gene changes
- Drugs that target cells with NTRK gene changes

11.2.6 Pharmacomics

Precision medicine also relies on individualized therapy, which has lagged behind targeted therapy. The only molecule applied in clinical pharmacomical practice is cytochrome p450 (CYP). CYP plays an important role in the pathogenesis of lung cancer (33). There are three major mechanisms that affect NSCLC development and treatment (Figure 11.2): 1) while CYP can metabolize carcinogenic smoke into inactive forms, it can also convert some substances in the smoke into carcinogens (34, 35); 2) CYP can convert some prodrugs to efficacious drugs targeting cancer cells (36, 37); 3) CYP decreases the half-life and thus the effects of some anticancer drugs (38). Oyama et al. reviewed and summarized CYP expression in both normal tissue and NSCLC and CYP effects on anti-cancer drugs (33). Since these data were obtained from population-based studies, the actual effects of CYP in each individual might be different. One CYP may have different effects with different drugs (39). Zanger and Schwab divided a group of 308 German individuals into four pharmacokinetic phenotypes: ultrarapid metabolizer (UM), extensive metabolizer (EM), intermediate metabolizer (IM), and poor metabolizer (PM). The majority of the individuals fell into the extensive metabolizer, and they are considered the "normal" phenotype. From the UM to PM, the urine metabolic ratios range from 0.1 to 100 (1,000 folds) for Sparteine, which accounts for the varied effects of Sparteine among those individuals.

11.3 Pulmonary Neuroendocrine Tumors

11.3.1 Small Cell Lung Cancer

Small cell lung cancer (SCLC) comprises around 15% of all the lung cancers. It is characterized by a neuroendocrine morphology

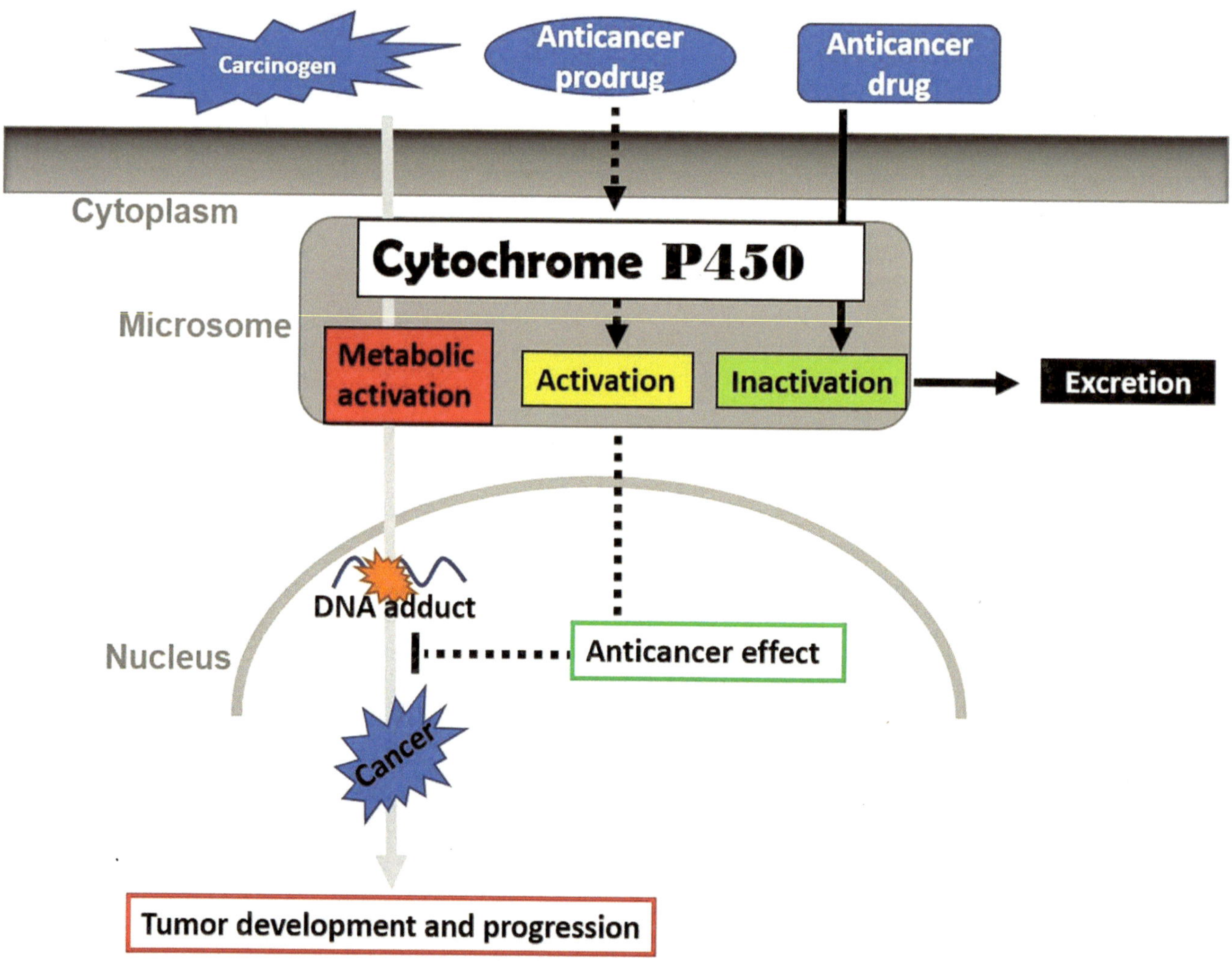

FIGURE 11.2 Major mechanisms of P450 on cancer development and treatment (modified from ref. 33). 1) Carcinogen precursors can be converted by P450 into a potent carcinogen that causes DNA damage to a normal cell and transforms the cell into a cancer cell; 2) anti-cancer prodrugs can also be converted by P450 into active forms to inhibit cancer development and cancer growth; 3) active anti-cancer drugs can also be quickly inactivated by P450 and excreted out of the body, so that the drug effects will be markedly reduced.

with a small amount of cytoplasm, round nuclei, salt-pepper chromatin, and occasional inconspicuous to conspicuous nucleoli (Figure 11.3). Mitotic figures and apoptosis are frequently identified, with a background of extensive tumor necrosis. In isolation it resembles small blue cell tumors, lymphoma, Merkel cell carcinoma, and carcinoid in small biopsy morphologically. The diagnosis of SCLC is centered in morphology. Immunostains for pancytokeratin, Ki67, and specific markers for small blue cell tumors can help differentiate SCLC from its morphologic mimics.

Compared to NSCLC, knowledge on the molecular targets of SCLC has lagged. A comprehensive genomic profile of 110 SCLC samples identified bi-allelic inactivating mutations of *TP53* and *RB1* in almost all the SCLC, suggesting that loss of tumor suppressor TP53 and RB1 is required for SCLC development (Table 11.7) (40). Interestingly, *TP73* also showed genetic abnormalities in place of *TP53* (41). Although TCGA has identified numerous genetic abnormalities, including amplification, deletions, and mutations (42, 43), there are no FDA-approved therapeutic agents yet for targeted therapy. Clinical trials with agents designed to target NSCLC proved ineffective for SCLC (44). Although genetic aberrations have been identified in several signal transduction or apoptosis pathways in SCLC, clinical trials targeting these pathways showed little effect (45). As cancer is cancer indeed and cancers have similarities in their molecular tumorigenesis, those small molecules may also be effective in treating SCLC (Table 11.8). Since imatinib, gefitinib, everolimus, thalidomide, and sunitinib may be readily available in most large medical centers, communication with the oncologist and enrollment of the patient in one of those clinical trials may be a treatment option if the tumor has failed to respond to the current standard combined chemoradiotherapy. Pathologists should provide information on the molecular targets required for the targeted therapy by either immunohistochemistry (IHC) and/or molecular diagnostics.

11.3.2 Large Cell Neuroendocrine Carcinoma

Large cell neuroendocrine carcinoma (LCNEC) clinically presents as and morphologically belongs to NSCLC, but it is biologically considered a variant of SCLC and should be managed similarly to SCLC (2). Therefore, it makes more sense to discuss this cancer together with SCLC. Except for the large cell morphology, the diagnosis of LCNEC requires at least one of the neuroendocrine markers. The majority of SCLC expresses TTF1 (90–95%), while only about 50% of LCNEC is positive for TTF1. Genetic studies also show a similar genetic profile between SCLC and LCNEC (46, 47) with *TP53* and *RB1* inactivating mutation being the predominant genetic abnormalities (Table 11.7).

Once the diagnosis of SCLC/LCNEC is confirmed, the patient with advanced limited disease (LD) will be subjected to combined-modality treatment with etoposide and cisplatin and thoracic radiation therapy (TRT). Only approximately 80% of patients respond, and the remission usually does not last long. For patients with

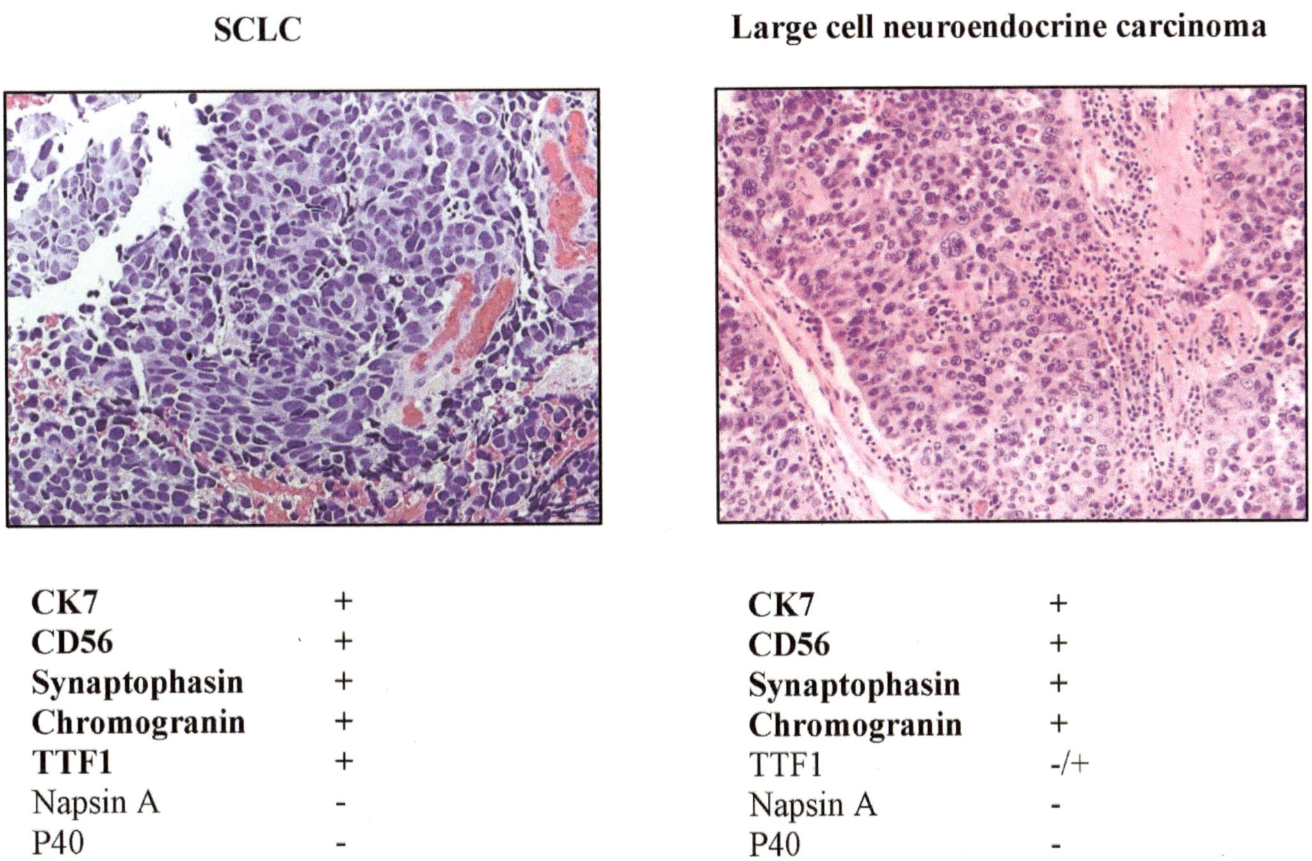

FIGURE 11.3 Pathologic diagnosis of pulmonary neuroendocrine tumors (PNETs). The typical morphology of the two major PNETs (from left to right: pulmonary small cell carcinoma; large cell neuroendocrine carcinoma). The immunophenotypes for differentiation of these cancers are underneath the photo of each tumor.

TABLE 11.7

Gene Alterations in SCLC

Genes	SCLC	LCNEC	Gene Alteration
TP53	98%	78%	Inactivating
RB1	91%	38%	Inactivating
TP73	13%		Activating
NOTCH	25%	33%	Inactivating
PTEN	9%	4–13%	Inactivating
PIK3CA	3%	3–4%	Activating
CREBBP	15%	6%	Inactivating
RBL1	6%		Inactivating
RBL2	6%		Inactivating
CDKN2A	5%		Inactivating
CCND1	2%		Activating
KIT	6%		Activating
FGFR1	6%		Activating
IRS2	2%		Activating
EP300	13%		Inactivating
MYC	6%		Activating
MYCL1	9%		Activating
MYCN	4%		Activating

TABLE 11.8

Novel Targeted Agents Investigated for Use in Treatment of Small Cell Lung Cancer

Target	Agent	Manufacturer
Inhibitors of cell signaling pathways controlling proliferation		
c-kit	Imatinib	Novartis
Src	AZD0530	AstraZeneca
Src	Dasatinib	Bristol-Myers Squibb
EGFR	Gefitinib	AstraZeneca
Farnesyl tranferase	Tipifarnib	Johnson & Johnson
mTOR	Temsirolimus	Wyeth
mTOR	Everolimus	Novartis
IGFR	IMC-A12	ImClone Systems
IGFR	CP-751, 871	Pfizer
IGFR	AMG 479	Amgen
c-MET	AMG 102	Amgen
Hedgehog	GDC-0449	Genentech
Hedgehog	IPI-926	Infinity Pharmaceuticals
Inhibitors of angiogenesis		
VEGF-A	Bevacizumab	Genentech
VEGFR-1, 2, 3	Cediranib	AstraZeneca
VEGFR, EGFR	Vandetanib	AstraZeneca
VEGFR, PDGFR, Raf-1	Sorafenib	Bayer Healthcare
	Thalidomide	Generic
VEGFR, PDGFR, FLT-3, RET, KIT	Sunitinib	Pfizer
VEGF-A, B	Aflibercept	Sanofi-Aventis
MMPIs	Marimastat	British Biotech
	Tanomastat	Bayer Healthcare
Apoptosis promoters		
Bcl-2	Oblimersen	Genta Inc.
Bcl-2	AT-101 (R-(-) gossypol)	Ascenta
Bcl-2, Mcl-1, Bcl-w, Bcl-XL, A-1	Obatoclax mesylate	Gemin X Pharmaceuticals
Bcl-2, Bcl-w, Bcl-XL	ABT-263	Abbott Laboratories
26S proteasome	Bortezomib	Janssen-Cilag

(Continued)

TABLE 11.8 (Continued)

Target	Agent	Manufacturer
Plk 1 serine/threonine kinase	PIK1 Inhibitor BI 2536	Boehringer Ingelheim
HDAC	Vorinostat	Merck & Co Inc
HDAC	Belinostat	Curagen & Topotarget
HDAC	Entinostat	Syndax Pharmaceuticals
Immune conjugates and vaccines		
CD56	BB-10901	British Biotech
GD3	BEC2/bCG adjuvant vaccine	ImClone Systems
p53	Autologous dendritic cell-adenovirus	Introgen Therapeutics
Multidrug resistance		
P-glycoprotein, MDR-1	Biricodar	Vertex Pharmaceuticals

Source: modified from ref. 44

Abbreviations: c-kit, c-kit cytokine receptor, c-MET, c-MET receptor tyrosine kinase, EGFR, epidermal growth factor receptor; FLT-3, FMS-like tyrosine kinase 3; HDAC, histone deacetylase; IGFR, insulin-like growth factor receptor; KIT, c-kit oncogene product; MMMPIs, matrix metalloproteinases; mTOR, mammaliam target of rapamycin; PDGFR, platelet-derived growth factor receptor; Plk 1, polo-like kinase 1; Raf-1, Raf-1 protein kinase; RET, Rearranged during transfection tyrosine kinase; Src, Src tyrosine kinase; VEGF(R), vascular endothelial growth factor (receptor).

extensive diseases, the survival rate is dismal. Thus, more effective treatment such as targeted therapy should be sought.

11.3.3 Current Targeted and Immuno-Therapeutic Agents

Several small molecules have been approved by FDA for the treatment of lung neuroendocrine tumors, but they are still in clinical trials (Table 11.9), and clinical use may not be far away.

11.3.4 Pharmacomics

Since cigarette smoking is the leading cause of small cell lung cancer (48), cytochrome p450 also plays an important role in the pathogenesis (33), like in NSCLC (Figure 11.2). Due to the fact that no targeted therapeutic agents are currently in clinical use for the treatment of SCLC, there are few reports on the pharmacogenomics of anti-SCLC agents. Some reported that cisplatin could decrease the clearance of etoposide (49), which could lead to increased drug effects or unwanted toxicity. Genetic polymorphic analysis of drug metabolism is recommended to optimize therapeutic efficacy and to avoid adverse effects (50).

11.4 Primary vs. Metastatic Pulmonary Carcinomas

The lung is not only one of the most common organs of primary cancer but also the most common site for metastatic diseases. Numerous studies have been dedicated to the differentiation of primary vs. metastatic pulmonary carcinomas, but currently there is no reliable biomarker to differentiate primary from metastatic lung cancers (51). Immunohistochemical markers combined with radiology have been used for identification of cancer origin. Advanced molecular techniques provide more help with differentiation of the cancer origin. When cancer has metastasized to the lung, it is already an advanced stage, and identification of molecular targets for precise therapy might be a better approach in the future.

11.5 Therapeutic Target Testing Strategies

How to rationalize testing strategies has been explored by various laboratories (52–54), and all the proposed strategies have their merits. Oberndorfer and Müllauer proposed using IHC to detect PD-L1 and EGFR in SCC and PD-L1, ROS1, ALK, and EGFR in adenocarcinoma and LCUC after morphological diagnosis assisted with IHC (52). Based on the IHC results obtained on adenocarcinoma and LCUC, mutation analysis of *EGFR* and FISH studies of *ALK*, *RET*, and *ROS1* would be performed. In certain types of adenocarcinoma, fusions of *NTRK1*, *NRG1*, *ERBB4*, *BRAF*, and *RET* were identified as targetable genetic alterations (53). Since *KRAS* and *EGFR* mutations are the most common genetic abnormalities in NSCLCs (mainly adenocarcinomas) (55), when NGS is readily available, simultaneous sequencing of both *EGFR* and *KRAS* can be performed. Our lab routinely uses a lung cancer panel to analyze mutations of *BRAF, EGFR*, *ERBB2*, *KRAS*, *HRAS*, *NRAS*, *PIK3A*, and *AKT1* by a targeted NGS panel and translocations of *ALK*, *ROS1*, *RET*, *MET*, and *NTRK1* by FISH (Figure 11.4).

For small laboratories or laboratories with limited resources, it may be more cost effective to detect *KRAS* mutation by polymerase chain reaction (PCR) or Sanger sequencing first to rule out adenocarcinoma/adenosquamous/LCUC with possible EGFR resistance. If activating mutations of *KRAS* are detected, it will be unnecessary to consider EGFR monoclonal antibodies and TKI inhibitors for EGFR mutations as treatment options in managing the patient and thus not necessary to pursue mutation studies on *EGFR* (Figures 11.4 and 5). FISH analysis for *ALK1*, *ROS1*, and *MET* translocation/amplification may be followed. If wild-type *KRAS* is detected, *EGFR* should be sequenced to identify targetable mutations. When no targetable mutations are

TABLE 11.9

Targeted Therapies in Treatment of Relapsed Small Cell Lung Cancer

Putative Target	Agent	Phase	Therapy	Setting	Outcome
Targeting Angiogenesis					
VEGF-A	Bevacizumab	II	Combination	R (M)	14.7 w PFS, 30 w OS
		II	Combination	R	17.4 w PFS, 31.6 w OS
		II	Combination	R	2.7 m PFS, 6.3 m OS
RAF-1, VEGFR-2, VEGFR-3 and PDGFRβ	Sorafenib	II	Monotherapy	R	6.7 m OS[PS], 5.3 m OS[PR]
VEGFR-1, VEGFR-2, VEGFR-3, PDGFR, c-KIT, FLT-3 and RET	Sunitinib	II	Monotherapy	R	1.4 m PFS, 5.6 m OS
VEGFR-1 and VEGFR-2	Aflibercept	II	Combination	R Ra	Negative
VEGFR-1, VEGFR-2 and VEGFR-3, PDGF and c-Kit	Pazopanib	II	Monotherapy	R	14.1 w PFS
Targeting cell signaling					
EGFR	Gefitinib	II	Monotherapy	R	50 d TTP
BCR-Abl, c-KIT and PDGFR	Imatinib	II	Monotherapy	R	1.2 m TTP
		II	Monotherapy	R	All PD by 4 w (n = 12)
mTOR	Everolimus	II	Monotherapy	R	1.3 m PFS, 6.7 m OS
Targeting apoptosis					
BCL-2, BCL-W, BCL-XL	Navitoclax	II	Monotherapy	R	1.5 m PFS, 3.2 m OS
BCL-2, BCL-XL, BCL-W, MCL-1	Gossypol	I/II	Combination	R	17.4 w PFS[PS], 11.7 w [PR]
Proteasome	Bortezomib	II	Monotherapy	R	1 m PFS, 3 m OS
HDAC	Panobinostat	II	Monotherapy	R	Negative
Targeting DNA repair defects					
PARP	BMN673	I	Monotherapy	R	18% RR
Targeting the immune system					
PD-1/CTLA-4	Nivolumab Ipilimumab	I/II	Combination	R	Nivolumab 18% ORR and 4.4 m OS, Combination 17% ORR and 8.2 m OS
Antibody-drug conjugates					
CD56	Lorvotuzumab mertansine	I	Monotherapy	R	25% PR/SD
DLL3	Rovalpituzumab tesirine	I	Monotherapy	R	22% ORR

Source: modified from ref. 45

Abbreviations: VEGF, Vascular endothelial growth factor; VEGFR, Vascular endothelial growth factor receptor; PDGFR, Platelet derived growth factor receptor; c-KIT, Stem cell factor receptor; FLT3, FMS-like tyrosine kinase 3; RET, Rearranged during transfection tyrosine kinase; mTOR, mammalian target of rapamycin; BCL-2, B-cell lymphoma; MCL-1, Myeloid cell leukaemia 1; HDAC, Histone deacetylase; CD56, Neural cell adhesion molecule; DLL3, delta-like 3; R, Relapsed; R (M), Relapsed followed by maintenance; Ra, Randomised; PFS, Progression free survival; TTP, Time to progression; OS, Overall survival; m, Months; [PR], Platinum resistant; [PS], Platinum sensitive; d, Days; PR, Partial response; SD, Stable disease; PARP, Poly-ADP ribose polymerase; CTLA, Cytotoxic T-lymphocyte-associated protein 4; EGFR, epidermal growth factor receptor; PD-1, programmed cell death protein-1; RR, Response rate; ORR, Overall response rate.

identified or wild-type *EGFR* is detected, FISH analysis for *ALK1* rearrangement should be performed, then FISH for *ROS1*, *MET*, *RET*, and *NTRK1* abnormalities. If none of these are abnormal, *BRAF*, *ERBB2*, *ERCC2*, and *HER*-2 should be sequenced for mutations that can be targeted. For FNA or core needle-biopsied specimens, the Emory approach is to do IHC for PD1/PD-L1, then a FISH panel for *ALK*, *ROS*, *MET*, and *RET*, and finally a targeted NGS panel. If NGS fails, use PCR/Sanger sequencing for *KRAS* and *BRAF* mutations.

Since *EGFR* mutations in pSCC are rare and, if detected, they are usually not targetable, it would be reasonable to stain for EGFR and PD-L1 with IHC first. If the results are positive, immunotherapy with antibodies might be an option for oncologists. If IHC results are negative, mutation analysis for the components of PI3K/AKT/mTOR, EGFR-mediated tyrosine kinases, and RAS/MAPK/ERK pathways may provide an option(s) for precision oncologists in managing late-stage pSCC patients.

At the time this chapter is being finalized, there are no FDA-approved therapeutic reagents for SCLC, LCNEC and other pulmonary malignancies. However, with the development of molecular assays and novel pharmaceutical reagents, this chapter will be updated in future editions.

11.6 Summary

Lung cancer remains the most fatal cancer in the world and costs most of the healthcare resources for patient management. Fortunately, significant progress in precision pathology and precision oncology has been made in NSCLCs and saved millions of

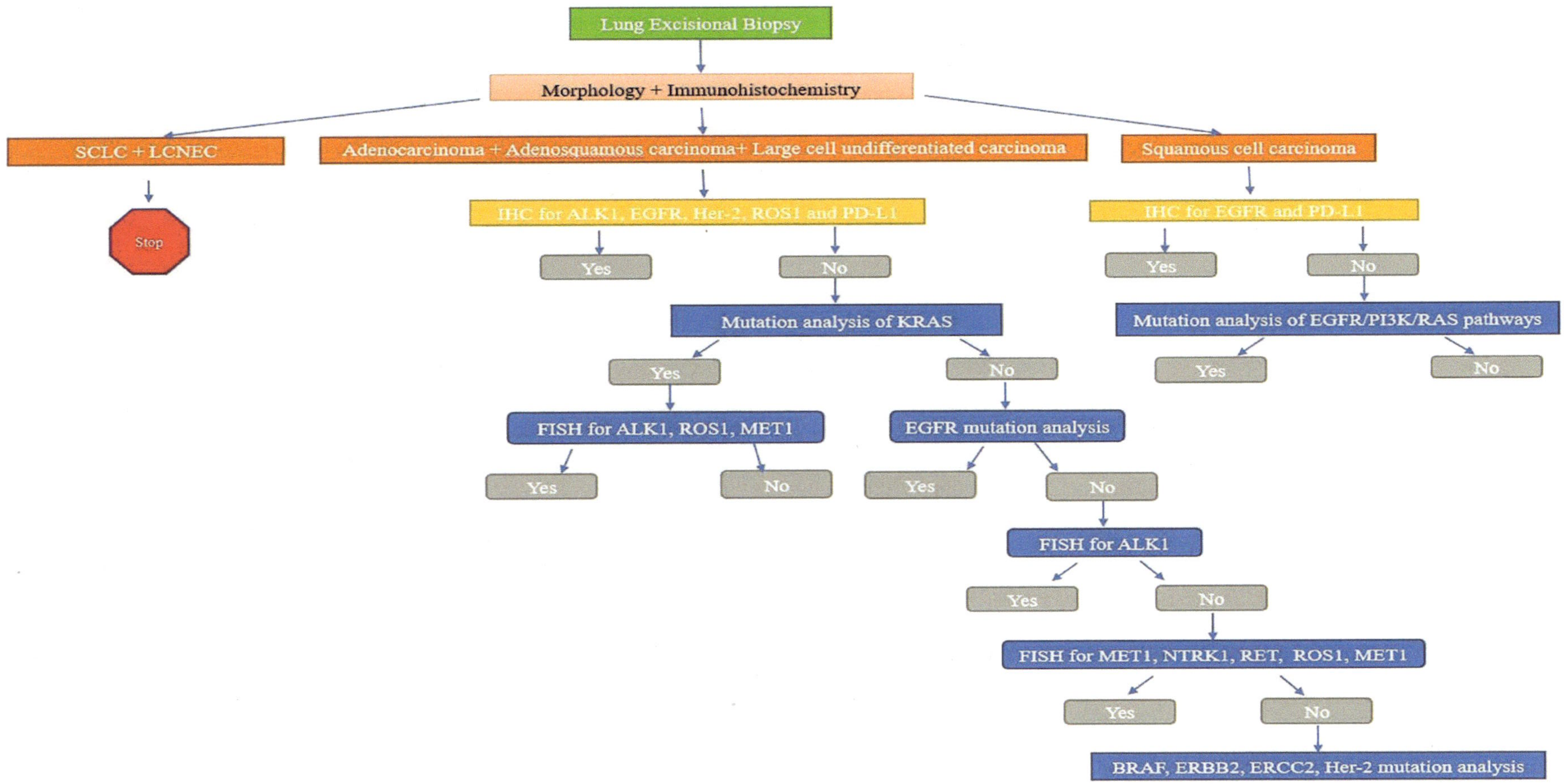

FIGURE 11.4 Proposed testing algorithm for lung cancer in excisional biopsy specimens. The first step is to separate the lung cancer into SCLC/LCNEC and NSCLC. SCLC/LCNEC will be managed with surgery and combined radiation/chemotherapy. NSCLC will be further classified into adenocarcinoma, pSCC, or LCUC, followed by molecular analysis of *KRAS*-activating mutations. If *KRAS* mutations are detected, skip *EGFR* and *BRAF* mutation analysis because they are mutually exclusive and proceed to FISH analysis for *ALK* and *ROS1* translocations and evaluate *MET* gene amplification. If *KRAS* mutations are not detected, proceed to *EGFR* mutation analysis. If *EGFR* drug-sensitive mutations are detected, stop here and treat with TKIs. If *EGFR* drug-resistant mutations or no mutations are detected, proceed to *ALK* FISH study. If *ALK* translocation is not detected, test *ROS1* translocation and *MET* amplification and sequence *BRAF* for activating mutations.

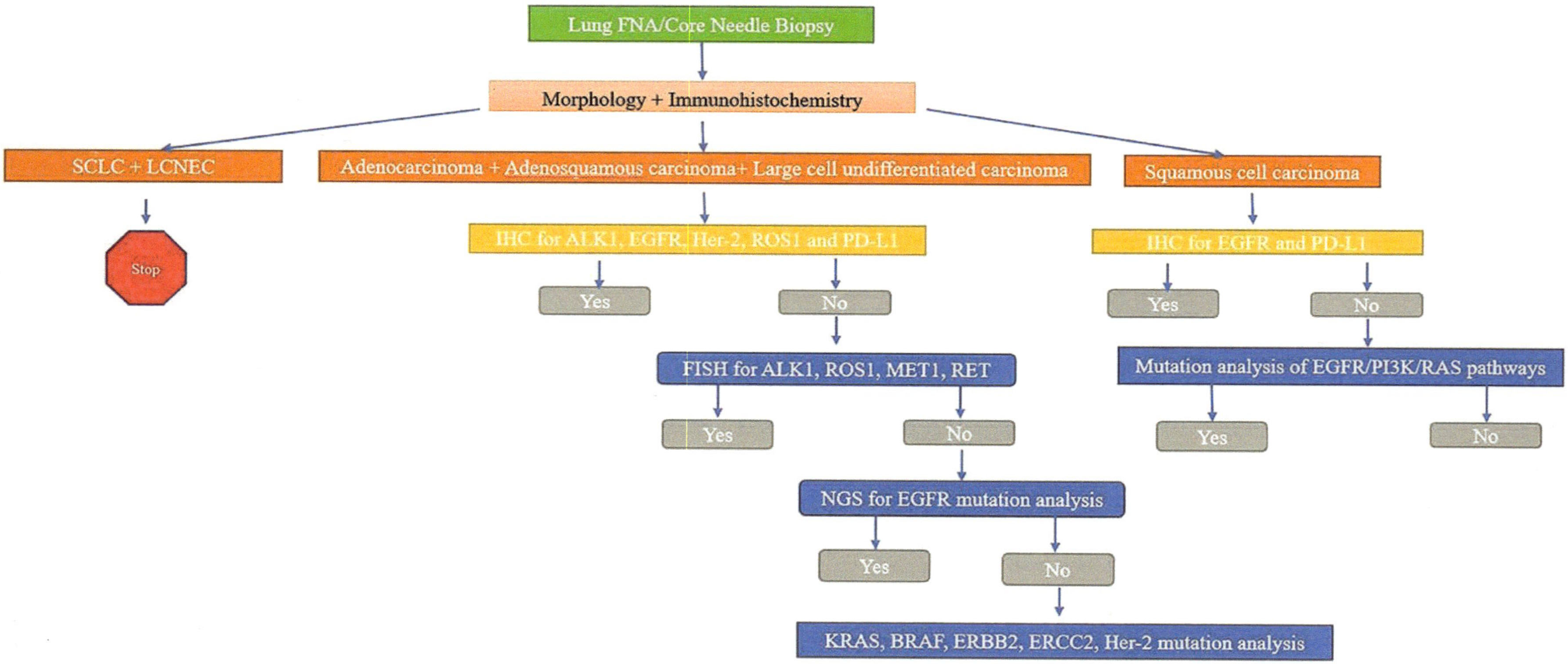

FIGURE 11.5 Proposed testing algorithm for lung cancer in FNA or core needle biopsy specimens (Emory approach). Similar to the algorithm for excisional biopsy specimens, the tumor will be separated into SCLC/LCNEC and NSCLC, and NSCLC will be further classified into adenocarcinoma, pSCC, or LCUC. Molecular analysis will be skipped to save the specimen for FISH analysis for *ALK*, *ROS1*, *MET1*, and *RET* translocations and evaluate *MET* gene amplification. If FISH analyses are negative, proceed to NGS for *EGFR* mutation analysis. If *EGFR* drug-resistant mutations or no mutations are detected, use *KRAS*, *BRAF*, *ERBB2*, *ERCC2*, and *HER-2* mutation analysis.

lives. Under the NCCN guidelines, molecular testing for EGFR and other oncogenic drivers and targetable genetic abnormalities has become a routine in all U.S. molecular diagnostic laboratories. This chapter summarizes the recent findings in molecular genomics/genetics on lung cancer and pharmacomics and provides guidelines for precision pathology diagnosis of lung cancers and strategies for precision therapy by oncologists. Progress on the precision pathology of SCLC was also discussed. With the discovery of more therapeutic targets and development of novel target drugs, precision pathology guidelines and strategies for precision therapy will be improved and revised.

REFERENCES

1. Key statistics for lung cancer. American Cancer Society. Retrieved on 23 February 2021. www.cancer.org/cancer/lung-cancer/about/key-statistics.html
2. Travis WD, Brambilla EW, Burke AP, et al. WHO Classification of Tumours of the Lung, Pleura, Thymus, and Heart, IARC Press, Lyon, 2015.
3. Non-Small Cell Lung Cancer Treatment (PDQ®)–Health Professional Version. National Cancer Institute. Retrieved on 13 February 2022. (www.cancer.gov/types/lung/hp/non-small-cell-lung-treatment-pdq).
4. Halliday PR, Blakely CM, Bivona TG. Emerging targeted therapies for the treatment of non-small cell lung cancer. Curr Oncol Rep. 2019;21(3):21.
5. Del Rivero J, Enewold L, Thomas A. Metastatic lung cancer in the age of targeted therapy: Improving long-term survival. Transl Lung Cancer Res. 2016;5(6):727–730.
6. The Cancer Genome Atlas Research Network. Comprehensive molecular profiling of lung adenocarcinoma. Nature. 2014;511 (7511):543–550.
7. NCCNGuidelines.Non-SmallCellLungCancer.Version1.2022. National Comprehensive Cancer Network. 2022. Retrieved on 13 February 2022. www.nccn.org/patients/guidelines/content/PDF/lung-metastatic-patient.pdf
8. Kris MG, Johnson BE, Kwiatkowski DJ, et al. Identification of driver mutations in tumor specimens from 1,000 patients with lung adenocarcinoma: The NCI's Lung Cancer Mutation Consortium (LCMC). J Clin Oncol. 2011;29:CRA7506.
9. da Cunha Santos G, Shepherd FA, Tsao MS. EGFR mutations and lung cancer. Ann Rev Pathol Mech Dis 2011;6:49–69.
10. Li AR, Chitale D, Riely GJ, et al. EGFR mutations in lung adenocarcinomas: Clinical testing experience and relationship to EGFR gene copy number and immunohistochemical expression. J Mol Diagn. 2008;10(3):242–248.
11. Sakurada A, Shepherd FA, Tsao MS. Epidermal growth factor receptor tyrosine kinase inhibitors in lung cancer: Impact of primary or secondary mutations. Clin Lung Cancer. 2006;7(Suppl 4):S138–S144.
12. Kobayashi S, Boggon TJ, Dayaram T, et al. EGFR mutation and resistance of non-small-cell lung cancer to gefitinib. N Engl J Med. 2005;352(8):786–792.
13. Zhou W, Ercan D, Chen L, et al. Novel mutant-selective EGFR kinase inhibitors against EGFR T790M. Nature. 2009;462(7276):1070–1074.
14. The Cancer Genome Atlas Research Network. Comprehensive genomic characterization of squamous cell lung cancers. Nature. 2012;489(7417):519–525.
15. Stransky N, Egloff AM, Tward AD, et al. The mutational landscape of head and neck squamous cell carcinoma. Science. 2011;333(6046):1157–1160.
16. Rekhtman N, Travis WD. Large no more: The Journey of Pulmonary large cell carcinoma from common to rare entity. J Thorac Oncol. 2019;14(7):1125–1127.
17. Wang Q, Mou J, Yang X, et al. EGFR mutations in patients with lung adenocarcinoma in southwest China: Are G719S/A and L861Q more likely detected in tumors derived from smokers? Lung Cancer (Auckl). 2013;4:27–33.
18. D'Angelo SP, Pietanza MC, Johnson ML, et al. Incidence of EGFR exon 19 deletions and L858R in tumor specimens from men and cigarette smokers with lung adenocarcinomas. J Clin Oncol. 2011;29(15):2066–2070.
19. Sun Y, Yin X, Wen M, et al. EGFR mutations subset in Chinese lung squamous cell carcinoma patients. Mol Med Rep. 2018;17(6):7575–7584.
20. Joshi A, Zanwar S, Noronha V, et al. EGFR mutation in squamous cell carcinoma of the lung: Does it carry the same connotation as in adenocarcinomas? Onco Targets Ther. 2017;10:1859–1863.
21. Wang R, Pan Y, Li C, et al. Analysis of major known driver mutations and prognosis in resected adenosquamous lung carcinomas. J Thorac Oncol. 2014;9(6):760–768.
22. Li C, Lu H. Adenosquamous carcinoma of the lung. Onco Targets Ther. 2018;11:4829–4835.
23. Fan L, Yang H, Yao F, et al. Clinical outcomes of epidermal growth factor receptor tyrosine kinase inhibitors in recurrent adenosquamous carcinoma of the lung after resection. Onco Targets Ther. 2017;10:239–245.
24. Chan AW, Chau SL, Tong JH, et al. The landscape of actionable molecular alterations in immunomarker-defined large-cell carcinoma of the lung. J Thorac Oncol. 2019;14(7):1213–1222.
25. Harrison PT, Vyse S, Huang PH. Rare epidermal growth factor receptor (EGFR) mutations in non-small cell lung cancer. Semin Cancer Biol. 2020;61:167–179.
26. D'Angelo SP, Pietanza MC, Johnson ML, et al. Incidence of EGFR exon 19 deletions and L858R in tumor specimens from men and cigarette smokers with lung adenocarcinomas. J Clin Oncol. 2011;29(15):2066–2070.
27. Morris SW, Kirstein MN, Valentine MB, et al. Fusion of a kinase gene, ALK, to a nucleolar protein gene, NPM, in non-Hodgkin's lymphoma. Science. 1994;263(5151):1281–1284.
28. Soda M, Choi YL, Enomoto M, et al. Identification of the transforming EML4–ALK fusion gene in non-small-cell lung cancer. Nature. 2007;448(7153):561–566.
29. Azelby CM, Sakamoto MR, Bowles DW. ROS1 targeted therapies: Current status. Curr Oncol Rep. 2012;23(8):94.
30. Cascetta P, Sforza V, Manzo A, et al. RET inhibitors in non-small-cell lung cancer. Cancers (Basel). 2021;13(17):4415.
31. Brahmer JR, Drake CG, Wollner I, et al. Phase I study of single-agent anti-programmed death-1 (MDX-1106) in refractory solid tumors: Safety, clinical activity, pharmacodynamics, and immunologic correlates. J Clin Oncol. 2010;28(19): 3167–3175.
32. Yu H, Boyle TA, Zhou C, et al. PD-L1 Expression in lung cancer. J Thorac Oncol. 2016;11(7):964–975.
33. Oyama T, Sugio K, Isse T, et al. Expression of cytochrome P450 in non-small cell lung cancer. Front Biosci Landmark. 2008;13(15):5787–5793.

34. McLemore TL, Adelberg S, Liu MC, et al. Expression of CYP1A1 gene in patients with lung cancer: Evidence for cigarette smoke-induced gene expression in normal lung tissue and for altered gene regulation in primary pulmonary carcinomas. J Natl Cancer Inst. 1990;82(16):1333–1339.
35. Spivack SD, Hurteau GJ, Fasco MJ, et al. Phase I and II carcinogen metabolism gene expression in human lung tissue and tumors. Clin Cancer Res. 2003;9(16 Pt 1):6002–6011.
36. Guengerich FP. Cytochrome P-450 3A4: Regulation and role in drug metabolism. Annu Rev Pharmacol Toxicol. 1999;39:1–17.
37. Kivisto KT, Kroemer HK, Eichelbaum M. The role of human cytochrome P450 enzymes in the metabolism of anticancer agents: Implications for drug interactions. Br J Clin Pharmacol. 1995;40(6):523–530.
38. Czerwinski M, McLemore TL, Gelboin HV, Gonzalez FJ. Quantification of CYP2B7, CYP4B1, and CYPOR messenger RNAs in normal human lung and lung tumors. Cancer Res. 1994;54(4):1085–1091.
39. Zanger UM, Schwab M. Cytochrome P450 enzymes in drug metabolism: Regulation of gene expression, enzyme activities, and impact of genetic variation. Pharmacol Ther. 2013;138(1):103–141.
40. George J, Lim JS, Jang SJ, et al. Comprehensive genomic profiles of small cell lung cancer. Nature. 2015;524(7563):47–53.
41. Kim KB, Dunn CT, Park KS. Recent progress in mapping the emerging landscape of the small-cell lung cancer genome. Exp Mol Med. 2019;51(12):1–13.
42. Peifer M, Fernandez-Cuesta L, Sos ML, et al. Integrative genome analyses identify key somatic driver mutations of small-cell lung cancer. Nat Genet. 2012;44(10):1104–1110.
43. Rudin CM, Durinck S, Stawiski EW, et al. Comprehensive genomic analysis identifies SOX2 as a frequently amplified gene in small-cell lung cancer. Nat Genet. 2012;44(10):1111–1116.
44. Abidin AZ, Garassino MC, Califano R, et al. Targeted therapies in small cell lung cancer: A review. Ther Adv Med Oncol. 2010;2(1):25–37.
45. Sharp A, Bhosle J, Abdelraouf F, et al. Development of molecularly targeted agents and immunotherapies in small cell lung cancer. Eur J Cancer. 2016;60:26–39.
46. Hiroshima K, Mino-Kenudson M. Update on large cell neuroendocrine carcinoma. Transl Lung Cancer Res. 2017; 6(5):530–539.
47. Rekhtman N, Pietanza MC, Hellmann MD, et al. Next-generation sequencing of pulmonary large cell neuroendocrine carcinoma reveals small cell carcinoma-like and non-small cell carcinoma-like subsets. Clin Cancer Res. 2016;22(14):3618–3629.
48. Osann KE, Lowery JT, Schell MJ. Small cell lung cancer in women: Risk associated with smoking, prior respiratory disease, and occupation. Lung Cancer. 2000;28(1):1–10.
49. Relling MV, McLeod HL, Bowman LC, Santana VM. Etoposide pharmacokinetics and pharmacodynamics after acute and chronic exposure to cisplatin. Clin Pharmacol Ther. 1994; 56(5):503–511.
50. Meyer UA. Pharmacogenetics and adverse drug reactions. Lancet. 2000; 356(9242):1667–1671.
51. Yatabe Y, Dacic S, Borczuk AC, et al. Best practices recommendations for diagnostic immunohistochemistry in lung cancer. J Thorac Oncol. 2019;14(3):377–407.
52. Oberndorfer F, Müllauer L. Molecular pathology of lung cancer: Current status and perspectives. Curr Opin Oncol. 2018;30(2):69–76.
53. Inamura K. Lung cancer: Understanding its molecular pathology and the 2015 WHO classification. Front Oncol. 2017;7:193.
54. Osmani L, Askin F, Gabrielson E, Li QK. Current WHO guidelines and the critical role of immunohistochemical markers in the subclassification of non-small cell lung carcinoma (NSCLC): Moving from targeted therapy to immunotherapy. Semin Cancer Biol. 2018;52(Pt 1):103–109.
55. Skoulidis F, Heymach JV. Co-occurring genomic alterations in non-small-cell lung cancer biology and therapy. Nat Rev Cancer. 2019;19(9):495–509.

12

Mesothelioma

Jian Jing

12.1 Introduction

Mesothelioma arises from the mesothelial surface of the pleural, peritoneal, and pericardial cavities that are covered by a monolayer of specialized cells (mesothelial cells). Mesothelioma in situ, well-differentiated papillary mesothelial tumor, and localized pleural mesothelioma have indolent behavior and are in a separate diagnostic category. Here, we focus on pleural mesothelioma with aggressive behavior.

Pleural mesothelioma constitutes less than 0.3% of all malignancies with a 5-year survival rate of 5% and a median survival of 7 to 9 months if untreated (1). The clinical symptoms are nonspecific, and most cases are in an advanced stage at the time of pathological diagnosis. Although the current progression on molecular mechanisms of mesothelioma is limited, molecular markers are helpful in making an accurate diagnosis between reactive vs. malignancy in challenging cases (2). Histological classification drives medical management; however, mesothelioma diagnosis and management are best addressed using the multidisciplinary approach in combination with clinical history, radiology, histology, immunohistochemical stains, and genetic analysis. This chapter will start with the histological subclassifications followed by current ancillary tests in practice. Therapy strategy based on histology classification will be discussed. Common genetic mutations with current clinical trials and future management will be briefly introduced.

12.2 Histology Subclassification and Diagnosis of Pleural Mesothelioma

Histology remains the gold standard for the diagnosis of mesothelioma. Mesothelioma has three histological subtypes with prognostic implications in the updated WHO 5th Edition: epithelioid, biphasic and sarcomatoid (3). Epithelioid mesothelioma is composed of cohesive tumor cells with eosinophilic cytoplasm, round nuclei, vesicular chromatin, and occasional prominent nucleoli (Figure 12.1). There are variable growth patterns in epithelioid mesothelioma, which can be helpful in diagnosis, with some patterns (discussed further subsequently) having prognostic value. Sarcomatoid mesothelioma is characterized by a clonal proliferation of more dyscohesive spindle cells arranged in fascicles or in haphazard patterns with true stromal invasion. Biphasic mesothelioma is composed of both epithelioid and sarcomatoid histomorphology with over 10% of each component in resection specimens. The methods and diagnostic accuracies for obtaining tissue, such as fluid cytology, thoracentesis, video-assisted thoracoscopic, or open thoracotomy will not be discussed in detail in this chapter; rather the associated cytological features and growth patterns with prognostic and therapeutic values will be emphasized.

Sarcomatoid and biphasic histologic subtypes have a worse prognosis when compared with epithelioid mesothelioma. Epithelioid mesothelioma should be graded in a two-tier grading system to demonstrate the predictive survival of patient. Nuclear grade (mitotic count and nuclear atypia) and presence of necrosis are integrated in the grading system. The growth patterns in epithelioid mesothelioma with aggressive clinical behavior are equal or over 50% tumor cells with solid and micropapillary pattern (3). The unfavorable cytologic features include rhabdoid, pleomorphic, and high nuclear grade (4) (Figure 12.2). In contrast, the favorable features of epithelioid mesothelioma include growth patterns of tubulopapillary, trabecular, and adenomatoid; cytologic features of lymphohistiocytoid and low nuclear grade; and predominantly myxoid stromal features.

Establishing a diagnosis of mesothelioma in a small biopsy is difficult due to limited tissue and variable stromal reactions. The key feature to differentiate between benign and malignant is true stromal invasion. However, this can be very difficult in practice, especially in small biopsies. Adipose tissue involvement is considered as a definite feature, but entrapment of benign mesothelial cells between fat lobules needs to be excluded (5). The entrapped mesothelial glands are usually linearly arranged in a trama frequently associated with perpendicularly oriented vessels. Other important features to support malignant mesothelioma include cellular heterogenous distribution without zonation, presence of necrosis, and marked cytological atypia with increased mitotic counts (at least 2 mitoses/2 mm^2). For cases with obscured features in cyto-histomorphology, ancillary tests can be helpful (Figure 12.3).

12.3 Ancillary Tests for Mesothelioma Diagnosis and Prognosis in Practice

The application of molecular tests in mesothelioma is limited due to a shortage of knowledge of molecular characteristics. The most common genetic alteration in mesothelioma is the homozygous deletion of the 9p21 locus including *CDKN2A* (cyclin-dependent kinase inhibitor 2A). Fluorescence *in situ* hybridization (FISH) for deletion of *P16* (*P16* FISH) and immunohistochemistry (IHC)

DOI: 10.1201/9781003513469-12

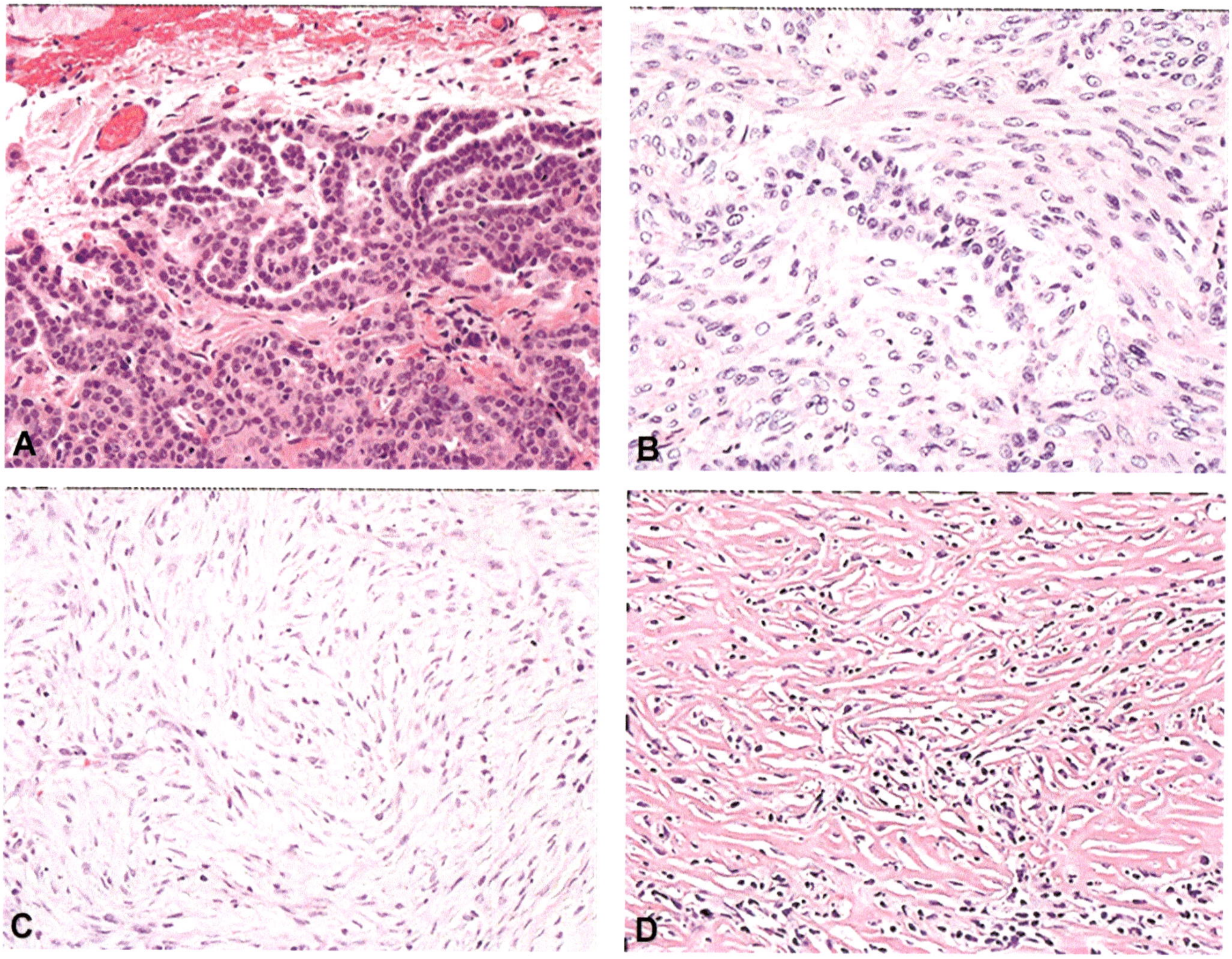

FIGURE 12.1 Histological subclassifications. (A) Epithelioid mesothelioma with tubule, trabecular, and focal solid pattern. Tumor cells are characterized by rounded cells with eosinophilic cytoplasm and round nuclei with inconspicuous to conspicuous nucleoli (H&E ×400). (B) Biphasic mesothelioma composed of rounded epithelioid cells in tubular formation and spindle neoplastic cells within a fibrous stroma (H&E ×400). (C) Sarcomatoid mesothelioma with fascicular arrangement. Tumor cells have variable pleomorphisms. (D) Desmoplastic mesothelioma with paucicellularity and haphazard slit-like space within dense hyaline fibrous stroma (H&E ×400).

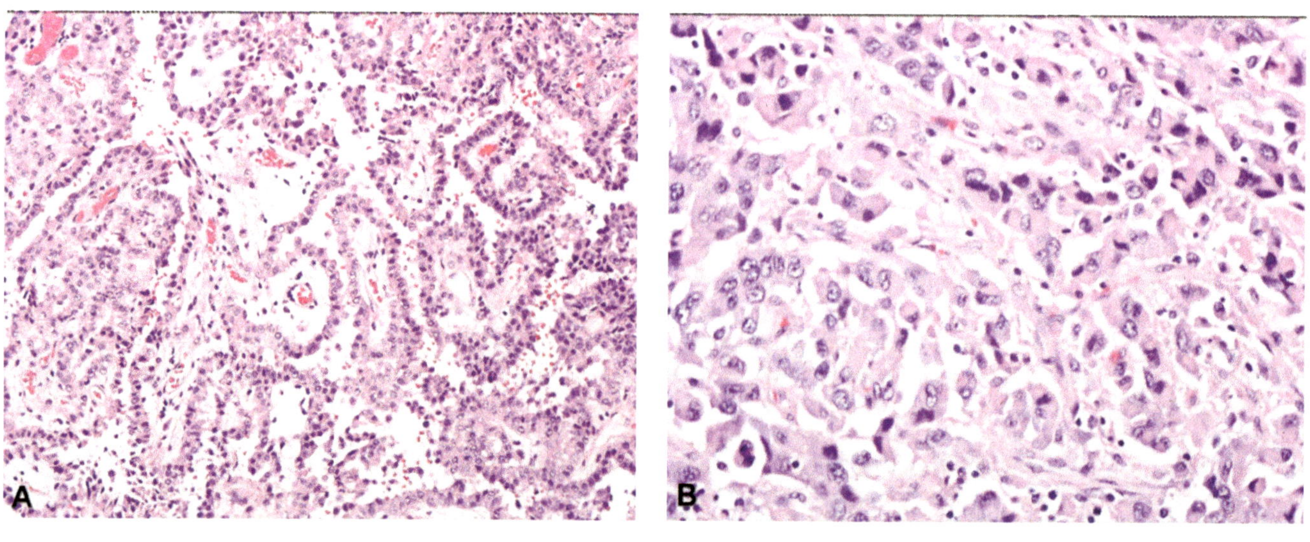

FIGURE 12.2 Prognostic features of epithelioid mesothelioma. (A) Favorable: tumor cells showing tubulopapillary pattern and low nuclear grade cytological features (H&E ×200). (B) Unfavorable: tumor cells showing rhabdoid and pleomorphic cytological features (H&E ×400).

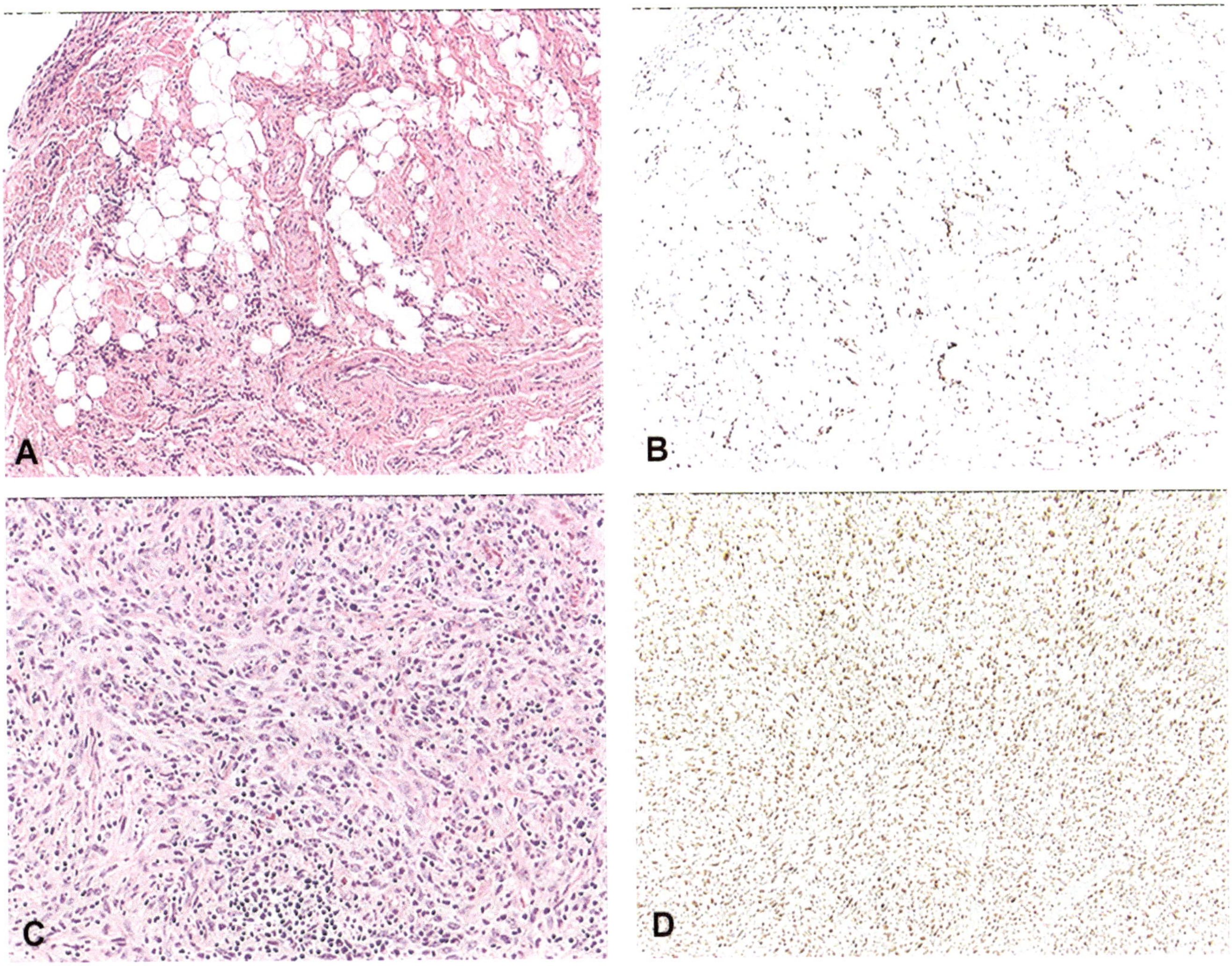

FIGURE 12.3 Challenge cases in small biopsy. (A) Epithelioid mesothelioma with true stromal invasion (fat involvement) (H&E ×100). (B) Diagnosis of mesothelioma is confirmed by loss of BAP-1 nuclear staining (H&E ×100). (C) Sarcomatoid mesothelioma with high-grade cytological features in a background of mixed inflammation and fibrosis (H&E ×200); no definite feature of stromal invasion. (D) BAP-1 nuclear staining is preserved (H&E ×100). Diagnosis of mesothelioma is confirmed by *P16* FISH analysis of "positive for homozygous deletion of *CDKN2A*".

for MTAP (methylthioadenosine phosphorylase) for *CDKN2A* deletion and IHC for BAP1 (BRCA-associated peptide-1) are used in practice to distinguish benign from malignant mesothelioma in both cytological cell block specimens and formalin-fixed paraffin-embedded (FFPE) tissue (6, 7).

The homozygous deletion of *CDKN2A* tested by *P16* FISH with a cutoff of 20% is only reported in malignant mesotheliomas (8, 9). This is particularly helpful in small biopsies including cytologic specimens with limited histological structure information. The overall sensitivity of *P16* FISH in the diagnosis of malignant mesothelioma has been shown to range from 56% to 79% with 100% positive predictive value (10). Homozygous *P16*/*CDKN2A* deletion is more frequently detected in sarcomatoid mesothelioma (approaching 100%) than epithelioid mesothelioma (67%–83%) and is a reliable marker to distinguish sarcomatoid mesothelioma from fibrous pleuritis (3, 11). The presence of a *P16* homozygous deletion is associated with shorter survival and briefer time to relapse in patients with mesothelioma (12, 13).

Although FISH assay is useful in both diagnosis and prognosis, it is not always as readily available as immunohistochemistry (IHC). *MTAP* is localized in the 9p21 chromosomal region and is correlated with the 9p21/*CNKD2A* deletion in FISH assay. Chapel et al. reported that MTAP IHC is an accurate and reproducible surrogate for *p16*/*CNKD2A* FISH in the diagnosis of pleural mesothelioma (14). Their study showed that MTAP cytoplasmic loss by IHC was 78% sensitive and 96% specific for *CDKN2A* homozygous deletion, with excellent interobserver agreement for all mesothelial lesions (kappa: 0.85). The other reliable immunomarker applied in practice is BAP1. BAP1 is a deubiquitinating enzyme and functions as a tumor suppressor. Germline *BAP1* mutations are observed in 1–2% of mesotheliomas and are associated with a favorable overall survival (15). Somatic mutations are more common in mesothelioma but have no clear prognostic significance. The somatic gene inactivating deletions or point mutations have been reported in neoplasms associated with *BAP1*-cancer syndrome (16). Loss of nuclear staining of BAP1 is specific for the diagnosis of malignancy, which is especially helpful in small biopsies. The sensitivity is around 42–67% in several studies with small numbers of biopsy cases and can be up to 77.8% when both BAP1 and MTAP are combined (14, 17–19). BAP1 loss is more often observed in epithelioid mesothelioma (42–65%) and less often in sarcomatoid mesothelioma (as few as 7%) (20) (Figure 12.3).

Histo-cytomorphology of reactive mesothelial cells can overlap with malignant cells, especially in the scenario of atypical mesothelial hyperplasia. Therefore, CDKN2A, BAP1, and MTAP play an important role in separating benign from malignant disease. Other markers have been reported to distinguish benign from malignant statistically but have not been generally applied in practice and require further validation (2).

The other important role of ancillary tests is to distinguish mesothelioma from metastatic carcinoma. Markers positive in mesothelioma with high sensitivity and specificity that are applied in practice include WT1 (nuclear staining), calretinin (nuclear and cytoplasmic), podoplanin (D2–40), and cytokeratin 5/6. Negative markers for mesothelioma commonly used in practice are MOC31, BER-EP4, and polyclonal CEA. A recent study has shown that Claudin4 has high sensitivity and specificity for metastatic adenocarcinoma compared with MOC-31 and Ber-EP4 (21).

Site-specific IHC markers are generally applied in inconclusive cases after the previous extensive workup. The most common metastatic carcinomas originate from the lung and breast. GATA3, though a marker of the mammary and urothelial systems, is sensitive (100%) and specific (85%) for sarcomatoid mesothelioma. GATA3 is useful to distinguish sarcomatoid mesothelioma from lung sarcomatoid carcinoma and organizing pleuritis (22, 23). For metastatic breast carcinoma, other mammary specific markers (ER, PR, GCDFP-15, SOX10) are preferred for differential diagnosis.

Unfortunately, no mesothelial markers are specific. Routine mesothelial markers can be focally and weakly positive in carcinomas, especially the poorly differentiated carcinoma. The International Mesothelioma Interest Group recommended an IHC panel with at least two positive and two negative markers in addition to cytokeratin (24). Pancytokeratin is useful in highlighting the infiltrating pattern in malignant carcinoma and nonsarcomatoid mesotheliomas. However, IHCs have a limited role in differentiating between sarcomatoid mesothelioma and metastatic sarcoma or sarcomatoid carcinoma (25). Cytokeratin can be negative or scant in sarcomatoid mesothelioma and some mesothelial markers can be expressed in metastatic sarcomatoid carcinoma. The combination of clinical history, radiologic information, *p16* FISH assay and an IHC panel of cytokeratin, calretinin, and GATA3 is invaluable in this challenging scenario.

It is important to emphasize that tumor stage and histology have a strong impact on the prognosis among patients with mesothelioma. Mesotheliomas with a sarcomatoid component (at least 10% in resection specimens) have worse outcomes compared with mesotheliomas with only an epithelioid component.

Several prognostic scoring systems emphasize either clinical characteristics or pathological features to support further management. Two validated systems emphasizing extent of disease and other clinical factors are the European Organization for Research and Treatment of Cancer (EORTC) and the Cancer and Leukemia Group B (CALGB) (26). A new grading system—the Mesothelioma Weighted Grading Scheme (MWGS)—has been proposed and includes more pathological features, including histological type and BAP1 expression, in addition to the criteria (necrosis, mitotic count, nuclear grade) in the current two-tier grading system for epithelioid mesothelioma (27) (Table 12.1). A study employed targeted next-generation sequencing to focus on major mesothelioma-mutated genes and the *TERT* promoter and showed that mutations in *TERT* promoter, *NF2*, and *TP53* were associated with poorer overall survival (28).

12.4 Management in Mesothelioma

Combined modalities (surgery, radiation therapy, chemotherapy, and immunotherapy) are applied in mesothelioma management. Small biopsy samples provide histology information and are correlated with clinical staging to determine management. It is generally acceptable that early-stage and localized mesothelioma will benefit from surgical removal, of which the goal is macroscopic complete resection (MCR). Pathological staging is accessed in maximal cytoreductive procedures, extended pleurectomy/decortication (EPD) and extrapleural pneumonectomy (EPP) and is more reliable than clinical staging. Virtually all patients with malignant mesothelioma, either non-surgical candidates or surgical candidates, will receive systemic therapy. All histological subtypes are candidates for chemotherapy; however, there is no clear evidence of correlation between histologic subtype and chemotherapy outcomes (29, 30). Nevertheless, histological subtypes play a role in guiding the initial treatment. For epithelioid mesothelioma, cisplatin and pemetrexed are suggested for front-line treatment. For nonepithelioid mesothelioma, immune checkpoint inhibitors targeting programmed death ligand 1 (PD-L1) and cytotoxic T lymphocyte antigen 4 (CTLA-4) have statistically significant overall survival compared with chemotherapy (31, 32). The combination of nivolumab plus ipilimumab is the suggested initial management for nonepithelioid mesothelioma (33, 34). The response assessment in practice includes radiological measurement (CT, PET/CT) and post-treatment pathological evaluation with cut-off of 50% viable tumor cells (35).

12.5 Future Management of Mesothelioma

To develop precision medicine for malignant mesothelioma, a comprehensive understanding of tumor heterogeneity is crucial. Recent study demonstrates that the current WHO classification only explains around 10% of the molecular differences between patients by utilizing whole-genome sequencing, transcriptomic, and epigenomic data to propose a new classification based on four dimensions: ploidy, tumor cell morphology, adaptive immune response, and CpG island methylator profile (36). This innovative classification system captures substantial molecular disparities among patients and is delineated by distinct phenotypes. Genetic alterations were diverse, with the most frequent changes observed in *BAP1*, *NF2*, and *CDKN2A/B* genes that could be potential targets (37). Gene expression profiling including miRNAs have demonstrated additional data to separate mesothelioma from benign lesions and to classify patients into distinct

TABLE 12.1

Summary of Mesotheliomas

Histology Subtype	Morphology		Axillary Tests				Prognosis		Treatment	
			Mesothelial vs. Non-Mesothelial Origin		Benign vs. Malignancy					
Epithelioid mesothelioma	Stromal invasion with adipose tissue involvement; cellular heterogeneous distribution without zonation	Cohesive tumor cells with eosinophilic cytoplasm, round nuclei, vesicular chromatin, and occasional prominent nucleoli.	IHCs: recommend panel of two positive markers and two negative markers Mesothelial origin: WT1 (nuclear), calretinin (cytoplasmic and nuclear), CK5/6, D2–40 Non-mesothelial origin: MOC31, BER-EP4, polyclonal CEA, Claudin4	WT1, calretinin, CK5/6, D2–40 are recommended. Negative pancytokeratins are suggestive of other tumors	High specificity in malignancy: Loss of BAP1 (nuclear) and MTAP (cytoplasmic); homozygous deletion of CDKN2A by P16 FISH	BAP1 more often observed in epithelioid component	Local involvement and early stage with better prognosis	High nuclear grading (pleomorphic cytology, mitosis, necrosis); solid and microscopic growth patterns are associated with unfavorable prognosis	Surgical resection for localized or early-stage mesothelioma	Front-line treatment: cisplatin and pemetrexed
Mesothelioma with sarcomatoid component		At least 10% of sarcomatoid component showing dyscohesive spindle cells arranged in fascicles or in haphazard patterns		Mesothelial markers are less sensitive in sarcomatoid component, while GATA3 shows high sensitivity and specificity.		BAP1 loss low sensitivity (7%); Homozygous deletion of CDKN2A common seen in sarcomatoid component		Generally poor prognosis		Initial management: immune checkpoint inhibitors (nivolumab + ipilimumab)

prognostic subgroups (38–41). These studies suggested that the molecular profile and the prognosis of mesothelioma are better fit in a continuous model rather than distinct groups. While the classification by gene expression does not perfectly match histological subtypes, they can complement each other and provide more information in future management. Currently, differentiating epithelioid and nonepithelioid histologic subtypes is practically feasible for further investigation in clinical trials. For example, antiangiogenic agents have been applied in clinical trials based on histological subtypes and show significant results (42). Blood-based biomarkers (soluble mesothelin/soluble mesothelin-related peptides, fibulin-3, calretinin, and osteopontin), generally with low sensitivity and high false-positive results, haven't been applied for diagnostic or prognostic purpose in practice for mesothelioma. Their role is limited to disease monitoring in the process of treatment (43). The likely predictive value in treatment requires further independent clinical trials and validation. In conclusion, these studies emphasize the complexity of malignant mesothelioma, underscoring the necessity of innovative classification systems and personalized treatment approaches. The intricate interplay between genetic mutations, tumor heterogeneity, and clinical outcomes is becoming clearer, offering hope for improved therapeutic strategies and better patient outcomes.

12.6 Summary

This chapter focuses on the pathological features of pleural mesothelioma. The discussion centers on histology, combined with ancillary tests in practice, guiding the diagnosis, prognosis, and management of mesothelioma (Table 12.1). Due to a lack of knowledge in genomic alterations in mesothelioma, the molecular pathology applications are limited. Some promising data are introduced, and further validations are expected in the future.

12.7 Acknowledgments

Thanks to Dr. Carlyne D. Cool for proofreading the article.

REFERENCES

1. Tsao AS, Lindwasser OW, Adjei AA, et al. Current and future management of malignant mesothelioma: A consensus report from the National Cancer Institute Thoracic Malignancy Steering Committee, International Association for the Study of Lung Cancer, and Mesothelioma Applied Research Foundation. J Thorac Oncol. 2018; 13:1655–1667.
2. Bruno R, Ali G, Fontanini G. Molecular markers and new diagnostic methods to differentiate malignant from benign mesothelial pleural proliferations: A literature review. J Thorac Dis. 2018;10: S342–S352.
3. WHO Classification of Tumours Editorial Board. WHO Tumours of the Lung, Pleura, Thymus and Heart. 5th ed. IARC; 2020.
4. Kadota K, Suzuki K, Sima CS, Rusch VW, Adusumilli PS, Travis WD. Pleomorphic epithelioid diffuse malignant pleural mesothelioma: A clinicopathological review and conceptual proposal to reclassify as biphasic or sarcomatoid mesothelioma. J Thorac Oncol. 2011;6:896–904.
5. Churg A, Naso JR. The separation of benign and malignant mesothelial proliferations: New markers and how to use them. Am J Surg Pathol. 2020; 44(11):e100–e112.
6. Illei PB, Ladanyi M, Rusch VW, Zakowski MF. The use of CDKN2A deletion as a diagnostic marker for malignant mesothelioma in body cavity effusions. Cancer. 2003;99(1):51–56.
7. Chiosea S, Krasinskas A, Cagle PT, Mitchell KA, Zander DS, Dacic S. Diagnostic importance of 9p21 homozygous deletion in malignant mesotheliomas. Mod Pathol. 2008;21(6):742–747.
8. Prins JB, Williamson KA, Kamp MM, et al. The gene for the cyclin dependent-kinase-4 inhibitor, CDKN2A, is preferentially deleted in malignant mesothelioma. Int J Cancer. 1998;75(4):649–653.
9. Cheng JQ, Jhanwar SC, Klein WM, et al. p16 alterations and deletion mapping of 9p21-P22 in malignant mesothelioma. Cancer Res. 1994;54(21):5547–5551.
10. Chaturvedi A, Holme J, Shah R, et al. P9 The utility of p16 fish in differentiating malignant mesothelioma and benign mesothelial proliferations. Thorax. 2016;71:A87–A88.
11. Wu D, Hiroshima K, Matsumoto S, et al. Diagnostic usefulness of p16/CDKN2A FISH in distinguishing between sarcomatoid mesothelioma and fibrous pleuritis. Am J Clin Pathol. 2013;139(1):39–46.
12. Dacic S, Kothmaier H, Land S, et al. Prognostic significance of p16/cdkn2a loss in pleural malignant mesotheliomas. Virchows Arch. 2008;453(6):627–635.
13. Jean D, Daubriac J, Le Pimpec-Barthes F, Galateau-Salle F, Jaurand MC. Molecular changes in mesothelioma with an impact on prognosis and treatment. Arch Pathol Lab Med. 2012;136(3):277–293.
14. Chapel DB, Schulte JJ, Berg K, et al. MTAP immunohistochemistry is an accurate and reproducible surrogate for CDKN2A fluorescence in situ hybridization in diagnosis of malignant pleural mesothelioma. Mod Pathol. 2020;33(2):245–254.
15. Baumann F, Flores E, Napolitano A, et al. Mesothelioma patients with germline BAP1 mutations have 7-fold improved long-term survival. Carcinogenesis. 2015;36(1):76–81.
16. Cigognetti M, Lonardi S, Fisogni S, et al. BAP1 (BRCA1-associated protein 1) is a highly specific marker for differentiating mesothelioma from reactive mesothelial proliferations. Mod Pathol. 2015;28(8):1043–1057.
17. Kinoshita Y, Hida T, Hamasaki M, et al. A combination of MTAP and BAP1 immunohistochemistry in pleural effusion cytology for the diagnosis of mesothelioma. Cancer Cytopathol. 2018;126(1):54–63.
18. Berg KB, Dacic S, Miller C, Cheung S, Churg A. Utility of methylthioadenosine phosphorylase compared with BAP1 immunohistochemistry, and CDKN2A and NF2 fluorescence in situ hybridization in separating reactive mesothelial proliferations from epithelioid malignant mesotheliomas. Arch Pathol Lab Med. 2018;142(12):1549–1553.
19. Hwang HC, Sheffield BS, Rodriguez SHT, et al. Utility of BAP1 immunohistochemistry and p16 (CDKN2A) FISH in the diagnosis of malignant mesothelioma in effusion cytology specimens. Am J Surg Pathol. 2016; 40(1):120–126.
20. Wang LM, Shi ZW, Wang JL, et al. Diagnostic accuracy of BRCA1-associated protein 1 in malignant mesothelioma: A meta-analysis. Oncotarget. 2017;8:68863–68872.
21. Najjar S, Gan Q, Stewart J, Sneige N. The utility of claudin-4 versus MOC-31 and Ber-EP4 in the

diagnosis of metastatic carcinoma in cytology specimens. Cancer Cytopathol. 2023;131(4):245–253.

22. Berg KB, Churg A. GATA3 Immunohistochemistry for distinguishing sarcomatoid and desmoplastic mesothelioma from sarcomatoid carcinoma of the lung. Am J Surg Pathol. 2017;41(9):1221–1225.
23. Piao ZH, Zhou XC, Chen JY. GATA3 is a useful immunohistochemical marker for distinguishing sarcomatoid malignant mesothelioma from lung sarcomatoid carcinoma and organizing pleuritis. Virchows Arch. 2021;479(2):257–263.
24. Husain AN, Colby TV, Ordóñez NG, et al. Guidelines for pathologic diagnosis of malignant mesothelioma 2017 update of the consensus statement from the international mesothelioma interest group. Arch Pathol Lab Med. 2018;142:89–108.
25. Lucas DR, Pass HI, Madan SK, et al. Sarcomatoid mesothelioma and its histological mimics: A comparative immunohistochemical study. Histopathol. 2003;42(3):270–279.
26. Edwards JG, Abrams KR, Leverment JN, et al. Prognostic factors for malignant mesothelioma in 142 patients: Validation of CALGB and EORTC prognostic scoring systems. Thorax. 2000;55:731.
27. Fuchs TL, Chou A, Aksoy Y, et al. A critical assessment of current grading schemes for diffuse pleural mesothelioma with a proposal for a novel mesothelioma weighted grading scheme (MWGS). Am J Surg Pathol. 2022;46(6):774–785.
28. Quetel L, Meiller C, Assié JB, et al. Genetic alterations of malignant pleural mesothelioma: Association with tumor heterogeneity and overall survival. Mol Oncol. 2020;14(6):1207–1223.
29. Vogelzang NJ, Rusthoven JJ, Symanowski J, et al. Phase III study of pemetrexed in combination with cisplatin versus cisplatin alone in patients with malignant pleural mesothelioma. J Clin Oncol. 2003;21:2636.
30. Kindler HL, Ismaila N, Armato SG III, et al. Treatment of malignant pleural mesothelioma: American Society of Clinical Oncology Clinical Practice Guideline. J Clin Oncol. 2018;36:1343–1373.
31. Baas P, Scherpereel A, Nowak AK, et al. First-line nivolumab plus ipilimumab in unresectable malignant pleural mesothelioma (CheckMate 743): A multicentre, randomised, open-label, phase 3 trial. Lancet. 2021; 397:375.
32. Peters S, Scherpereel A, Cornelissen R, et al. First-line nivolumab plus ipilimumab versus chemotherapy in patients with unresectable malignant pleural mesothelioma: 3-year outcomes from CheckMate 743. Ann Oncol. 2022;33:488.
33. Nivolumab injection. United States Prescribing Information. US National Library of Medicine. www.accessdata.fda.gov/drugsatfda_docs/label/2020/125554s089lbl.pdf (Accessed on October 5, 2020).
34. Ipilimumab injection. United States Prescribing Information. US National Library of Medicine. www.accessdata.fda.gov/drugsatfda_docs/label/2020/125377s115lbl.pdf (Accessed on October 5, 2020).
35. Amin MB, Edge SB, Greene FL, et al., eds. AJCC Cancer Staging Manual. 8th ed. New York, NY: Springer; 2017.
36. Mangiante L, Alcala N, Sexton-Oates A, et al. Multiomic analysis of malignant pleural mesothelioma identifies molecular axes and specialized tumor profiles driving intertumor heterogeneity. Nat Genet. 2023;55:607–618.
37. Hiltbrunner S, Fleischmann Z, Sokol ES, et al. Genomic landscape of pleural and peritoneal mesothelioma tumours. Br J Cancer. 2022;127:1997–2005.
38. Gordon GJ, Jensen RV, Hsiao LL, et al. Using gene expression ratios to predict outcome among patients with mesothelioma. J Natl Cancer Inst. 2003;95:598.
39. Andersen M, Grauslund M, Ravn J, et al. Diagnostic potential of miR-126, miR-143, miR-145, and miR652 in malignant pleural mesothelioma. J Mol Diagn. 2014;16:418–430.
40. Micolucci L, Akhtar MM, Olivieri F, et al. Diagnostic value of microRNAs in asbestos exposure and malignant mesothelioma: Systematic review and qualitative metaanalysis. Oncotarget. 2016;7:58606–58637.
41. Bruno R, Alì G, Giannini R, et al. Malignant pleural mesothelioma and mesothelial hyperplasia: A new molecular tool for the differential diagnosis. Oncotarget. 2017;8:2758–2770.
42. Zalcman G, Mazieres J, Margery J, et al. Bevacizumab for newly diagnosed pleural mesothelioma in the Mesothelioma Avastin Cisplatin Pemetrexed Study (MAPS): A randomised, controlled, open-label, phase 3 trial. Lancet. 2016;387(10026):1405–1414.
43. Scherpereel A, Lee YC. Biomarkers for mesothelioma. Curr Opin Pulm Med. 2007;13(4):339–443.

13

Breast Cancers

Fatemeh Derakhshan, Dara S. Ross and Fresia Pareja

13.1 Introduction

Breast cancer displays profound heterogeneity at the transcriptomic, genetic, and histologic levels (1, 2). Within this intricate molecular landscape, various transcriptomic subtypes have been recognized, each characterized by distinct biology, further distributed across the clinical subtypes of breast cancer, which show transcriptomic heterogeneity within each subtype (3–5). Notably, the recent recognition of HER2-low breast cancer has introduced an additional layer of heterogeneity to this complex disease (6, 7). The assessment of predictive biomarkers, such as estrogen receptors (ER), progesterone receptors (PR), and HER2, is conducted routinely in breast cancer, following the guidelines put forward by the American Society of Clinical Oncology/College of American Pathologists (ASCO/CAP) (8, 9). Beyond these biomarkers, an array of additional prognostic and predictive biomarkers are assessed through various methods, including immunohistochemistry (IHC), *in situ* hybridization, multigene expression assays, and genetic profiling.

From a genetic standpoint, various mutational processes are operative in breast cancer, among which the most predominant prevalent mutational signatures are aging/clock-like, homologous recombination deficiency (HRD) signatures, apolipoprotein B mRNA editing enzyme, and catalytic polypeptide (APOBEC) mutagenesis (10). ER-positive and ER-negative breast cancers are categorically different, with different mutational profiles (10). Large scale genomic studies that encompass all breast cancer subtypes irrespective of their histology revealed *TP53* and *PIK3CA* are the most frequently mutated genes, with *TP53* mutations being enriched in ER-negative breast cancer and *PIK3CA* in ER-positive disease (10, 11). There are, however, over 20 histologic subtypes of breast cancer, within both ER-positive and ER-negative subgroups (12). These subtypes are characterized by distinctive phenotypes and different behavior (2, 12, 13). Furthermore, unlike invasive ductal carcinoma of no special type (IDC-NST), the most common form of breast cancer, a subset of special histologic subtypes are characterized by specific or even pathognomonic genetic alterations (1, 2, 13). These unique associations give rise to key genotypic-phenotypic correlations in breast cancer, and their recognition and understanding are pivotal for refining the taxonomy of breast cancer and for identifying potential therapeutic targets. Other special histologic subtypes of breast cancer, while lacking pathognomonic genetic alterations, display distinct molecular profiles compared to IDC-NSTs (2, 12–14).

Furthermore, genetic profiling of breast cancer can serve as a valuable tool to identify actionable genetic alterations, as well as alterations associated with therapeutic resistance. Taken together, the genetic analysis of breast cancer is critical to overcome diagnostic challenges in breast pathology and to refine the breast cancer taxonomy, tailoring it towards the principles of precision medicine.

13.2 Genotypic-Phenotypic Correlations in Breast Cancer

Breast cancer exhibits vast histologic heterogeneity. In fact, IDC-NST is regarded as a diagnosis of exclusion when histologic criteria of a special histologic subtype are not met. The histologic complexity of breast cancer is underscored by the existence of over 20 special histologic subtypes, collectively constituting about 20% of all breast cancer cases (12). Special subtypes of breast cancers are characterized by distinctive histologic features, and a subset of them harbor specific or even pathognomonic genetic alterations (Figure 13.1 and Table 13.1). Notably, these genetic alterations are used to facilitate the diagnosis of these uncommon and challenging entities and can also be utilized as therapeutic targets (13).

13.2.1 Genotypic-Phenotypic Correlations in ER-Positive Breast Cancer

Several special histologic subtypes of breast cancer fall under the ER-positive umbrella of breast cancer, including tubular, mucinous, micropapillary, papillary, and lobular breast cancers and neuroendocrine tumors (12). While most of these subtypes lack a pathognomonic genetic alteration and do not constitute genotypic-phenotypic correlations, they are characterized by an array of genetic alterations that set them apart from common forms of breast cancer (1, 13). For instance, tubular breast cancers are characterized by a high frequency of *PIK3CA* mutations (13). Mucinous breast cancers lack concurrent 1q gains and 16q losses that characterize common forms of ER-positive breast cancer and rarely harbor mutations in *PIK3CA* and *TP53*, the most frequently altered genes in breast cancer (15, 16). Neuroendocrine tumors are genomically similar to mucinous carcinomas, lacking concurrent 1q gains/16q losses and *TP53* and *PIK3CA* mutations, and, in addition, they display enrichment in genetic alterations affecting chromatin remodeling genes (17, 18). In contrast,

DOI: 10.1201/9781003513469-13

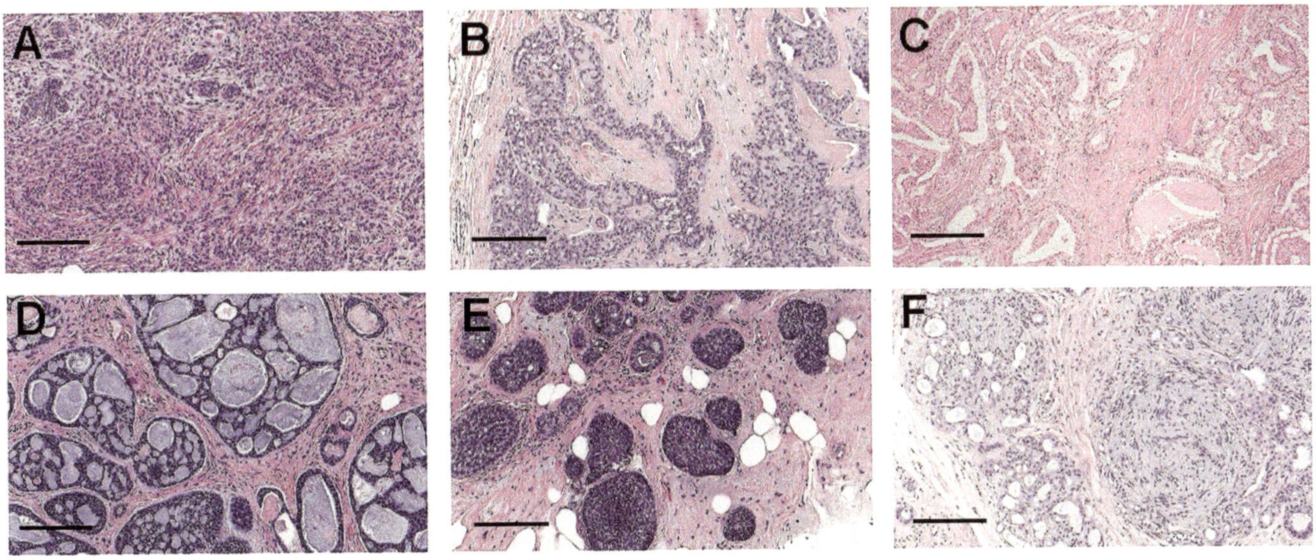

FIGURE 13.1 Representative hematoxylin and eosin (H&E) micrographs of (A) invasive lobular carcinoma, (B) secretory carcinoma, (C) tall cell carcinoma with reversed polarity, (D) classic adenoid cystic carcinoma, (E) solid and basaloid adenoid cystic carcinoma, and (F) adenomyoepithelioma. Scale bar, 200 micrometers.

TABLE 13.1

Genotypic-Phenotypic Correlations in Breast Cancer

Breast Cancer Special Histologic Subtype	Key Histologic Features	Pathognomonic Genetic Alteration	Other Genetic Characteristics
Invasive lobular carcinoma	Discohesive phenotype; composed of single cells or single cell files	*CDH1* bi-allelic inactivation (loss-of-function mutations, homozygous deletions, promoter methylation)	Enrichment in genetic alterations targeting the PI3K pathway, *ERBB2*, and *ERBB3* and transcription factors, such as *FOXA1* and *TBX3*
Secretory carcinoma	Abundant intracellular and extracellular secretions	*ETV6::NTRK3* fusion gene	Few copy number alterations, few genetic alterations affecting other cancer genes
Breast adenoid cystic carcinoma (AdCC)	–Classic: Composed of epithelial and myoepithelial cells arranged in cribriform, tubular or trabecular patterns –Solid-basaloid: Solid basaloid nests composed predominantly of epithelial cells	–Classic: *MYB::NFIB* fusion gene, *MYBL1* fusion genes, *MYB* amplifications –Solid basaloid: Lower frequency of *MYB/MYBL1* alterations. Enrichment in genetic alterations in *NOTCH* and chromatin remodeling genes	Genetic alterations in *NOTCH* genes and chromatin remodelers enriched in recurrent and metastatic AdCCs
Breast adenomyoepitheliomas (AME)	Biphasic proliferation of epithelial and myoepithelial cells; myoepithelial component is usually dominant	*HRAS* Q61 or G12/G13 hotspot mutations, coexisting with *PIK3CA* mutations in ER-negative AMEs	Recurrent genetic alterations in the PI3K pathway in ER-positive AMEs
Tall cell carcinoma with reversed polarity	Solid, papillary, and follicular growth pattern. Composed of tall cells with reversed polarization and nuclei resembling those of cells in the tall cell variant of papillary thyroid carcinoma	*IDH2* R172 hotspot mutations, coexisting with PI3K pathway genetic alterations	*TET2* loss-of-function mutations in cases lacking *IDH2* R172 hotspot mutations

invasive lobular carcinoma (ILC) is characterized by a hallmark genetic alteration and represents a strong genotypic-phenotypic correlation in breast cancer (12).

ILC is the second most common histologic subtype of breast cancer after IDC-NST, making up roughly 15% of all breast cancer cases (12). The histologic hallmark of ILC is its discohesive phenotype (12) (Figure 13.1A), caused by bi-allelic inactivation of *CDH1*, a tumor suppressor gene that maps to 16q22.1 and encodes E-cadherin, a critical component of the epithelial adhesion complex (19, 20). *CDH1* inactivation most commonly results from inactivating mutations associated with loss of heterozygosity (LOH) of the wild-type allele but can also be due to *CDH1* homozygous deletions or *CDH1* promoter methylation (19, 21, 22) (Table 13.1). E-cadherin protein expression is usually assessed in the diagnostic workup of ILC, and although most ILCs display loss or marked reduction in E-cadherin expression, a subset of cases display aberrant immunoreactivity, characterized by retention of E-cadherin expression or cytoplasmic expression (23, 24). Therefore, the identification of *CDH1* inactivating genetic alterations by next-generation sequencing (NGS) can aid in diagnosing ILC. NGS studies have shown that up to 15% to 20% of ILCs may lack *CDH1* inactivating genetic alterations despite displaying a distinctive lobular phenotype. At least a subset of these cases harbor genetic alterations affecting other key proteins playing crucial roles in the cell-cell adhesion process and interacting directly with E-cadherin, such as alpha-catenin (CTNNA1), suggesting that ILC constitutes a convergent phenotype (25).

ILCs harbor a repertoire of genetic alterations that differ from that of IDC-NSTs. ILCs are characterized by an enrichment of genetic alterations affecting the PI3K pathway, such as *PIK3CA* and *PTEN*; mutations affecting receptor tyrosine kinases, such as *ERBB2* and *ERBB3*; and genetic alterations affecting transcription factors such as *FOXA1*, *RUNX1*, and *TBX3* (19, 21, 22) (Table 13.1). Compared to primary ILCs, metastatic cases display a higher tumor mutation burden (TMB) and a statistically significantly higher frequency of genetic alterations affecting *ESR1*, *FAT1*, *RFWD2*, and *NF1*, as well as a numerically higher frequency of alterations affecting *ERBB2* (21, 26). Notably, *NF1* alterations have been reported arising in the setting of relapse following endocrine therapy, suggesting that these genetic alterations drive endocrine resistance (26). Metastatic ILCs also show enrichment in APOBEC mutagenesis, a process implicated in tumor hypermutation (27) that likely plays a role in resistance to endocrine therapy (28).

Notably, ILCs show a lower rate of pathologic complete response (pCR) following neoadjuvant chemotherapy (NACT) compared to IDC-NST (29). Moreover, when adjusted for covariates, no differences in survival were observed between neoadjuvant endocrine treatment (NET) and NACT in patients with node-positive ILC (30). Similarly, the combination of NET and CDK4/6 inhibitors did not show a clear efficacy specific to ILC (31). Novel therapies leveraging synthetic lethal interactions associated with E-cadherin deficiency, such as ROS1 inhibitors, are being investigated in ILC (32, 33).

13.2.2 Genotypic Phenotypic Correlations in ER-Negative Breast Cancer

ER-negative breast cancer encompasses an array of entities, including high-grade and low-grade neoplasms. High-grade ER-negative special histologic subtypes include entities such as high-grade forms of metaplastic breast cancer and apocrine breast cancer (12). These entities are characterized by high levels of genetic instability and lack of a pathognomonic genetic alteration (12). Low-grade forms of ER-negative breast cancer include various entities that histologically resemble their salivary gland counterparts and are characterized by pathognomonic or disease-defining genetic alterations (12, 34).

13.2.2.1 Secretory Carcinoma

Secretory carcinoma, previously called juvenile carcinoma, constitutes an exceedingly rare subtype of ER-negative breast cancer, with usually favorable clinical outcomes (12, 13). Secretory carcinomas display microcystic, solid, and/or tubular architectures and are composed of tumor cells with vacuolated cytoplasm and abundant intracellular and extracellular secretions (12) (Figure 13.1B). In contrast to common forms of breast cancer, secretory carcinomas have simple genomes, few copy number alterations, and a paucity of mutations affecting cancer genes, akin to other entities harboring highly recurrent or pathognomonic fusion genes (13, 34, 35). Like their counterparts in the salivary gland, mammary analogue secretory carcinomas of the salivary gland (MASC), secretory carcinomas of the breast are characterized by the translocation t(12;15) resulting in the *ETV6::NTRK3* fusion (36, 37) (Table 13.1). This pathognomonic genetic alteration can be detected by fluorescence in situ hybridization (FISH) or NGS. *NTRK1*, *NTRK2*, and *NTRK3* encode the tropomyosin receptor kinase A (TRKA), TRKB and TRKC, respectively. Upon binding of their cognate ligands, receptors phosphorylate and activate the oncogenic MAPK and PI3K pathways. Notably, immunohistochemical (IHC) assays using pan-TRK antibodies can be used diagnostically in a sensitive and specific manner to detect *NTRK* fusion genes (38, 39).

13.2.2.2 Tall Cell Carcinoma with Reversed Polarity

Tall cell carcinomas with reversed polarity (TCCRPs) are vanishingly rare breast cancers, now included in the WHO classification (12). TCCRPs display distinctive histologic features that resemble those of the tall cell variant of papillary thyroid carcinomas (Figure 13.1C). These neoplasms show a solid, papillary, and follicular architecture and are composed of tall columnar cells showing reversed polarization, that is, apical location of their nuclei. Notably, akin to papillary thyroid carcinoma, TCCRPs show clear nuclei, nuclear grooves, and intranuclear inclusions (13, 40). TCCRPs have a unique genetic makeup, as they harbor recurrent *IDH2* R172 hotspot mutations that in most cases coexist with genetic alterations affecting the PI3K pathway (41–43) (Table 13.1). Notably, TCCRPs lacking *IDH2* R172 mutations were found to harbor loss-of-function mutations affecting *TET2* (41) (Table 13.1). Importantly, *IDH2* R172 mutations are extremely rare in other breast cancers (13), and their detection by NGS can facilitate the diagnosis of this rare and challenging entity. Notably, IHC assays using mutation-specific antibodies can detect the presence of *IDH2* R172 hotspot mutations in a highly sensitive and specific manner (44).

13.2.2.3 Breast Adenoid Cystic Carcinoma

Breast adenoid cystic carcinomas (AdCCs) are vanishingly rare, accounting for less than 0.1% of all breast cancers (45). These are biphasic epithelial-myoepithelial tumors that histologically resemble AdCCs from other anatomic locations (12). The classic form of AdCC displays various architectures, such as cribriform, tubular, or trabecular (12) (Figure 13.1D). Akin to AdCCs arising in other organ systems, the majority of breast classic AdCCs are underpinned by the translocation t(6;9), resulting in the *MYB::NFIB* gene fusion (46, 47) (Table 13.1). Notably, breast AdCCs lacking the *MYB::NFIB* fusion gene have alternative genetic alterations affecting the MYB pathway, such as fusion genes affecting *MYBL1*, a paralog of *MYB*, or harbor *MYB* gene amplification (48) (Table 13.1), indicating that these tumors might represent a convergent phenotype (13). *MYB* or *MYBL1* fusion genes are detectable by fluorescence in situ hybridization

(FISH) or NGS. Notably, AdCCs display MYB overexpression, detectably by IHC (13).

Solid and basaloid AdCC (SB-AdCC) is an aggressive form of AdCC featuring a solid-basaloid architecture, a higher histologic grade, and more frequent nodal and distant metastases than classic AdCC(12) (Figure 13.1E). In comparison to classic AdCCs that have *MYB* or *MYBL1* rearrangements in over 80% of cases, SB-AdCCs less frequently harbor these genetic alterations (~20%) (49) (Table 13.1). In addition, SB-AdCCs display enrichment in genetic alterations affecting *NOTCH* genes and chromatin remodelers (49–51) (Table 13.1). Although classic breast AdCCs are usually indolent, recurrences and distant metastases have been documented (46, 52–54). Notably, the overall survival and disease-free survival of patients with SB-AdCC are markedly shorter than those of patients with breast classic AdCC (49). Recurrences and metastasis in breast AdCC have been associated with an enrichment in mutations targeting *NOTCH* genes and chromatin remodelers, and the identification of these genetic alterations in the recurrent and metastatic setting predicts a poor outcome (55). The utility of CB-103, an oral pan-Notch inhibitor that downregulates the transcriptional activity of the oncogenic Notch pathway, is currently being investigated in AdCC in the advanced clinical setting, with promising results (56).

The Food and Drug Administration (FDA) has approved the use of selective TRK inhibitors, such as larotrectinib and entrectinib, for the treatment of patients with pediatric or adult solid tumors harboring *NTRK* gene fusions, irrespective of anatomic location (57, 58). The use of TRK inhibitors in patients with recurrent or metastatic breast secretory carcinomas has been shown to result in profound and long-lasting effects (58–61).

13.2.2.4 Adenomyoepitheliomas of the Breast

Adenomyoepitheliomas of the breast are rare epithelial-myoepithelial neoplasms that encompass ER-positive and ER-negative tumors (12, 62) (Figure 13.1F). Although most adenomyoepitheliomas are benign, atypical and malignant lesions exist and can be associated with recurrences or distant metastasis (12). The mutational repertoire of adenomyoepitheliomas varies with their ER status (63). Adenomyoepitheliomas that express ER are usually of lower histologic grade and harbor recurrent genetic alterations affecting the PI3K pathway, such as *PIK3CA* or *AKT1* mutations (63) (Table 13.1). In contrast, ER-negative adenomyoepitheliomas, usually of higher histologic grade, are characterized by recurrent *HRAS* Q61 hotspot mutations that often co-occur with PI3K pathway genetic alterations, such as *PIK3CA* or *PIK3R1* mutations (63) (Table 13.1). Notably, in a breast-specific context, *HRAS* mutations are pathognomonic for adenomyoepitheliomas, and therefore their detection by NGS or other molecular tests can be used to facilitate the diagnosis of this challenging entity. In addition, *HRAS* Q61 mutations can be detected by IHC in a highly specific and moderately sensitive manner using mutation-specific antibodies (64).

Malignant adenomyoepitheliomas also harbor oncogenic driver mutations in *HRAS* Q61 hotspot mutations and *PIK3CA* mutations (65). In addition, *HRAS* G13 and G12 hotspot mutations have also been reported in these tumors (66). Chemotherapy has been used to treat patients with malignant adenomyoepitheliomas at advanced stages, with poor outcomes (66). Preclinical studies using patient-derived xenografts (PDX) from *HRAS*-mutant adenomyoepitheliomas showed that targeting the Ras/RAF/MEK/ERK signaling pathway with the FDA-approved MEK inhibitor trametinib exhibited significant anti-tumor activity, illustrating how *HRAS* mutations might constitute a rational therapeutic target in these neoplasms (66).

13.2.2.5 Clinically Relevant Biomarkers in Breast Cancer

The most significant genetic alterations in breast cancer from a clinical perspective are described and reviewed in the following sections.

13.2.3 Targetable Genetic Alterations in Breast Cancer

ERBB2 encodes the transmembrane tyrosine kinase receptor HER2 and is amplified and overexpressed in about a fourth of all breast cancers (67, 68). Following the ASCO/CAP guidelines (9), *ERBB2*/HER2 assessment is conducted using IHC and/or FISH or other *in situ* hybridization (ISH) (69). It is worth noting that *ERBB2* copy number alterations can be robustly assessed using NGS (70). *ERBB2* amplification in breast cancer predicts response to anti-HER2 therapy, in the primary and metastatic settings (9). FDA-approved agents for the management of HER2-positive disease include trastuzumab, pertuzumab, the antibody-drug conjugates (ADC) trastuzumab emtansine (T-DM1), trastuzumab deruxtecan (T-DXd), and the tyrosine kinase inhibitors lapatinib and neratinib (71). They all have shown marked improvements in disease-free and overall survival of these patients (72–79). Mutations affecting *ERBB2* occur in a small subset of breast cancer but appear to be enriched in invasive lobular breast cancer (80, 81), and are associated with HER2-positive, HER2-negative, and HER2-low status (80, 82–85). *ERBB2* mutations are enriched in exon 8 affecting the extracellular domain and exons 19–20, affecting the tyrosine kinase domain (80). *ERBB2* L755S mutations were found to be causative of resistance to the reversible tyrosine kinase inhibitor lapatinib and associated with sensitivity to the irreversible inhibitor neratinib (80). In the SUMMIT basket trial, neratinib showed remarkable activity in breast patients with *ERBB2* mutations in the extracellular and kinase domains (86).

Genetic alterations affecting key members of the PI3K pathway constitute actionable alterations in breast cancer. *PIK3CA* mutations result in activation of the oncogenic AKT/mTOR signaling pathway (87) and are a prevalent genetic alteration in breast cancer, being found particularly enriched in luminal and HER2-enriched molecular subtypes (11). Mutations in *PIK3CA* affect primarily exon 9 (helical domain) and exon 20 (kinase domain) (1). The use of Alpelisib, a PI3K inhibitor, is FDA approved in combination with the selective estrogen receptor degrader fulvestrant for post-menopausal patients with ER-positive/HER2-negative advanced or metastatic breast cancer harboring *PIK3CA* mutations that progressed upon treatment with hormonal therapy (88). Detection of *PIK3CA* mutations can be conducted by NGS or using the FDA-cleared companion diagnostic test based on the *PIK3CA* Rotor Gene Q (RGQ) PCR Kit for FFPE tissue and/or a liquid biopsy (69). *AKT* and *PTEN* genetic alterations also result in activation of the PI3K signaling pathway. Genetic alterations in *AKT1* and *PTEN* are found in approximately 5% of breast cancers each (89–92). AZD5363, an AKT1, -2, and -3 inhibitor, showed promising results for breast cancers harboring *AKT1*, *PIK3CA*, or *PTEN* mutations in the advanced or metastatic setting (93). Notably, inactivating *PTEN* mutations have been identified as causative of resistance to the PI3K inhibitor alpesilib (94).

A subset of breast cancers harbor genetic alterations affecting homologous recombination deficiency (HRD) genes, such as *BRCA1* and *BRCA2* (12). Blocking the function of polyadenosine diphosphate-ribose polymerase (PARP) with PARP inhibitors (PARPi) results in the selective targeting of *BRCA1/2*-deficient cancer cells, and PARPi have shown antitumor activity in patients with early and advanced breast cancer with *BRCA1/2* germline mutations (95). Mutational signature analysis can aid in the detection of HRD in breast cancer. HRDetect (96) is a bioinformatic tool that predicts BRCA1 and BRCA2 deficiency and could facilitate the triage of tumors that would be sensitive to PARPi (97).

13.2.4 Genetic Alterations Associated with Therapeutic Resistance in Breast Cancer

ESR1 encodes ER-alpha that is expressed in approximately 75% of breast cancers (12). Hormone therapy in the form of estrogen deprivation therapy, such as aromatase inhibitors or gonadotropin-releasing hormone agonists, and direct ER inhibitors, such as selective ER modulators and degraders, is effective for patients with ER-positive breast cancer (98, 99). *ESR1* mutations, detectable in tissues or liquid biopsies, however, can result in its constitutive activation and resistance to these therapies (100–103). *ESR1* D538G and Y537S mutations are the most common ones and are associated with worse outcomes (103). Other molecular mechanisms of endocrine resistance include mutations in *ERBB2* and *NF1*; in other MAPK genes, such as *KRAS* and *EGFR*; and in ER transcriptional regulators, such as *FOXA1*, *TBX3*, *MYC*, and *CTCF* (104).

FGFR1 amplification has also been implicated in resistance to endocrine therapies (105). CDK4/6 inhibitors, such as palbociclib, ribociclib, and abemaciclib, are routinely used for ER-positive breast cancer. Inactivating *RB1* genetic alterations, however, results in resistance to these agents.

13.3 Conclusions and Future Perspectives

Breast cancer is a complex and multifaceted disease. The recognition of genotypic-phenotypic correlations in breast cancer carries profound implications not only for diagnosis but also for the development of targeted therapeutic approaches. Precision medicine strategies are constantly evolving, and the discovery of actionable genetic alterations has transformed therapeutic paradigms. The integration of artificial intelligence (AI) in pathology holds great potential for refining breast cancer taxonomy and unearthing novel therapeutic targets. AI-based approaches are poised to revolutionize how we practice breast pathology and inform therapeutic decision making.

In recent years, we have witnessed a surge in efforts to harness AI-based approaches for a broad range of applications in breast pathology, such as the development of breast cancer classification systems, histologic grading, the automation of biomarker expression assessment from IHC, prediction of biomarker expression, and genetic alterations from hematoxylin and eosin (H&E) whole slide images, among others (106–111). Deployment of AI-based solutions as a real-time tool in diagnostic practice routine holds promise to enhance the robustness of pathologic diagnosis and simplify the workflow of breast pathology practice (112, 113). For instance, AI-based assessment of tumor infiltrating lymphocytes (TILs), a robust biomarker in breast cancer associated with increased overall survival and response to chemotherapy (114), shows promising results (106). Another example pertains to the detection of HER2-low breast cancer, whose recognition has unlocked new therapeutic opportunities and reshaped the landscape of breast cancer treatment through the utilization of ADCs (7). Efforts to develop algorithms for reducing interobserver variability in the identification of HER2-low cases through the assessment of immunohistochemically stained slides and to predict the expression of HER2 from H&E whole slide images are ongoing (115–117).

REFERENCES

1. Ross DS, Pareja F. Molecular pathology of breast tumors: Diagnostic and actionable genetic alterations. Surg Pathol Clin. 2021;14(3):455–471.
2. Rakha EA, Pareja FG. New advances in molecular breast cancer pathology. Semin Cancer Biol. 2021;72:102–113.
3. Zagami P, Carey LA. Triple negative breast cancer: Pitfalls and progress. NPJ Breast Cancer. 2022;8(1):95.
4. Anderson WF, Rosenberg PS, Prat A, et al. How many etiological subtypes of breast cancer: Two, three, four, or more? J Natl Cancer Inst. 2014;106(8):dju165.
5. Prat A, Adamo B, Cheang MC, et al. Molecular characterization of basal-like and non-basal-like triple-negative breast cancer. Oncologist. 2013;18(2):123–133.
6. Nicolo E, Tarantino P, Curigliano G. Biology and treatment of HER2-low breast cancer. Hematol Oncol Clin North Am. 2023;37(1):117–132.
7. Tarantino P, Viale G, Press MF, et al. ESMO expert consensus statements (ECS) on the definition, diagnosis, and management of HER2-low breast cancer. Ann Oncol. 2023;34(8):645–659.
8. Allison KH, Hammond MEH, Dowsett M, et al. Estrogen and progesterone receptor testing in breast cancer: ASCO/CAP guideline update. J Clin Oncol. 2020;38(12):1346–1366.
9. Wolff AC, Hammond MEH, Allison KH, et al. Human epidermal growth factor receptor 2 testing in breast cancer: American Society of Clinical Oncology/College of American Pathologists Clinical Practice Guideline Focused Update. J Clin Oncol. 2018;36(20):2105–2122.
10. Nik-Zainal S, Davies H, Staaf J, et al. Landscape of somatic mutations in 560 breast cancer whole-genome sequences. Nature. 2016;534(7605):47–54.
11. Cancer Genome Atlas N. Comprehensive molecular portraits of human breast tumours. Nature. 2012;490(7418):61–70.
12. WHO Classification of Tumors Editorial Board. Breast tumours. WHO Classification of Tumors. 5th ed. Lyon: IARC, 2019.

13. Pareja F, Weigelt B, Reis-Filho JS. Problematic breast tumors reassessed in light of novel molecular data. Mod Pathol. 2021;34(Suppl 1):38–47.
14. Ross DS, Liu B, Schram AM, et al. Enrichment of kinase fusions in ESR1 wild-type, metastatic breast cancer revealed by a systematic analysis of 4854 patients. Ann Oncol. 2020;31(8):991–1000.
15. Pareja F, Lee JY, Brown DN, et al. The Genomic Landscape of Mucinous Breast Cancer. J Natl Cancer Inst. 2019;111(7):737–741.
16. Nguyen B, Veys I, Leduc S, et al. Genomic, transcriptomic, epigenetic, and immune profiling of mucinous breast cancer. J Natl Cancer Inst. 2019;111(7):742–746.
17. Pareja F, D'Alfonso TM. Neuroendocrine neoplasms of the breast: A review focused on the updated World Health Organization (WHO) 5th Edition morphologic classification. Breast J. 2020;26(6):1160–1167.
18. Pareja F, Vahdatinia M, Marchio C, et al. Neuroendocrine tumours of the breast: A genomic comparison with mucinous breast cancers and neuroendocrine tumours of other anatomic sites. J Clin Pathol. 2022;75(1):10–17.
19. Ciriello G, Gatza ML, Beck AH, et al. Comprehensive molecular portraits of invasive lobular breast cancer. Cell. 2015;163(2):506–519.
20. Caldeira JR, Prando EC, Quevedo FC, et al. CDH1 promoter hypermethylation and E-cadherin protein expression in infiltrating breast cancer. BMC Cancer. 2006;6:48.
21. Pareja F, Ferrando L, Lee SSK, et al. The genomic landscape of metastatic histologic special types of invasive breast cancer. NPJ Breast Cancer. 2020;6:53.
22. Desmedt C, Zoppoli G, Gundem G, et al. Genomic characterization of primary invasive lobular breast cancer. J Clin Oncol. 2016;34(16):1872–1881.
23. Da Silva L, Parry S, Reid L, et al. Aberrant expression of E-cadherin in lobular carcinomas of the breast. Am J Surg Pathol. 2008;32(5):773–783.
24. Grabenstetter A, Mohanty AS, Rana S, et al. E-cadherin immunohistochemical expression in invasive lobular carcinoma of the breast: Correlation with morphology and CDH1 somatic alterations. Hum Pathol. 2020;102:44–53.
25. de Groot JS, Ratze MA, van Amersfoort M, et al. alphaE-catenin is a candidate tumor suppressor for the development of E-cadherin-expressing lobular-type breast cancer. J Pathol. 2018;245(4):456–467.
26. Sokol ES, Feng YX, Jin DX, et al. Loss of function of NF1 is a mechanism of acquired resistance to endocrine therapy in lobular breast cancer. Ann Oncol. 2019;30(1):115–123.
27. Roberts SA, Gordenin DA. Hypermutation in human cancer genomes: Footprints and mechanisms. Nat Rev Cancer. 2014;14(12):786–800.
28. Sammons S, Raskina K, Danziger N, et al. APOBEC mutational signatures in hormone receptor-positive human epidermal growth factor receptor 2-negative breast cancers are associated with poor outcomes on CDK4/6 inhibitors and endocrine therapy. JCO Precis Oncol. 2022;6:e2200149.
29. Straver ME, Rutgers EJ, Rodenhuis S, et al. The relevance of breast cancer subtypes in the outcome of neoadjuvant chemotherapy. Ann Surg Oncol. 2010;17(9):2411–2418.
30. Thornton MJ, Williamson HV, Westbrook KE, et al. Neoadjuvant endocrine therapy versus neoadjuvant chemotherapy in node-positive invasive lobular carcinoma. Ann Surg Oncol. 2019;26(10):3166–3177.
31. Cottu P, D'Hondt V, Dureau S, et al. Letrozole and palbociclib versus chemotherapy as neoadjuvant therapy of high-risk luminal breast cancer. Ann Oncol. 2018;29(12):2334–2340.
32. Van Baelen K, Geukens T, Maetens M, et al. Current and future diagnostic and treatment strategies for patients with invasive lobular breast cancer. Ann Oncol. 2022;33(8):769–785.
33. Bajrami I, Marlow R, van de Ven M, et al. E-cadherin/ROS1 inhibitor synthetic lethality in breast cancer. Cancer Discov. 2018;8(4):498–515.
34. Pareja F, Geyer FC, Marchio C, et al. Triple-negative breast cancer: The importance of molecular and histologic subtyping, and recognition of low-grade variants. NPJ Breast Cancer. 2016;2:16036.
35. Krings G, Joseph NM, Bean GR, et al. Genomic profiling of breast secretory carcinomas reveals distinct genetics from other breast cancers and similarity to mammary analog secretory carcinomas. Mod Pathol. 2017;30(8):1086–1099.
36. Tognon C, Knezevich SR, Huntsman D, et al. Expression of the ETV6-NTRK3 gene fusion as a primary event in human secretory breast carcinoma. Cancer Cell. 2002;2(5):367–376.
37. Skalova A, Vanecek T, Sima R, et al. Mammary analogue secretory carcinoma of salivary glands, containing the ETV6-NTRK3 fusion gene: A hitherto undescribed salivary gland tumor entity. Am J Surg Pathol. 2010;34(5):599–608.
38. Harrison BT, Fowler E, Krings G, et al. Pan-TRK immunohistochemistry: A useful diagnostic adjunct for secretory carcinoma of the breast. Am J Surg Pathol. 2019;43(12):1693–1700.
39. Hechtman JF, Benayed R, Hyman DM, et al. Pan-Trk immunohistochemistry is an efficient and reliable screen for the detection of NTRK fusions. Am J Surg Pathol. 2017;41(11):1547–1551.
40. Masood S, Davis C, Kubik MJ. Changing the term "breast tumor resembling the tall cell variant of papillary thyroid carcinoma" to "tall cell variant of papillary breast carcinoma". Adv Anat Pathol. 2012;19(2):108–110.
41. Chiang S, Weigelt B, Wen HC, et al. IDH2 mutations define a unique subtype of breast cancer with altered nuclear polarity. Cancer Res. 2016;76(24):7118–7129.
42. Zhong E, Scognamiglio T, D'Alfonso T, et al. Breast tumor resembling the tall cell variant of papillary thyroid carcinoma: Molecular characterization by next-generation sequencing and histopathological comparison with tall cell papillary carcinoma of thyroid. Int J Surg Pathol. 2019;27(2):134–141.
43. Bhargava R, Florea AV, Pelmus M, et al. Breast tumor resembling tall cell variant of papillary thyroid carcinoma: A solid papillary neoplasm with characteristic immunohistochemical profile and few recurrent mutations. Am J Clin Pathol. 2017;147(4):399–410.
44. Pareja F, da Silva EM, Frosina D, et al. Immunohistochemical analysis of IDH2 R172 hotspot mutations in breast papillary neoplasms: Applications in the diagnosis of tall cell carcinoma with reverse polarity. Mod Pathol. 2020;33(6):1056–1064.
45. Marchio C, Weigelt B, Reis-Filho JS. Adenoid cystic carcinomas of the breast and salivary glands (or 'The strange case of Dr Jekyll and Mr Hyde' of exocrine gland carcinomas). J Clin Pathol. 2010;63(3):220–228.
46. D'Alfonso TM, Mosquera JM, MacDonald TY, et al. MYB-NFIB gene fusion in adenoid cystic carcinoma of the breast with special focus paid to the solid variant with basaloid features. Hum Pathol. 2014;45(11):2270–2280.
47. Persson M, Andren Y, Mark J, et al. Recurrent fusion of MYB and NFIB transcription factor genes in carcinomas of the breast and head and neck. Proc Natl Acad Sci U S A. 2009;106(44):18740–18744.

48. Kim J, Geyer FC, Martelotto LG, et al. MYBL1 rearrangements and MYB amplification in breast adenoid cystic carcinomas lacking the MYB-NFIB fusion gene. J Pathol. 2018;244(2):143–150.
49. Schwartz CJ, Brogi E, Marra A, et al. The clinical behavior and genomic features of the so-called adenoid cystic carcinomas of the solid variant with basaloid features. Mod Pathol. 2022;35(2):193–201.
50. Masse J, Truntzer C, Boidot R, et al. Solid-type adenoid cystic carcinoma of the breast, a distinct molecular entity enriched in NOTCH and CREBBP mutations. Mod Pathol. 2020;33(6):1041–1055.
51. Shamir ER, Bean GR, Schwartz CJ, et al. Solid-basaloid adenoid cystic carcinoma of the breast: An aggressive subtype enriched for Notch pathway and chromatin modifier mutations with MYB overexpression. Mod Pathol. 2023;36(12):100324.
52. Derakhshan F, Reis-Filho JS. Pathogenesis of triple-negative breast cancer. Annu Rev Pathol. 2022;17:181–204.
53. Fusco N, Geyer FC, De Filippo MR, et al. Genetic events in the progression of adenoid cystic carcinoma of the breast to high-grade triple-negative breast cancer. Mod Pathol. 2016;29(11):1292–1305.
54. Solek JM, Braun M, Kalwas M, et al. Adenoid cystic carcinoma of the breast—an uncommon malignancy with unpredictable clinical behaviour. A case series of three patients. Contemp Oncol (Pozn). 2020;24(4):263–265.
55. Ho AS, Ochoa A, Jayakumaran G, et al. Genetic hallmarks of recurrent/metastatic adenoid cystic carcinoma. J Clin Invest. 2019;129(10):4276–4289.
56. Hanna GJ, Stathis A, Lopez-Miranda E, et al. A phase I study of the pan-Notch inhibitor CB-103 for patients with advanced adenoid cystic carcinoma and other tumors. Cancer Res Commun. 2023;3(9):1853–1861.
57. Amatu A, Sartore-Bianchi A, Siena S. NTRK gene fusions as novel targets of cancer therapy across multiple tumour types. ESMO Open. 2016;1(2):e000023.
58. Drilon A, Laetsch TW, Kummar S, et al. Efficacy of larotrectinib in TRK fusion-positive cancers in adults and children. N Engl J Med. 2018;378(8):731–739.
59. Laetsch TW, DuBois SG, Mascarenhas L, et al. Larotrectinib for paediatric solid tumours harbouring NTRK gene fusions: Phase 1 results from a multicentre, open-label, phase 1/2 study. Lancet Oncol. 2018;19(5):705–714.
60. Drilon A, Siena S, Ou SI, et al. Safety and antitumor activity of the multitargeted pan-TRK, ROS1, and ALK inhibitor entrectinib: Combined results from two Phase I trials (ALKA-372-001 and STARTRK-1). Cancer Discov. 2017;7(4):400–409.
61. Shukla N, Roberts SS, Baki MO, et al. Successful targeted therapy of refractory pediatric ETV6-NTRK3 fusion-positive secretory breast carcinoma. JCO Precis Oncol. 2017;2017: PO.17.00034.
62. Nadelman CM, Leslie KO, Fishbein MC. "Benign," metastasizing adenomyoepithelioma of the breast: A report of 2 cases. Arch Pathol Lab Med. 2006;130(9):1349–1353.
63. Geyer FC, Li A, Papanastasiou AD, et al. Recurrent hotspot mutations in HRAS Q61 and PI3K-AKT pathway genes as drivers of breast adenomyoepitheliomas. Nat Commun. 2018;9(1):1816.
64. Pareja F, Toss MS, Geyer FC, et al. Immunohistochemical assessment of HRAS Q61R mutations in breast adenomyoepitheliomas. Histopathology. 2020;76(6):865–874.
65. Baum JE, Sung KJ, Tran H, et al. Mammary epithelial-myoepithelial carcinoma: Report of a case with HRAS and PIK3CA mutations by next-generation sequencing. Int J Surg Pathol. 2019;27(4):441–445.
66. Bieche I, Coussy F, El-Botty R, et al. HRAS is a therapeutic target in malignant chemo-resistant adenomyoepithelioma of the breast. J Hematol Oncol. 2021;14(1):143.
67. Slamon DJ, Clark GM, Wong SG, et al. Human breast cancer: Correlation of relapse and survival with amplification of the HER-2/neu oncogene. Science. 1987;235(4785):177–182.
68. Slamon DJ, Godolphin W, Jones LA, et al. Studies of the HER-2/neu proto-oncogene in human breast and ovarian cancer. Science. 1989;244(4905):707–712.
69. U.S. Food and Drug Administration. List of cleared or approved companion diagnostic devices (in vitro and imaging tools). Accessed on November 1, 2023: www.fda.gov/medical-devices/vitro-diagnostics/list-cleared-or-approved-companion-diagnostic-devices-vitro-and-imaging-tools.
70. Ross DS, Zehir A, Cheng DT, et al. Next-generation assessment of human epidermal growth factor receptor 2 (ERBB2) amplification status: Clinical validation in the context of a hybrid capture-based, comprehensive solid tumor genomic profiling assay. J Mol Diagn. 2017;19(2):244–254.
71. U.S. Food and Drug Administration. Drugs@FDA: FDA-approved drugs. Accessed on November 1, 2023: www.accessdata.fda.gov/scripts/cder/daf/index.cfm.
72. Piccart-Gebhart MJ, Procter M, Leyland-Jones B, et al. Trastuzumab after adjuvant chemotherapy in HER2-positive breast cancer. N Engl J Med. 2005;353(16):1659–1672.
73. Romond EH, Perez EA, Bryant J, et al. Trastuzumab plus adjuvant chemotherapy for operable HER2-positive breast cancer. N Engl J Med. 2005;353(16):1673–1684.
74. Slamon D, Eiermann W, Robert N, et al. Adjuvant trastuzumab in HER2-positive breast cancer. N Engl J Med. 2011;365(14):1273–1283.
75. Perez EA, Romond EH, Suman VJ, et al. Trastuzumab plus adjuvant chemotherapy for human epidermal growth factor receptor 2-positive breast cancer: Planned joint analysis of overall survival from NSABP B-31 and NCCTG N9831. J Clin Oncol. 2014;32(33):3744–3752.
76. von Minckwitz G, Procter M, de Azambuja E, et al. Adjuvant pertuzumab and trastuzumab in early HER2-positive breast cancer. N Engl J Med. 2017;377(2):122–131.
77. von Minckwitz G, Huang CS, Mano MS, et al. Trastuzumab emtansine for residual invasive HER2-positive breast cancer. N Engl J Med. 2019;380(7):617–628.
78. Tapia M, Hernando C, Martinez MT, et al. Clinical impact of new treatment strategies for HER2-positive metastatic breast cancer patients with resistance to classical anti-HER therapies. Cancers (Basel). 2023;15(18):4522.
79. Antonarelli G, Corti C, Tarantino P, et al. Management of patients with HER2-positive metastatic breast cancer after trastuzumab deruxtecan failure. ESMO Open. 2023;8(4):101608.
80. Bose R, Kavuri SM, Searleman AC, et al. Activating HER2 mutations in HER2 gene amplification negative breast cancer. Cancer Discov. 2013;3(2):224–237.
81. Gaibar M, Beltran L, Romero-Lorca A, et al. Somatic mutations in HER2 and implications for current treatment paradigms in HER2-positive breast cancer. J Oncol. 2020;2020:6375956.
82. Kurozumi S, Alsaleem M, Monteiro CJ, et al. Targetable ERBB2 mutation status is an independent marker of adverse prognosis in estrogen receptor positive, ERBB2 non-amplified primary lobular breast carcinoma: A retrospective in silico analysis of public datasets. Breast Cancer Res. 2020;22(1):85.

83. Petrelli F, Tomasello G, Barni S, et al. Clinical and pathological characterization of HER2 mutations in human breast cancer: A systematic review of the literature. Breast Cancer Res Treat. 2017;166(2):339–349.
84. Subramanian J, Katta A, Masood A, et al. Emergence of ERBB2 mutation as a biomarker and an actionable target in solid cancers. Oncologist. 2019;24(12):e1303–e1314.
85. Berrino E, Annaratone L, Bellomo SE, et al. Integrative genomic and transcriptomic analyses illuminate the ontology of HER2-low breast carcinomas. Genome Med. 2022;14(1):98.
86. Hyman DM, Piha-Paul SA, Won H, et al. HER kinase inhibition in patients with HER2- and HER3-mutant cancers. Nature. 2018;554(7691):189–194.
87. Bader AG, Kang S, Zhao L, et al. Oncogenic PI3K deregulates transcription and translation. Nat Rev Cancer. 2005;5(12):921–929.
88. Andre F, Ciruelos E, Rubovszky G, et al. Alpelisib for PIK3CA-mutated, hormone receptor-positive advanced breast cancer. N Engl J Med. 2019;380(20):1929–1940.
89. Bleeker FE, Felicioni L, Buttitta F, et al. AKT1(E17K) in human solid tumours. Oncogene. 2008;27(42):5648–5650.
90. Kim MS, Jeong EG, Yoo NJ, et al. Mutational analysis of oncogenic AKT E17K mutation in common solid cancers and acute leukaemias. Br J Cancer. 2008;98(9):1533–1535.
91. Rudolph M, Anzeneder T, Schulz A, et al. AKT1 (E17K) mutation profiling in breast cancer: Prevalence, concurrent oncogenic alterations, and blood-based detection. BMC Cancer. 2016;16:622.
92. Bazzichetto C, Conciatori F, Pallocca M, et al. PTEN as a prognostic/predictive biomarker in cancer: An unfulfilled promise? Cancers (Basel). 2019;11(4):435.
93. Hyman DM, Smyth LM, Donoghue MTA, et al. AKT inhibition in solid tumors with AKT1 mutations. J Clin Oncol. 2017;35(20):2251–2259.
94. Razavi P, Dickler MN, Shah PD, et al. Alterations in PTEN and ESR1 promote clinical resistance to alpelisib plus aromatase inhibitors. Nat Cancer. 2020;1(4):382–393.
95. Litton JK, Rugo HS, Ettl J, et al. Talazoparib in patients with advanced breast cancer and a germline BRCA mutation. N Engl J Med. 2018;379(8):753–763.
96. Davies H, Glodzik D, Morganella S, et al. HRDetect is a predictor of BRCA1 and BRCA2 deficiency based on mutational signatures. Nat Med. 2017;23(4):517–525.
97. Lord CJ, Ashworth A. BRCAness revisited. Nat Rev Cancer. 2016;16(2):110–120.
98. Early Breast Cancer Trialists' Collaborative Group. Effects of chemotherapy and hormonal therapy for early breast cancer on recurrence and 15-year survival: An overview of the randomised trials. Lancet. 2005;365(9472):1687–1717.
99. Mouridsen H, Gershanovich M, Sun Y, et al. Phase III study of letrozole versus tamoxifen as first-line therapy of advanced breast cancer in postmenopausal women: Analysis of survival and update of efficacy from the International Letrozole Breast Cancer Group. J Clin Oncol. 2003;21(11):2101–2109.
100. Toy W, Shen Y, Won H, et al. ESR1 ligand-binding domain mutations in hormone-resistant breast cancer. Nat Genet. 2013;45(12):1439–1445.
101. Robinson DR, Wu YM, Vats P, et al. Activating ESR1 mutations in hormone-resistant metastatic breast cancer. Nat Genet. 2013;45(12):1446–1451.
102. Fribbens C, O'Leary B, Kilburn L, et al. Plasma ESR1 mutations and the treatment of estrogen receptor-positive advanced breast cancer. J Clin Oncol. 2016;34(25):2961–1968.
103. Chandarlapaty S, Chen D, He W, et al. Prevalence of ESR1 mutations in cell-free DNA and outcomes in metastatic breast cancer: A secondary analysis of the BOLERO-2 clinical trial. JAMA Oncol. 2016;2(10):1310–1315.
104. Razavi P, Chang MT, Xu G, et al. The genomic landscape of endocrine-resistant advanced breast cancers. Cancer Cell. 2018;34(3):427–438.e6.
105. Turner N, Pearson A, Sharpe R, et al. FGFR1 amplification drives endocrine therapy resistance and is a therapeutic target in breast cancer. Cancer Res. 2010;70(5):2085–2094.
106. Thagaard J, Broeckx G, Page DB, et al. Pitfalls in machine learning-based assessment of tumor-infiltrating lymphocytes in breast cancer: A report of the International Immuno-Oncology Biomarker Working Group on Breast Cancer. J Pathol. 2023;260(5):498–513.
107. Verghese G, Lennerz JK, Ruta D, et al. Computational pathology in cancer diagnosis, prognosis, and prediction—present day and prospects. J Pathol. 2023;260(5):551–563.
108. Liu Y, Han D, Parwani AV, Li Z. Applications of artificial intelligence in breast pathology. Arch Pathol Lab Med. 2023;147(9):1003–1013.
109. Rakha EA, Vougas K, Tan PH. Digital technology in diagnostic breast pathology and immunohistochemistry. Pathobiology. 2022;89(5):334–342.
110. Yousif M, van Diest PJ, Laurinavicius A, et al. Artificial intelligence applied to breast pathology. Virchows Arch. 2022;480(1):191–209.
111. Ibrahim A, Lashen A, Toss M, et al. Assessment of mitotic activity in breast cancer: Revisited in the digital pathology era. J Clin Pathol. 2022;75(6):365–372.
112. Sandbank J, Bataillon G, Nudelman A, et al. Validation and real-world clinical application of an artificial intelligence algorithm for breast cancer detection in biopsies. NPJ Breast Cancer. 2022;8(1):129.
113. Rakha EA, Toss M, Shiino S, et al. Current and future applications of artificial intelligence in pathology: A clinical perspective. J Clin Pathol. 2021;74(7):409–414.
114. Savas P, Salgado R, Denkert C, et al. Clinical relevance of host immunity in breast cancer: From TILs to the clinic. Nat Rev Clin Oncol. 2016;13(4):228–241.
115. Garberis I, Andre F, Lacroix-Triki M. [L'intelligence artificielle pourrait-elle intervenir dans l'aide au diagnostic des cancers du sein?—L'exemple de HER2] Could artificial intelligence play a role in breast cancer diagnosis?—The example of HER2]. Bull Cancer. 2021;108(11S):11S35–11S45.
116. Wu S, Yue M, Zhang J, et al. The role of artificial intelligence in accurate interpretation of HER2 immunohistochemical scores 0 and 1+ in breast cancer. Mod Pathol. 2023;36(3):100054.
117. Ivanova M, Porta FM, D'Ercole M, et al. Standardized pathology report for HER2 testing in compliance with 2023 ASCO/CAP updates and 2023 ESMO consensus statements on HER2-low breast cancer. Virchows Arch. 2024;484(1):3–14.

14

Gastrointestinal System Carcinomas

Wen-Yu Hsiao, Arron Sohn, Eunice Chou, Maria Diab, and Wei Zheng

14.1 Introduction

Gastrointestinal (GI) cancers, including carcinomas of the esophagus, stomach, small intestine, and colorectum, account for at least one-fifth of global cancer diagnoses and contribute to more than one-third of cancer-related deaths. Revolutionary changes have transformed GI cancer management in the past two decades owing to advances in molecular mechanisms involving GI carcinogenesis and clinical application of next-generation DNA/RNA sequencing technology. GI cancer treatment is being based more and more on integrated histomolecular pathology that yields integrated morphologic and molecular information leading to targeted therapy, that is, morphological classification of the histological type of the cancer, molecular characterization of the tumor profile, and identification of actionable genomic alterations. Molecular targeted therapy utilizing therapeutic monoclonal antibodies and small molecule agents has been established as a fundamental backbone in precision medicine for GI cancer treatment. Clinicians can now choose from a substantial list of personalized therapeutic interventions that are associated with higher response rates, less toxicity, and longer survival. This chapter aims to provide an up-to-date overview of the histomolecular classifications of GI cancers, key molecular pathways in carcinogenesis as well as therapeutically relevant molecular targets, agents, and clinical trials in colorectal and gastric cancers.

14.2 Colorectal Cancer

14.2.1 Histopathology Classification

Colorectal cancer predominantly comprises adenocarcinomas and is further classified into nine histopathological subtypes by the 2019 WHO classification (5th edition) (1). These subtypes include mucinous adenocarcinoma, signet ring cell adenocarcinoma, medullary carcinoma, undifferentiated carcinoma, carcinoma with sarcomatoid components, micropapillary adenocarcinoma, serrated adenocarcinoma, adenoma-like adenocarcinoma, and adenosquamous carcinoma (Table 14.1).

Mucinous adenocarcinoma is the most common subtype and is defined as adenocarcinoma with over 50% extracellular mucin (Figure 14.1A). This subtype is associated with a higher rate of microsatellite instability (MSI-H) and shows a relatively poor response to systemic chemotherapy. Signet-ring cell carcinoma is defined as a subtype with over 50% of the cancer cells showing prominent intracytoplasmic mucin/signet ring appearance (Figure 14.1B). This subtype has a worse prognosis and is often detected at advanced stages with distant metastasis. Serrated adenocarcinoma shares morphological similarities with serrated polyps (Figure 14.1C) and exhibits a serrated neoplastic pathway with a higher frequency of *BRAF* or *KRAS* mutations. Adenoma-like adenocarcinoma is another newly recognized subtype, characterized by a low-grade morphology that mimics adenoma but with invasive growth into deeper colonic tissue (Figure 14.1D). This subtype has a low rate of metastasis and a good prognosis. Micropapillary adenocarcinoma is defined as a subtype with over 5% of cancer showing a micropapillary architecture and is associated with a poor prognosis.

Medullary carcinoma is characterized by poorly differentiated or undifferentiated sheets of malignant epithelial cells with a solid/medullary growth pattern (Figure 14.1E). The medullary subtype has prominent intratumoral infiltration of lymphocytes and/or neutrophilic granulocytes. This subtype often shows an aberrant immunohistochemical pattern, with loss of CDX2 and CK20 and intact SATB2 expression. It often shows MSI-H and is commonly associated with the *BRAF* V600E mutation. Adenosquamous carcinoma is a very rare subtype characterized by the presence of both mucin-producing glandular elements and squamous components (with at least 30% of squamous component, Figure 14.1F).

In contrast to adenocarcinomas, adenosquamous carcinoma, and medullary carcinoma, undifferentiated carcinoma often has greater nuclear pleomorphism and lacks prominent lymphocytic infiltrates and MSI-H (Figure 14.1H). Carcinoma with sarcomatoid components is a newly recognized subtype in the WHO 2019 classification. This subtype may also show partly undifferentiated histology but often has spindle cell components (Figure 14.1G) or rhabdoid features with loss of nuclear immunostaining for SMARCB1 (INI1), SMARCA4, SMARCA2, or other SWI/SNF family proteins.

The 5th edition WHO Classification recommends grading colorectal carcinoma using a two-tier system based on gland formation and epithelial maturation, i.e., low-grade (formerly well- to moderately differentiated) and high-grade (formerly poorly differentiated). Grading should be based on the least differentiated component away from the invasive front. Understanding these histologic subtypes can help us with the diagnosis, treatment, and prognosis of colorectal cancer.

DOI: 10.1201/9781003513469-14

TABLE 14.1

WHO Histological Subtypes of Colorectal Adenocarcinoma

Subtypes	Prognosis	Histological Features
Mucinous adenocarcinoma	Adverse	> 50% of tumor composed of pools of extracellular mucin with malignant glands or cells
Signet-ring cell adenocarcinoma	Adverse	> 50% of the tumor cells containing prominent intracytoplasmic mucin with nuclear displacement
Serrated adenocarcinoma		Glandular serration with tumor cells showing a low nuclear-to-cytoplasmic ratio
Adenoma-like adenocarcinoma	Favorable	≥ 50% of the invasive components showing adenoma-like villous structures and a pushing growth pattern
Medullary carcinoma	Favorable	Sheets of malignant epithelial cells with a solid or medullary growth pattern and prominent intratumoral infiltration of lymphocytes and/or neutrophilic granulocytes
Micropapillary adenocarcinoma	Adverse	≥ 5% of the tumor showing small clusters of tumor cells infiltrating stroma and forming lacunar-like spaces
Adenosquamous carcinoma		Showing features of both adenocarcinoma and squamous cell carcinoma
Carcinomas with sarcomatoid components	Adverse	Partially undifferentiated component with spindle cell or rhabdoid features
Undifferentiated carcinoma	Adverse	Malignant epithelial cells with diffuse sheets growth pattern and scant stroma, and lacking morphological and immunohistochemical evidence of definite lineage differentiation

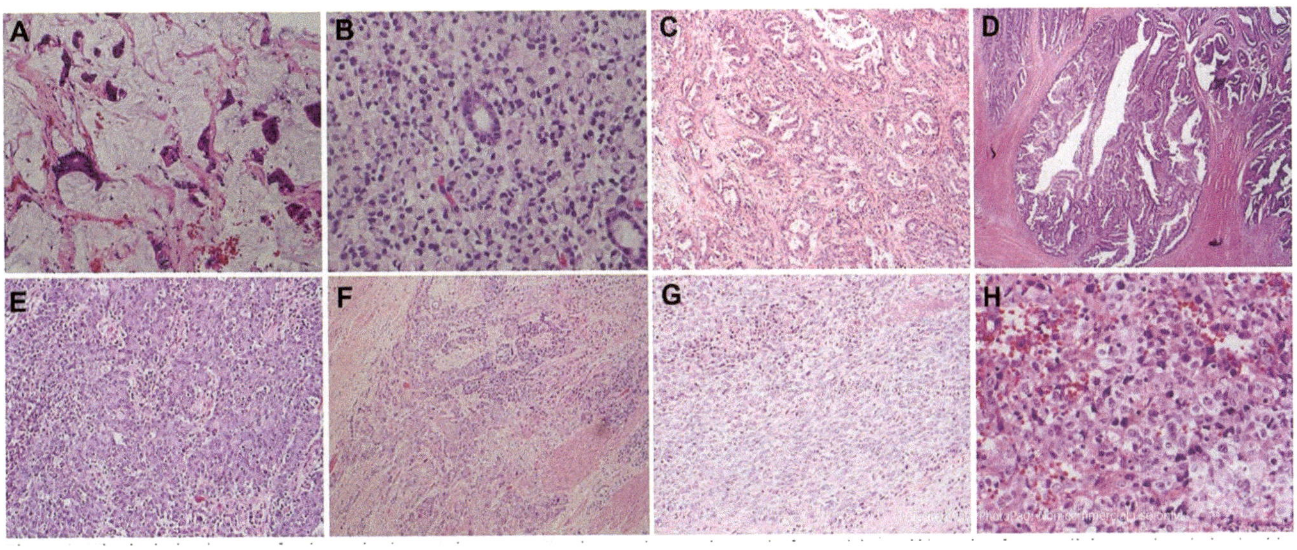

FIGURE 14.1 Histological subtypes of colorectal adenocarcinoma. (A) Mucinous adenocarcinoma is featured by >50% pools of extracellular mucin admixed with malignant glands and cells. (B) Signet-ring cell adenocarcinoma shows >50% discohesive signet-ring cells. (C) Serrated adenocarcinoma shows glandular serration with tumor cells showing a low nuclear-to-cytoplasmic ratio. (D) Adenoma-like adenocarcinoma has >50% of the invasive components showing adenoma-like villous structures and a pushing growth pattern. (E) Medullary carcinoma consists of sheets of malignant epithelial cells with a solid or medullary growth pattern and prominent intratumoral infiltration of lymphocytes. (F) Adenosquamous carcinoma shows features of both adenocarcinoma and squamous cell carcinoma. (G) Carcinomas with sarcomatoid components shows sarcomatoid spindle cells and focal glandular differentiation (right upper). (H) Undifferentiated carcinoma consists of sheets of malignant epithelial cells with scant stroma, lacking morphological and immunohistochemical evidence of definite lineage differentiation.

14.2.2 Molecular (Genomic and Transcriptomic) Classification

Genetic profiling has provided important insights into the genetic landscape of colorectal cancer and greatly advanced our understanding of the disease. Two major classifications have been established: the Cancer Genome Atlas (TCGA) and the Colorectal Cancer Subtyping Consortium (CRCSC) classifications (Table 14.2), both of which have important therapeutic implications.

The Cancer Genome Atlas first categorized colorectal cancers into two groups: hypermutated/ultramutated (16%) and non-hypermutated (84%) groups, based on mutation rates and chromosomal instability (2).

The hypermutated group demonstrated MSI-H, primarily caused by hypermethylation and *MLH1* silencing. A small number of cases were resulted from inherited Lynch syndrome. In contrast, the ultramutated group exhibited a distinct nucleotide base change spectrum due to mutations in DNA polymerase ε (POLE) and mismatch-repair genes. On the other hand, the non-hypermutated group had a low mutation rate and was microsatellite stable. However, it displayed significant chromosomal instability characterized by a high frequency of somatic copy number alterations (SCNAs), chromosomal segment gains and losses, and extensive chromosome imbalances (aneuploidy). Significant mutated genes were identified in this group, including *APC*, *TP53*, *KRAS*, *SMAD4*, and *PIK3CA*. These genes were linked to the

TABLE 14.2

Molecular Classifications of Colorectal Adenocarcinoma

The Cancer Genome Atlas			The Colorectal Cancer Subtyping Consortium		
Classifications	**Frequency**	**Molecular Features**	**Classifications**	**Frequency**	**Molecular Features**
Ultramutated/ hypermutated	16%	POLE proofreading mutations/dMMR/MSI-high (hypermethylation and *MLH1*-silencing), CIMP-high, *BRAF*-mut, SCNA-low	CMS1: MSI-Immune	14%	MSI, CIMP-high, hypermutation, *BRAF*-mut, immune infiltration and activation
Non-hypermutated	84%	Chromosomal instability, SCNA-high, MSS, WNT-pathway deregulation, *APC, TP53, KRAS, PIK3CA, SMAD4, NRAS, CTNNB1* mutation(s)	CMS2: Canonical	37%	SCNA-high, WNT and MYC activation
			CMS3: Metabolic	13%	Mixed MSI status, SCNA-low, CIMP-low, *KRAS*-mut, metabolic deregulation
			CMS4: Mesenchymal	23%	SCNA-high, stromal infiltration, TGFβ activation, angiogenesis
			Mixed or indeterminate	13%	Transitional phenotype/ Intratumoral heterogeneity

Abbreviations: dMMR: deficient mismatch repair, MSI: microsatellite instability, CIMP: CpG island methylator phenotype, SCNA: somatic copy number alterations, CMS: consensus molecular subtype, MSS: microsatellite stability.

dysregulation of WNT, MAPK, and PI3K signaling pathways, as well as the inactivation of the TGFβ inhibitory pathway.

The Colorectal Cancer Subtyping Consortium subsequently developed a transcriptomics-based molecular classification algorithm, resulting in four distinct consensus molecular subtypes (CMS): CMS1, CMS2, CMS3, and CMS4. This classification was reported to be most closely linked to tumor phenotype and clinical behavior (3).

CMS1, also known as the MSI-immune subtype, comprised 14% of cases and was characterized by MSI-H with hypermutation, *BRAF* mutations, and strong immune activation. These tumors were frequently located on the right side of the colon and had a higher histopathological grade.

CMS2, also known as the canonical subtype, comprised 37% of cases and was chromosomally unstable with high levels of SCNAs. These tumors exhibited WNT and MYC pathway activation and had higher expression of *EGFR* and *ERBB2*. CMS2 tumors were mainly located on the left side of the colon.

CMS3, also known as the metabolic subtype, comprised 13% of cases and was genomically stable with *KRAS* mutations and metabolic dysregulation. These tumors were also located on the left side of the colon.

CMS4, also known as the mesenchymal subtype, comprised 23% of cases and was chromosomally unstable with high levels of SCNAs. These tumors showed strong upregulation of genes associated with epithelial-mesenchymal transition, prominent transforming growth factor β activation, stromal invasion, and angiogenesis. CMS4 tumors were diagnosed at more advanced stages (III and IV) and had worse overall survival and relapse-free survival. CMS1 cancers had very poor survival after relapse, while CMS2 cases showed superior survival after relapse. Both CMS1 and CMS3 showed nearly universal genetic activations of receptor tyrosine kinase (RTK)/MAPK pathways.

14.2.3 Established Actionable Genomic Targets and Companion Pathologic Tests

Molecular studies have provided valuable insights into the genetic and molecular complexity of colorectal cancer. The identification of key molecular pathways, including the DNA repair pathway, RTK/RAS/RAF, and PI3K/AKT/mTOR pathways, has opened new avenues for precision therapy. Clinical trials have established multiple genomic alterations that can be targeted with precision therapy, such as MSI-H/dMMR, *KRAS* mutation, *BRAF* V600E mutation, *HER2* amplification, *NTRK* fusion, and *EGFR* alteration. Consequently, the U.S. Food and Drug Administration (FDA) has granted accelerated approval to four molecularly targeted therapies for advanced colorectal cancer since 2020.

For example, pembrolizumab has been approved as the first-line therapy for MSI-H/dMMR metastatic colorectal cancer (mCRC) (4). Additionally, several other agents have been approved as second-line or subsequent therapies for chemotherapy-refractory mCRC, including combinational tucatinib and trastuzumab for *RAS* wild-type and *HER2*-positive mCRC (5), adagrasib plus cetuximab for *KRAS* G12C–mutated mCRC (6), and encorafenib in combination with cetuximab for *BRAF* V600E-mutated mCRC (7).

To identify appropriate candidates for these precision therapies, pathologic assay methods and testing recommendations are also evolving rapidly. These advancements offer significant hope for more effective and personalized treatments for patients with colorectal cancer.

14.2.3.1 DNA Repair Pathway: MSI-H/dMMR

The DNA mismatch repair (MMR) pathway is a critical mechanism for repairing DNA damage and consists primarily of four enzymes: MLH1, MSH2, MSH6, and PMS2. When deficient MMR (dMMR) proteins occur due to genetic or epigenetic events, it results in hypermutation and MSI-H. Hypermutation-generated neoantigens lead to tumor immunogenicity, which is associated with high CD8+ T cell infiltration and a response to immune checkpoint inhibitors (8).

In primary colorectal cancers, the prevalence of MSI-immune type is approximately 14% per CRCSC molecular classification. Recently, the NICHE trial has demonstrated that short-term neoadjuvant immunotherapy (six weeks of anti-PD-1 antibody nivolumab and anti-CTLA4 antibody ipilimumab) before surgery achieved unprecedented responses in clinical stage I-III, resectable MSI-H/dMMR colon cancers and exhibited a high percentage of pathologic complete response. The patients had a 3-year disease-free survival (DFS) of 93% (9).

In metastatic colorectal cancer, MSI-H/dMMR has a prevalence of 3%-5% and predicts a poor response to standard chemotherapy. Several phase II clinical trials, such as KEYNOTE-164, CheckMate-142 and KEYNOTE-177 [NCT02460198, NCT02060188, NCT02563002], have demonstrated that immunotherapy with immune-checkpoint inhibitors, such as pembrolizumab and nivolumab, led to a significant improvement in progression-free survival (PFS). Notably, the KEYNOTE-177 trial showed that pembrolizumab doubled PFS compared with chemotherapy in patients with MSI-H/dMMR mCRC (10). Consequently, the FDA has approved pembrolizumab as a first-line treatment for patients with unresectable or metastatic MSI-H/dMMR colorectal cancer.

Most clinical guidelines recommend universal screening of colorectal cancer for defects in the MMR pathway. To detect MSI, the three most used pathological assays are immunohistochemistry (IHC), polymerase chain reaction (PCR), and next-generation sequencing (NGS).

The MMR-IHC approach is a cost-effective technique widely used in anatomical pathological laboratories. It assesses four MMR protein expressions (MLH1, MSH2, MSH6, and PMS2) in formalin-fixed paraffin-embedded (FFPE) tissue. If there is a complete loss of nuclear staining of at least one of the four MMR proteins, this is defined as dMMR. There are four common dMMR patterns: MLH1-/PMS2-, MSH2-/MSH6-, PMS2-only, and MSH6-only. If abnormal MLH1 IHC results are found, further testing for *BRAF* V600E mutation or *MLH1* promoter hypermethylation can help determine whether the tumor is sporadic or related to Lynch syndrome. If abnormal MSH2 IHC results or MSH6- or PSM2-only IHC patterns are found, genetic counseling/germline testing is recommended to screen for Lynch syndrome.

MSI-PCR is a molecular test that assesses the number of nucleotide repeats in a defined panel of microsatellites, such as BAT-25, BAT-26, MONO-27, NR-21, and NR-24 (11, 12). If two or more unstable loci of a panel of microsatellite markers are found, this is defined as a high frequency of MSI (MSI-H). PCR is the gold standard for confirming the MMR status and is suitable for equivocal/indeterminate MMR IHC results, such as heterogeneous or subclonal loss of MMR protein expression or retained MMR IHC stains with truncated MMR mutations in the setting of familial cancer syndrome.

NGS-MSI directly analyzes the coding exons and flanking intronic regions of *MLH1*, *MSH2*, *MSH6*, *PMS2*, and *EPCAM* genes to identify their pathologic mutations for MSI detection. Although MMR-IHC, MSI-PCR, and MSI-NGS have comparable performance metrics in CRC patients, IHC and PCR are the preferred screening methods due to their fast turnaround time, according to the guideline from the College of American Pathologists (CAP) (13, 14).

14.2.3.2 RTKs and RAS/RAF Pathway

RTKs are a family of cell-surface receptors with tyrosine kinase activity which receive and transduce signals to trigger downstream cell proliferation and survival pathways. Pathogenic RTK mutations and amplification/fusion have been identified as established or potential molecular targets for advanced CRC such as epidermal growth factor receptor (EGFR), human epidermal growth factor receptor 2 (HER2), neurotrophic tropomyosin receptor kinase (NTRK), fibroblast growth factor receptor (FGFR), tyrosine-protein kinase c-Met/hepatocyte growth factor receptor (MET), and insulin-like growth factor receptor (IGFR), among others (15). Therapies targeting RTKs are small-molecule inhibitors and monoclonal antibodies.

14.2.3.2.1 EGFR Alteration

EGFR, also known as human epidermal growth factor receptor 1 (HER1), is overexpressed in 60–80% of CRCs. Functional activation of EGFR via mutation or amplification plays an important role in carcinogenesis of CRC. Targeting *EGFR* alteration with therapeutic monoclonal antibodies, such as cetuximab and panitumumab, was one of the first successful precision medicine strategies exploited in mCRC in the early years in the 21st century.

Based on CRYSTAL (**C**etuximab combined with i**R**inotecan in first-line therap**Y** for meta**ST**atic colorect**AL** cancer), PRIME, and ASPECCT trials, the FDA approved cetuximab and panitumumab for use in *RAS* wildtype mCRC as a first-line therapy in combination with FOLFOX and as monotherapy following disease progression after prior treatment with fluoropyrimidine, oxaliplatin, and irinotecan-containing chemotherapy. The application of anti-EGFR antibodies can prolong survival for 10–20% in *RAS* wildtype mCRC patients (16–18).

14.2.3.2.2 HER2 Amplification

HER2 alteration is a well-known oncogenic driver in different tumors and has rapidly become an actionable target over the past few years in advanced CRC. The prevalence of *HER2* amplification is ~2–3% in CRC overall, but it is higher in metastatic *RAS/BRAF*-wildtype CRC (~5%) (19).

Several phase II clinical trials, such as HERACLES (NCT03225937), MyPathway (NCT02091141), DESTINY-CRC01 (NCT03384940), and MOUNTAINEER (NCT03043313), have demonstrated that dual HER2 inhibition strategies, such as combinational antibody-TKI or antibody-drug conjugates, were effective in chemotherapy-refractory, HER2-positive mCRC, with an objective response rate (ORR) ranging from 15–45% (20–22). In particular, the MOUNTAINEER study showed 38% ORR with complete responses observed in 3.6% of patients and partial responses seen in 35%. Based on these emerging efficacy data, FDA granted accelerated approval to tucatinib a TKI in combination with trastuzumab for HER2-positive unresectable or metastatic colorectal cancer that has progressed following chemotherapy.

To identify patients who may benefit from HER2-targeted therapy, the current (2022–2023) National Comprehensive Cancer Network (NCCN) colon cancer guideline recommends testing all metastatic colon cancers for HER2, except for those with *RAS/BRAF* mutations. This is due to the mutual exclusivity of *HER2* amplification and *KRAS*, *NRAS*, and *BRAF* mutations.

HER2 overexpression can be detected by IHC for HER2 protein, fluorescence in situ hybridization (FISH) for *ERBB2* gene amplification, or NGS. Among these methods, IHC is recommended as the initial test for *HER2* overexpression.

It is important to note that the IHC scoring system (HERACLES criteria) adopted by the NCCN colon cancer guideline differs from those used in breast and gastric cancers. This is due to the homogeneous cellularity of *HER2* amplification and staining patterns of colorectal cancer. According to the HERACLES criteria, HER2 IHC positivity (no confirmatory FISH needed) is defined as > 50% tumor cells showing intense (3+) membrane staining with circumferential, basolateral, or lateral patterns. Cases with > 10% but < 50% tumor cells showing intense (3+) membrane staining and those with ≥ 50% of tumor cells showing moderate (2+) membrane staining should undergo reflex FISH testing (23). *HER2* amplification by FISH is considered positive (amplified) when the HER2:CEP17 ratio is ≥ 2 in more than 50% of tumor cells.

NGS is another important methodology for testing for *HER2* amplification, which could provide a definite answer for a small percentage of cases with discordant HER2 IHC and FISH results.

14.2.3.2.3 NTRK Fusions

NTRK fusions are very rare in colorectal carcinomas, with a reported incidence from 0.2% to 1%. A small cohort of studies showed that CRCs harboring *NTRK* fusions were frequently present in female patients, associated with pan-wild type *KRAS*, *NRAS*, and *BRAF*; dMMR/MSI-H; and high tumor mutation burden (TMB) (24).

Several clinical trials (LOXO-195–001, NAVIGATE, ALKA-372–001, and TAK-659–302) have shown that TRK inhibitors produced clinically meaningful tumor response in metastatic solid tumors with *NTRK* fusions (25). These trials have led to FDA approval of larotrectinib (a first-generation TRK inhibitor) and entrectinib (another panTRK inhibitor) for the treatment of advanced solid tumors including colorectal carcinoma with NTRK fusions in the non-first-line setting.

Current pathologic assays in assessment of *NTRK* fusions include IHC, in situ hybridization (typically FISH), RT-PCR, and NGS (RNA-based, DNA-based, or mixed DNA/RNA-based). Pan-TRK IHC only detects NTRK protein expression but does not directly detect *NTRK* fusions; thus it is only recommended for screening but not for confirmatory. FISH and PCR are also not recommended for the routine detection of *NTRK* fusions in all patients because both FISH and PCR are only designed to identify limited, known fusion partners and many unreported fusion partners exist. NGS assays identify rearrangements (fusions) involving targeted regions of the *NTRK1*, *NTRK2*, and *NTRK3* genes regardless of fusion partners and have been established as the optimal way to detect *NTRK* fusions.

14.2.3.2.4 KRAS/NRAS Mutation

RAS proteins belong to small GTPase and are downstream effectors of EGFR. *RAS*-activating mutations lead to deregulated proliferative signaling through the MAPK pathway (also known as the Ras-Raf-MEK-ERK pathway) and occur in ~ 30–40% of mCRC. *KRAS* mutation predominantly occurs in codons 12 or 13 of exon 2. KRAS mutations show three major hotspots (codons 12, 13, and 61), with dominant codon 12 accounting for ~65% of KRAS mutations (26). The frequent mutation sites of *NRAS* are located in exons 2, 3, and 4. *KRAS/NRAS* exon 2, 3, and 4 mutations have been recognized as a predictor of negative response to anti-EGFR antibody treatments (i.e., patients with any *RAS* mutations should not be treated with either cetuximab or panitumumab).

Several small molecular inhibitors targeting the *KRAS* pG12C mutation (present in ~3% of mCRC), such as sotorasib and adagrasib, have been developed and have shown encouraging preclinical studies and early clinical data in mCRC. In particular, the KRYSTAL-1 trial (NCT03785249) showed a combination of adagrasib and cetuximab elicited an objective response rate (ORR) of 46% and median response duration of 7.6 months in a small cohort of patients with chemotherapy-refractory, *KRAS* G12C-mutated mCRC (27). Although adagrasib plus cetuximab is undergoing further evaluation in the ongoing phase 3 KRYSTAL-10 trial (NCT04793958), the FDA has granted accelerated approval to its application in patients with *KRAS* G12C–mutated mCRC in the second-line setting. Testing for the *RAS* mutations can be performed by PCR or NGS.

14.2.3.2.5 BRAF V600E Mutation

BRAF is a serine/threonine kinase, and activating mutations result in unregulated proliferative signaling via the MAPK pathway. *BRAF* V600E mutations are present in ~8–12% of mCRCs and are mutually exclusive with *KRAS* mutations. *BRAF* mutations are associated with worse prognosis and predict a poor response to anti-EGFR treatment (28). Although monotherapy with a BRAF inhibitor did not achieve disease control (NCT01524978), the BEACON CRC trial (NCT02928224) has shown that combination of a BRAF inhibitor (encorafenib) with EGFR inhibitor (cetuximab) led to significant improvements in OS, ORR, and PFS when compared with treatment with standard chemotherapy (29). These results led to FDA approval for the usage of encorafenib in combination with cetuximab in the chemotherapy-refractory setting of *BRAF* V600E-mutated mCRC. Testing for the *BRAF* V600E mutation can be performed by PCR or NGS.

14.2.4 Emerging Targetable Genomic Alterations

14.2.4.1 Tumor Mutational Burden High Status

Tumor mutational burden (TMB), also known as mutation load, is a measure of the total amount of somatic protein-coding mutations within a tumor genome. It is determined by NGS assay and reported as the total number of DNA mutations per one million bases (megabase) (30). The KEYNOTE-158 trial (NCT02628067) defined tumor mutational burden high status (TMB-H) as ≥ 10 mutations per megabase and showed that immunotherapy with pembrolizumab treatment elicited an ORR of 29% in unresectable or metastatic TMB-H solid tumors, in comparison to 6% of non-TMB-H tumors (31). Based on the efficacy data from the trial, FDA approved the use of pembrolizumab for treatment-refractory, unresectable or metastatic TMB-H solid tumors.

The companion NGS TMB assay approved by the FDA includes FoundationOne CDx, FoundationOne Liquid CDx, and MSK-IMPACT. However, the current 2022–2023 NCCN guideline does not recommend routine TMB testing in CRC patients due to limited clinical data.

14.2.4.2 *PIK3CA* Mutation

Activating mutations of *PIK3CA* (phosphatidylinositol-4,5-bisphosphate 3-kinase catalytic subunit alpha) are oncogenic and lead to deregulation of downstream AKT/mTOR signaling pathway. *PIK3CA* mutation is present in 10–18% of CRCs and is a negative predictor for response to anti-EGFR therapy (32). Several clinical trials for use of PIK3CA inhibitor in *PIK3CA*-mutated mCRC are ongoing, such as ALCAP (NCT04753203) and C-PRECISE-01(NCT04495621).

14.2.4.3 *MET* Alteration

Mesenchymal-epithelial transition (MET) factor is a receptor tyrosine kinase, and activation of MET leads to downstream activation of MAPK and PI3K/AKT pathways. MET amplification occurs in ~12.5% of CRC and drives resistance to anti-EGFR therapies due to the crosstalk between the MET and MAPK pathways (33). MET inhibitors tepotinib and capmatinib have been approved by FDA for treating patients with metastatic non-small cell lung cancer harboring *MET* exon 14–skipping alterations based on the GEOMETRY mono-1 and VISION trials (NCT02414139 and NCT02864992) (34), but their efficacy in *MET*-amplified mCRC is under investigation by several clinical trials, such as NCT03592641 and NCT04515394.

14.2.4.4 *FGFR* Alteration

The fibroblast growth factor receptor (FGFR) family consists of four isoforms (FGFR1–4), and their activation leads to the activation of both the RAS-MAPK and PI3K/AKT pathways. A small subset (~4–5%) of colorectal cancers harbors *FGFR* genetic alterations such as amplifications, mutations, and fusions. Pemigatinib, a selective FGFR 1–3 inhibitor, has been FDA approved for the treatment of previously treated metastatic cholangiocarcinoma harboring *FGFR2* fusions based on FIGHT-202 trial (NCT02924376) (35, 36). Clinical efficacy studies of pemigatinib are ongoing in patients with mCRC harboring *FGFR* alterations, including mutations, translocations, and amplifications (NCT05202236 and NCT04096417).

14.3 Gastric Cancer

14.3.1 Histopathology Classification

Gastric cancer is a heterogeneous group of malignant epithelial tumors, with 90–95% being adenocarcinoma. Historically, gastric carcinoma was divided into two histomorphologic subtypes by Laurén classification. The intestinal type (glandular architecture) and diffuse type (discohesive cells) exhibit distinct morphologic appearance, pathogenesis, and genetic profile. Today the 2019 WHO classification has further subdivided the Laurén types into five main histologic subtypes (tubular, papillary, poorly cohesive including signet-ring cell type and other cell types, mucinous, mixed adenocarcinomas) and other rare histological subtypes (Table 14.3) (1).

Tubular adenocarcinoma is the most common subtype and composed of tubules of variable diameter (Figure 14.2A). Clear cell change and solid components can also be present in this subtype. Papillary adenocarcinoma is relatively uncommon but has a higher frequency of liver metastasis and poor prognosis.

TABLE 14.3

WHO Histological Subtypes of Gastric Adenocarcinoma

Subtypes	Relative Frequency	Histological Features
Tubular adenocarcinoma	45% (Europe) to 64% (Japan)	Composed of predominant tubules of variable diameter; clear cell change and solid component classified in this subtype
Papillary adenocarcinoma	2.7 to 9.9%	Well differentiated tumor with filiform, finger-like processes with readily identifiable fibrovascular cores; higher frequency of liver metastasis and worse prognosis
Mucinous adenocarcinoma	2.1 to 8.1%	Substantial amount of extracellular mucin admixed with malignant glands and floating signet-ring cell nests
Poorly cohesive carcinoma	20 to 54%	Composed predominantly of signet-ring cell (signet-ring type) and of poorly cohesive cells of non-signet-ring cells (< 10% signet-ring cells, non-signet ring cell type)
Mixed adenocarcinoma	6 to 22%	Showing two or more histological components such as tubular, papillary, mucinous, signet-ring cells, or poorly cohesive cells; worse prognosis than tumors with a single component
Gastric adenocarcinoma with lymphoid stroma	1 to 7%, more common in males	Poorly formed tubular structures or syncytia of polygonal cells with prominent lymphocytic infiltration or a lymphocyte-rich stroma; association with EBV infection or MSI-H/dMMR
Hepatoid adenocarcinoma and related entities	2.6 to 5.4%	Hepatoid carcinoma showing trabecular or sheets of hepatoid polygonal cells with eosinophilic cytoplasm; enteroblastic adenocarcinoma with sheets or tubulopapillary growth of neoplastic columnar/cuboidal cells with clear cytoplasm resembling the primitive gut
Micropapillary	Rare	Small clusters of tumor cells infiltrating stroma and forming lacunar-like spaces without fibrovascular cores; poor prognosis with frequent lymph node metastasis
Paneth cell carcinoma	Rare	Malignant Paneth cell-like tumor cells containing brightly eosinophilic, coarse granules in cytoplasm with lysozyme immunoreactivity
Gastric adenocarcinoma of fundic-gland type	1% of early GCs	Three subtypes: chief cell–predominant, parietal cell–predominant, and mixed phenotype; submucosal invasion observed in 60% of cases and slow-growing tumor with rare lymph node metastasis

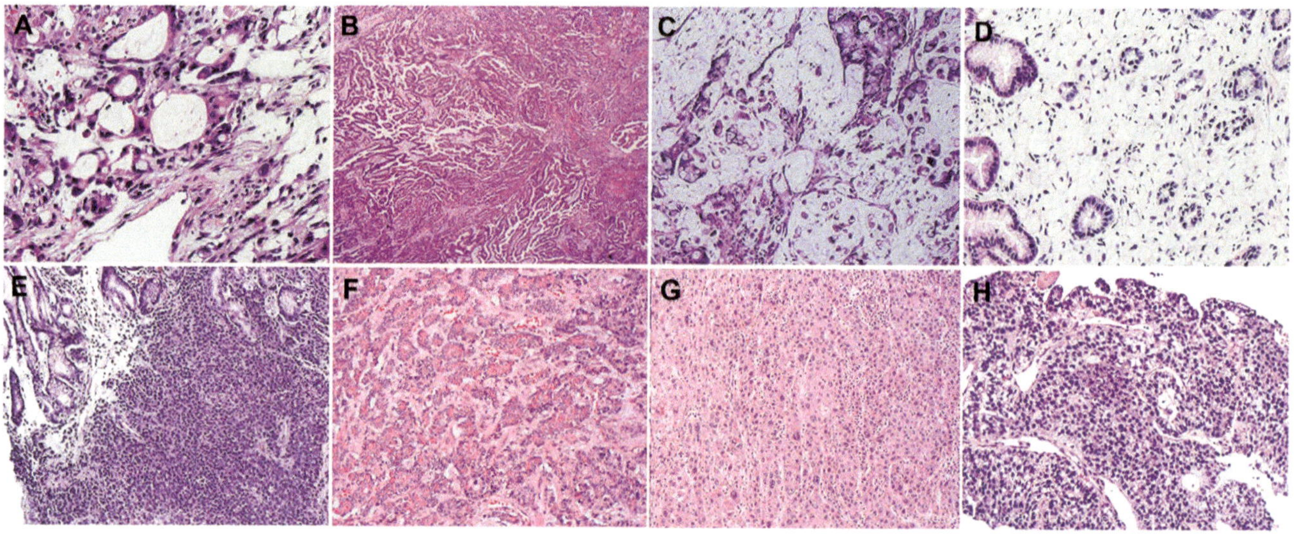

FIGURE 14.2 Histological subtypes of gastric adenocarcinoma. (A) Tubular adenocarcinoma is composed of tubules of variable diameter. (B) Papillary adenocarcinoma has filiform, finger-like processes with readily identifiable fibrovascular cores. (C) Mucinous adenocarcinoma is featured by substantial amount of extracellular mucin admixed with malignant glands and floating signet-ring cell nests. (D) Poorly cohesive carcinoma (signet-ring cell type) is composed predominantly of signet-ring cells infiltrating the stomach. (E) Gastric (adeno) carcinoma with lymphoid stroma is characterized by poorly formed tubular structures or syncytia of polygonal cells admixed with a lymphocyte-rich stroma. (F) Paneth cell carcinoma is featured by predominant Paneth cell-like tumor cells containing brightly eosinophilic, coarse granules in cytoplasm with lysozyme immunoreactivity. (G) Hepatoid adenocarcinoma consists of trabecular or sheets of hepatoid polygonal cells with eosinophilic cytoplasm. (H) Gastric adenocarcinoma with enteroblastic differentiation consists of sheets or tubulopapillary growth of neoplastic columnar/cuboidal cells with clear cytoplasm resembling the primitive gut.

This subtype has a well-differentiated morphology characterized by filiform, finger-like processes with readily identifiable fibrovascular cores (Figure 14.2B). A tubular component can also be present (termed tubulopapillary). Both tubular and papillary adenocarcinoma are graded by a two-tiered system: low grade (well or moderately differentiated) and high grade (poorly differentiated).

Poorly cohesive carcinoma is corresponding to the diffuse type of Lauren's classification and has signet-ring cell type and other-cell type (Figure 14.2D). Signet-ring cell type is composed predominantly of signet-ring cell component (often > 90% signet-ring cells), while other-cell type often consists mainly of poorly cohesive cells of non-signet-ring cell type (< 10% signet-ring cells). Limited tubular differentiation can also be present. This subtype often shows a poor response to standard chemoradiation therapy. Mucinous adenocarcinoma is featured by substantial amount of extracellular mucin (≥ 50% of tumor volume) and has two main growth patterns, i.e., glands/tubules admixed with extracellular mucin pools and floating signet-ring cell nests in extracellular mucin (Figure 14.2C). It is noteworthy that mucinous adenocarcinoma containing nests of signet-ring cells is different from poorly cohesive carcinoma of signet-ring cell type morphologically and genetically. Mixed adenocarcinoma contains two or more distinct histological components (tubular/papillary/poorly cohesive/mucinous) and has a worse prognosis than those with only one component. The phenotypic divergence has been reportedly to be associated with *CDH1* mutation.

Other rare histological subtypes include gastric (adeno)carcinoma with lymphoid stroma, hepatoid adenocarcinoma with related entities, Paneth cell carcinoma, micropapillary adenocarcinoma, and adenocarcinoma of fundic-gland type, among others. Gastric (adeno) carcinoma with lymphoid stroma, also known as medullary carcinoma or lymphoepithelioma-like carcinoma, is characterized by poorly formed tubular structures or syncytia of polygonal cells admixed with a lymphocyte-rich stroma (Figure 14.2E). This subtype is more common in males and often found at the proximal stomach. Many of these tumors are Epstein–Barr virus (EBV) positive and microsatellite stable, while some others are EBV negative but MSI-H/dMMR. Both tumors often express PD-L1 and show good response to immune checkpoint inhibitors. Paneth cell carcinoma is composed predominantly of malignant Paneth cell-like tumor cells containing brightly eosinophilic, coarse granules in cytoplasm with lysozyme immunoreactivity (Figure 14.2F). Hepatoid adenocarcinoma with related entities is gastric adenocarcinoma with hepatoid differentiation (Figure 14.2G), which often coexists with enteroblastic differentiation (Figure 14.2H) and a yolk sac tumor-like component. All components are alpha-fetoprotein (AFP)-producing and thus grouped together as "related entities". Immunochemical staining for oncoproteins (AFP, SALL4 and glypican-3) is frequently positive.

14.3.2 Molecular Classification

Two landmark studies, one by TCGA and the other by the Asian Cancer Research Group (ACRG), have proposed molecular classifications for gastric cancer based on multi-omic analyses (Table 14.4).

The Cancer Genome Atlas conducted a study that analyzed 295 cases of treatment-naïve primary gastric cancers from the USA, Western Europe, and Asia using six molecular platforms: whole-exome sequencing, DNA methylation profiling, messenger RNA sequencing, microRNA sequencing, microarray-based somatic copy number analysis, and reverse-phase protein array. TCGA classified gastric cancers into four groups based on the integrated results: Epstein–Barr virus (EBV), MSI, genomically stable (GS), and chromosomal instability (CIN) (37).

The EBV group comprised 9% of the cases and was enriched for high EBV burden. Histologically, the group displayed

TABLE 14.4

Molecular Classifications of Gastric Adenocarcinoma

The Cancer Genome Atlas			The Asian Cancer Research Group		
Classifications	Frequency	Molecular Features	Classifications	Frequency	Molecular Features
MSI	22%	Hypermutations and hypermethylation, including *MLH1* promoter methylation; *RAS* and *PIK3CA* mutations, lacking *BRAF* V600E mutations	MSI	23%	Hypermutation, loss of MLH1 expression, and frequent mutations in *KRAS*, PI3K-PTEN-mTOR pathway, *ALK*, and *ARID1A*; PD-L1 overexpression
Genomically stable (GS)	20%	*CDH1* and *RHOA* mutations or fusions involving RHO-family GTPase-activating proteins such as *CLDN18::ARHGAP26* fusion	Microsatellite stable with epithelial to mesenchymal transition features (MSS/EMT)	15%	Loss of CDH1, loss of cellular adhesions, angiogenesis, motility
Chromosomal instability (CIN)	50%	Frequent TP53 mutations, extensive DNA copy-number abnormalities, including frequent amplification of genes involving cell cycle mediators (*CCNE1*, *CCND1*, and *CDK6*) and receptor tyrosine kinase (RTKs), RAS and PI(3)-kinase signaling such as *KRAS/NRAS*, *PIK3CA*, *MET*, and *FGFR2*	MSS with functional loss of TP53 (MSS/TP53-)	36%	*TP53* mutations and significant recurrent focal amplification in genes such as *HER2*, *EGFR*, *CCNE1*, *CCND1*, *MDM2*, *ROBO2*, *GATA6*, and *MYC*
Epstein–Barr virus (EBV)	9%	DNA promoter hypermethylation, frequent *PIK3CA* and *ARID1A* mutations, amplification of *JAK2*, *ERBB2* (*HER2*), *PD-L1*, and *PD-L2*	MSS with TP53 activity (MSS/TP53+)	26%	Frequent mutations in *APC*, *ARID1A*, *KRAS*, *PIK3CA*, and *SMAD4*, frequent EBV infection

Abbreviations: MSI, microsatellite instability; MSS: microsatellite stability

carcinoma with lymphoid stroma and extensive DNA promoter hypermethylation. Additionally, the EBV group showed frequent *PIK3CA* and *ARID1A* mutations and amplification of *JAK2*, *ERBB2* (*HER2*), *PD-L1*, and *PD-L2*.

The MSI group comprised 22% of the cases and showed hypermutations and hypermethylation, including *MLH1* promoter methylation. Although this group shared many mutations at hotspot sites seen in other cancers such as *RAS* and *PIK3CA*, it lacked *BRAF* V600E mutations (commonly seen in MSI colorectal cancer) and targetable amplifications.

The GS group comprised 20% of the cases and often had diffuse type histology. This group showed *CDH1* and *RHOA* mutations or fusions involving RHO-family GTPase-activating proteins such as *CLDN18:ARHGAP26* fusion.

The CIN group comprised 50% of the cases and was mainly intestinal-type histology. The group showed frequent *TP53* mutations and extensive DNA copy-number abnormalities, including frequent amplification of genes involving cell cycle mediators (CCNE1, CCND1, and CDK6) and receptor tyrosine kinase (RTKs), RAS, and PI(3)-kinase signaling such as *KRAS/NRAS*, *PIK3CA*, *MET*, and *FGFR2*.

Although TCGA did not report prognostic association in the original study, a subsequent prediction model developed from the TCGA cohort ($n = 262$) showed that the EBV group had the best prognosis, the GS group had the worst prognosis, and the MSI and CIN groups had poorer overall survival than the EBV group but better overall survival than the GS group (38).

The Asian Cancer Research Group conducted a study on primary gastric cancers in Korean patients, utilizing mRNA sequencing, targeted gene sequencing, and copy number microarrays to identify potential molecular subtypes. The study comprised 300 cases and proposed a molecular classification of four subtypes, namely MSI, microsatellite stable with epithelial to mesenchymal transition features (MSS/EMT), MSS with TP53 activity (MSS/TP53+), and MSS with functional loss of TP53 (MSS/TP53-). The subtypes exhibited good prognostic correlations (39).

MSI cases accounted for 23% of the study population and demonstrated hypermutation, loss of MLH1 expression, and mutations in genes such as *KRAS*, PI3K-PTEN-mTOR pathway, *ALK*, and *ARID1A*. This subtype had the best prognosis and lowest recurrence rate.

The MSS/EMT group accounted for 15% of the population and exhibited a predominant diffuse histology with loss of *CDH1* expression. This group was mutually exclusive with the MSI group and had a higher recurrence rate, a higher probability of peritoneal seeding at recurrence, and the worst survival rate.

The remaining non-MSI and non-EMT gastric carcinomas were stratified into two distinct subtypes based on the status of TP53 activation, using a two-gene (*CDKN1A* and *MDM2*)/TP53-activity signature. The MSS/TP53+ subtype, which accounted for 26% of cases, was characterized by mutations in genes such as *APC*, *ARID1A*, *KRAS*, *PIK3CA*, and *SMAD4* and was associated with EBV infection. On the other hand, the MSS/TP53- subtype, which represented 36% of cases, was enriched for *TP53* mutations and exhibited significant recurrent focal amplification in genes such as *HER2*, *EGFR*, *CCNE1*, *CCND1*, *MDM2*, *ROBO2*, *GATA6*, and *MYC*. The MSS/TP53- subtype was found to have a worse prognosis than the MSI and MSS/TP53+ subtypes but a better prognosis than the MSS/EMT subtype.

The two molecular classifications highlight the complexity and heterogeneity of gastric cancer, dividing tumors into subgroups with enrichment of targetable molecules. These genomic and transcriptomic characterizations have significant implications for the development of tailored therapy but do not entirely overlap. Furthermore, these molecular classifiers have significant implications for developing clinically applicable pathological assays that stratify patients using formalin-fixed paraffin-embedded tissue. For instance, an immunohistochemical analysis of MLH1, E-cadherin, and p53, as well as EBV-ISH, were utilized to classify a cohort of 349 gastric carcinomas into five subtypes: EBV+, MSI-H/MLH1 expression loss, aberrant E-cadherin expression/EMT or GS, aberrant p53 expression, and normal p53 expression. These immunohistochemical subtypes presented distinct clinicopathologic characteristics and corresponded to the TCGA and ACRG subtypes, indicating their potential to be utilized in routine pathology practice (40).

14.3.3 Established Actionable Genomic Targets and Companion Pathologic Tests

At present, four therapeutically relevant molecular targets have been established in gastric cancer: *HER2* amplification, PD-L1 expression, MSI-H/dMMR, and *NTRK* fusion. Multiple corresponding therapeutic agents, such as trastuzumab, pembrolizumab/nivolumab, and entrectinib/larotrectinib, have been approved by the FDA for use in first- or second-line or subsequent therapy of advanced or metastatic gastric cancer. Current 2022–2023 NCCN guideline recommends that pathologic testing of these genomic alterations should be first based on IHC/ISH/targeted PCR assays followed by additional NGS testing as appropriate.

14.3.3.1 HER2 Amplification

HER2 amplification occurs in ~10–20% of gastric cancer and results in overexpression of *HER2*. The Trastuzumab for Gastric Cancer (ToGA) trial (41) and HERXO trial (42) added trastuzumab into standard chemotherapy and demonstrated significantly improved OS and PFS in patients with previously untreated, HER2-positive advanced gastroesophageal carcinoma. This led to FDA approval of trastuzumab in combination with chemotherapy as a first-line treatment for patients with unresectable or metastatic HER2-positive gastroesophageal carcinoma.

However, intratumor heterogeneity of *HER2* expression/amplification exists in up to 30% of HER2-positive gastric cancers and causes anti-Her2 resistance. To overcome this, combinations of anti-HER2 antibody with other drugs with various mechanisms of action have been developed. Recently, the KEYNOTE-811 trial (NCT03615326) showed that adding pembrolizumab to trastuzumab and chemotherapy markedly reduces tumor size and significantly improves objective response rate (43). Given the synergistic antitumor effect of dual PD-1 and HER2 blockade, FDA approved pembrolizumab plus trastuzumab and chemotherapy as first-line therapy for unresectable or metastatic, HER2-positive gastric or gastroesophageal junction carcinoma.

In addition, based on the DESTINY-Gastric 01/02 trials (44), the FDA has approved fam-trastuzumab-deruxtecan-nxki (an antibody-drug conjugate consisting of trastuzumab covalently linked to the topoisomerase I inhibitor deruxtecan) to be used as a second-line treatment for patients with HER2-positive gastric carcinoma following failure of prior treatment with a trastuzumab-based regimen. All of these have opened a new era of HER2-targeted therapy in gastric cancer.

IHC is recommended to be the initial testing methodology for assessment of HER2 overexpression in gastric cancer. The four-tiered scoring algorithm (3+, 2+, 1+, and 0 based on staining intensity and percentage cutoff) is different from colon and breast cancers. The percentage cutoff is ≥ 10% stained cancer cells in resection specimens and cluster of five tumor cells or more in biopsies. HER2 IHC positivity is defined as strong (3+) complete, basolateral, or lateral membranous staining. Moderate (2+, equivocal) membrane staining should be reflexed to FISH testing. *HER2*:*CEP17* ratio ≥ 2 or an average *HER2* copy number ≥ 6.0 signals/cell are considered FISH positive/amplified. Weak (1+) or negative (0) membranous staining is considered negative *HER2* overexpression and do not require further FISH testing (45). NGS may play an important role in determination of *HER2* status in liquid biopsies.

14.3.3.2 PD-L1 Expression

The programmed cell death protein 1 (PD-1)/programmed death ligand-1 (PD-L1) pathway is a key signaling pathway that regulates immune tolerance within the tumor microenvironment. By blocking the interaction between PD-1 and PD-L1, anti-PD-1 monoclonal antibodies, such as nivolumab, pembrolizumab, and dostarlimab, can reactivate the immune system and boost T cells to attack cancer cells.

Several clinical trials have demonstrated the efficacy of combining immune checkpoint inhibitors with chemotherapy in the treatment of advanced gastric or gastroesophageal cancer with PD-L1 expression. In particular, the Checkmate-649 trial showed significant improvements in OS and PFS with the addition of nivolumab to chemotherapy in previously untreated patients with advanced HER2-negative gastric or gastroesophageal cancer with PD-L1 expression (defined as a combined positive score (CPS) ≥ 5 using PD-L1 IHC 28-8 pharmDx assay) (46, 47).

Other trials, including the KEYNOTE-012 (48) and KEYNOTE-059 (49) trials, have also demonstrated significant treatment responses with pembrolizumab plus chemotherapy in patients with advanced gastric cancer with PD-L1 positivity (defined as CPS ≥1 using the Dako 22C3 pharmDx IHC assay). Additionally, the recent phase 3 KEYNOTE-859 trial (NCT03675737) has shown a significant improvement in OS, PFS, and ORR for pembrolizumab plus chemotherapy as first-line therapy for patients with advanced HER2-negative gastric or gastroesophageal cancer. Based on the efficacy data, the FDA has approved nivolumab or pembrolizumab, in combination with chemotherapy, for the first or second-line treatment of patients with advanced or metastatic gastric cancer with PD-L1 expression.

To determine PD-L1 expression, the FDA has approved PD-L1 IHC 22C3 pharmDx as a companion diagnostic assay for the use of pembrolizumab. The scoring system used to assess PD-L1 expression is CPS. To calculate the CPS, the number of PD-L1-positive cells (i.e., tumor cells, macrophages, and lymphocytes) is counted and divided by the total number of viable tumor cells. The resulting value is then multiplied by 100 to obtain the CPS score (50).

14.3.3.3 MSI-H/dMMR

MSI-H/dMMR occurs in ~22% of gastric cancers according to TCGA molecular classification. Among patients with MSI-H advanced gastric or gastroesophageal junction cancer, the anti–PD-L1 antibody pembrolizumab alone or in combination with chemotherapy has been reported to be associated with prolonged OS and PFS in KEYNOTE-059 (2 or more previous lines of therapy), 061 (1 previous line of therapy) and 062 (no previous therapy) (51). Current 2022–2023 NCCN guideline has included Pembrolizumab as options for second-line or subsequent therapy for patients with metastatic gastric cancer (52, 53) and recommended universal testing of MSI-H/dMMR in newly diagnosed gastric cancer patients. Pathologists should use MMR-IHC and/or MSI by PCR over NGS-MSI for the detection of DNA mismatch repair defects.

14.3.3.4 NTRK Fusions

NTRK fusions are extremely uncommon in gastric cancer with only rare case reports (54). Given the antitumor activity and manageable safety profiles of TRK inhibitors in unresectable or metastatic solid tumors harboring an *NTRK* gene fusion, entrectinib and larotrectinib are also recommended as second-line or subsequent treatment options for metastatic gastric cancer by NCCN guideline. For pathologic assays for *NTRK* fusion, see colorectal carcinoma section.

14.3.4 Emerging Targetable Genomic Alterations

14.3.4.1 Claudin18.2 (CLDN18.2) Expression

CLDN18.2 is an isoform of the tight junction protein of CLDN18 and only has limited expression in normal gastric mucosa. It is highly expressed in the genomically stable (GS) subgroup of gastric cancer, particularly carcinomas with *CLDN18*::*ARHGAP26* fusion (55).

A monoclonal antibody for CLDN18, Zolbetuximab, has been reported to selectively kill CLDN18.2-positive cancer cells through immune effector mechanisms. Two clinical trials (phase II FAST study and phase III SPOTLIGHT study) have showed that the addition of zolbetuximab to chemotherapy significantly improved PFS and OS in advanced gastric and esophageal adenocarcinoma patients with CLDN18.2 expression (defined by moderate-to-strong membrane immunohistochemical staining in ≥ 70% of tumor cells in FAST study (56) and at least 75% of tumor cells in SPOTLIGHT study).

In addition, clinical trials on chimeric antigen receptor (CAR) T-cell immunotherapy in advanced gastric adenocarcinoma are ongoing, which evaluate anti-tumor responses to autologous T cells with a CLDN18.2-targeted chimeric antigen receptor, such as NCT03159819 and NCT04404595. The anti-CLND18.2 therapy appears promising to become a new potential first-line treatment for patients with metastatic gastric cancers with CLDN18.2 expression.

14.3.4.2 Tumor Mutational Burden High Status (TMB-H)

Given FDA approval of pembrolizumab for the treatment of patients with metastatic TMB-H solid tumors (31), current NCCN guideline has recommended pembrolizumab as the second-line or subsequent treatment of advanced TMB-H (≥ 10 mutations/megabase) gastric cancers, though routine TMB testing in gastric cancer patients is not yet recommended.

14.3.4.3 Tumor Epstein-Barr Virus Status

Epstein-Barr virus (EBV) positivity occurs in ~9% of gastric cancer according to TCGA molecular study. EBV-positive gastric cancers show PD-L1 overexpression due to high focal amplification of *CD274*, indicating increased sensitivity to PD-1/PD-L1 immunotherapy (57). An early phase 1/2 study (NCT02951091) has reported that nivolumab in combination with paclitaxel showed antitumor activity and a manageable safety profile when used as second-line therapy for patients with EBV-related, MSI-H or PD-L1-positive advanced gastric cancer. Testing for EBV status is not currently recommended for routine clinical care in gastric cancer.

14.3.4.4 Homologous Recombination Pathway

Homologous recombination (HR) is one of the major repair mechanisms of DNA double-strand breaks and involves many genes such as *BRCA1/2*, *RAD51*, *PALB1/2*, *CHEK1*, *FANCs*, and *DNMT3*. HR deficiency (HRD) due to inactivation of such genes results in impaired double strand break repair and is a frequent driver of carcinogenesis (58). HRD has been largely explored in ovarian and breast cancers and HRD targeted therapy with poly ADP-ribose polymerase inhibitors (PARPi, such as olaparib and niraparibare) has advanced treatment paradigm (59).

Clinical trials investigating the efficacy of PARPi alone (NCT03840967, niraparib monotherapy) and in combination with chemotherapy (NCT01924533, olaparib+paclitaxel) or other targeted therapy (NCT05379972, olaparib+pembrolizumab) in metastatic gastric cancer are ongoing. Although FDA has approved several companion assays for HRD determination in ovarian cancer, such as FoundationOne CDx, and Myriad myChoice CDx, there are no standardized methods to define, measure, and report HR status in gastric cancers.

14.4 Summary

The past decade has witnessed remarkable progress in molecular targeted therapy for gastrointestinal cancers, which has been largely propelled by the advances in larger-scale genomic profiling technologies and the emergence of commercial vendors such as Foundation One, Caris, and Tempus. These advancements have underscored the need for precision pathology diagnosis, prompting a paradigm shift in pathology from traditional histology to histomolecular characterization of GI cancers based on integrated histomorphologic subtypes and genomic aberrations. The integrated diagnosis and precision pathology will provide clinicians with the ability to customize treatment plans according to the unique characteristics of each patient's tumor, holding great promise for improving patient care.

Another area that has experienced significant progress is the molecular profiling of circulating tumor DNA (ctDNA) and cell-free DNA (cfDNA), commonly known as liquid biopsy. This approach provides the ability to monitor disease progression and track genetic changes in response to treatment in GI cancers. Compared to tumor tissue analyses, ctDNA profiling offers significant advantages in characterizing intratumoral heterogeneity and evolutionary processes of cancer (60–62). While its clinical utility is still being studied in various settings, future integration of ctDNA profiling with histomolecular characterization has the potential to further improve the accuracy of diagnosis and guide targeted therapy for different treatment stages of GI cancers. This integration could significantly contribute to improving patient outcomes and advancing the field of GI precision pathology.

REFERENCES

1. WHO Classification of Tumours Editorial Board. WHO Classification of Tumors: Digestive System Tumours. Lyon: International Agency for Research on Cancer. 2019; 5th edition.
2. Cancer Genome Atlas N. Comprehensive molecular characterization of human colon and rectal cancer. Nature. 2012;487(7407):330–337.
3. Guinney J, Dienstmann R, Wang X, et al. The consensus molecular subtypes of colorectal cancer. Nat Med. 2015;21(11):1350–1356.
4. U.S. Food and Drug Administration. FDA Approves Pembrolizumab for First-Line Treatment of MSI-H/dMMR Colorectal Cancer. 2020. Available at: www.fda.gov/drugs/drug-approvals-and-databases/fda-approves-pembrolizumab-first-line-treatment-msi-hdmmr-colorectal-cancer.
5. U.S. Food and Drug Administration. FDA Grants Accelerated Approval to Tucatinib with Trastuzumab for Colorectal Cancer. 2023. Available at: www.fda.gov/drugs/resources-information-approved-drugs/fda-grants-accelerated-approval-tucatinib-trastuzumab-colorectal-cancer.
6. U.S. Food and Drug Administration. FDA Approves Adagrasib in Combination with Cetuximab in Patients with KRASG12C-Mutated Advanced Colorectal Cancer. 2022. Available at: www.onclive.com/view/fda-grants-breakthrough-therapy-designation-to-adagrasib-plus-cetuximab-for-kras-g12c-mutated-advanced-crc.
7. U.S. Food and Drug Administration. FDA Approves Encorafenib in Combination with Cetuximab for Metastatic Colorectal Cancer with a BRAF V600E Mutation. 2020. Available at: www.fda.gov/drugs/resources-information-approved-drugs/fda-approves-encorafenib-combination-cetuximab-metastatic-colorectal-cancer-braf-v600e-mutation.
8. Ganesh K, Stadler ZK, Cercek A, et al. Immunotherapy in colorectal cancer: Rationale, challenges and potential. Nat Rev Gastroenterol Hepatol. 2019;16(6):361–375.
9. Chalabi M, Fanchi LF, Dijkstra KK, et al. Neoadjuvant immunotherapy leads to pathological responses in MMR-proficient and MMR-deficient early-stage colon cancers. Nat Med. 2020;26(4):566–576.
10. Andre T, Shiu KK, Kim TW, et al. Pembrolizumab in microsatellite-instability-high advanced colorectal cancer. N Engl J Med. 2020;383(23):2207–2218.
11. Suraweera N, Duval A, Reperant M, et al. Evaluation of tumor microsatellite instability using five quasimonomorphic mononucleotide repeats and pentaplex PCR. Gastroenterology. 2002;123(6):1804–1811.
12. Buhard O, Suraweera N, Lectard A, Duval A, Hamelin R. Quasimonomorphic mononucleotide repeats for high-level microsatellite instability analysis. Dis Markers. 2004;20(4–5):251–257.
13. Bartley AN, Mills AM, Konnick E, et al. Mismatch repair and microsatellite instability testing for immune checkpoint inhibitor therapy: Guideline from the College of American Pathologists in collaboration with the Association for Molecular Pathology and Fight Colorectal Cancer. Arch Pathol Lab Med. 2022;146(10):1194–1210.
14. Vikas P, Messersmith H, Compton C, et al. Mismatch repair and microsatellite instability testing for immune checkpoint inhibitor therapy: ASCO endorsement of College of American Pathologists guideline. J Clin Oncol. 2023:JCO2202462.
15. Saraon P, Pathmanathan S, Snider J, et al. Receptor tyrosine kinases and cancer: Oncogenic mechanisms and therapeutic approaches. Oncogene. 2021;40(24):4079–4093.
16. Heinemann V, von Weikersthal LF, Decker T, et al. FOLFIRI plus cetuximab or bevacizumab for advanced colorectal cancer: Final survival and per-protocol analysis of FIRE-3, a randomised clinical trial. Brit J Cancer. 2021;124(3):587–594.
17. Van Cutsem E, Kohne CH, Hitre E, et al. Cetuximab and chemotherapy as initial treatment for metastatic colorectal cancer. N Engl J Med. 2009;360(14):1408–1417.
18. Price TJ, Peeters M, Kim TW, et al. Panitumumab versus cetuximab in patients with chemotherapy-refractory wild-type KRAS exon 2 metastatic colorectal cancer (ASPECCT): A randomised, multicentre, open-label, non-inferiority phase 3 study. Lancet Oncol. 2014;15(6):569–579.
19. Takegawa N, Yonesaka K. HER2 as an emerging oncotarget for colorectal cancer treatment after failure of anti-epidermal growth factor receptor therapy. Clin Colorectal Cancer. 2017;16(4):247–251.
20. Sartore-Bianchi A, Lonardi S, Martino C, et al. Pertuzumab and trastuzumab emtansine in patients with HER2-amplified metastatic colorectal cancer: The phase II HERACLES-B trial. ESMO Open. 2020;5(5):e000911.
21. Meric-Bernstam F, Hurwitz H, Raghav KPS, et al. Pertuzumab plus trastuzumab for HER2-amplified metastatic colorectal cancer (MyPathway): An updated report from a multicentre, open-label, phase 2a, multiple basket study. Lancet Oncol. 2019;20(4):518–530.
22. Siena S, Di Bartolomeo M, Raghav K, et al. Trastuzumab deruxtecan (DS-8201) in patients with HER2-expressing metastatic colorectal cancer (DESTINY-CRC01): A multicentre, open-label, phase 2 trial. Lancet Oncol. 2021;22(6):779–789.
23. Valtorta E, Martino C, Sartore-Bianchi A, et al. Assessment of a HER2 scoring system for colorectal cancer: Results from a validation study. Mod Pathol. 2015;28(11):1481–1491.
24. Gatalica Z, Xiu J, Swensen J, Vranic S. Molecular characterization of cancers with NTRK gene fusions. Mod Pathol. 2019;32(1):147–153.

25. Doebele RC, Drilon A, Paz-Ares L, et al. Entrectinib in patients with advanced or metastatic NTRK fusion-positive solid tumours: Integrated analysis of three phase 1–2 trials. Lancet Oncol. 2020;21(2):271–282.
26. Punekar SR, Velcheti V, Neel BG, Wong KK. The current state of the art and future trends in RAS-targeted cancer therapies. Nat Rev Clin Oncol. 2022;19(10):637–655.
27. Ou SI, Janne PA, Leal TA, et al. First-in-human phase I/IB dose-finding study of adagrasib (MRTX849) in patients with advanced KRAS(G12C) solid tumors (KRYSTAL-1). J Clin Oncol. 2022;40(23):2530–2538.
28. Kopetz S, Grothey A, Yaeger R, et al. Encorafenib, binimetinib, and cetuximab in BRAF V600E-mutated colorectal cancer. N Engl J Med. 2019;381(17):1632–1643.
29. Tabernero J, Grothey A, Van Cutsem E, et al. Encorafenib plus cetuximab as a new standard of care for previously treated BRAF V600E-mutant metastatic colorectal cancer: Updated survival results and subgroup analyses from the BEACON study. J Clin Oncol. 2021;39(4):273–284.
30. Fancello L, Gandini S, Pelicci PG, Mazzarella L. Tumor mutational burden quantification from targeted gene panels: Major advancements and challenges. J Immunother Cancer. 2019;7(1):183.
31. Marabelle A, Fakih M, Lopez J, et al. Association of tumour mutational burden with outcomes in patients with advanced solid tumours treated with pembrolizumab: Prospective biomarker analysis of the multicohort, open-label, phase 2 KEYNOTE-158 study. Lancet Oncol. 2020;21(10):1353–1365.
32. Ogino S, Lochhead P, Giovannucci E, et al. Discovery of colorectal cancer PIK3CA mutation as potential predictive biomarker: Power and promise of molecular pathological epidemiology. Oncogene. 2014;33(23):2949–2955.
33. Bardelli A, Corso S, Bertotti A, et al. Amplification of the MET receptor drives resistance to anti-EGFR therapies in colorectal cancer. Cancer Discov. 2013;3(6):658–673.
34. Wolf J, Seto T, Han JY, et al. Capmatinib in MET exon 14-mutated or MET-amplified non-small-cell lung cancer. N Engl J Med. 2020;383(10):944–957.
35. Bibeau K, Feliz L, Lihou CF, Ren H, Abou-Alfa GK. Progression-free survival in patients with cholangiocarcinoma with or without FGF/FGFR alterations: A FIGHT-202 post hoc analysis of prior systemic therapy response. JCO Precis Oncol. 2022;6:e2100414.
36. Abou-Alfa GK, Sahai V, Hollebecque A, et al. Pemigatinib for previously treated, locally advanced or metastatic cholangiocarcinoma: A multicentre, open-label, phase 2 study. Lancet Oncol. 2020;21(5):671–684.
37. Cancer Genome Atlas Research N. Comprehensive molecular characterization of gastric adenocarcinoma. Nature. 2014;513(7517):202–209.
38. Sohn BH, Hwang JE, Jang HJ, et al. Clinical significance of four molecular subtypes of gastric cancer identified by The Cancer Genome Atlas project. Clin Cancer Res. 2017;23(15):4441–4449.
39. Cristescu R, Lee J, Nebozhyn M, et al. Molecular analysis of gastric cancer identifies subtypes associated with distinct clinical outcomes. Nat Med. 2015;21(5):449–456.
40. Ahn S, Lee SJ, Kim Y, et al. High-throughput protein and mRNA expression-based classification of gastric cancers can identify clinically distinct subtypes, concordant with recent molecular classifications. Am J Surg Pathol. 2017;41(1):106–115.
41. Bang YJ, Van Cutsem E, Feyereislova A, et al. Trastuzumab in combination with chemotherapy versus chemotherapy alone for treatment of HER2-positive advanced gastric or gastro-oesophageal junction cancer (ToGA): A phase 3, open-label, randomised controlled trial. Lancet. 2010; 376(9742):687–697.
42. Rivera F, Romero C, Jimenez-Fonseca P, et al. Phase II study to evaluate the efficacy of Trastuzumab in combination with capecitabine and oxaliplatin in first-line treatment of HER2-positive advanced gastric cancer: HERXO trial. Cancer Chemother Pharmacol. 2019;83(6):1175–1181.
43. Janjigian YY, Kawazoe A, Yanez P, et al. The KEYNOTE-811 trial of dual PD-1 and HER2 blockade in HER2-positive gastric cancer. Nature. 2021;600(7890):727–730.
44. Shitara K, Bang YJ, Iwasa S, et al. Trastuzumab deruxtecan in previously treated HER2-positive gastric cancer. N Engl J Med. 2020;382(25):2419–2430.
45. Bartley AN, Washington MK, Ventura CB, et al. HER2 testing and clinical decision making in gastroesophageal adenocarcinoma: Guideline from the College of American Pathologists, American Society for Clinical Pathology, and American Society of Clinical Oncology. Arch Pathol Lab Med. 2016;140(12):1345–1363.
46. Janjigian YY, Shitara K, Moehler M, et al. First-line nivolumab plus chemotherapy versus chemotherapy alone for advanced gastric, gastro-oesophageal junction, and oesophageal adenocarcinoma (CheckMate 649): A randomised, open-label, phase 3 trial. Lancet. 2021;398(10294):27–40.
47. Shitara K, Ajani JA, Moehler M, et al. Nivolumab plus chemotherapy or ipilimumab in gastro-oesophageal cancer. Nature. 2022;603(7903):942–948.
48. Muro K, Chung HC, Shankaran V, et al. Pembrolizumab for patients with PD-L1-positive advanced gastric cancer (KEYNOTE-012): A multicentre, open-label, phase 1b trial. Lancet Oncol. 2016;17(6):717–726.
49. Fuchs CS, Doi T, Jang RW, et al. Safety and efficacy of pembrolizumab monotherapy in patients with previously treated advanced gastric and gastroesophageal junction cancer: Phase 2 clinical KEYNOTE-059 trial. JAMA Oncol. 2018;4(5):e180013.
50. Kalpakoff M, Hund S, Musser J, et al. Intrapatient tumor heterogeneity in IHC interpretation using PD-L1 IHC 22C3 pharmDx. Appl Immunohistochem Mol Morphol. 2021;29(9):667–673.
51. Chao J, Fuchs CS, Shitara K, et al. Assessment of pembrolizumab therapy for the treatment of microsatellite instability-high gastric or gastroesophageal junction cancer among patients in the KEYNOTE-059, KEYNOTE-061, and KEYNOTE-062 clinical trials. JAMA Oncol. 2021;7(6):895–902.
52. Le DT, Uram JN, Wang H, et al. PD-1 blockade in tumors with mismatch-repair deficiency. N Engl J Med. 2015; 372(26):2509–2520.
53. Marabelle A, Le DT, Ascierto PA, et al. Efficacy of pembrolizumab in patients with noncolorectal high microsatellite instability/mismatch repair-deficient cancer: Results from the phase II KEYNOTE-158 study. J Clin Oncol. 2020;38(1):1–10.
54. Shinozaki-Ushiku A, Ishikawa S, Komura D, et al. The first case of gastric carcinoma with NTRK rearrangement: Identification of a novel ATP1B-NTRK1 fusion. Gastric Cancer. 2020;23(5):944–947.

55. Singh P, Toom S, Huang Y. Anti-claudin 18.2 antibody as new targeted therapy for advanced gastric cancer. J Hematol Oncol. 2017;10(1):105.
56. Sahin U, Tureci O, Manikhas G, et al. FAST: A randomised phase II study of zolbetuximab (IMAB362) plus EOX versus EOX alone for first-line treatment of advanced CLDN18.2-positive gastric and gastro-oesophageal adenocarcinoma. Ann Oncol. 2021;32(5):609–619.
57. Nakano H, Saito M, Nakajima S, et al. PD-L1 overexpression in EBV-positive gastric cancer is caused by unique genomic or epigenomic mechanisms. Sci Rep. 2021;11(1):1982.
58. Takamatsu S, Brown JB, Yamaguchi K, et al. Utility of homologous recombination deficiency biomarkers across cancer types. JCO Precis Oncol. 2022;6:e2200085.
59. Gonzalez-Martin A, Pothuri B, Vergote I, et al. Niraparib in patients with newly diagnosed advanced ovarian cancer. N Engl J Med. 2019;381(25):2391–2402.
60. Parikh AR, Leshchiner I, Elagina L, et al. Liquid versus tissue biopsy for detecting acquired resistance and tumor heterogeneity in gastrointestinal cancers. Nat Med. 2019;25(9):1415–1421.
61. Nakamura Y, Taniguchi H, Ikeda M, et al. Clinical utility of circulating tumor DNA sequencing in advanced gastrointestinal cancer: SCRUM-Japan GI-SCREEN and GOZILA studies. Nat Med. 2020;26(12):1859–1864.
62. Hsiehchen D, Bucheit L, Yang D, et al. Genetic features and therapeutic relevance of emergent circulating tumor DNA alterations in refractory non-colorectal gastrointestinal cancers. Nat Commun. 2022;13(1):7477.

15

Hepatobiliary and Pancreatic Cancers

Zaid Mahdi and Haider A. Mejbel

15.1 Introduction

Hepatocellular carcinoma (HCC) and cholangiocarcinoma are the two major primary malignant neoplasms of the liver. The molecular oncogenesis of HCC is often complex and occurs in multistep progression. In HCC, *TP53*, *CTNNB1*, *AXIN1*, and *RB1* are the most commonly mutated genes in which several signaling pathways are involved including WNT-β catenin, RAS, and PI3K/AKT/mTOR. In contrast, the molecular basis of cholangiocarcinoma is remarkably less complex including pathogenic mutations in *KRAS*, *BRAF*, and *IDH1*/*IDH2* as followed by mutations in *BAP1* and *ARID1A* as well as *FGFR2* gene fusion.

Alternatively, pancreatic ductal adenocarcinoma represents the most common cancer type comprising approximately 90% of all pancreatic malignant tumors. The reminder encompasses intraductal and cystic neoplasms, followed by neuroendocrine tumors, acinar cell carcinoma, and other less common neoplasms. Since the first recognition of *KRAS* as a major driver gene, several other genes were found to be a key genetic element in the oncogenesis of pancreatic neoplasms. *TP53* and *CDKN2A* were initially recognized in neoplasms of the uterine cervix and found to be pathogenically altered in several types of pancreatic tumors, followed by the recognition of *SMAD4*. These four genes are considered the major genes of pancreatic neoplasm oncogenesis. Nonetheless, recent whole-exome and whole-genome sequencing have yielded an extended list of genetic alterations and uncovered novel pathways.

Herein we discuss the clinicopathologic and molecular features of the most common and major liver and pancreatic malignant neoplasms, highlighting the essential role of molecular testing that alters the disease stage and informs therapy.

15.2 Hepatocellular Carcinoma

15.2.1 Diagnosis and Molecular Classification

Hepatocellular carcinoma (HCC) is the most common primary liver malignant neoplasm and is the fourth most common cause of cancer-related death worldwide (1). Currently, the most common risk factor is the hepatitis B virus while cases of hepatitis C virus infection have substantially decreased. Alternatively, non-alcoholic steatohepatitis has become the fastest-growing cause of HCC especially in Western countries (2). According to the American Association For The Study Of Liver Disease guidelines, the current diagnosis of HCC does not require a histological confirmation due to the excellent reported diagnostic performance of imaging procedures, and therefore confirmation of tissue diagnosis is not necessarily needed unless the radiological features are not classic (3). Histologically, the tumor cells show hepatocytic morphology with loss of normal hepatocyte architecture, thickened trabeculae with cells showing mild atypia and increase cell density in well to moderately differentiated HCCs. In poorly differentiated tumors, the atypia is marked, and the cells lose its resemblance to hepatocytes. In addition, HCC usually demonstrates various growth patterns such as pseudo-glandular, solid, and macro-trabecular pattern (Figure 15.1A).

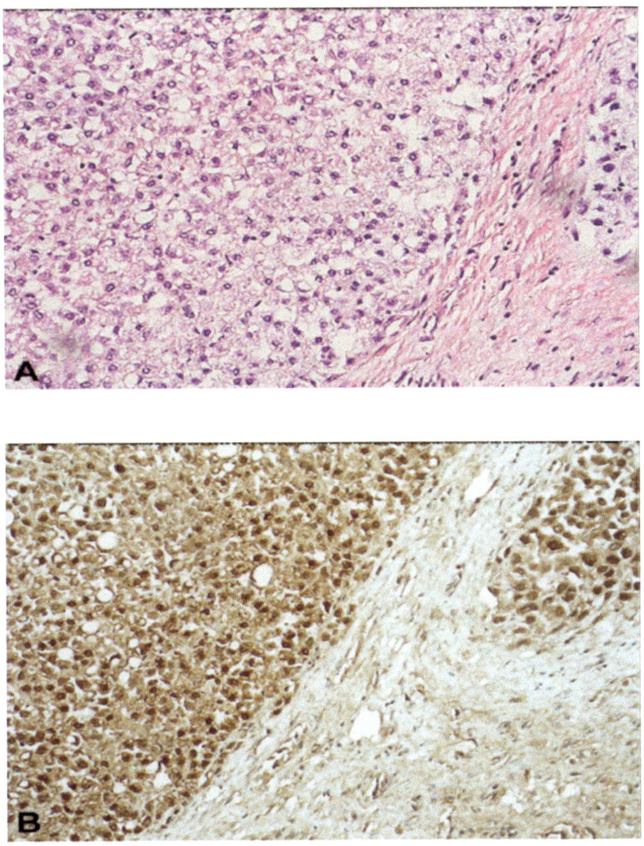

FIGURE 15.1 Moderately differentiated hepatocellular carcinoma. (A) Neoplastic cells infiltrating with a trabecular and solid growth pattern and demonstrating moderate cytological atypia (H&E, 200×); (B) Tumor cells strongly positive for arginase (IHC, 200×).

DOI: 10.1201/9781003513469-15

By immunohistochemistry, HCC is typically positive for arginase (85%) (Figure 15.1B), Hep-Parl (70%), and glypican-3 (only in poorly differentiated HCC). CA10 and polyclonal CEA usually show a characteristic canalicular pattern of staining in 75–80% of tumors (4, 5). Most HCCs develop in patients with cirrhosis that occurs due to an etiological factor that is also responsible for carcinogenesis. In up to 85% of the cases, HCCs appear to follow an evolution starting from chronic liver disease providing the basis for premalignant lesions (also known as dysplastic nodules) that eventually evolve into carcinomas while acquiring and accumulating clonal molecular alterations and activating different pathways during the process (6). Many oncogenic mutations have recently been identified in HCCs using the already-established technology of next-generation sequencing (NGS) (7). The most common somatic mutation in HCC is the one that affects the promoter region of the gene encoding telomerase reverse transcriptase (*TERT*), a master regulator of telomerase length, and occurs in approximately 60% of tumors. It has been reported that high levels of telomerase contribute to liver carcinogenesis by preventing senescence in chronically injured cells (8, 9). The second most common mutated gene in HCCs is known to be *CTNNB1* (30–35%) which is involved in the WNT pathway (10). Other mutations that are involved in chromatin remodeling such as *ARID1A*, *ARID1B*, and *ARID2* have been reported. In addition, other not-so-common mutations like *AXIN1*, *AXL*, and *BAP1*, as well as mutations in receptor tyrosine kinase pathways including *VEGFR*, *PDGFRA*, *EGFR*, and *PIK3CA* have also been reported (11, 12). A recently discovered *FGF19* mutation has also been described (13). The latter is known to be a protein that regulates bile acid synthesis and hepatocyte proliferation via activation of its receptor FGFR4. Besides the clonal mutations mentioned previously, carcinogenesis of HCC includes the involvement of several signaling pathways including telomere stability, TP53/cell cycle, chromatin remodeling, WNT signaling, PI3K/RAS/mTOR, oxidative stress, and MAPK/ERK pathways (13–17).

About 30% of HCCs can be further divided into distinctive subtypes and some of which show specific molecular alterations; the most common is the fibrolamellar carcinoma that usually presents in the young age group and has been only described in non-cirrhotic livers. Usually, fibrolamellar carcinoma shows a fusion transcript of exon 1 of the heat shock protein *DNAJB1* and *PRKACA* genes located on exons 2–10 forming a 400-kb fusion transcript of *DNAJB1::PRKACA*. This fusion protein retains the catalytic activity of protein kinase A (PKA) from *PRKACA*. Currently, patients with fibrolamellar carcinoma of the liver are included in the Pediatric Hepatic Malignancy International Therapeutic Trial, receiving surgery plus cisplatin and doxorubicin combination therapy. Since the oncogenic activity of the fusion transcript is driven by PKA, uprosertib, a PKA inhibitor has been used currently in xenograft cell lines (18). Other inhibitors like capivasertib have also been tested recently *in vitro* and showed a uniform activity against several cell lines. Transcriptomic analysis of the fibrolamellar carcinoma revealed upregulation in various tumor oncogenic pathways including Aurora Kinase A and members of the epidermal growth factor receptor (EGFR) pathway such as ERBB2. However, none of their inhibitors seems to be tested in clinical trials for fibrolamellar carcinoma (23).

15.2.2 Current Targeted Therapy

Given the several molecular alterations present in HCCs, there are currently already some established therapeutic approaches that are in use for patients with advanced HCC while others are being tested and in progress. In the following, we summarize the main molecular targeted monotherapies in Table 15.1.

TABLE 15.1

Targeted Therapy for HCC

Therapy Line	Agent	Molecular Target	Clinical Application
First line	Sorafenib	Multi-tyrosine kinase inhibitor targeting RAF kinases of the MAPK/ERK pathway, and thus inhibits angiogenic activity of VEGFR, PDGFR, BRAF and KIT (18).	Considered the standard of care for patients with advanced unresectable HCC since 2007.
	Lenvatinib	Multi-tyrosine kinase inhibitor targeting VEGFR1–3, FGFR1–4, PDGFR-α, RET and c-Kit (19, 20).	FDA approved in 2018 as first-line treatment for advanced HCC as it showed significant improvement in progression-free survival (7.4 months vs. 3.7 months; Hazard ratio 0.66; $p < 0.0001$) and positive objective response rate when compared to sorafenib (21).
	Donafenib	Targets VEGFR, PDGFR, and various RAF kinases; thereby inhibiting tumor angiogenesis and proliferation.	Significantly enhances overall survival when compared to Sorafenib (12.1 months vs. 10.3 months) in addition to an overall improvement in safety and tolerability (22).
Second line	Regorafenib	Similar in structure to Sorafenib; exhibits strong binding affinity towards VEGFR.	Given its known side effects, the FDA approved it as a second-line therapy for patients with progressing disease while on Sorafenib therapy (24).
	Cabozantinib	Targets VEGFR1–3, MET, and AXL, which are implicated in the progression of hepatocellular carcinoma and the development of resistance to sorafenib (25).	In the randomized phase 3 clinical trial, the drug showed longer overall survival and progression-free survival than placebo, but the high-grade adverse events were approximately twice that observed in placebo group (25).
	Ramucirumab	Anti-VEGFR2 monoclonal antibody that inhibit VEGF binding to VEGFR2 receptor and therefore inhibits angiogenesis.	Tested in a phase 3 clinical trial but didn't significantly improve survival over placebo except in patients with serum AFP levels > 400 (26).

In addition, other agents with selective targets, including selective MET, fibroblast growth factor receptor 4 (FGFR4), transforming growth factor-β (TGFβ), and phosphoinositide 3-kinase (PI3K)–AKT–mammalian target of rapamycin (mTOR) inhibitors, have also shown therapeutic potential for HCC in ongoing clinical trials (NCT02325739, NCT01246986, and NCT01177397).

15.3 Cholangiocarcinoma

15.3.1 Diagnosis and Molecular Classification

Cholangiocarcinoma is the second most common primary hepatic malignancy after HCC that arises from the biliary epithelia (lining epithelia and peribiliary glands) and accounts for about 10–15% of primary liver cancers (27). In general, it is classified by location into intrahepatic, perihilar, and extrahepatic cholangiocarcinoma. Intrahepatic cholangiocarcinoma, which will be described in this chapter, is further subclassified into large duct and small duct types. Large duct type arises in the large intrahepatic bile ducts near the hepatic hilum (proximal to the right and left hepatic ducts) and resembles perihilar and extrahepatic cholangiocarcinoma while small duct subtype occurs in the hepatic periphery. Small duct-type cholangiocarcinoma is composed of non-mucin-producing cuboidal cells, whereas large duct type is composed of mucin-producing columnar cells, reflecting different cells of origin (Figure 15.2).

Both types of intrahepatic cholangiocarcinoma show an increase in incidence in the last few decades in different parts of the world while the incidence of perihilar and extrahepatic counterparts show a stable or relatively decreased incidence (28–30). The risk factors for the small duct type show a similar trend to the risk factors that are involved in the pathogenesis of HCC (i.e., viral hepatitis, alcoholic liver disease, metabolic syndrome, and chemical exposure) while the large duct-type etiology is mainly related to risk factors similar to perihilar and extrahepatic cholangiocarcinoma such as primary sclerosing cholangitis, infection, hepatolithiasis and other rare biliary tracts malformations (30, 31). Interestingly, this classification has been shown to have clinicopathologic, molecular, therapeutic as well as prognostic significance (31). The prognosis of small duct type was shown to be generally favorable compared to that of large duct type. Cholangiocarcinoma in general is positive for CK7 and CK19 (Figure 15.3) and negative for CDX2 and generally negative for CK20. This pattern of staining can differentiate it from low gastrointestinal tract/colorectal carcinoma but unfortunately, there isn't any specific immunophenotype to exclude it from upper gastrointestinal malignancy and pancreatic ductal adenocarcinoma. Currently, there is no routine staining that is being used to separate large duct type from small duct type in intrahepatic cholangiocarcinoma but few studies have shown that large duct type is usually positive for S100p and TFF1, while small duct type shows positive staining for N-cadherin and CD56 (32).

Interestingly, the molecular profiles for these two subtypes can be different. Large duct type shows *KRAS* mutation in 20–30% of cases, and they usually carry *TP53* and *SMAD4* mutations. In contrast, small duct type exhibits frequent *IDH1/2* hotspot mutations, *FGFR2* fusions, and *BAP1* mutations (31). In addition to the molecular mutations, few signaling pathways have been reported to be dysregulated and hence involved in the carcinogenesis of cholangiocarcinoma. Interleukin-6 signal transducer and activator of transcription 3 (STAT3) signaling has been shown to be dysregulated in cholangiocarcinoma due to the associated chronic inflammatory process and fibrosis associated with the tumor (33). It has been additionally reported that high expression of IL-6 in

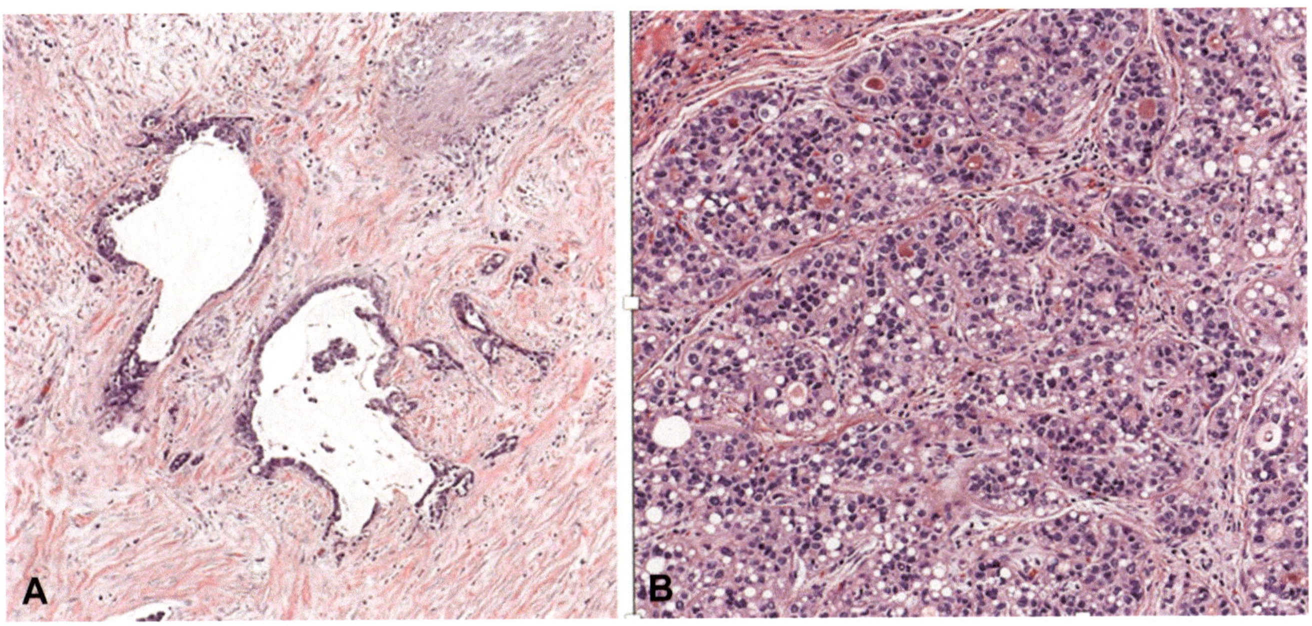

FIGURE 15.2 Cholangiocarcinoma, large duct type vs. small duct type. (A) Large duct type showing dilated neoplastic glands with desmoplastic stroma (H&E, ×100); (B) Small duct type showing packed small neoplastic glands with cuboidal cells (H&E, ×100).

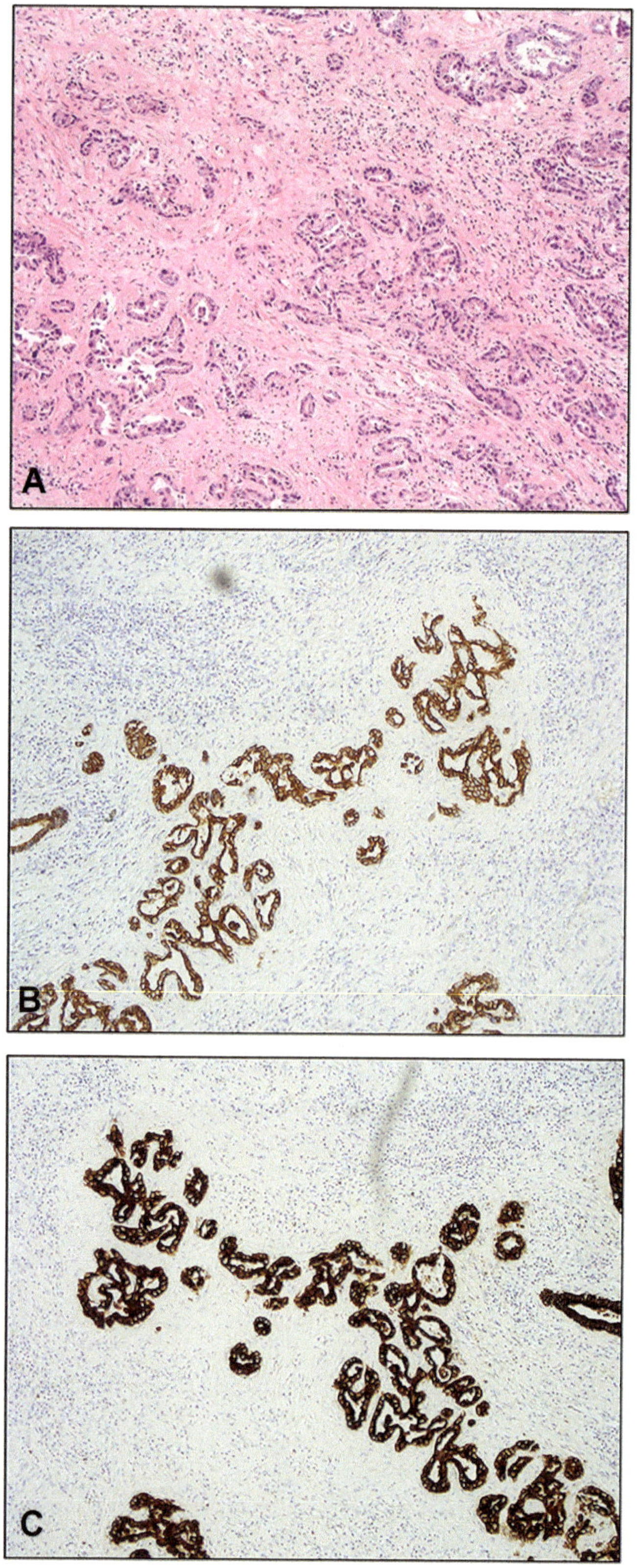

FIGURE 15.3 Cholangiocarcinoma. (A) Infiltrating neoplastic glands with desmoplastic stroma, with tumor cells exhibiting moderate cytologic atypia (H&E, 100×); (B) Neoplastic cells positive for CK7 (IHC, 100×); (C) Neoplastic cells positive for CK19 (IHC, 100×).

fibrotic stromal cells is associated with poor prognosis and resistance to chemotherapy in cholangiocarcinoma (34). Dysregulation in receptor tyrosine kinase pathways is another common feature among all cholangiocarcinoma subtypes. Any abnormal signaling through epidermal growth factor receptor (EGFR), vascular endothelial growth factor receptor (VEGFR), and fibroblast growth factor receptor (FGFR2) leads to proliferation and survival through RAS/MAPK and PIK3/AKT pathways (35). Another pathway found to be involved in cholangiocarcinoma is NOTCH signaling. It has been found that up to 75% of *NOTCH* genes are aberrantly expressed in cholangiocarcinoma (36).

Importantly, *FGFR2* being the prevalent gene that undergoes fusion, is harbored in approximately 25–30% of all cholangiocarcinomas (37). They are more common in small duct type and frequently show *FGFR::BACC1* fusion (38). Key downstream signaling pathways altered by FGFR activation are the Ras-Raf-MEK-ERK and the PI3-AKT-mTOR pathways (39, 40).

15.3.2 Current Targeted Therapy

Despite our increased understanding for the carcinogenesis of cholangiocarcinoma that has led to the discovery of novel targets amenable to therapeutic intervention, the outlook for cholangiocarcinoma remains disappointing. The aggressive nature of the tumor tends to be asymptomatic in its early stages and would lead to a late diagnosis. The latter may compromise the efficacy of surgical resection which currently represents the only curative option. For patients with unresectable tumors, palliative chemotherapy with gemcitabine plus cisplatin is the first-line treatment. For advanced tumors, so far, the main and the most clinically significant molecular targets that have been tested are summarized in Table 15.2.

15.4 Pancreatic Carcinoma

15.4.1 Ductal Adenocarcinoma

Pancreatic ductal adenocarcinoma (PDAC) is an invasive carcinoma with ductal/glandular differentiation. The majority of PDACs are solitary tumors and arise in the pancreatic head of adult individuals. PDAC is the most common primary malignant epithelial neoplasm of the pancreas accounting for approximately 90% of all pancreatic neoplasms with an estimated age-dependent incidence rate ranging from 1.5–6.2 new cases per 100,000 individuals per year (42). Histologically, conventional types of PDACs are characterized by infiltrating adenocarcinoma with duct-like glandular formation and desmoplastic reaction (Figure 15.4).

PDAC typically exhibits a pancreatobiliary immunophenotype with positive expression for CK7, CK8, CK18, CK19, and CEA, and loss of SMAD4 immunostain in 50% of the cases. Histologic subtypes of PDAC include adenosquamous, colloid, medullary, poorly cohesive signet-ring cell, hepatoid, and undifferentiated carcinomas. Molecular profiling of PDACs revealed genetic alteration in four major genes, which include *KRAS, TP53, CDKN2A*, and *SMAD4*. *KRAS* activation by point mutation and/or gene copy number changes is detected in up to 95% of PDACs (42), whereas *TP53, CDKN2A*, and *SMAD4* are each

TABLE 15.2

Targeted Therapy for Cholangiocarcinoma

Agent	Molecular Target	Clinical Application
Ivosidenib	IDH1 inhibitor	Used in a randomized, double-blind, phase III trial and shows an enhanced progression-free survival when compared with a placebo alone (38, 41). In August 2021, the FDA approved ivosidenib for patients with locally advanced or metastatic cholangiocarcinoma harboring *IDH1* mutation (38).
Pemigatinib	ATP- competitive FGFR kinase inhibitor	Shows marked difference in response rate between patients with *FGFR2* fusions compared with those with other or no *FGFR* alterations (median overall survival for patients with *FGFR2* fusions was 21.1 month with 35.5% of *FGFR2* fusion-positive patients reached an objective response while no objective response was seen in patients with other or no *FGFR* mutations (38, 39).

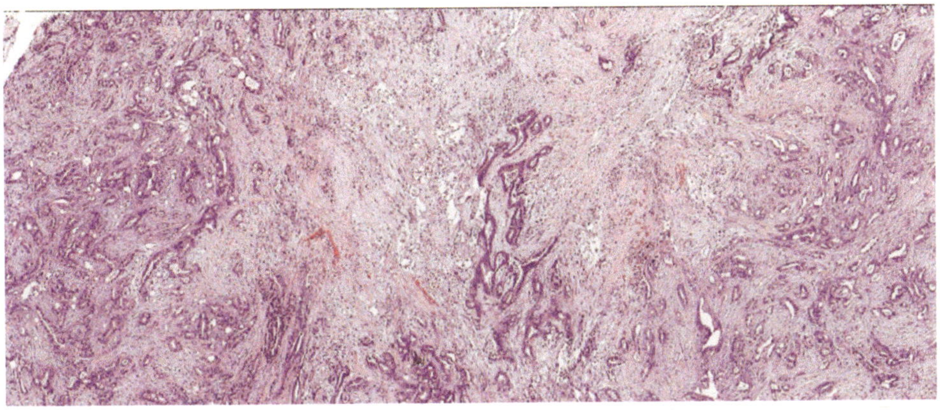

FIGURE 15.4 Conventional type of PDAC. Neoplastic cells infiltrating with duct-like glandular formation and associated desmoplastic reaction (H&E, 20×).

inactivated in approximately 50% of PDACs (43). Among the four major genes of PDACs, *SMAD4* is considered prognostically significant and associated with poor outcomes. Furthermore, germline mutations in several genes including DNA mismatch repair genes (*MLH1*, *MLH3*, *MSH2*, *MSH6*, and *PMS2*), *BRCA1*, *BRCA2*, *PALB2*, *CDKN2A*, *ATM*, and *STK11* have been found to provide genetic evidence of PDAC association with familial cancer syndromes (44).

15.4.2 Adenosquamous Carcinoma

Pancreatic adenosquamous carcinoma (AdSCC) is a rare subtype of PDAC that accounts for less than 4% of malignant epithelial neoplasms of the pancreas. AdSCC is defined by its glandular and squamous differentiation, where each constitutes at least 30% of the tumor (5). The squamous component is recognized histologically by exhibiting keratinizing and/or non-keratinizing squamous differentiation with cells exhibiting intracellular bridges and expressing squamous immunophenotypes such as p40 positive expression. In addition to the four main genes detected in PDACs, up to 80% of AdSCC harbor inactivating mutations in the *UPF1* gene (45). In comparison to conventional PDAC, AdSCC is associated with a worse prognosis with a median survival of 6 months. Several studies suggested an inverse correlation between the tumor percentage of squamous cell component and overall survival; however, due to the tumor rarity and the coexistence of several potential confounders such as smoking, obesity, patient general health, and socioeconomic status, the prognostic significance of squamous cell component is yet to be explored.

15.4.3 Colloid Carcinoma

Pancreatic colloid carcinoma is a rare subtype of PDAC accounting for less than 3% of all malignant pancreatic epithelial neoplasms and is characterized by its abundant mucin production forming large pools that comprise at least 80% of the tumor (44). In addition to sharing the same genetic characteristic with conventional PDAC, molecular testing of colloid carcinoma revealed additional genetic alterations including mutations in *GNAS* and *RNF43* genes (45). In contrast to AdSCC, colloid carcinoma is associated with a good prognosis with an estimated 5-year survival rate of 60%.

15.4.4 Medullary Carcinoma

Pancreatic medullary carcinoma is another rare subtype of PDAC that is histologically characterized by its pushing borders, poor epithelial differentiation, syncytial growth pattern, and associated lymphoplasmacytic reaction. Medullary carcinoma is a genetically distinct subtype as it is predominantly MMR-deficient, mostly *KRAS* wild-type, and about a third of this cancer is *BRAF* mutated. Compared to the conventional type of PDAC, medullary carcinoma has a better prognosis (46).

15.4.5 Acinar Cell Carcinoma

Pancreatic acinar cell carcinoma (PACC) is an exceedingly rare malignant epithelial neoplasm with acinar cell differentiation and significant exocrine enzyme production. In comparison to PDAC, PACC has a distinct molecular profile that includes a significantly higher detection rate of *BRAF* mutation, amplification, and rearrangements. Additionally, up to a third of PACC harbor a pathogenic mutation in one or more of the following genes *BRCA2*, *JAK1*, *ATM*, *PALB2*, and *BAP1* (47). In contrast to PDAC, PACC has a lower rate of genetic alteration in *KRAS*, *TP53*, and *SMAD4* (48).

15.4.6 Neuroendocrine Neoplasms

Pancreatic neuroendocrine neoplasms (PanNEN) are defined as malignant epithelial neoplasms with strong neuroendocrine differentiation and lack of other cell line differentiation. PanNEN is classified as pancreatic neuroendocrine tumors (PanNET) and pancreatic neuroendocrine carcinoma (PanNEC)

Histologically (Figure 15.5A and B), PanNETs typically exhibit the characteristic "salt and pepper" nuclei with nested, lobular, tubular/pseudoglandular, and/or trabecular pattern of growth and are graded based on its proliferative index as estimated by Ki-67 immunostaining into grade 1 (< 2 mitoses/10 HPF, < 3% Ki-67), grade 2 (2–20 mitoses/10 HPF, 3–20% Ki-67), and grade 3 (> 20 mitoses/10 HPF, > 20% Ki-67). Alternatively, NECs are poorly differentiated, high grade, and composed of atypical cells exhibiting nuclear molding and variable expression of neuroendocrine (NE) markers including synaptophysin and chromogranin (49) (Figure 15.5 C&D). Although both PanNET and PanNEC are immunophenotypically similar, they are genetically distinct. Extended molecular profiling of PanNET revealed four main molecular drivers including *MEN1*, *ATRX*, *DAXX*, and *mTOR* (50). In contrast, PanNEC lacks these mutations and harbors late event mutations such as *TP53* and *RB* in PDAC.

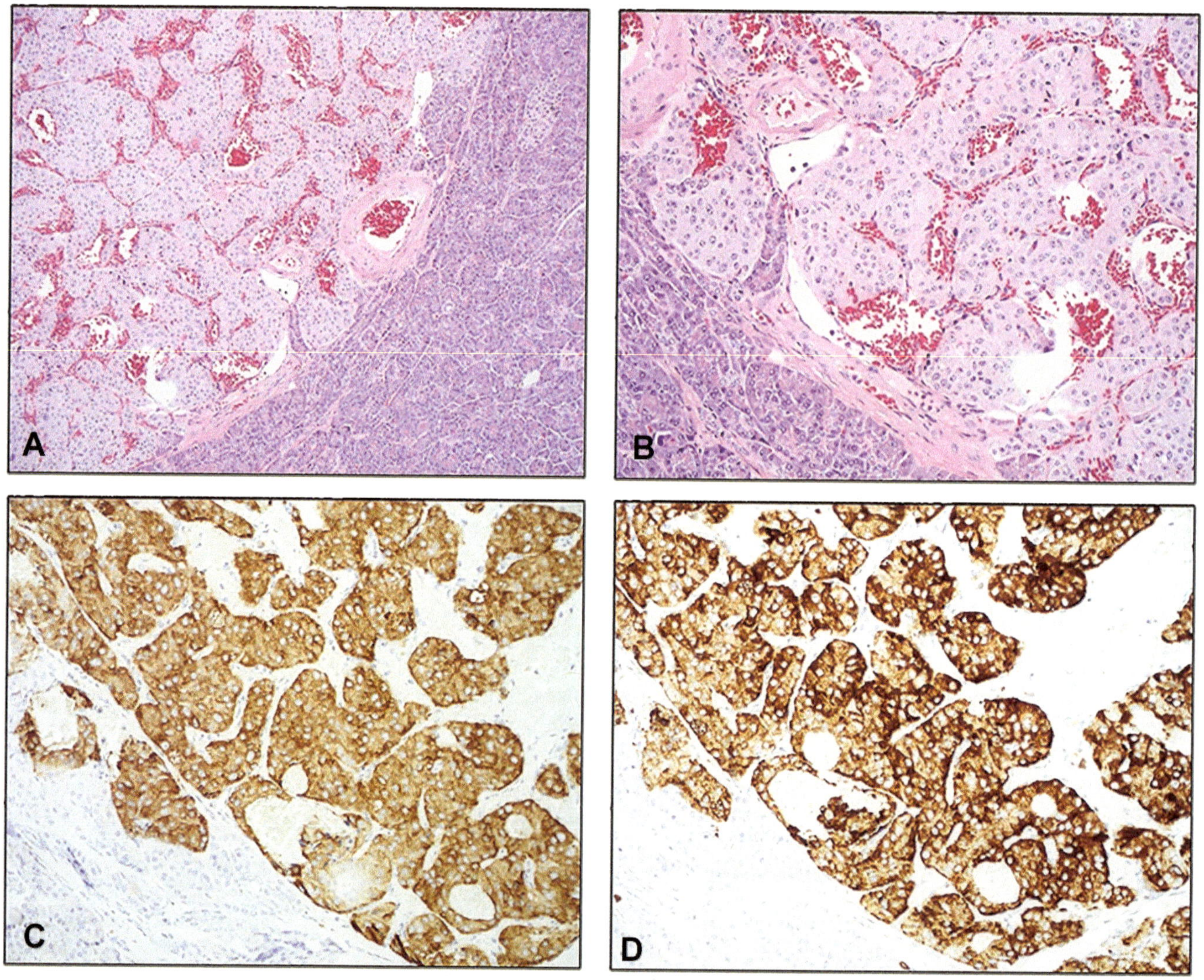

FIGURE 15.5 Pancreatic well-differentiated neuroendocrine tumor. (A) Neoplastic cells growing in lobular or nesting pattern (H&E, 100×); (B) Cytomorphology showing the characteristic "salt and pepper" appearance of nuclear chromatin (H&E, 200×); Neoplastic cells diffusely positive for synaptophysin (C, IHC, 200×) and chromogranin (D, IHC, 200×).

15.4.7 Current Targeted Therapy

Due to the complex pancreatic cancer network and microenvironment encompassing tumor cells, endothelial cells, immune cells, and tumor-associated fibroblasts, the medical treatment of pancreatic carcinoma can be challenging. Alternatively, advanced molecular testing of whole-genome and whole-exome sequencing have expanded our understating of the molecular profile of pancreatic carcinomas to design personalized targeted therapy. Genetic analysis of PDACs revealed several targeted genes including *BRCA2* and mismatch repair genes. *BRCA2* biallelic inactivation is found to be sensitive to PARP inhibitors (51). Studies have shown that AdSCC may respond to platinum-based therapy, in which, the addition of a single platinum agent to the adjuvant regimen plan shows an improvement in survival rate (HR = 2.4; 95% CI, 1.0–5.8; P = 0.04) (52). PDAC with microsatellite instability high (MSI-H) has been shown to have a durable response to immunotherapy, including pembrolizumab and nivolumab, whereas *BRAF* rearrangement in PACCs provides a therapeutic target for BRAF/MEK inhibition with a good response rate reported for dabrafenib and trametinib (53). In PanNET, a mutation in *mTOR* poses a therapeutic target for mTOR inhibitors such as everolimus (54).

15.5 Testing Strategies in Pancreatic Carcinoma

The ideal personalized oncologic treatment plans starts with a patient visit to the oncology clinic, obtaining tissue by image-guided core needle biopsy, and rendering a definitive diagnosis, followed by mutational and transcriptional tumor profiling. In about 30% of pancreatic carcinoma, up to 20 actionable somatic mutations were detected. These include *ARID1A* (8%), *CDK4/6* (7%), *PIK3CA* (7%), *PTEN* (5%), *RNF43* (3%), and *BRAF* (2%) (55). In addition, genetic analysis of PACCs for *BRAF* rearrangement can be performed using a single-probe FISH or RNA-based NGS fusion gene panel. The latter may help detect *BRAF* fusion and thus provide an additional option for therapeutic targets. However, fast disease progression as well as tumor inherited characteristics including intertumor and intratumor heterogeneity, are considered the major challenges that limit designing the perfect personalized oncologic therapeutic module.

REFERENCES

1. Vij M, Calderaro J. Pathologic and molecular features of hepatocellular carcinoma: An update. World J Hepatol. 2021;13(4):393–410.
2. McGlynn KA, Petrick JL, El-Serag HB, Epidemiology of hepatocellular Carcinoma. Hepatology 2021;73(Suppl 1):4–13.
3. Tan CH, Low SC, Thng CH. APASL and AASLD consensus guidelines on imaging diagnosis of hepatocellular carcinoma: A review. Int J Hepatol. 2011;2011:519783.
4. Takahashi Y, Dungubat E, Kusano H, et al. Application of immunohistochemistry in the pathological diagnosis of liver tumors. Int J Mol Sci. 2021;22(11):5780.
5. WHO Classification of Tumours Editorial Board. WHO Classification of Tumors: Digestive System Tumours. 5th ed. Lyon, France: International Agency for Research on Cancer; 2019.
6. Llovet JM, Kelley RK, Villanueva A, et al. Hepatocellular carcinoma. Nat Rev Dis Primers. 2021;7(1):6.
7. Dominguez DA, Wang XW. Impact of next-generation sequencing on outcomes in hepatocellular carcinoma: How precise are we really? J Hepatocell Carcinoma. 2020;7:33–37.
8. Ozturk M, Arslan-Ergul A, Bagislar S, et al. Senescence and immortality in hepatocellular carcinoma. Cancer Lett. 2009;286(1):103–13.
9. Nault JC, Ningarhari M, Rebouissou S, Zucman-Rossi J. The role of telomeres and telomerase in cirrhosis and liver cancer. Nat Rev Gastroenterol Hepatol. 2019;16(9):544–558.
10. Xu C, Xu Z, Zhang Y, et al. β-Catenin signaling in hepatocellular carcinoma. J Clin Invest. 2022;132(4).
11. Xiao Y, Liu G, Ouyang X, et al. Loss of ARID1A promotes hepatocellular carcinoma progression via up-regulation of MYC transcription. J Clin Transl Hepatol. 2021;9(4):528–536.
12. Liu L, Tian N, Zhou C, et al. A potentially functional variant of ARID1B interacts with physical activity in association with risk of hepatocellular carcinoma. Oncotarget. 2017;8(19):31057–31064.
13. Raja A, Park I, Haq F, Ahn SM. *FGF19-FGFR4* signaling in hepatocellular carcinoma. Cells. 2019 4;8(6):536.
14. Loesch R, Chenane L, Colnot S. ARID2 chromatin remodeler in hepatocellular carcinoma. Cells. 2020;9(10):2152.
15. Ding XX, Zhu QG, Zhang SM, et al. Precision medicine for hepatocellular carcinoma: Driver mutations and targeted therapy. Oncotarget. 2017;8(33):55715–55730.
16. Khemlina G, Ikeda S, Kurzrock R. The biology of Hepatocellular carcinoma: Implications for genomic and immune therapies. Mol Cancer. 2017;16(1):149.
17. Moon H, Ro SW. MAPK/ERK Signaling pathway in hepatocellular carcinoma. Cancers (Basel). 2021;13(12):3026.
18. Llovet JM, Ricci S, Mazzaferro V, et al. Sorafenib in advanced hepatocellular carcinoma. N Engl J Med. 2008; 359(4):378–390.
19. Zschäbitz S, Grüllich C. Lenvantinib: A tyrosine kinase inhibitor of VEGFR 1–3, FGFR 1–4, PDGFRα, KIT and RET. Recent Results Cancer Res. 2018:211:187–198.
20. Yamamoto Y, Matsui J, Matsushima T, et al. Lenvatinib, an angiogenesis inhibitor targeting VEGFR/FGFR, shows broad antitumor activity in human tumor xenograft models associated with microvessel density and pericyte coverage. Vasc Cell. 2014;6:18.
21. Kudo M, Finn RS, Qin S, et al. Lenvatinib versus sorafenib in first-line treatment of patients with unresectable hepatocellular carcinoma: A randomised phase 3 non-inferiority trial. Lancet. 2018;391(10126):1163–1173.
22. Qin S, Bi F, Gu S, et al. Donafenib versus Sorafenib in first-line treatment of unresectable or metastatic hepatocellular carcinoma: A randomized, open-label, parallel-controlled Phase II-III trial. J Clin Oncol. 2021; 39(27):3002–3011.
23. Lalazar G, Requena D, Ramos-Espiritu L, et al. Identification of novel therapeutic targets for fibrolamellar carcinoma using patient-derived xenografts and direct-from-patient screening. Cancer Discov. 2021;11(10):2544–2563.
24. Yang C, Zhang H, Zhang L, et al. Evolving therapeutic landscape of advanced hepatocellular carcinoma. Nat Rev Gastroenterol Hepatol. 2023;20(4):203–222.
25. Abou-Alfa GK, Meyer T, Cheng AL, et al. Cabozantinib in patients with advanced and progressing hepatocellular carcinoma. N Engl J Med. 2018;379(1):54–63.

26. Zhu AX, Finn RS, Kang YK, et al. Serum alpha-fetoprotein and clinical outcomes in patients with advanced hepatocellular carcinoma treated with ramucirumab. Br J Cancer. 2021;124(8):1388–1397.
27. Tyson GL, Ilyas JA, Duan Z, et al. Secular trends in the incidence of cholangiocarcinoma in the USA and the impact of misclassification. Dig Dis Sci. 2014;59(12):3103–3110.
28. Palmer WC, Patel T. Are common factors involved in the pathogenesis of primary liver cancers? A meta-analysis of risk factors for intrahepatic cholangiocarcinoma. J Hepatol. 2012;57(1):69–76.
29. Liau JY, Tsai JH, Yuan RH, et al. Morphological subclassification of intrahepatic cholangiocarcinoma: Etiological, clinicopathological, and molecular features. Mod Pathol. 2014;27(8):1163–1173.
30. Nakanuma Y, Sato Y, Harada K, et al. Pathological classification of intrahepatic cholangiocarcinoma based on a new concept. World J Hepatol. 2010;2(12):419–427.
31. Chung T, Park YN. Up-to-date pathologic classification and molecular characteristics of intrahepatic cholangiocarcinoma. Front Med (Lausanne). 2022;9:857140.
32. Krasinskas AM. Cholangiocarcinoma. Surg Pathol Clin. 2018;11(2):403–429.
33. Yang R, Song Y, Shakoor K, et al. Insights into the role of STAT3 in intrahepatic cholangiocarcinoma (review). Mol Med Rep. 2022;25(5):171.
34. Kittirat Y, Suksawat M, Thongchot S, et al. Interleukin-6-derived cancer-associated fibroblasts activate STAT3 pathway contributing to gemcitabine resistance in cholangiocarcinoma. Front Pharmacol. 2022;13:897368.
35. Chen C, Nelson LJ, Ávila MA, Cubero FJ. Mitogen-activated protein kinases (MAPKs) and cholangiocarcinoma: The missing link. Cells. 2019;8(10):1172.
36. O'Rourke CJ, Matter MS, Nepal C, et al. Identification of a pan-gamma-secretase inhibitor response signature for Notch-driven cholangiocarcinoma. Hepatology. 2020;71(1):196–213.
37. Vogel A, Segatto O, Stenzinger A, Saborowski A. FGFR2 inhibition in cholangiocarcinoma. Annu Rev Med. 2023:74: 293–306.
38. Param NJ, Bramel ER, Sia D. The molecular pathogenesis and targeted therapies for cholangiocarcinoma. Surg Pathol Clin. 2022;15(3):529–539.
39. Jusakul A, Cutcutache I, Yong CH, et al. Whole-genome and epigenomic landscapes of etiologically distinct subtypes of cholangiocarcinoma. Cancer Discov. 2017;7(10):1116–1135.
40. Goyal L, Kongpetch S, Crolley VE, et al. Targeting FGFR inhibition in cholangiocarcinoma. Cancer Treat Rev. 2021; 95:102170.
42. Bray F, Ferlay J, Soerjomataram I, et al. Global cancer statistics 2018: GLOBOCAN estimates of incidence and mortality worldwide for 36 cancers in 185 countries. CA Cancer J Clin. 2018;68(6):394–424.
43. Witkiewicz AK, McMillan EA, Balaji U, et al. Whole-exome sequencing of pancreatic cancer defines genetic diversity and therapeutic targets. Nat Commun. 2015;6:6744.
44. Pihlak R, Valle JW, McNamara MG. Germline mutations in pancreatic cancer and potential new therapeutic options. Oncotarget. 2017;8(42):73240–73257.
45. Liu C, Karam R, Zhou Y, et al. The UPF1 RNA surveillance gene is commonly mutated in pancreatic adenosquamous carcinoma. Nat Med. 2014;20(6):596–598.
46. Lee JH, Kim Y, Choi JW, et al. KRAS, GNAS, and RNF43 mutations in intraductal papillary mucinous neoplasm of the pancreas: A meta-analysis. Springerplus. 2016;5(1):1172.
47. Humphris JL, Patch AM, Nones K, et al. Hypermutation in pancreatic cancer. Gastroenterology. 2017;152(1):68–74.e2.
48. Chmielecki J, Hutchinson KE, Frampton GM, et al. Comprehensive genomic profiling of pancreatic acinar cell carcinomas identifies recurrent RAF fusions and frequent inactivation of DNA repair genes. Cancer Discov. 2014;4(12):1398–1405.
49. Jiao Y, Yonescu R, Offerhaus GJ, et al. Whole-exome sequencing of pancreatic neoplasms with acinar differentiation. J Pathol. 2014;232(4):428–435.
50. Heaphy CM, de Wilde RF, Jiao Y, et al. Altered telomeres in tumors with ATRX and DAXX mutations. Science. 2011;333(6041):425.
51. Lowery MA, Kelsen DP, Stadler ZK, et al. An emerging entity: Pancreatic adenocarcinoma associated with a known BRCA mutation: Clinical descriptors, treatment implications, and future directions. Oncologist. 2011;16(10):1397–1402.
52. Busch E, Kreutzfeldt S, Agaimy A, et al. Successful BRAF/MEK inhibition in a patient with *BRAF*^{V600E}-mutated extrapancreatic acinar cell carcinoma. Cold Spring Harb Mol Case Stud. 2020;6(4):a005553.
53. Cramer S, Marcus MA, Ramkissoon S, et al. Pediatric *BRAF* (V600E)-mutated pancreatic acinar cell carcinoma with complete and durable response to Dabrafenib and Trametinib. JCO Precis Oncol. 2020;4:801–805.
54. Yao JC, Shah MH, Ito T, et al. Everolimus for advanced pancreatic neuroendocrine tumors. N Engl J Med. 2011;364(6): 514–523.
55. Aung KL, Fischer SE, Denroche RE, et al. Genomics-driven precision medicine for advanced pancreatic cancer: Early results from the COMPASS trial. Clin Cancer Res. 2018;24(6):1344–1354.

16

Urinary and Male Genital Tract Tumors

Lara Harik, Faisal Saeed, Sara Wobker, and Yingbei Chen

16.1 Introduction

Precision medicine and targeted therapy are increasingly incorporated into treatment regimens for genitourinary tumors. As these treatment modalities become more refined, there may be a bigger role for the general pathologist in influencing therapy, as part of the multi-disciplinary care unit. In this chapter we will discuss the molecular alterations of the various histologic subtypes by organ systems and provide an overview of treatments beyond traditional chemotherapy for those tumors.

16.2 Prostate Cancer

Prostatic adenocarcinoma (PC) is the second most common cancer in men, with an estimated 268,490 new cases and an estimated 34,500 deaths in the United States in 2022 (1). Neoplasms other than adenocarcinoma are exceptionally uncommon, accounting for ~1% of prostatic tumors (Table 16.1). PC can be grouped into early-stage and advanced-stage disease (Table 16.2). Localized PC is often initially managed with active surveillance or curative-intent strategies (radical prostatectomy or radiation therapy +/- androgen deprivation therapy (ADT)), depending on initial risk stratification (Table 16.3) including Gleason grade (Figure 16.1 and Table 16.4), and has an excellent prognosis. Androgen receptor (AR) signaling plays a crucial role in PC initiation and progression and remains the key therapeutic target. ADT has been the backbone of systemic therapy in advanced PC for several decades. Recently, data has shown that addition of novel AR-signaling inhibitors (ARSIs) or docetaxel to ADT improves patient outcome in metastatic castration-sensitive PC (mCSPC). While these agents have had successful outcomes, most cases ultimately progress to castration-resistant PC (CRPC) with an average time of onset of 2–3 years after AR-directed therapy (2) (Figure 16.2). Chemotherapy, novel ARSIs, and

TABLE 16.1

Clinical and Molecular Characteristics of Prostatic Tumors Other Than Adenocarcinoma

Histologic Type	Description	Association	Molecular Alterations
Prostatic squamous cell carcinoma	Squamous histology (keratinization, keratin pearls, intercellular bridges) with no glandular elements	Association with previous hormone or radiation therapy	Recent case reports have shown *TMPRSS2::ERG* fusion (fusion presence confirms prostatic origin)
Prostatic adenosquamous carcinoma	Both glandular and squamous components	Association with previous hormone or radiation therapy	Show *TMPRSS2::ERG* fusions, *PTEN* deletions, and *SPOP* mutations
Prostatic adenoid cystic (basal cell) carcinoma	Prostatic basal cell origin		17–47% show *MYB::NFIB* fusion >90% overexpress ERBB2 (HER2) *TMPRSS2::ERG* fusions have not been identified
Prostatic stromal tumor of uncertain malignant potential (PST- UMP)	Arises from specialized prostatic stroma and has uncertain clinical behavior	Coexist with PSS	Similar alterations in PSS and PST-UMP (including deletions of chromosomes 13 and 14) Higher mutation burden and more disorganized aberrations in PSS No convincing reports of progression from PST-UMP to PSS PST-UMP and PSS are molecularly heterogeneous with largely non-recurrent alterations
Prostatic stromal sarcoma (PSS)	Arises from specialized prostatic stroma and has the potential to act aggressively and metastasize to distant sites such as bone and lung	Coexist with PST-UMP	

Source: ref. 4, 5

DOI: 10.1201/9781003513469-16

TABLE 16.2

Prostate Cancer Stages and 5-Year Relative Survival Rates for Different Stages

Stage at Diagnosis		Definition (TNM Stage)	% of Cases Diagnosed at This Stage	SEER 5-Year Relative Survival* Rates, 2012–2018
Early-stage	Localized	Confined to primary site (any T, N0, M0)	73%	100%
Advanced-stage	Regional	Spread to regional lymph nodes (any T, N1, M0)	14%	100%
	Distant	Cancer has metastasized (any T, any N, M1)	7%	32.3%
	Unknown/unstaged		6%	85.8%
All stages			100%	96.8%

Note: *Relative survival is an estimate of the percentage of patients who would be expected to survive the effects of their cancer (https://seer.cancer.gov/news/SEER-Relative-Survival-Overview.pdf).

TABLE 16.3

Initial Risk Stratification of Localized Prostate Cancer (NCCN risk groups)

Risk Group	Clinical/Pathological Features		
Very low risk	Has all of the following: • cT1c • Grade group 1 • PSA < 10 ng/mL • < 3 prostate needle cores/fragments involved; ≤ 50% cancer in each core/fragment • PSA density < 0.15 ng/mL/g		
Low risk	Has all of the following but does not qualify for very low risk: • cT1—cT2a • Grade group 1 • PSA < 10 ng/mL		
Intermediate risk	Has all of the following: • No high-risk group features • No very high-risk group features • Has one or more of the following intermediate risk factors (IRFs): • cT2b—cT2c • Grade group 2 or 3 • PSA 10–20 ng/mL	Favorable intermediate	Has all of the following: • 1 IRF • Grade group 1 or 2 • < 50% biopsy cores involved
		Unfavorable intermediate	Has one or more of the following: • 2 or 3 IRFs • Grade group 3 • ≥ 50% biopsy cores involved
High risk	Has no very high-risk features and has only one of the following high-risk features: • cT3a • Grade group 4 or 5 • PSA > 20 ng/mL		
Very high risk	Has at least one of the following: • cT3b—cT4 • Primary Gleason pattern 5 • 2 or 3 high risk features • > 4 cores with Grade group 4 or 5		

Source: adapted from ref. 83

radiopharmaceuticals have significantly improved the management of metastatic (m)CRPC; however, median survival remains less than 2 years (3). In recent years, success of PROfound, IPATential150, and TheraP trials has been instrumental in transitioning from sequential to precision treatment, based on therapeutic targets. Several FDA approved drugs are available for treatment of advanced PC (Table 16.5).

16.2.1 Molecular Findings

Advances in genomic sequencing have expanded the molecular landscape of PC, leading to identification of actionable targets and emerging resistance mechanisms. In early-stage PC, ETS gene fusions (e.g. *TMPRSS2::ERG*) are the most frequent genomic alteration. TCGA cohort of 333 primary PC cases reported seven main molecular subtypes for 74% of the cases,

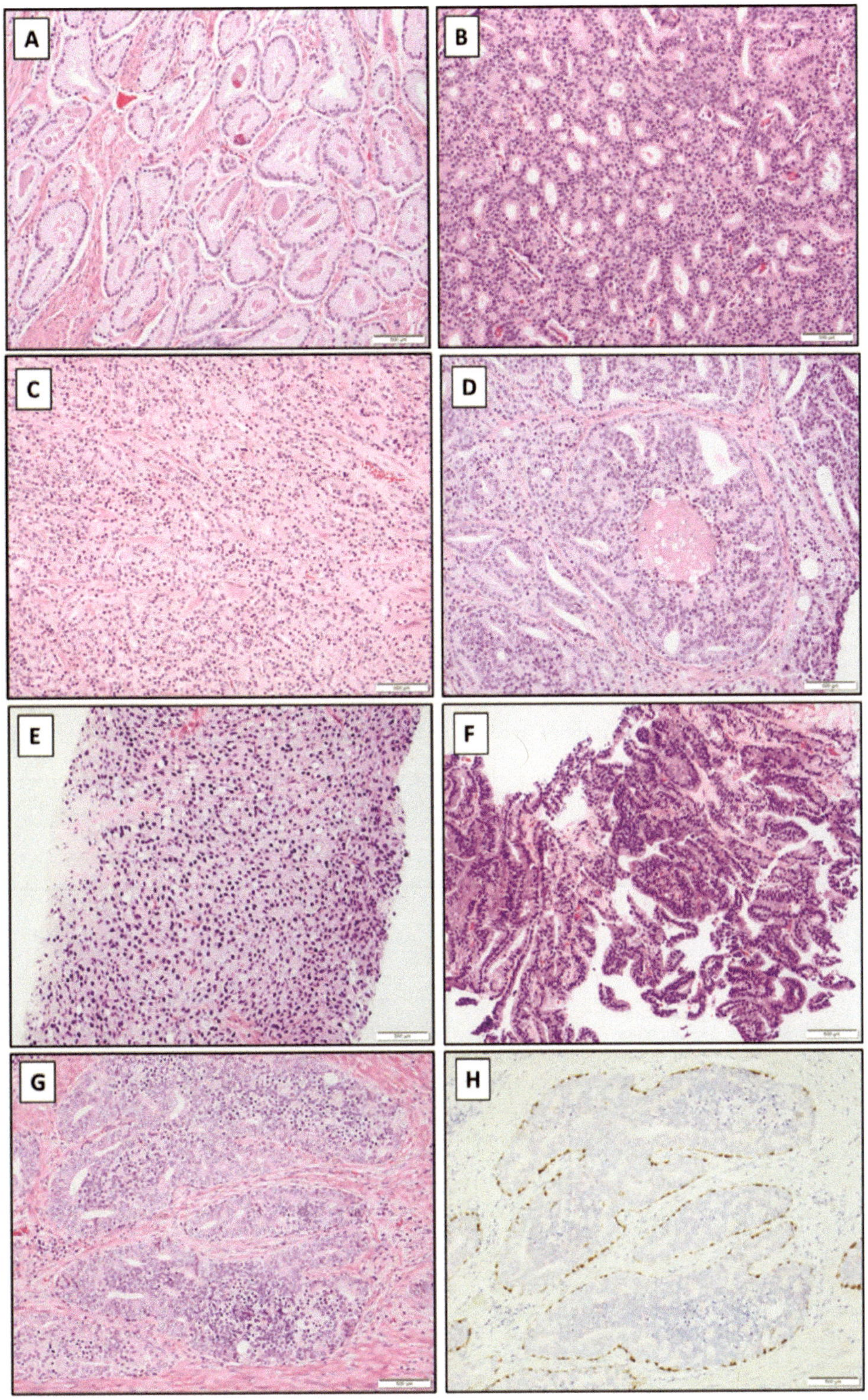

FIGURE 16.1 Morphology of different Gleason patterns. (A) Gleason pattern 3 (hematoxylin and eosin, ×200). (B) Gleason pattern 4, cribriform morphology (hematoxylin and eosin, ×200). (C) Gleason pattern 4, poorly formed and fused glands (hematoxylin and eosin, ×200). (D) Gleason pattern 5, comedonecrosis (hematoxylin and eosin, ×200). (E) Gleason pattern 5, sheets of cells with signet ring cells (hematoxylin and eosin, ×200). (F) Ductal morphology (hematoxylin and eosin, ×200). (G) Intraductal carcinoma of the prostate (hematoxylin and eosin, ×200). (H) PIN3 stain highlighting basal cells in intraductal carcinoma of the prostate (×200).

TABLE 16.4

Prostate Cancer Grade Groups[a]

Grade Group	Total Gleason Score	Gleason Patterns[b]
1	≤ 6	≤ 3+3
2	7	3+4
3	7	4+3
4	8	3+5, 4+4, 5+3
5	9 or 10	4+5, 5+4, 5+5

Notes:

[a]Adapted from reference (6).

[b]Gleason pattern 3: Individual discrete well-formed glands;

Gleason pattern 4: Poorly-formed/fused/cribriform glands, glomeruloid forms;

Gleason pattern 5: Comedo necrosis, cords, sheets, solid nests, single cells.

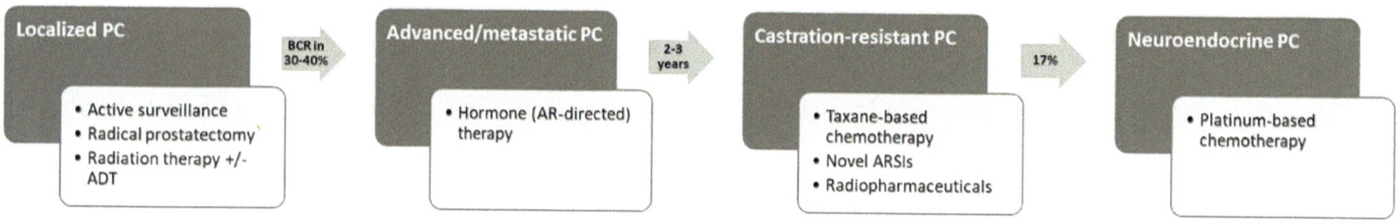

FIGURE 16.2 Evolution and standard of care for different stages of prostate cancer.

TABLE 16.5

FDA-Approved Drugs for Advanced/Metastatic Prostate Cancer in the Last 15 Years and Their Mechanism of Action and Clinical Indications

Drug	Initial FDA Approval Date	Mechanism of Action	Clinical Trial (NCT #)	Clinical Indications
Abiraterone acetate [a]	April 2011	Androgen synthesis inhibitor—inhibits 17 α-hydroxylase/C17,20-lyase (CYP17)	COU-AA-301 (NCT00638690) COU-AA-302 (NCT00887198) LATITUDE (NCT01715285) STAMPEDE (NCT00268476)	In combination with prednisone for treatment of patients with mCRPC and mCSPC
Enzalutamide	August 2012	AR inhibitor—competitively inhibits androgen binding to AR; inhibits nuclear translocation of AR and its interaction with DNA	AFFIRM (NCT00974311) PREVAIL (NCT01212991) TERRAIN (NCT01288911) PROSPER (NCT02003924) ENZAMET (NCT02446405) ARCHES (NCT02677896)	Treatment of patients with mCRPC and nmCRPC Treatment of patients with mCSPC
Apalutamide	September 2019	AR inhibitor—competitively inhibits androgen binding to AR; inhibits nuclear translocation of AR and its interaction with DNA	SPARTAN (NCT01946204) TITAN (NCT02489318)	Treatment of patients with nmCRPC if PSADT is less than or equal to 10 months Treatment of patients with mCSPC
Darolutamide	July 2019	AR inhibitor—competitively inhibits androgen binding to AR; inhibits nuclear translocation of AR and its interaction with DNA	ARAMIS (NCT02200614)	Treatment of patients with nmCRPC if PSADT is less than or equal to 10 months Treatment of patients with mCSPC
Cabazitaxel	June 2010	Microtubule inhibitor (binds to tubulin and promotes its assembly into microtubules while simultaneously inhibiting disassembly)	TROPIC (NCT00417079) PROSELICA (NCT01308580) CARD (NCT02485691) FIRSTANA (NCT01308567)	In combination with prednisone or dexamethasone for treatment of patients with mCRPC previously treated with a docetaxel-containing treatment regimen
Denosumab	November 2010	RANK ligand (RANKL) inhibitor	Trial 3	Prevent or delay disease-associated skeletal-related events in patients with mCRPC and bone metastases To prevent bone loss and fractures during ADT

(Continued)

TABLE 16.5 (Continued)

Drug	Initial FDA Approval Date	Mechanism of Action	Clinical Trial (NCT #)	Clinical Indications
Relugolix	December 2020	GnRH/LHRH receptor antagonist (competitively binds to pituitary GnRH receptors)	HERO (NCT03085095)	Treatment of patients with advanced prostate cancer
Olaparib	May 2020	Poly (ADP-ribose) polymerase (PARP) inhibitor	PROfound (NCT02987543)	Treatment of patients with mCRPC and deleterious or suspected deleterious germline and/or somatic HRR gene mutations in at least one of 14 genes (*BRCA1, BRCA2, ATM, BARD1, BRIP1, CDK12, CHEK1, CHEK2, FANCL, PALB2, RAD51B, RAD51C, RAD51D*, or *RAD54L*) and who had previously received treatment with enzalutamide or abiraterone
Rucaparib	May 2020	Poly (ADP-ribose) polymerase (PARP) inhibitor	TRITON2 (NCT02952534)	Treatment of patients with mCRPC and deleterious or suspected deleterious germline and/or somatic HRR gene mutations in *BRCA1* or *BRCA2*, who have been previously treated with a novel hormonal agent and a taxane-based chemotherapy
Sipuleucel-T	April 2010	Autologous cellular immunotherapy (induces an immune response targeted against PAP, an antigen expressed in most PC cells)	D9902B (NCT00065442)	Treatment of asymptomatic or minimally symptomatic mCRPC with no visceral metastasis
Lutetium Lu 177 vipivotide tetraxetan (Lu-177-PSMA-617)	March 2022	Radioligand therapeutic agent (radionuclide which delivers radiation directly to PSMA-expressing cells)	VISION (NCT03511664)	Treatment of patients with PSMA-positive mCRPC who have been treated with AR pathway inhibition and taxane-based chemotherapy
Radium-223	May 2013	Alpha particle-emitting radioactive therapeutic agent (mimics calcium and forms complexes with the bone mineral hydroxyapatite at areas of increased bone turnover, such as bone metastases)	ALSYMPCA (NCT00699751)	Treatment of patients with mCRPC, symptomatic bone metastases and no known visceral metastatic disease
Pembrolizumab	May 2017	Programmed death receptor-1 (PD-1)-blocking antibody	KEYNOTE-199 (NCT02787005) KEYNOTE-158 (NCT02628067)	Treatment of patients with unresectable or metastatic, MSI-H or dMMR solid tumors, or TMB-H [≥ 10 mutations/megabase (mut/Mb)] solid tumors, as determined by an FDA-approved test, that have progressed following prior treatment and who have no satisfactory alternative treatment options

Note:

[a] Patients receiving novel ARSIs (abiraterone, enzalutamide, apalutamide, or darolutamide) should also receive GnRH/LHRH analog concurrently or should have had bilateral orchiectomy.

Abbreviation: ADT, androgen deprivation therapy; AR, androgen receptor; dMMR, deficient mismatch repair; HRR, homologous recombination repair; GnRH, gonadotrophin-releasing hormone; LHRH, luteinizing hormone-releasing hormone; mCRPC, metastatic castration-resistant prostate cancer; mCSPC, metastatic castration-sensitive prostate cancer; MSI-H, microsatellite instability-high; nmCRPC, non-metastatic castration-resistant prostate cancer; PAP, prostatic acid phosphatase; PSADT, prostate-specific antigen doubling time; PSMA, prostate-specific membrane antigen; TMB-H, tumor mutational burden-high.

with heterogeneous genomic alterations in the remaining 26% cases (7) (Figure 16.3). Gain of 8q24 (including *MYC*), *PTEN* loss, *TP53* inactivation, and additional mutations and hypermethylation events are linked to disease progression. Table 16.6 summarizes the most common recurrent genomic alterations in localized PC, mCSPC, and mCRPC (7–10).

The transition of CSPC to CRPC is associated with *AR* gene amplification, mutation, and/or activation of *AR* splice variants (12) (Figure 16.4), indicating that *AR* is a key driver of late-stage disease as well. A small subset of CRPC is the result of *trans*-differentiation into an AR-negative phenotype (13) (Figures 16.5 and 16.6). Finally, ~20–30% of PC appear

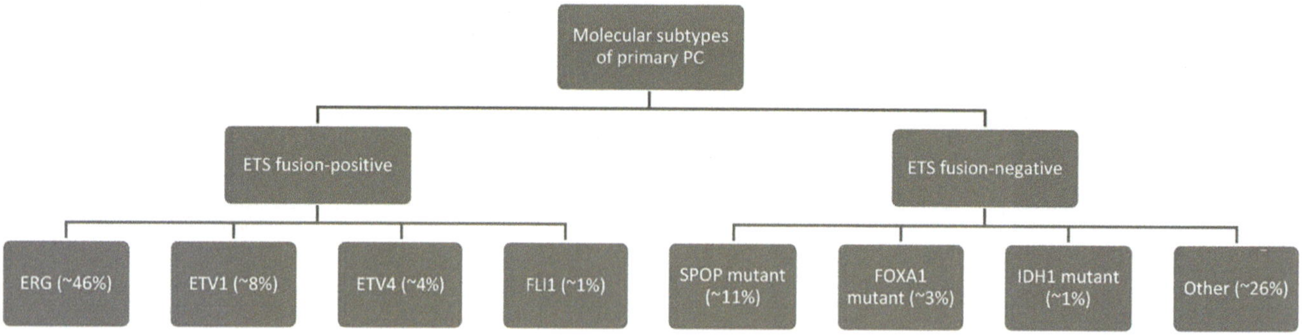

FIGURE 16.3 Molecular subtypes of primary prostate cancer (TCGA cohort of 333 cases).

TABLE 16.6

Frequency of Recurrent Genetic Alterations in Localized PC, mCSPC and mCRPC

Genes	Localized PC (n = 333)	mCSPC (n = 424)	mCRPC (n = 444)
ERG	46%	26%	32%
ETV1/ETV4/FLI1	13%	2.4%	10%
AR	1.2%	6%	59%
PTEN	17%	25%	33%
TP53	8%	33%	40%
RB1	0.9%	5%	13%
SPOP	11%	13%	11%
FOXA1	3%	15%	14%
MYC	8%	8%	25%
CHD1	7%	N/P	7%
BRCA2	3%	7%	12%
BRCA1	1.2%	0.5%	5%
ATM	7%	8%	8%
CDK12	2.4%	7%	10%
APC	5%	12%	8%
CTNNB1	2.7%	6%	9%

Note: Castration-resistant prostate cancer (CRPC) is defined as PC that progresses clinically, radiographically, or biochemically despite castrate levels of serum testosterone (< 50 ng/dL) (ref. 11). PC, prostate cancer; mCSPC and mCRPC, metastatic castration-sensitive and -resistant prostate cancer

to harbor germline or somatic alterations in DNA repair genes involved in homologous recombination repair (HRR), mismatch repair (MMR), and others (10, 14).

16.2.2 Predictive and Prognostic Biomarkers

Several genomic tests (Decipher (15), Oncotype DX Prostate (16), and Polaris (17)) are commercially available to improve risk stratification of patients with PC (Table 16.7). The ProMark Proteomic Prognostic Test (18) is a biopsy-based prognostic test that evaluates formalin-fixed paraffin-embedded tissue to differentiate indolent from aggressive PC. Several biomarkers are available and others are emerging owing to the recent advances in metabolomic, genomic, and transcriptomic analysis, which can be utilized in the prediction of PC outcome and response to therapy (Table 16.8) (19).

16.2.3 Targeting Signaling Pathways

Molecular and genetic profiles are increasingly being used to subtype cancers and guide selection of more precisely targeted therapeutic interventions. Chung et al. (14) in 2019 performed comprehensive genomic profiling on 3476 PCs and found that 57% of cases had genomic alterations in pathways that were investigational biomarkers for targeted therapies (Table 16.9). Armenia et al. (20) also reported genomic alterations in similar pathways and that they were more frequently altered in metastatic compared to primary tumors (Table 16.10). Figure 16.7 summarizes the clinically actionable targets in PC.

16.2.4 Targeting AR-Signaling Pathway

The AR-signaling pathway can be targeted via multiple approaches (Table 16.11). In recent years, several novel ARSIs

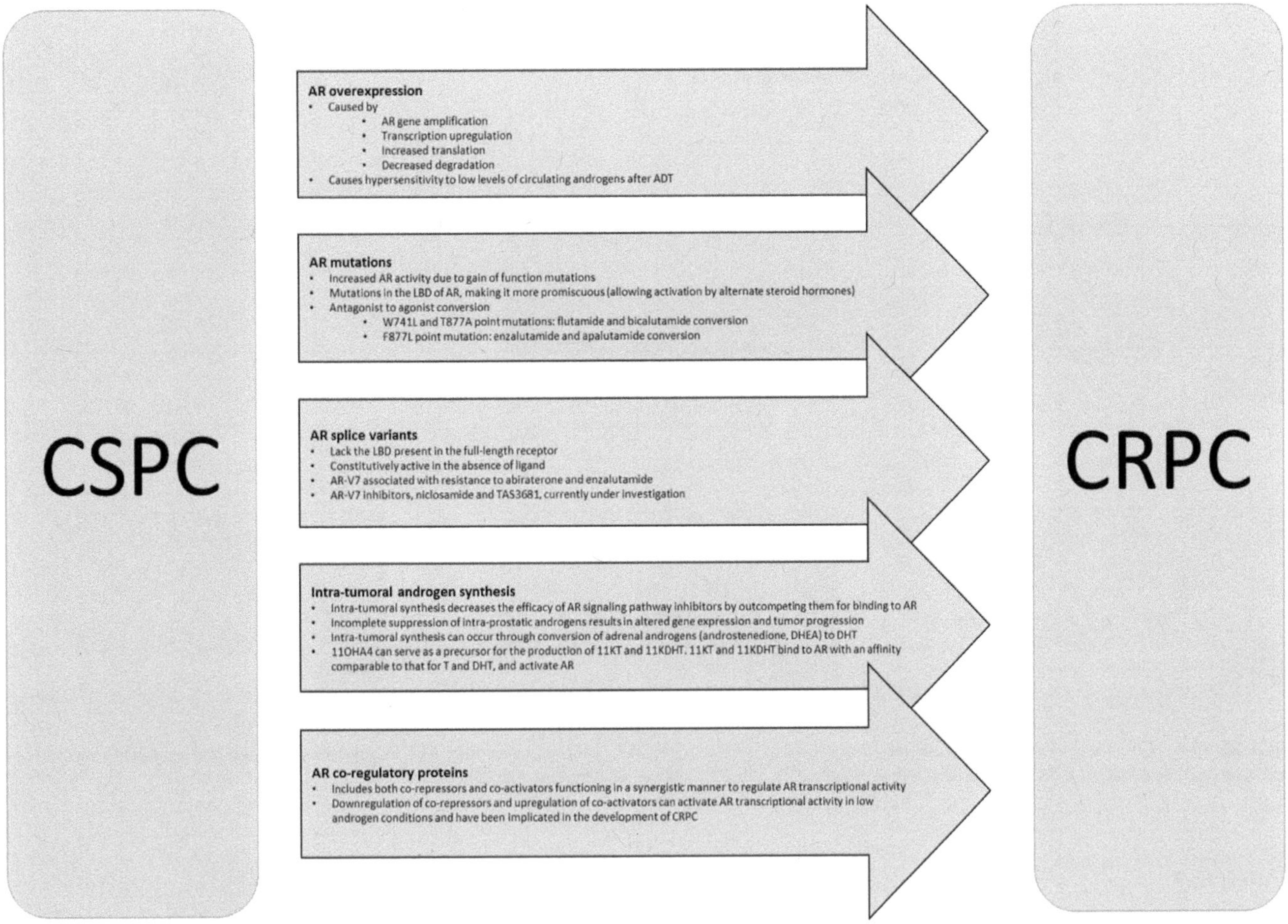

FIGURE 16.4 AR-dependent mechanisms driving castration-resistant prostate cancer.

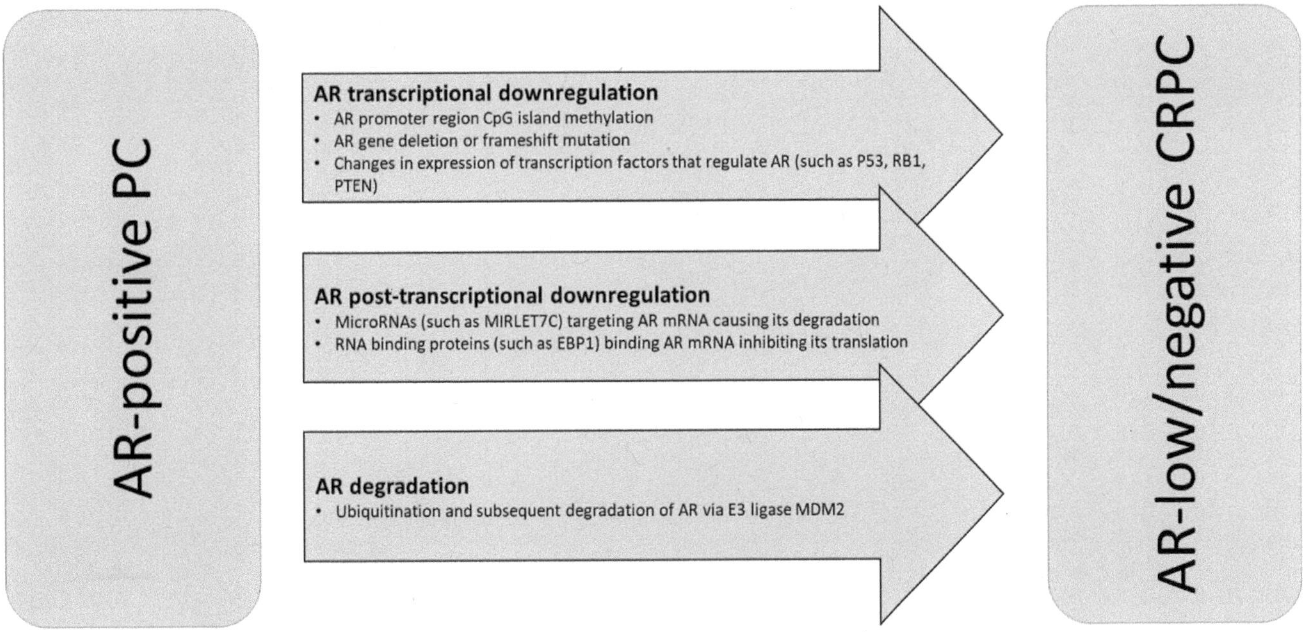

FIGURE 16.5 Mechanisms mediating loss of AR expression in castration-resistant prostate cancer.

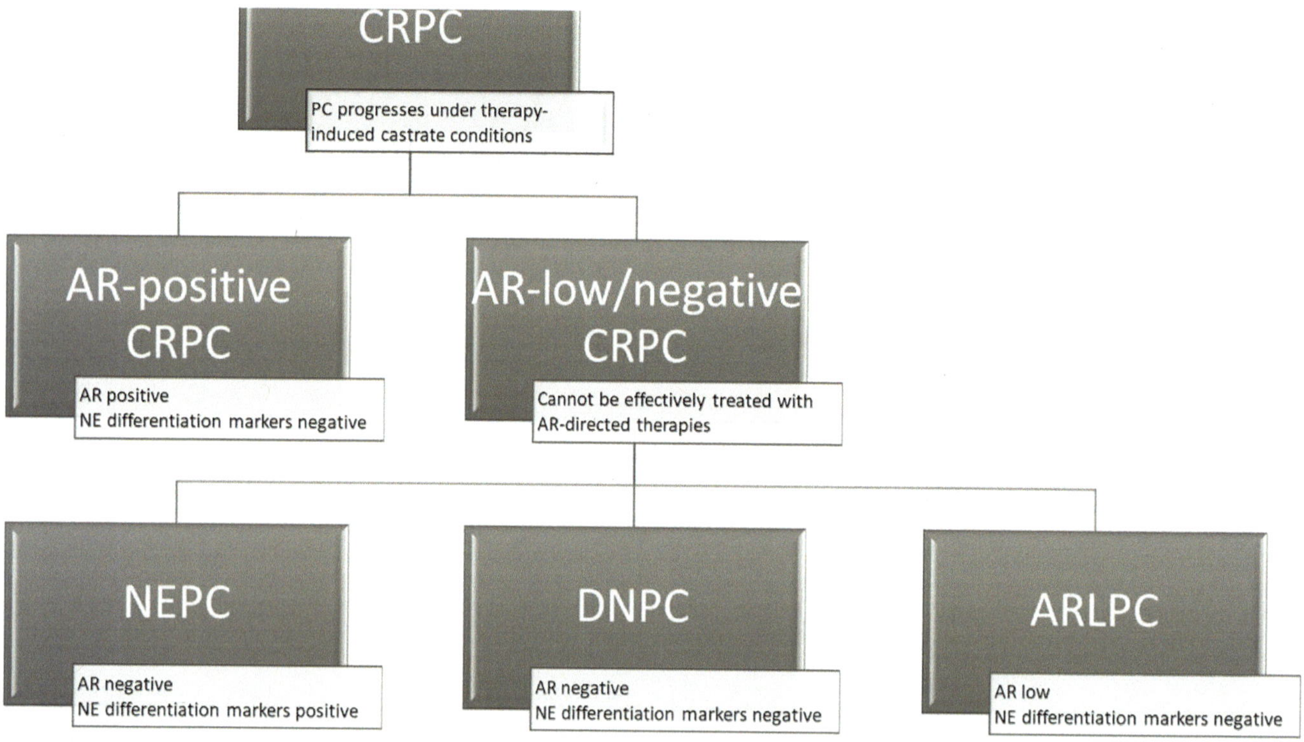

FIGURE 16.6 Overview of subtypes of castration-resistant prostate cancer. AR, androgen receptor; ARLPC, AR-low prostate cancer; CRPC, castration-resistant prostate cancer; DNPC, double negative prostate cancer; NEPC, neuroendocrine prostate cancer.

TABLE 16.7

Gene Expression Testing for Risk Stratification of Patients with Prostate Cancer

Genomic Classifier	Decipher	Oncotype DX Prostate	Prolaris
Platform	Whole-transcriptome microarray RNA	Quantitative RT-PCR	Quantitative RT-PCR
Tissue biomarkers	22 cancer-related genes	12 cancer-related genes + 5 housekeeping genes	31 cell-cycle-related genes + 15 housekeeping genes
Tested genes	*LASP1* *IQGAP3* *NFIB* *S1PR4* *THBS2* *ANO7* *PCDH7* *MYBPC1* *EPPK1* *TSBP* *PBX1* *NUSAP1* *ZWILCH* *UBE2C* *CAMK2N1* *RABGAP1* *PCAT-32* *GLYATL1P4* *PCAT-80* *TNFRSF19*	*AZGP1* *KLK2* *SRD5A2* *FAM13C* *FLNC* *GSN* *TPM2* *GSTM2* *TPX2* *BGN* *COL1A1* *SFRP4*	*FOXM1* *CDC20* *CDKN3* *CDC2* *KIF11* *KIAA0101* *NUSAP1* *CENPF* *ASPM* *BUB1B* *RRM2* *DLGAP5* *BIRC5* *KIF20A* *PLK1* *TOP2A* *TK1* *PBK* *ASF1B* *C18orf24* *RAD54L* *PTTG1* *CDCA3* *MCM10*

(Continued)

TABLE 16.7 (Continued)

Genomic Classifier	Decipher	Oncotype DX Prostate	Prolaris
			PRC1 *DTL* *CEP55* *RAD51* *CENPM* *CDCA8* *ORC6L*
Score	Genomic Classifier Score Ranges from 0–1	Genomic Prostate Score Ranges from 0–100	Cell-cycle Progression Score Ranges from 0–10
Target population	Low-risk or favorable/unfavorable intermediate-risk or high-risk disease and life expectancy ≥ 10 years	Low-risk or favorable intermediate-risk disease and life expectancy ≥ 10 years	Low-risk or favorable/unfavorable intermediate-risk or high-risk disease and life expectancy ≥ 10 years
Clinical utility	Predict the 5-yr probability of metastases after RP Guide adjuvant therapy when adverse features found after RP GC score > 0.6 have a high-risk of developing metastatic disease	Predict the probability of adverse pathological features (grade group ≥ 3 or extracapsular extension) at RP	Predict the 10-yr prostate cancer-specific mortality with watchful waiting Predict the 10-yr risk of metastases after definitive therapy

Note: Decipher, Oncotype DX Prostate, and Prolaris are tissue-based mRNA genomic classifiers. GC, Genomic Classifier; RP, radical prostatectomy

TABLE 16.8

Predictive and Prognostic Biomarkers That Are Available and Emerging in the Management of Prostate Cancer

Biomarker	Predictive vs. Prognostic	Clinical Utility
Androgen receptor (AR)	Predictive	Detection of *AR* amplification and heavily mutated *AR* in plasma cell-free DNA is associated with worse progression free survival (PFS) in mCRPC patients treated with enzalutamide. Circulating *AR* copy number variations in plasma DNA are associated with a worse outcome in mCRPC patients treated with ARSIs. *AR* gain in plasma DNA is also associated with a worse outcome in docetaxel-treated mCRPC patients, but *AR*-gained patients seem to derive greater benefit from treatment with taxanes than with ARSIs.
AR splice variant 7 (AR-V7)	Predictive/ prognostic	*AR-V7* levels in primary tumors can be used as a predictive marker for the development of CRPC and as a prognostic marker in CRPC patients. AR-V7 expression is associated with shorter survival in CRPC patients. *AR-V7* in circulating tumor cells is a predictor for resistance to novel ARSIs, but not to taxane-based chemotherapy in mCRPC.
Bone metabolic markers (BMMs)	Predictive/ prognostic	BMMs may have a role as predictive and prognostic indicators in mCRPC with bone metastases. Possible predictive role for BMMs in patients treated with radium-223.
Bone scan index (BSI)	Prognostic	Bone scan index has been studied as a prognostic indicator of overall survival (OS). mCRPC patients with a lower BSI (≤ 5) have better OS compared to patients with higher BSI (> 5).
Circulating cell-free DNA (cf-DNA) or circulating tumor-DNA (ct-DNA)	Predictive	In November 2020, the FDA approved the NGS-based FoundationOne Liquid CDx test that uses cf-DNA isolated from plasma of cancer patients for use in mCRPC to identify mutations in the *BRCA1*, *BRCA2* and *ATM* genes.
Circulating tumor cell (CTC) enumeration	Prognostic	CTC assessment using CellSearch has been approved by the FDA as a prognostic tool in PC. Presence of ≥ 5 CTCs is prognostic for shorter survival in men with mCRPC. Presence of < 5 CTCs at baseline prior to start of cabazitaxel therapy is a prognostic indicator of better PFS and OS. CTC may be used to monitor the effects of different treatments in CRPC when measured before and after treatment.
ERG and SOX9	Predictive	ERG and SOX9 positivity correlate with a lower PSA-PFS, rPFS, and OS following docetaxel treatment in mCRPC patients and may help decide which patients are less likely to benefit from chemotherapy. *ERG* fusion status may be a biomarker of docetaxel resistance.
Homologous recombination repair (HRR) mutations	Predictive/ prognostic	Germline *BRCA2* mutations have been associated with aggressive disease and poor clinical outcomes. The PROREPAIR-B study has shown that the detection of germline *BRCA2* alterations has negative prognostic significance. Predictive of response to PARP inhibitors. May be predictive of response to platinum-based chemotherapy and ICIs.

(Continued)

TABLE 16.8 (Continued)

Biomarker	Predictive vs. Prognostic	Clinical Utility
HSD3B1 genotype	Predictive/ prognostic	*HSD3B1* gene encodes HSD3B1 enzyme that catalyzes the conversion of DHEA to testosterone and DHT in prostatic tissue. *HSD3B1(1245A)* is an adrenal-restrictive allele that encodes an enzyme that is more rapidly degraded, limiting conversion of DHEA to DHT. *HSD3B1(1245C)* is an adrenal-permissive allele, encoding a more stable enzyme and resulting in more DHT production. In patients with low volume mCSPC who received ADT with or without docetaxel, OS at 5 years was worse and progression to CRPC was higher in adrenal-permissive genotypes (inheritance of at least one copy of *HSD3B1 (1245C)* compared to adrenal-restrictive genotypes. *HSD3B1* genotype may serve as a prognostic marker for patients with mCSPC with low volume disease and as a predictive marker for response to ADT in this population.
Microsatellite instability (MSI) and deficient mismatch repair (dMMR)	Predictive	dMMR and MSI-H can serve as a biomarker for PD-1 blockade. May predict response to pembrolizumab.
Neutrophil-to-lymphocyte ratio (NLR)	Predictive	Patients with NLR of ≥ 2.5 had lower 2-year cause-specific survival (CSS) and 1-year rPFS compared to those with NLR < 2.5, receiving docetaxel before or after AR-directed therapy. For patients with NLR < 2.5, better CSS and rPFS was seen in patients who received docetaxel followed by ARSIs rather than vice versa. NLR can be potentially used in guiding sequencing of therapy in CRPC where the NLR is < 2.5.
Prostate-specific antigen (PSA)	Predictive/ prognostic	PC screening, risk stratification, monitoring of recurrence, and monitoring of therapy response. Lower PSA nadir and a longer time to PSA nadir (>9 months) after ADT associated with improved OS in PC patients with bone metastasis receiving primary ADT. PSA of ≤ 4 ng/mL after 7 months of ADT is a strong predictor of survival in mCSPC, with patients with a PSA of ≤ 0.2 ng/mL having the greatest survival advantage.
PSA doubling time (PSADT)	Predictive/ prognostic	PSADT > 10 months in nmCRPC patients predicts a relatively indolent disease course; however, patients with PSADT ≤ 10 months are at high risk for metastases. PSADT is currently used to select nmCRPC patients for additional therapy with a novel ARSI such as enzalutamide, apalutamide, or darolutamide.
PSMA expression and PET tracers	Predictive/ prognostic	PSMA expression in primary tumor is not predictive of metastatic disease, but a higher expression is associated with a more aggressive tumor, particularly in CRPC. A 68Ga-PSMA-11 PET/CT may allow the selection of patients expected to respond best to Lutetium-177-PSMA radionuclide therapy.
PTEN loss	Predictive/ prognostic	*PTEN* loss or inactivation is considered a biomarker for aggressive prostate cancer. *PTEN* loss predicts improved clinical outcomes with ipatasertib/abiraterone combination in mCRPC.
RB1 loss	Predictive/ prognostic	Alterations in *RB1* have the strongest association with poor outcome in mCRPC patients. mCRPC patients treated with enzalutamide and concurrent *RB1* alterations show worse clinical outcomes and worse PFS. Alterations in *RB1* and *TP53* are associated with shorter time on treatment with abiraterone or enzalutamide. Cooperative loss of two or more tumor suppressor genes, including *TP53*, *PTEN*, and *RB1*, may derive more aggressive disease and an increased risk of relapse.
Serum testosterone	Predictive/ prognostic	Higher serum testosterone (≥ 13 ng/dL) was a significant prognostic factor in CRPC patients treated with docetaxel therapy. The high-testosterone group had significantly shorter OS and PFS than the low-testosterone group. Testosterone levels of ≤25 ng/dL after the first month of ADT was significantly associated with a lower risk of progression to CRPC. Pre-treatment serum testosterone levels may have predictive value in the selection of AR-targeted therapy vs. chemotherapy in patients with mCRPC.
Schlafen family member-11 (SLFN11) expression	Predictive	DNA/RNA helicase SLFN11 expression may have a role in selecting patients who may benefit from platinum-based chemotherapy.
Tumor mutation burden (TMB) and PD-L1 expression	Predictive	PD-L1 expression may not be a useful marker of response to ICI monotherapy. High TMB may predict response to ICIs in mCRPC.
Total alkaline phosphatase (tALP)	Predictive	For patients treated with Radium-223, a normal pre-treatment tALP is associated with longer OS than with an elevated tALP. A reduction of 10% or greater in an elevated baseline tALP at 4 weeks or beyond from treatment is also associated with improved OS. tALP is not specifically used to clinically select patients for radium-223 at this time.

Source: adapted from ref. 19

Note: The list of biomarkers is compiled from literature search and review, and not all of them are validated as prognostic/predictive biomarkers. Adapted from Asif et al. (19).

TABLE 16.9

Frequency of Genomic Alterations in Pathways That Are Investigational Biomarkers for Targeted Therapies

Pathway	% of Cases
ETS gene fusions	35.5%
AR genomic alterations	22.5%
PI3K/AKT/mTOR	40.8%
HRR	23.4%
MMR	4.3%
G1/S-cell cycle	23.4%
WNT	16.2%
RAS/RAF/MEK	5.7%

Source: adapted from ref. 14

TABLE 16.10

Frequency of Genetic Alterations in Clinically Actionable Pathways in Metastatic Disease Compared to Primary Disease

Pathway	Primary Samples (n = 680); % of Samples	Metastatic Samples (n = 333); % of Samples
PI3K	17	40
DNA repair	10	27
Epigenetic regulators	17	27
Cell cycle	9	24
WNT/CTNNB1	6	19
RAS/RAF/MAPK	4	8
Splicing	2	7

Source: adapted from ref. 20

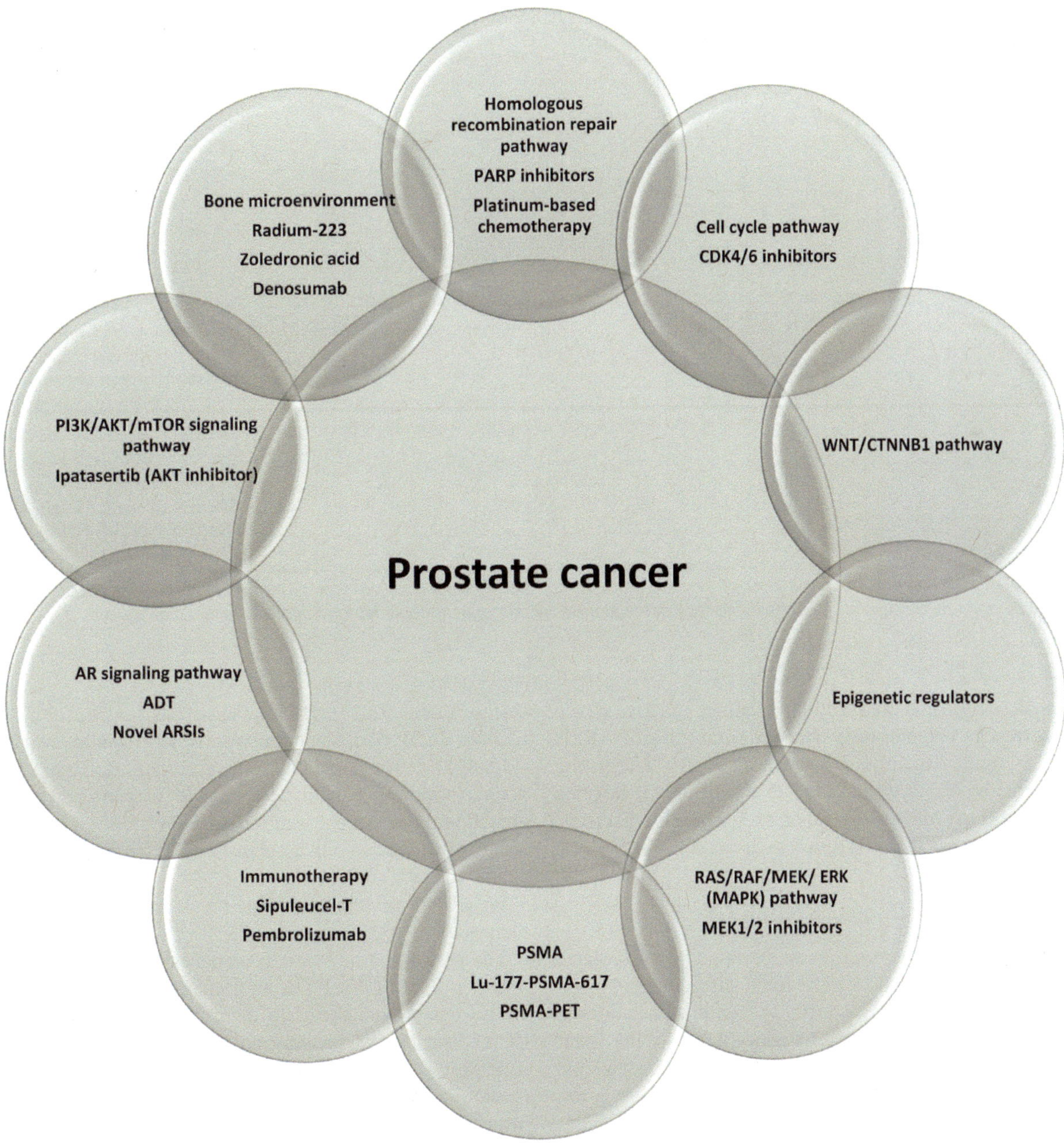

FIGURE 16.7 Clinically actionable targets in prostate cancer.

TABLE 16.11

Drugs Targeting AR Signaling Pathway

Target	Drug Class	Drug Name	FDA Approved	Mechanism of Action	
Targeting GnRH/ LHRH	GnRH/LHRH agonists	Leuprolide	Yes	Stimulate the GnRH/LHRH receptor, creating a temporary surge in LH and testosterone levels followed by downregulation of the receptor, with a subsequent reduction in LH and suppression of testosterone production by the testes	Initially produce a rapid and transient increase in LH and testosterone levels, called the "flare-up" phenomenon; may lead to side effects, such as bone pain and cardiovascular complications
		Goserelin	Yes		
		Triptorelin	Yes		
	GnRH/LHRH antagonists	Degarelix	Yes	Competitively bind to the GnRH/LHRH receptor, inhibiting downstream LH signaling and suppressing testosterone secretion from the testes	Reduces the risk of "flare-up" phenomenon
		Relugolix	Yes		
Directly targeting AR	Antiandrogens (1st generation)	Bicalutamide	Yes	Inhibit binding of dihydrotestosterone (DHT) to the androgen receptor (AR)	
		Flutamide	Yes		
		Nilutamide	Yes		
	Antiandrogens (2nd generation)	Enzalutamide	Yes	Competitively binds to AR Inhibits nuclear translocation of AR Inhibits both DNA binding to AR and recruitment of coactivators	Binds to AR with a greater relative affinity than 1st generation antiandrogens
		Apalutamide	Yes		Greater efficacy than enzalutamide
		Darolutamide	Yes		Antagonizes mutated *AR*, such as F877L and T878A, which confer resistance to enzalutamide and apalutamide
	Proteolysis targeting chimera (PROTAC)	ARV-110	No	AR protein degrader that degrades more than 95% of AR	Overcomes enzalutamide resistance in xenograft models
Targeting CY-P17A1	Androgen synthesis inhibitor	Abiraterone	Yes	Selective and irreversible inhibition of the enzyme 17α-hydroxylase/C17,20-lyase (CYP17)	Suppression of 17α-hydroxylase activity leads to overproduction of mineralocorticoids, which can result in adverse events, these side effects are largely prevented by the co-administration of prednisone
		Seviteronel	No	Selectively inhibits CYP17 lyase (C17,20-lyase). Also has dual function as an AR inhibitor	Competitive antagonist in both wild type and certain mutated forms of *AR* Decreases AR transactivation and offers an advantage over abiraterone because it does not require combination with prednisone

Note: The goal of ADT is to achieve castrate levels of serum testosterone (< 50 ng/dL) and this can be accomplished either surgically or chemically. LHRH agonists and antagonists used as monotherapy. Antiandrogens and androgen synthesis inhibitors used as combination therapy.

have been developed and used in clinical settings and have shown promising results (Figure 16.8). The sequential use of ARSIs in CRPC is limited by cross-resistance between AR-targeting drugs. Furthermore, early and long exposure to AR-targeted therapies results in evolving downstream resistance mechanisms, leading to an increase in non-AR-driven disease.

16.2.5 Targeting DNA Repair Pathways

HRR gene defects, either somatic or germline, are associated with aggressive disease and are more frequently altered in metastatic rather than primary tumors (10, 14). Germline mutations in DNA repair genes (21) (Table 16.12, Figure 16.9) have important implications for patients and their family members. The National Comprehensive Cancer Network (NCCN) recommends germline and/or somatic testing for DNA repair defects in patients with aggressive primary tumors and those with metastatic disease (Table 16.13). HRR gene defects sensitize PC patients to poly (ADP-ribose) polymerase (PARP) inhibitors (PARPi) (Figure 16.10) and platinum chemotherapy through a mechanism of synthetic lethality. Two PARPi, olaparib and rucaparib, are currently FDA approved for use in PC. Several other PARPi are being investigated in combination therapy with AR-targeting agents and radium-223.

PARP is a protein that helps repair DNA when it becomes damaged.

The prevalence of MMR gene deficiency in mCRPC is estimated at 2–5% (23). PC is an immune "cold" tumor that generally remains unresponsive to immune checkpoint inhibitors (ICIs). The NCCN recommends testing for MSI-H/dMMR in metastatic PC, as these patients may potentially respond to ICIs. Pembrolizumab, an anti-PD1 antibody, is FDA approved for treatment of patients with unresectable or metastatic MSI-H/dMMR solid tumors, including PC. Several phase 3 clinical trials are

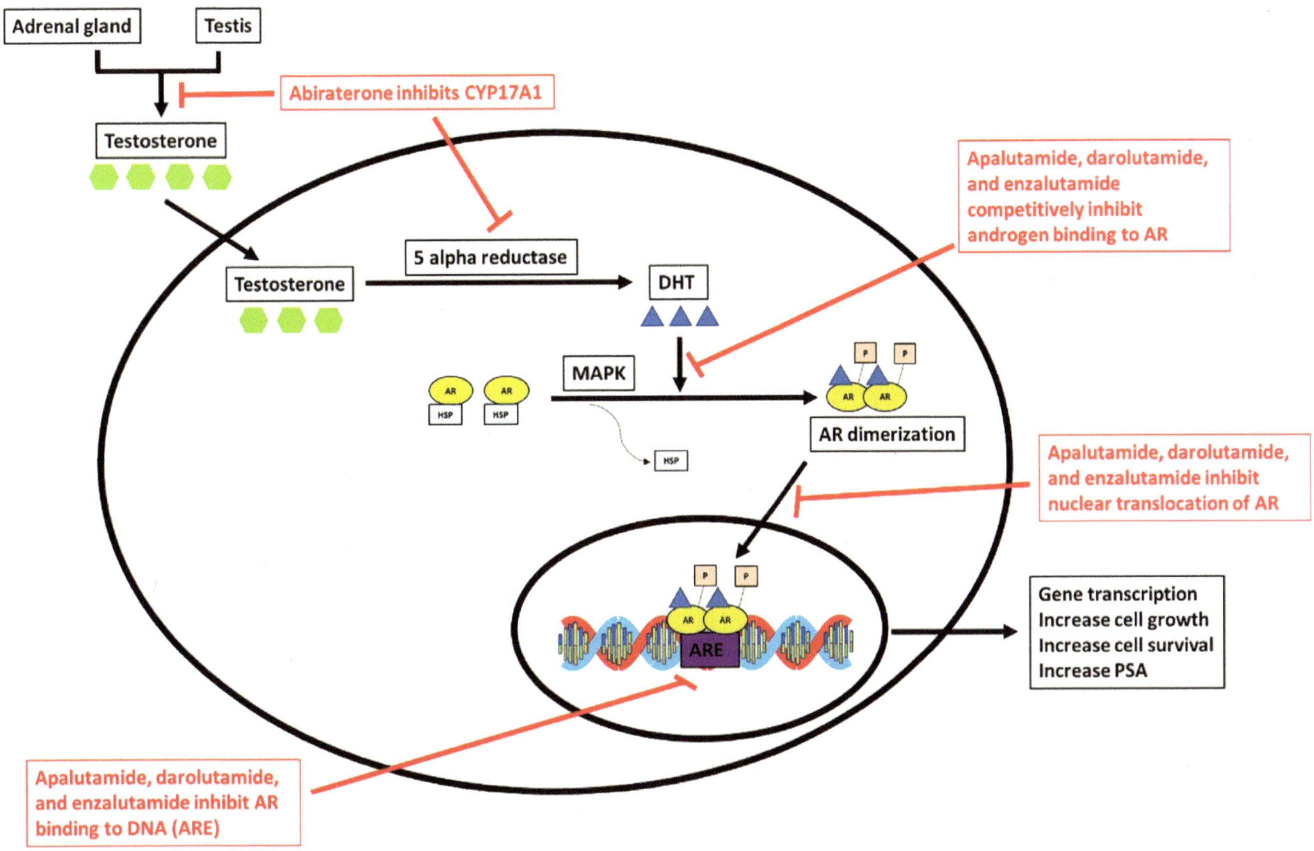

FIGURE 16.8 Mechanism of action of novel ARSIs (abiraterone, enzalutamide, darolutamide, and apalutamide).

TABLE 16.12

Frequency of Deleterious Germline DNA Repair Gene Mutations in Metastatic Prostate Cancer vs. Localized Prostate Cancer

Gene	Metastatic Prostate Cancer (n = 692)	Primary Prostate Cancer (n = 499)
BRCA2	5.35%	0.20%
CHEK2	1.87%	0.40%
ATM	1.59%	1.00%
BRCA1	0.87%	0.60%
GEN1	0.46%	0%
PALB2	0.43%	0.40%
RAD51D	0.43%	0.20%
ATR	0.29%	0%
NBN	0.29%	0.20%
PMS2	0.29%	0.20%
BRIP1	0.18%	0.20%
FAM175A	0.18%	0%
MRE11A	0.14%	0.20%
MSH2	0.14%	0.20%
MSH6	0.14%	0.20%
RAD51C	0.14%	0.40%
BARD1	0%	0.20%

Source: adapted from ref. 21

currently underway to evaluate the efficacy of pembrolizumab in combination with docetaxel, enzalutamide, and olaparib. Tables 16.14 and 16.15 summarize the ongoing phase 3 clinical trials for CRPC and CSPC, respectively.

Cyclin-dependent kinase 12 (CDK12) is inactivated in ~7–10% of mCRPC and is associated with expression of high levels of neoantigens, implicating it in immunotherapy sensitivity (24). CDK12's role in homologous recombination repair (HRR) also implicates it in PARPi sensitivity. Antonarakis et al. (25) reported that *CDK12*-mutated PCs are aggressive with poor response to hormonal therapy, taxane therapy, and PARPi; however, some of these patients may benefit from anti-PD-1 ICIs.

Sipuleucel-T, approved by FDA in April 2010, is an autologous cancer "vaccine", and can be used in certain patients with mCRPC who have not had prior therapy with docetaxel or novel ARSIs.

16.2.6 Targeting Prostate-Specific Membrane Antigen

Prostate-specific membrane antigen (PSMA) is expressed at high levels on the surface of PC cells and at very low levels in normal and non-prostatic tissue. Hence, it is an excellent theranostic target. PSMA-targeted radionuclide therapy uses radiopharmaceuticals to deliver radiation directly to cancer cells. 177Lu-PSMA-617 (Figure 16.11) is FDA approved for treatment of PSMA-positive mCRPC that has been previously with ARSI

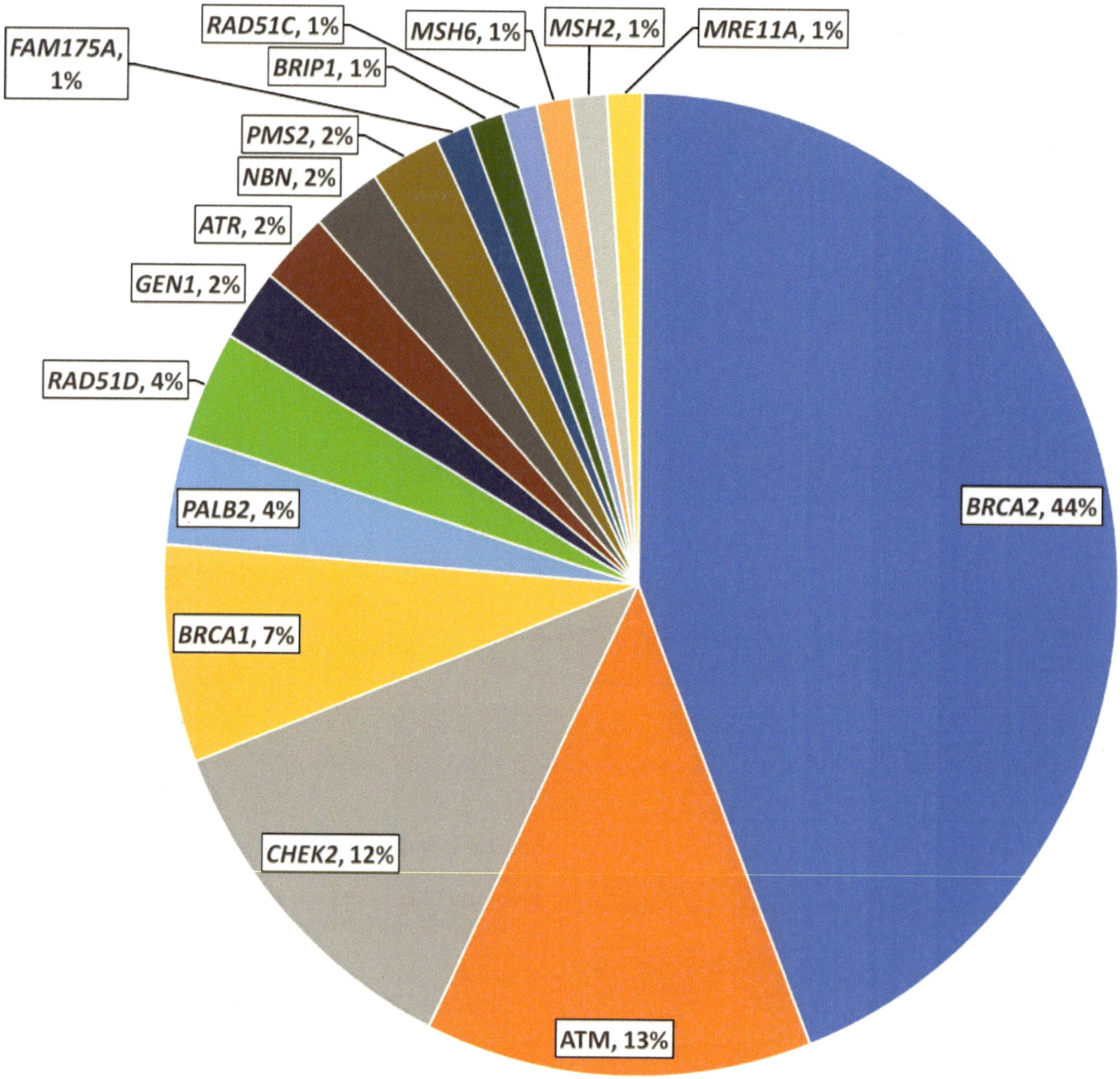

FIGURE 16.9 Distribution of deleterious germline DNA repair gene mutations in metastatic prostate cancer (adapted from ref. 21)

and taxane chemotherapy (26). PSMA can also be targeted via several novel methods, and these are being investigated in clinical trials (Table 16.16). PSMA is also utilized in a new imaging procedure called PSMA-PET that involves injecting a radioactive tracer that attaches to PSMA, followed by detection of the concentrated PSMA tracer by PET scan, thus pinpointing PSMA-positive tumors. Two PSMA tracers Ga-68 PSMA-11 and F-18 piflufolastat are FDA approved for patients at initial staging with suspected metastatic disease.

16.2.7 Targeting Bone Microenvironment

Bone metastasis is very common in PC and occurs in ~90% of patients with advanced disease. Multiple FDA approved agents target the bone microenvironment to treat bone metastasis in PC patients (Table 16.17).

16.2.8 Targeting Cell Cycle Pathway

Cell cycle regulators, RB1 and/or cyclin-dependent kinases (CDKs), are altered in up to 24% of metastatic PCs (14). Loss of *RB1* and/or amplification of CDKs causes cell transition from G1-to-S phase and uncontrolled cell proliferation. CDK4/6 inhibitors block the proliferation of cancer cells by inducing G1 cell cycle arrest in *RB1*-wild-type patients. Several CDK4/6 inhibitors have entered early phase clinical trials in *RB1*-wild-type metastatic PC as monotherapy and in combination therapy.

TABLE 16.13

NCCN Guidelines for Germline and/or Somatic Mutation Testing in Patients with Prostate Cancer

Germline Mutation Testing	Somatic Mutation Testing
Recommended in patients with PC in the following scenarios: • High-risk localized PC, very high-risk localized PC, regional (N1) PC, metastatic PC • Positive family history (see NCCN specific guidelines) • Ashkenazi Jewish ancestry • History of breast cancer	Recommended in patients with PC in the following scenarios: • Testing for somatic homologous recombination gene mutations (eg, *BRCA1*, *BRCA2*, *ATM*, *PALB2*, *FANCA*, *RAD51D*) in metastatic PC • Testing for MSI or dMMR in mCRPC • Decipher molecular assay to inform adjuvant treatment if adverse features are found post-radical prostatectomy
May be considered in patients with PC in the following scenarios: • Intermediate-risk PC with cribriform histology and/or intraductal carcinoma of the prostate • History of exocrine pancreatic cancer, breast cancer, colorectal cancer, gastric cancer, melanoma, upper tract urothelial cancer, glioblastoma, biliary tract cancer, and small intestinal cancer	**May be considered in patients with PC in the following scenarios:** • Testing for somatic homologous recombination gene mutations (eg, *BRCA1*, *BRCA2*, *ATM*, *PALB2*, *FANCA*, *RAD51D*) in regional (N1) PC • Testing for MSI or dMMR in regional or mCSPC • Testing for TMB in patients with mCRPC • Multigene molecular testing in patients with low-, intermediate-, and high-risk prostate cancer and life expectancy ≥ 10 years • Decipher molecular assay as part of counseling for risk stratification in patients with PSA resistance/recurrence after radical prostatectomy
Genes tested should include: • *MLH1*, *MSH2*, *MSH6*, and PMS2 (for Lynch syndrome) • Homologous recombination genes *BRCA1*, *BRCA2*, *ATM*, *PALB2*, and *CHEK2* • *HOXB13*	

Source: adapted from ref. 22

Abbreviations: PC, prostate cancer; TMB, tumor mutation burden.

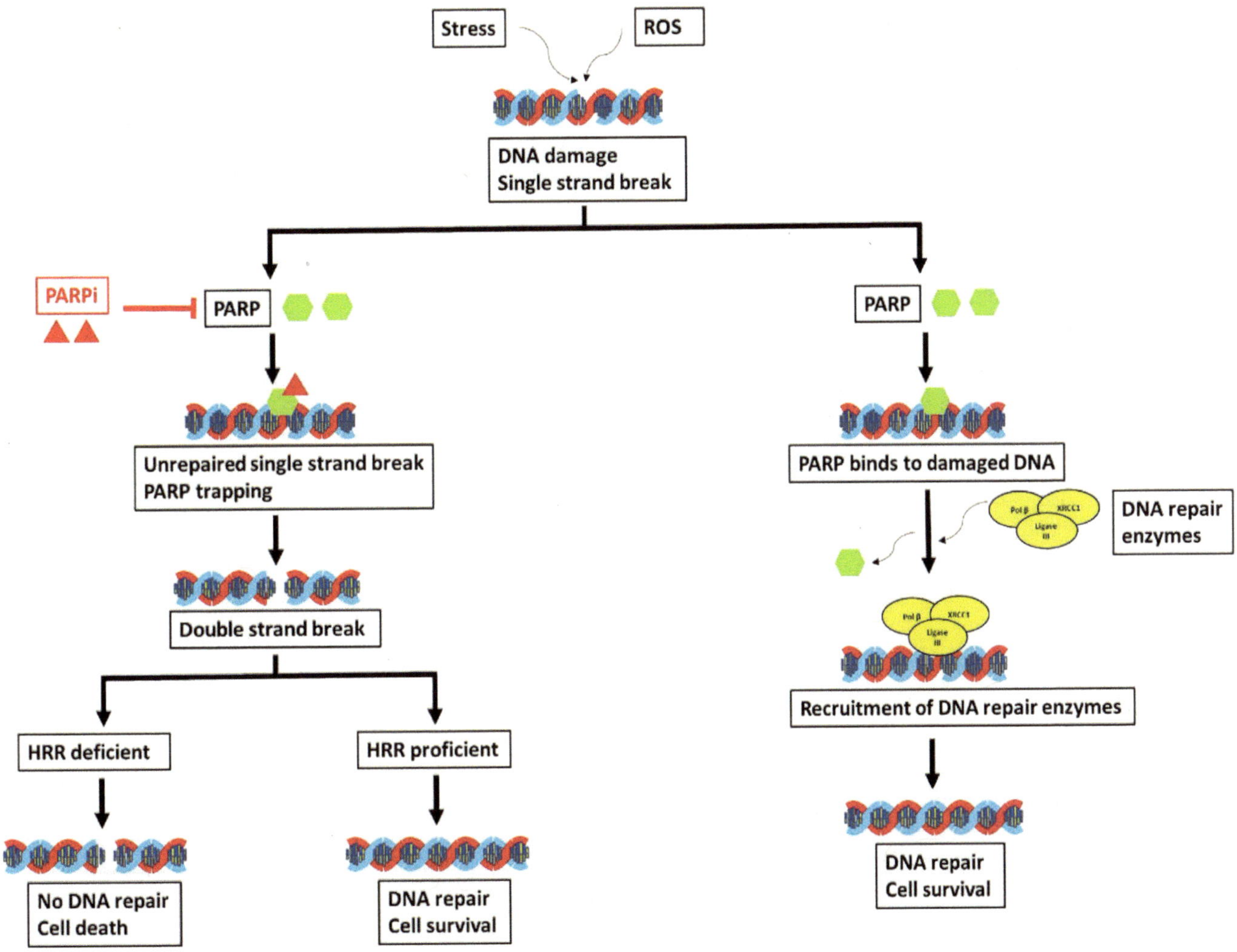

FIGURE 16.10 Mechanism of action of PARP inhibitors.

TABLE 16.14

Ongoing Phase 3 Clinical Trials for Castration-Resistant Prostate Cancer

NCT Number	Acronym	Phase	Conditions	Intervention Arm	Control Arm	Primary Outcome Measure
NCT03732820	PROpel	Phase 3	First-line therapy in mCRPC	Olaparib plus abiraterone	Placebo plus abiraterone	rPFS
NCT02987543	PROfound	Phase 3	mCRPC in patients who have failed prior NHT and have HRR gene mutations	Olaparib	Enzalutamide or abiraterone acetate	rPFS
NCT02975934	TRITON3	Phase 3	mCRPC associated with HRR deficiency (have a deleterious mutation in a *BRCA1/2* or *ATM* gene)	Rucaparib	Abiraterone acetate or enzalutamide or docetaxel	rPFS
NCT04691804		Phase 3	First-line therapy in mCRPC	Fuzuloparib plus abiraterone acetate plus Prednisone	Placebo plus abiraterone acetate plus prednisone	rPFS
NCT03850795		Phase 3	mCRPC. Prior NHT not permitted	HC-1119 (deuterated form of enzalutamide)	Enzalutamide	ORR
NCT02288247	PRESIDE	Phase 3	mCRPC (chemotherapy naïve mCRPC patients treated with docetaxel plus prednisolone who have progressed on enzalutamide alone)	Period 1: enzalutamide; Period 2: enzalutamide plus docetaxel plus prednisolone	Period 1: placebo; Period 2: placebo plus docetaxel plus prednisolone	PFS
NCT02003924	PROSPER	Phase 3	nmCRPC	Enzalutamide	Placebo	MFS
NCT04647526	SPLASH	Phase 3	mCRPC in patients who have progressed following NHT	PSMA [Lu-177]-PNT2002	Abiraterone or enzalutamide	rPFS
NCT04844749	VERACITY	Phase 3	mCRPC in patients who have failed at least one NHT	VERU-111 (Sabizabulin)	Abiraterone or enzalutamide	rPFS
NCT02685397	PCS IX	Phase 2/3	CRPC with oligometastases	LHRH agonist plus enzalutamide plus SBRT	LHRH agonist plus enzalutamide	rPFS
NCT01946204	SPARTAN	Phase 3	nmCRPC	Apalutamide	Placebo	MFS
NCT05348577	CAPItello-280	Phase 3	mCRPC	Capivasertib plus docetaxel	Placebo plus docetaxel	OS
NCT05204927		Phase 3	mCRPC	Lu-177-PSMA-I&T	Abiraterone plus prednisone or enzalutamide	rPFS
NCT04100018	CheckMate 7DX	Phase 3	mCRPC	Nivolumab plus docetaxel plus prednisone	Placebo plus docetaxel plus prednisone	rPFS
NCT03834493	KEYNOTE-641	Phase 3	mCRPC	Pembrolizumab plus enzalutamide	Placebo plus enzalutamide	OS
NCT03834506	KEYNOTE-921	Phase 3	Chemotherapy-naïve mCRPC who have progressed on NHT	Pembrolizumab plus docetaxel	Placebo plus docetaxel	OS
NCT03834519	KEYLYNK-010	Phase 3	mCRPC who have failed prior treatment with one NHT (either abiraterone or enzalutamide) and chemotherapy	Pembrolizumab plus olaparib	Abiraterone plus prednisone or enzalutamide	rPFS and OS
NCT02257736		Phase 3	Chemotherapy-naïve mCRPC	Apalutamide plus abiraterone acetate plus prednisone	Placebo plus abiraterone acetate plus prednisone	rPFS
NCT03851640		Phase 3	mCRPC who have failed treatments with Abiraterone acetate and Docetaxel	HC-1119 (deuterated form of enzalutamide)	Placebo	OS
NCT03903835	ProBio	Phase 3	mCRPC and mCSPC	Treatments based on a biomarker signature inferred from diagnostic tissue or liquid biopsy profiling	SOC	PFS
NCT03511664	VISION	Phase 3	PSMA-positive mCRPC	177Lu-PSMA-617 plus best supportive/best SOC	Best supportive/best SOC	rPFS and OS

(Continued)

TABLE 16.14 (Continued)

NCT Number	Acronym	Phase	Conditions	Intervention Arm	Control Arm	Primary Outcome Measure
NCT04876651	PROSTACT	Phase 3	PSMA-positive mCRPC progressing despite prior NHT	177Lu-DOTA-rosopatamab plus best SOC	Best SOC	rPFS
NCT03072238	IPATential150	Phase 3	Asymptomatic or mildly symptomatic, and previously untreated mCRPC	Ipatasertib plus abiraterone plus prednisone	Placebo plus abiraterone plus prednisone	rPFS (PTEN loss population vs. intent to treat population)
NCT05551117	Tamarack	Phase 2/3	mCRPC	Vobramitamab duocarmazine (MGC018)	Abiraterone or enzalutamide	rPFS
NCT05627752		Phase 2/3	First-line treatment of mCRPC previously treated with Abiraterone	Docetaxel plus enzalutamide	Docetaxel plus placebo	rPFS
NCT04446117	CONTACT-02	Phase 3	mCRPC	Cabozantinib plus atezolizumab	Abiraterone plus prednisone or enzalutamide	PFS and OS
NCT04455750	CASPAR	Phase 3	mCRPC	Enzalutamide plus rucaparib	Enzalutamide plus placebo	rPFS and OS
NCT03395197	TALAPRO-2	Phase 3	mCRPC	Talazoparib plus enzalutamide	Placebo plus enzalutamide	Talazoparib dose confirmation. rPFS in unselected patients and patients with HRRm
NCT04689828	PSMAfore	Phase 3	Taxane naïve progressive mCRPC	177Lu-PSMA-617 plus best supportive care	Androgen receptor-directed therapy plus best supportive care	rPFS
NCT03819101	PEACE-4	Phase 3	CRPC	SOC plus acetylsalicylic acid; or SOC plus atorvastatin; or SOC plus acetylsalicylic acid plus atorvastatin	SOC	OS
NCT03016312	IMbassador250	Phase 3	mCRPC after failure of an Androgen synthesis inhibitor and failure of, ineligibility for, or refusal of a Taxane regimen	Atezolizumab plus enzalutamide	Enzalutamide	OS
NCT03706365	CYCLONE 2	Phase 2/3	mCRPC	Abiraterone plus prednisone plus abemaciclib	Abiraterone plus prednisone plus placebo	rPFS
NCT02043678	ERA 223	Phase 3	Asymptomatic or mildly symptomatic, chemotherapy-naïve, bone predominant mCRPC	Radium-223 dichloride plus abiraterone plus prednisone	Placebo plus abiraterone plus prednisone	SSE-FS
NCT03574571		Phase 3	mCRPC	Docetaxel plus radium-223	Docetaxel	OS
NCT03458559	RaRe	Phase 3	mCRPC	Rhenium-188-HEDP	Radium-223-chloride	OS
NCT02194842	PEACE III	Phase 3	Asymptomatic or mildly symptomatic CRPC with metastases to bone	Enzalutamide plus Radium-223	Enzalutamide	rPFS
NCT03748641	MAGNITUDE	Phase 3	mCRPC	Niraparib plus abiraterone acetate plus prednisone	Placebo plus abiraterone acetate plus prednisone	rPFS in cohort 1 (HRR gene alterations) and cohort 3 (open label)
NCT01949337		Phase 3	mCRPC	Enzalutamide plus abiraterone plus prednisone	Enzalutamide	OS

Abbreviations: ADT, androgen deprivation therapy; HRR, homologous recombination repair; LHRH, luteinizing hormone-releasing hormone; mCRPC, metastatic castration-resistant prostate cancer; mCSPC, metastatic castration-sensitive prostate cancer; MFS, metastasis free survival; NHT, novel hormonal therapy; nmCRPC, non-metastatic castration-resistant prostate cancer; ORR, overall response rate; OS, overall survival; PARPi, poly (ADP-ribose) polymerase inhibitor; PSA, prostate-specific antigen; PSMA, prostate-specific membrane antigen; PTEN, phosphatase and tensin homolog; rPFS, radiological progression-free survival; SBRT, stereotactic body radiation therapy; SOC, standard of care; SSE-FS, symptomatic skeletal event-free survival.

TABLE 16.15

Ongoing Phase 3 Clinical Trials for Castration-Sensitive Prostate Cancer

NCT Number	Acronym	Phases	Conditions	Intervention Arm	Control Arm	Primary Outcome Measures
NCT04497844	AMPLITUDE	Phase 3	mCSPC with deleterious germline or somatic HRR gene mutations	Niraparib plus abiraterone acetate plus prednisone	Placebo plus abiraterone acetate plus prednisone	rPFS
NCT02799602	ARASENS	Phase 3	mCSPC	Darolutamide (ODM-201) plus standard ADT plus docetaxel	Placebo plus standard ADT plus docetaxel	OS
NCT02677896	ARCHES	Phase 3	mCSPC	Enzalutamide plus ADT	Placebo plus ADT	rPFS
NCT04493853	CAPItello-281	Phase 3	Denovo mCSPC with PTEN deficiency	Capivasertib plus abiraterone	Placebo plus abiraterone	rPFS
NCT04191096	KEYNOTE-991	Phase 3	mCSPC	Pembrolizumab plus enzalutamide plus ADT	Placebo plus enzalutamide plus ADT	rPFS and OS
NCT03879122		Phase 2/3	mCSPC	ADT plus docetaxel plus nivolumab or ADT plus Ipilimumab alternating with docetaxel and followed by nivolumab	ADT plus docetaxel	OS
NCT04736199	ARANOTE	Phase 3	mCSPC	Darolutamide plus ADT	Placebo plus ADT	rPFS
NCT00309985	CHAARTED	Phase 3	mCSPC	ADT plus docetaxel	ADT	OS
NCT03520478		Phase 3	CSPC	Rezvilutamide (SHR3680)	Bicalutamide	rPFS and OS
NCT04115007	PRESTO	Phase 3	Oligometastatic CSPC	SOC plus SBRT for oligometastases	SOC	CRPC-FS
NCT04983095	METRO	Phase 3	Oligometastatic CSPC	SBRT plus standard treatment	Standard treatment	Failure (CRPC) free survival
NCT05288166	CYCLONE 3	Phase 3	mCSPC	Abemaciclib plus abiraterone plus prednisone/prednisolone	Placebo plus abiraterone plus prednisone/prednisolone	rPFS
NCT04409288		Phase 3	Recurrent or mCSPC	Apalutamide followed by enzalutamide; or Enzalutamide followed by apalutamide		Patient preference questionnaire
NCT04557059	PRIMORDIUM	Phase 3	High-risk patients with PSMA-PET-positive CSPC	RT plus LHRH agonist plus apalutamide	RT plus LHRH agonist	ppMPFS
NCT04821622		Phase 3	DDR-deficient mCSPC	Talazoparib plus enzalutamide	Placebo plus enzalutamide	rPFS
NCT03903835	ProBio	Phase 3	mCRPC and mCSPC	Treatments based on a biomarker signature inferred from diagnostic tissue or liquid biopsy profiling	Standard of care	PFS
NCT02319837	EMBARK	Phase 3	High-risk non-metastatic prostate cancer	Enzalutamide monotherapy or enzalutamide plus leuprolide	Placebo plus leuprolide	MFS
NCT04720157	PSMAddition	Phase 3	mCSPC	177Lu-PSMA-617 plus SOC (NHT plus ADT)	SOC (NHT plus ADT)	rPFS
NCT02489318	TITAN	Phase 3	mCSPC	Apalutamide plus ADT	Placebo plus ADT	rPFS and OS
NCT05352178	SPARKLE	Phase 3	Oligorecurrent mCSPC	MDT (surgery and/or SBRT) plus 1 month of ADT; or MDT (surgery and/or SBRT) plus 6 months of ADT + enzalutamide	MDT (surgery and/or SBRT) alone	PMFS
NCT05209243	START-MET	Phase 3	Oligometastatic CSPC	SOC plus SBRT (all metastatic lesions). ADT plus RT to the primary tumor plus NHT	SOC. ADT plus RT to the primary tumor plus NHT	rPFS

Abbreviation: ADT, androgen deprivation therapy; CRPC, castration-resistant prostate cancer; CSPC, castration-sensitive prostate cancer; DDR, DNA damage repair; HRR, homologous recombination repair; LHRH, luteinizing hormone-releasing hormone; mCSPC, metastatic castration-sensitive prostate cancer; MDT, metastasis-directed therapy; MFS, metastasis free survival; NHT, novel hormonal therapy; nmCRPC, non-metastatic castration-resistant prostate cancer; ORR, overall response rate; OS, overall survival; PET, positron emission tomography; PMFS, poly-metastatic free survival; ppMPFS, Prostate-specific membrane antigen (PSMA)-positron emission tomography (PET) metastatic progression-free survival; PSA, prostate-specific antigen; PTEN, phosphatase and tensin homolog; RT, radiation therapy; rPFS, radiological progression-free survival; SBRT, stereotactic body radiation therapy; SOC, standard of care.

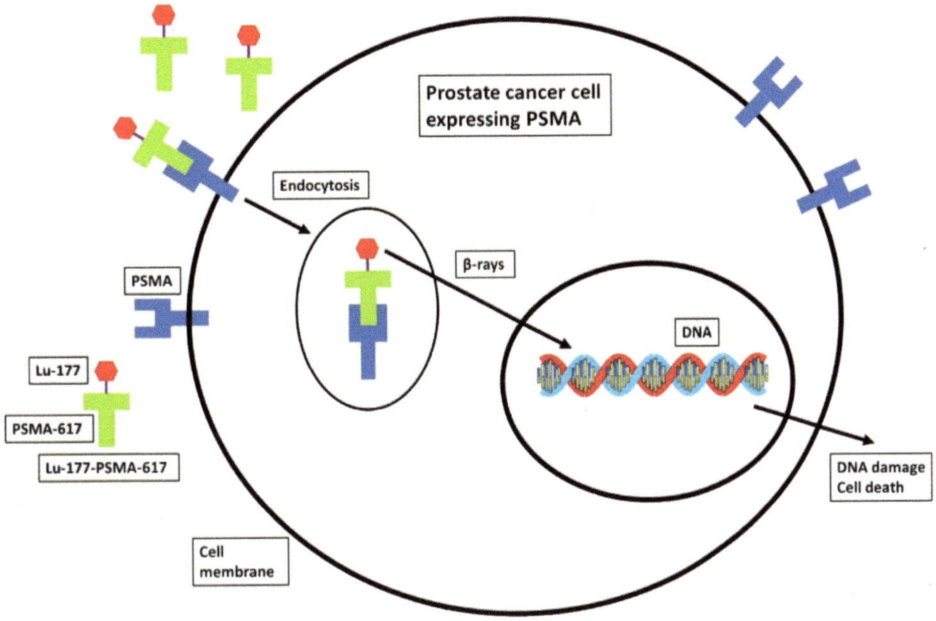

FIGURE 16.11 Mechanism of action of Lu-177-PSMA-617. PSMA-targeted ligand (PSMA-617) is conjugated with a radionuclide 177Lu (beta-emitter).

TABLE 16.16

Targeting PSMA via Novel Methods

Drug Class	Drug Name	Mechanism of Action	Future
PSMA-directed antibody drug conjugates (PSMA-ADC)	BIND-014	PSMA-specific antibodies are used to bind cytotoxic drugs	BIND-014, a novel PSMA-ADC conjugated with docetaxel nanoparticles, was active and well tolerated in a phase 2 clinical trial in chemotherapy-naïve mCRPC
PSMA-directed immunotherapy	Bispecific T-cell-engager (BiTE) molecules (e.g. pasotuximab)	Engage CD3 on T cells and PSMA on PC cells, thereby activating a patient's own T cells to eliminate PSMA-expressing PC cells	Pasotuximab demonstrated safety and preliminary efficacy in a recent phase I dose-escalation study
	Chimeric antigen receptor (CAR)-T cells	Genetically engineered by modifying a patient's own T cells to target PSMA; thus, delivering immune cells to the tumor	Several clinical trials are underway to test their safety and efficacy

Abbreviations: PSMA: prostate-specific membrane antigen; PC, prostate cancer; mCRPC, metastatic castration-resistant prostate cancer

TABLE 16.17

Agents Targeting the Bone Microenvironment and Their Mechanism of Action and Clinical Indications

Drug Class	Drug Name	Mechanism of Action	Clinical Use
Radiopharmaceuticals	Strontium-89	Calcium-mimetic and form complexes with the bone mineral hydroxyapatite at areas of increased bone turnover, such as bone metastases. The radiation emitted by these agents causes double-strand DNA breaks leading to cell death.	Beta-emitter. Palliative treatment of bone pain with no impact on survival.
	Samarium-153		Beta-emitter. Palliative treatment of bone pain with no impact on survival.
	Radium-223		Alpha-emitter. Short tissue penetration, which reduces bone marrow toxicity.
Bisphosphonates	Zoledronic acid	Inhibits osteoclastic activity and induces osteoclast apoptosis.	Prevent skeletal-related events in patients with mCRPC.
RANKL inhibitors	Denosumab	RANKL is a transmembrane or soluble protein essential for the formation, function, and survival of osteoclasts. Denosumab induces osteoclast apoptosis and impairs osteoclast activity.	Prevent or delay disease-associated SREs in patients with mCRPC and bone metastases. Also used to prevent bone loss and fractures in patients receiving hormone therapy.

Abbreviation: mCRPC, metastatic castration-resistant prostate cancer

16.2.9 Targeting PTEN/PI3K/AKT/mTOR Pathway

PTEN gene inactivation is identified in ~20% of primary PCs and in as many as 40–50% of mCRPC. Functional PTEN loss results in activation of PI3K/AKT/mTOR pathway (Figure 16.12) and is associated with poor prognosis, making PTEN a potentially useful marker to distinguish indolent from aggressive disease. Several drugs targeting PI3K/AKT/mTOR signaling pathway are being evaluated in combination therapy in clinical trials. IPATential150 (27), a phase 3 clinical trial, showed improved radiological progression-free survival with ipatasertib (AKT inhibitor) plus abiraterone compared to abiraterone alone in patients with mCRPC with PTEN loss by IHC. PTEN status can be helpful in identifying patients who are more likely to benefit from these therapies (28).

16.2.10 Targeting RAS/RAF/MEK/ERK Pathway

Extracellular signal-regulated kinase (ERK)/mitogen-activated protein kinase (MAPK) signaling is activated by upstream activating mutations in RAS, RAF, growth factor receptors and their ligands (Figure 16.12). Increased activation of ERK/MAPK pathway is found in mCRPC and is associated with poor prognosis and androgen independence. Trametinib, a MEK1/2 inhibitor, is currently being tested in a phase 2 trial of mCRPC patients.

16.2.11 Targeting Epigenetic Modifications

Epigenetic alterations may upregulate oncogenes or reduce the expression of tumor suppressor genes, promoting PC progression and metastasis. Thus, epigenetic modifications provide exciting potential as PC biomarkers and therapeutic targets. Several epigenetic modifying drugs are being tested in clinical trials, either alone or in combination therapy (8). EZH2, a histone methyltransferase, plays an important role in promoting lineage plasticity, which is highly associated with neuroendocrine PC (NEPC). Thus, EZH2 is an attractive target, and many EZH2 inhibitors have emerged in early clinical studies.

16.2.12 Other Targets

Several other drugs, including vascular endothelial growth factor inhibitors, endothelin type-A receptor inhibitors, transforming growth factor-beta inhibitors, tyrosine kinase inhibitors, and WNT/β-catenin signaling inhibitors have been tested in early phase clinical trials and several clinical trials are ongoing. Further studies are needed to evaluate their clinical efficacy as monotherapy or in combination therapy.

16.3 Treatment-Related Neuroendocrine Prostate Cancer

Treatment-related neuroendocrine prostate cancer (t-NEPC) (Figure 16.13) occurs in CRPC patients after AR-directed therapy and is more common than *de novo* small cell/NEPC occurring in untreated patients. Aggarwal et al. (29) identified t-NEPC in 17% of mCRPC patients that had progressed after prior ARSI therapy and was associated with shortened overall survival. Emerging evidence suggests that lineage plasticity (characterized

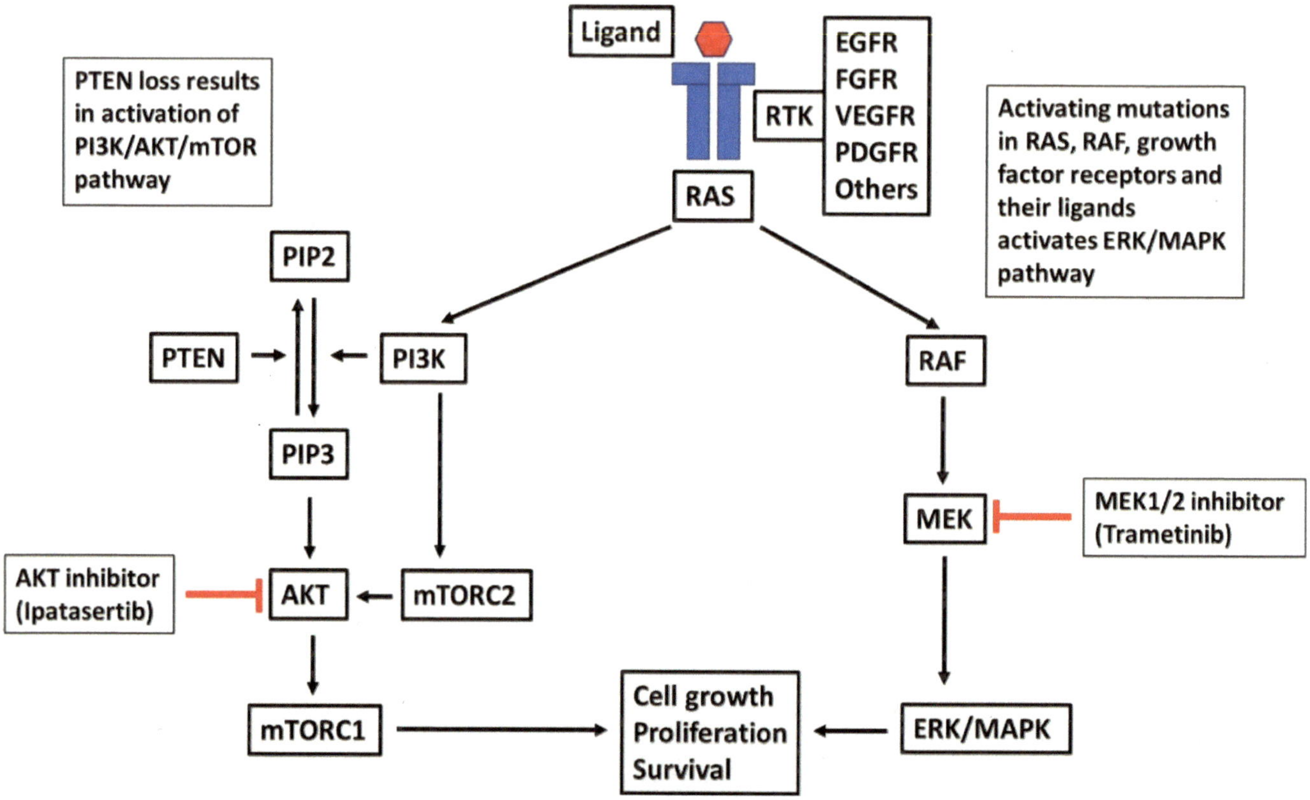

FIGURE 16.12 Targeting the PTEN/PI3K/AKT/mTOR and RAS/RAF/MEK/ERK (MAPK) pathways.

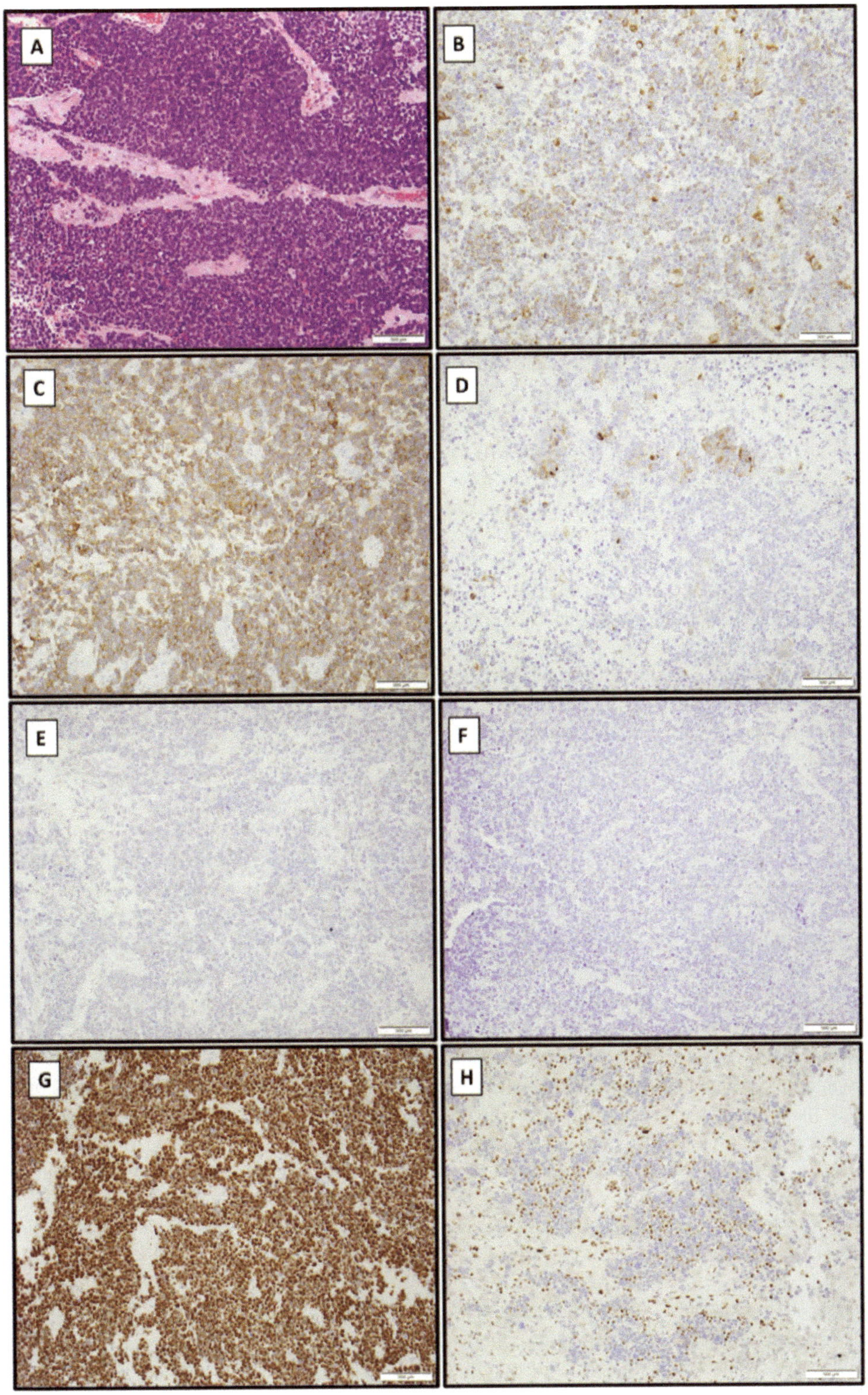

FIGURE 16.13 Treatment-related neuroendocrine prostate cancer. (A) Hematoxylin and eosin (×200). (B) AE1/3 (×200). (C) Synaptophysin (×200). (D) Chromogranin (×200). (E) NKX3.1 (×200). (F) PSA (×200). (G) P53 (×200). (H) Rb1 (×200).

by AR-indifference) plays an important role in progression of advanced PC to t-NEPC while undergoing AR-directed therapy (30). Lineage plasticity is driven by epigenetic changes (overexpression of EZH2 and specific DNA methylation profile) that arise in specific genomic context, including (but not limited to) *TP53*, *RB1*, and *PTEN* loss (31). t-NEPC no longer responds to AR-directed therapy and is managed with platinum-based chemotherapy. N-MYC and Aurora kinase A (AURKA) are also overexpressed in the majority of NEPC tumors and cooperate to induce a neuroendocrine phenotype and drive lineage plasticity (32). Emerging therapies include drugs that target AURKA and EZH2.

16.4 Bladder Cancer

Bladder cancer is the sixth most common malignancy in the United States, with an estimated 81,180 new cases and 17,100 deaths predicted in 2022 (1). It more commonly occurs in men than women and is usually diagnosed in the seventh to eighth decade of life. Bladder cancer includes tumors of varying histologic types and origins including the most common types: urothelial carcinoma (> 90% of bladder tumors), squamous cell carcinoma and adenocarcinoma (approximately 5% combined). Rare tumors arise from the mesenchymal components of the bladder (sarcomas) and embryologic remnants (Müllerian carcinoma). Urothelial carcinomas may occur anywhere there is urothelium, with bladder sites being the most common, followed by upper urinary tract (ureter, renal pelvis) and urethra (31). Tumors involving the urinary tract frequently present with hematuria, prompting evaluation of the bladder *via* cystoscopy.

16.4.1 Urothelial Carcinoma

As the most common type of bladder cancer, urothelial carcinoma is characterized by several clinical presentations—non-invasive tumor, non-muscle invasive tumor, muscle invasive tumor, and metastatic disease. Smoking is the leading risk factor for development of urothelial carcinoma. Prognosis is directly related to depth of invasion and cytologic grade, which is categorized as low-grade or high-grade based on the degree of atypia, architectural disorganization, and mitotic rate. Historically, the primary treatment modality for non-metastatic muscle invasive urothelial carcinoma was radical cystectomy; however, over the past two decades, there has been a paradigm shift to the use of neoadjuvant chemotherapy prior to radical cystectomy with evidence of improved survival over cystectomy alone.

For metastatic disease, the standard first-line treatment is systemic therapy with combination agents, typically gemcitabine and cisplatin in eligible patients. Currently, the role for immunotherapy is largely as second-line treatment or in patients who are ineligible for cisplatin therapy.

16.4.2 Molecular Findings

Based on the Cancer Genome Atlas (TCGA), the most common genetic alterations in urothelial carcinoma are *CDKN2A*, *FGFR3*, *PIK3CA*, and *ERBB2 (HER2)* (33). Many of these mutations represent potential targets for therapy; however, proof of efficacy and approval of targeted drugs for urothelial carcinoma remains elusive. A consensus classification for molecular subtypes of muscle invasive urothelial carcinoma includes six different classes including: luminal papillary, luminal non-specified, luminal unstable, stroma-rich, basal/squamous, and neuroendocrine-like. Each class is defined by a mutational or expression profile that broadly corresponds to cellular differentiation within the urothelium (basal versus luminal) (34). Our understanding of molecular classes of non-muscle invasive bladder cancer is still developing, but there do appear to be four distinct classes based on gene expression and mutational profile (35).

Mutations in the cell surface receptor tyrosine kinase fibroblast growth factor receptor 2/3 (FGFR2/3) gene are more frequently identified in low-grade tumors, as well as the luminal papillary class of tumors. The luminal papillary group has generally favorable outcomes, are generally low stage and with low risk of recurrence; however, they may be identified in high-grade, high stage tumors as well, occurring in up to 20% in one study (36, 37).

PIK3CA is involved in cell growth and survival, and approximately 25% of urothelial carcinomas demonstrated activating mutations in the TCGA cohort, along with other mutations of the PI3K-AKT-mTOR pathway. These mutations are also enriched in low-grade and low stage tumors, frequently co-existing with *FGFR3* mutations.

TP53 is a tumor suppressor gene that is one of the most frequently mutated in urothelial carcinoma, specifically tumors on the carcinoma in situ (CIS)/high-grade pathway. Mutations in *TP53* are associated with higher stage disease, with approximately 50% of muscle-invasive tumors harboring *TP53* mutations, compared with 25% in non-invasive tumors (37).

RB1 is another tumor suppressor gene that is frequently altered in urothelial carcinoma, seen in approximately 15% of tumors. *RB1* loss is strongly associated with aggressive disease and mutations are overrepresented in basal and neuroendocrine subtypes. Combined *TP53/RB1* mutations were seen in 72% of small cell bladder cancer in one series of 132 cases of urothelial cancer with small cell/neuroendocrine features (38). These co-mutations are associated with higher response rates to immune checkpoint inhibitors, based on the data from IMVigor 210 (39).

ERBB2/3 amplifications have been identified in around 13% conventional urothelial carcinomas but occur at higher rates in the micropapillary subtype of urothelial carcinoma. While *ERBB2* (*HER2/NEU*) amplification presents a potential target for anti-HER2 therapy, clinical trials of lapatinib in urothelial carcinoma have so far failed to show benefit, along with significant toxicities for patients taking the drug.

16.4.3 Current Targeted and Immuno-Therapeutic Agents

In patients with locally advanced or metastatic muscle-invasive urothelial carcinoma, erdafitinib a receptor tyrosine-kinase FGFR inhibitor, has been approved for use in patients with *FGFR2/3* mutations. The NCCN recommends testing for *FGFR2* and *FGFR3* mutations in advanced stage patients, and a diagnostic PCR test (Therascreen, Qiagen) is approved as a companion assay for erdafitinib. Immune checkpoint therapy is also approved for patients who are cisplatin-ineligible or platinum-refractory (40).

Antibody-drug conjugates (ADCs) pair an antibody against a protein located on the tumor with a chemotherapeutic agent.

For locally advanced or metastatic urothelial carcinoma, there are two ADCs currently approved by the FDA—EV (Nectin-4-monomethyl auristatin E) and SG (Trop-2-SN38). A biomarker is not necessary for the use of these drugs, as both ADCs target proteins that are essentially ubiquitous on urothelial carcinomas (41).

Given the relatively frequent mutations identified in *ERBB2/HER2* in urothelial carcinoma, multiple clinical trials have evaluated the efficacy of anti-HER2 drugs in this setting. Assessment of HER2 status is not straightforward, with imperfect concordance between HER2 IHC, *HER2* FISH and genetic testing, which limits our current understanding of efficacy of anti-HER2 therapy. While numerous trials are ongoing, there is no HER2 therapy currently approved in urothelial carcinoma (42). Newer antibody drug conjugates that combine cytotoxic drugs with antibodies directed at tumor-specific antigens show promise for the treatment of HER2-expressing urothelial carcinomas. The majority of these drugs are still in early clinical trials.

Immune checkpoint inhibitors play an increasing role in the treatment of advanced and metastatic urothelial carcinoma with PD-L1 used as a predictive biomarker for response to treatment. Specifically, the drugs atezolizumab, avelumab, durvalumab, pembrolizumab, and nivolumab have received approval for second-line treatment in advanced/metastatic disease, whereas pembrolizumab and atezolizumab were later approved for first-line therapy of cisplatin-ineligible patients. For non-muscle invasive urothelial carcinoma and metastatic urothelial carcinoma, immune checkpoint inhibitor therapy is approved for therapy. The KEYNOTE-057 clinical trial demonstrated a durable response of at least one year in patients with CIS with or without papillary tumors when treated with pembrolizumab (43). Specific companion diagnostic PD-L1 assays are paired with the FDA approved drugs, with scoring algorithms differing by assay. The utility of PD-L1 expression as a predictive biomarker for response to therapy remains unclear with mixed results from several studies. Given the limited reliability of PD-L1 expression in urothelial carcinoma, inclusion of tumor mutational burden (TMB) has been evaluated to improve performance. Similarly, studies have demonstrated increased numbers of tumor infiltrating lymphocytes (TILs) may correlate with response to immune checkpoint inhibitors.

Upper urinary tract urothelial carcinoma is associated with Lynch syndrome and is the third most common tumor type after colorectal and endometrial carcinoma in this patient population. As a result, screening for Lynch syndrome using mismatch repair protein immunohistochemistry is performed in many institutions on a universal, or selected, basis in upper urinary tract urothelial carcinoma (44, 45).

16.5 Non-Urothelial Bladder Carcinoma

There are several non-urothelial carcinomas of the bladder, primarily represented by squamous cell carcinoma, adenocarcinoma, and neuroendocrine carcinoma. It is important to distinguish these primary bladder tumors from divergent differentiation arising within a urothelial carcinoma that exhibits squamous, glandular, or neuroendocrine features.

16.5.1 Squamous Cell Carcinoma

Pure squamous cell carcinoma (SCC) of the bladder is the second most common type of cancer involving the bladder, although remains rare overall compared to urothelial histology. In areas where *Schistosoma* parasites are endemic, SCC is far more common. SCCs unrelated to *Schistosoma* are associated with chronic irritation and stasis including, urinary tract infections, chronic catheterization, stones, and neurogenic bladder (31).

The most common genetic alterations identified in squamous cell carcinoma are *TP53* and *CDKN2A*. Unlike urothelial carcinoma, there is no established benefit of neoadjuvant chemotherapy for SCC. Standard treatment is radical cystectomy.

16.5.2 Adenocarcinoma

Primary bladder adenocarcinoma is the third most common type of bladder carcinoma, comprising approximately 1% of total bladder tumors. It is a challenging diagnosis to make, as histologic overlap exists with urothelial carcinoma with glandular differentiation, urachal carcinoma, and secondary involvement by colorectal adenocarcinoma.

There are mutational differences between pure bladder adenocarcinoma and its histologic mimics. Bladder adenocarcinoma harbors mutations most frequently in *TP53, KRAS, PIK3CA, CTNNB1, APC, TERT, FBXW7, IDH2, RB1, ARID1A, BRAF, PTEN*, and *SMAD4* (46, 47). Like squamous cell carcinoma, adenocarcinoma of the bladder is treated by radical cystectomy, with no targeted therapy approved at this time.

16.6 Kidney Cancer

Kidney cancer accounts for approximately 2% of all cancers globally, and its incidence has been increasing (48, 49). Renal cell carcinoma (RCC) is the main type of kidney cancer, and there are approximately 80,000 new cases and 14,000 deaths from RCC in the United States each year (50). Risk factors related to developing RCC include obesity, cigarette smoking, hypertension, acquired cystic kidney disease, occupational exposure, and genetic susceptibility (31); however, the mechanisms by which these risk factors underlying RCC tumorigenesis largely remain obscure.

Importantly, RCC is a heterogeneous disease and encompasses a wide spectrum of tumors with distinctive clinical behaviors, pathologic characteristics, and oncogenic pathways. While overall RCC is a male-predominant (M:F = 2:1) disease typically presentating in the sixth and seventh decades of life, the age and gender distribution could differ significantly among the histologic and molecular types of RCC recognized in the current classification system (31). Clear cell RCC (ccRCC), papillary (pRCC), and chromophobe RCC (chRCC) are the three most common histologic types, with ccRCC being most prevalent and accounting for approximately 70% of all RCC; pRCC, chRCC, and other less common types of RCC are often referred to as "non-clear cell RCC" (nccRCC) to distinguish them from ccRCC for clinical management purposes; however, nccRCC remains a highly diverse group and includes many new and emerging entities that have been identified in recent years.

The management of RCC has undergone a major transformation in the last two decades. While surgery remains the mainstay of curative treatment for localized disease, nephron-sparing surgery, active surveillance, and minimally invasive procedures have reduced the morbidity and the need for surgery while preserving oncological effectiveness. For advanced diseases, systemic therapy options have moved beyond tyrosine kinase inhibitors (TKIs) that target the vascular endothelial growth factor (VEGF) and related pathways to include check point inhibitor immunotherapy as well as various combination approaches and have significantly enhanced the clinical effects in the treatment of metastatic RCC, including producing long-term durable response in some patients (51).

16.6.1 Molecular Findings

While the majority of RCCs occur as sporadic cases, an estimated 2–5% cases present as part of hereditary syndromes (Table 16.18). Genetic alterations discovered in these familial/hereditary forms of RCC provide the foundation for our current understanding of the molecular basis of kidney cancer and implicate genes such as von Hippel-Lindau (*VHL*), mesenchymal epithelial transition (*MET*), fumarate hydratase (*FH*), folliculin (*FLCN*), hamartin and tuberin (*TSC1* and *TSC2*), and succinate dehydrogenase B (*SDHB*) in the pathogenesis of various subtypes of sporadic and familial types of RCC (52, 53). Understanding the underlying molecular biology in RCC has helped link histomorphology with specific molecular alterations and served as a major driving force for the continued discovery of new and emerging entities and a knowledge base for tumor classification schemes. Compared to other cancer types with oncogenes driving tumorigenesis, the vast majority of somatic mutations identified in RCC involve tumor suppressor genes, posing a critical challenge for direct therapeutic targeting.

Clear cell RCC (ccRCC): Common molecular alterations identified in ccRCC are 3p loss and *VHL* (3p25) mutation (54, 55). The 3p loss is detected in approximately 90% of ccRCC and is considered the first event of tumorigenesis (56). *VHL* inactivation via mutation or methylation and concurrent 3p loss leads to a loss of VHL complex-mediated protein degradation of hypoxia-inducible factor (HIF) and results in the

TABLE 16.18

Hereditary Renal Cell Carcinoma: Molecular Alterations, Clinical Manifestations, and Histologic Features

Syndrome	Gene (Locus)—Protein	Clinical Manifestations	Histologic Features of Renal Tumors
von Hippel-Lindau (VHL) disease	*VHL* (3p25)—pVHL	Clear cell RCC, pheochromocytoma, pancreatic endocrine tumors, CNS and retinal hemangioblastomas	Clear cell RCC
Hereditary papillary RCC	*MET* (7q31)—MET	Papillary RCC	Papillary RCC, classic morphology (type 1)
Hereditary leiomyomatosis and RCC (HLRCC)	*FH* (1q42.1)—Fumarate hydratase	Renal cell carcinoma, cutaneous leiomyomas uterine leiomyomas pheochromocytoma-paraganglioma	FH-deficient RCC
Birt-Hogg-Dubé (BHD) syndrome	*FLCN* (17p11.2)—Folliculin	Renal tumors, fibrofolliculomas and other skin lesions, pulmonary cysts	Hybrid oncocytic tumors, oncocytoma, chromophobe and other RCCs
Tuberous sclerosis complex (TSC)	*TSC1* (9q34)—Hamartin *TSC2* (16p13.3)—Tuberin	Multiple renal AML, RCCs, cardiac rhabdomyomas, hamartomas, neurologic disorders/seizures	AML, renal cysts, RCCs with a spectrum of morphology
Succinate dehydrogenase (SDH)-associated pheochromocytoma/paraganglioma syndrome type 4	*SDHB* (1p36), *SDHA* (5p15), *SDHC* (1q23.3), *SDHD* (11q23), and *SDHAF2* (11q12.2)—Succinate dehydrogenase complex	Bilateral and extra-adrenal pheochromocytoma/paraganglioma, RCC and other malignancies	SDH-deficient RCC
BAP1 tumor predisposition syndrome	*BAP1* (3p21.1)—BRCA1 Associated Protein 1	BAP1-inactivated melanocytic tumors, mesothelioma, RCCs	RCC, renal cysts
PTEN hamartoma tumor syndromes (Cowden syndrome etc.)	*PTEN* (10q23.3)—Phosphatidylinositol 3,4,5-triphosphate 3-phosphatase and dual-specificity protein phosphatase PTEN	Increased risk for breast, thyroid, endometrial, and other cancers; benign breast, thyroid, and uterine lesions; neurodevelopmental disorders	RCC
Hyperparathyroidism-jaw tumor syndrome	*CDC73* (1q31.2)—Parafibromin	Hyperparathyroidism, ossifying fibromas of maxilla and mandible, renal and uterine tumors	Renal cyst, renal mixed epithelial and stromal tumors (MEST)

Abbreviations: CNS, central nerve system; RCC, renal cell carcinoma; AML, angiomyolipoma.

activation of various downstream targets of HIF pathway that regulate angiogenesis, cell proliferation and survival, glucose metabolism, and extracellular matrix remodeling, such as vascular endothelial growth factor (VEGF), platelet-derived growth factor (PDGF), epidermal growth factor receptor (EGFR), glucose transporter (GLUT1), and CA-IX. Additionally, 3p21 also harbors the three other most commonly mutated genes in ccRCC, *PBRM1*, *SETD2*, and *BAP1*, which encode proteins regulating chromatin modifying processes. Other less commonly mutated but well-established cancer-related genes such as *TP53*, *MTOR*, *TSC1*, *TSC2*, *PIK3CA*, and *PTEN* also contribute to the disease progression. Aside from 3p loss, recurrent somatic copy number alterations most commonly involve losses on chromosomes 1p, 4q, 6q, 8p, 9p, and 14q, as well as gains on chromosomes 1q, 2q, 5q, 7q, 8q, 12p, and 20q. Intertumoral heterogeneity, chromosomal complexity, and different evolutional trajectories revealed by multiregional genomic characterization highlight the diverse and complex genetic landscape of ccRCC, which has important implications in effective therapeutic strategies (57, 58).

The molecular characterization of ccRCC has also discovered a subtype of RCC with wildtype *VHL* gene and intact 3p but harboring recurrent hotspot mutations of *ELOC* (8q21) and chromosome 8 loss of heterozygosity (LOH). *ELOC* (formerly known as *TCEB1*) is a component of the VHL E3 ligase complex, and biallelic inactivation of *ELOC* provides another mechanism to disrupt VHL complex and activate the HIF pathway. These tumors are now recognized as *ELOC*-mutated RCC, a distinct molecular entity in the WHO classification (31).

Papillary RCC (pRCC): Sporadic pRCC is characterized by nearly universal gains or trisomy of chromosomes 7 and 17 and less frequently gain of chromosomes 2, 3, 12, 16, and 20 (59). Mutations of *MET* gene (7q31), identified from hereditary pRCC patients, have been reported in 10–13% of sporadic type 1 or classic pRCC cases. Mutations in *TP53* and *PBRM1*, as well as alterations of *CDKN2A*, are associated with poor survival in pRCC. An important conceptual change in pRCC is that many tumors that have been considered "type 2" pRCC are found to have distinct molecular features and are now classified as molecular entities such as FH-deficient RCC, *TFE3*-rearranged RCC, *TFEB*-altered RCC, and *ALK*-rearranged RCC (31).

Chromophobe RCC (chRCC): chRCCs have a characteristic loss of chromosomes 1, 2, 6, 10, 13, and 17 in approximately 80% of cases; additional less frequent loss of chromosomes 3, 5, 8, 9, 11, 18, and 21q occurs in 12–58% of cases (60). However, this classic pattern of chromosomal losses is less common in eosinophilic chRCC. Compared to ccRCC or pRCC, chRCC has a lower mutation burden, with only *TP53* and *PTEN* frequently mutated in about 30% and 8% of cases, respectively. A recent genomic analysis of localized and metastatic chRCC found enrichment of *TP53* and *PTEN* mutations, as well as imbalanced chromosome duplication (duplication of ≥ 3 chromosomes) in metastatic chRCC (61). Meanwhile, *PTEN* mutations were associated with worse survival in the TCGA chRCC cohort (60).

Other Histologic and Molecularly Defined Subtypes of RCC: A number of other uncommon histologic subtypes of RCC can also be encountered and include mucinous tubular and spindle cell carcinoma (MTSCC), tubulocystic carcinoma, and acquired cystic disease-associated RCC. While lacking frequent mutations, MTSCC has a characteristic pattern of chromosomal losses involving 2, 4, 6, 8, 13, 14, 15, and 22. Importantly, with the utilization of molecular assays such as immunohistochemical biomarkers (e.g. TFE3, FH, SDHB, SMARCB1), fluorescence in-situ hybridization (FISH), and next-generation sequencing (NGS) based-DNA and RNA analyses, molecularly defined subtypes of RCC, tumors primarily characterized by specific molecular alterations, are increasingly being recognized in clinical diagnostic settings. In the current WHO classification (31) for renal cell tumors, the diagnosis of seven entities would rely on evidence of specific molecular alteration (Table 16.19). Intriguingly, somatic *TSC1*/*TSC2* or mTOR complex 1 (mTOC1) gene mutations (e.g. *MTOR*) have been found to be the primary driver of tumorigenesis in a heterogenous group of tumors with distinctive histologic features, including eosinophilic solid and cystic (ESC) carcinoma, eosinophilic and vacuolated tumors (EVTs), low-grade oncocytic tumors (LOTs), and some cases of RCC with fibromyomatous stroma. These sporadic cases appear to share similar morphology to renal tumors in tuberous sclerosis complex (TSC) patients. Limited genetic information is available for the remaining histologic types of RCC.

16.6.2 Systemic Therapies

The management of metastatic RCC has been transformed in the last two decades by the advances in agents targeting biologically important VEGF and related pathways in RCC and by immunotherapy utilizing immune checkpoint inhibitors (ICIs). There are now 17 approved agents with varying molecular mechanisms for treating ccRCC. These agents can be categorized as follows: (1) cytokines such as IL-2 and alpha-Interferon; (2) inhibitors of the VEGF pathway including sorafenib, sunitinib, pazopanib, axitinib, bevacizumab, and tivozanib; (3) TKIs targeting multiple tyrosine kinase receptors such as cabozantinib, which inhibits VEGFR2, cMET, and AXL, and lenvatinib, inhibiting VEGFR2 and FGFR; (4) mTORC1 inhibitors such as everolimus and temsirolimus; (5) PD-1/L1 blocking antibodies like nivolumab, avelumab, and pembrolizumab; (6) an anti-CTLA-4 antibody known as ipilimumab; and (7) the latest addition of HIF2α inhibitor belzutifan for patients with previously treated advanced ccRCC [PMID 38420616]. Combination approaches incorporating ipilimumab plus nivolumab, or a TKI agent with PD-1/PD-L1 have been adopted as a standard of care (62). With this new paradigm, some patients can achieve a prolonged and/or complete remission; however, most still do not derive a durable

TABLE 16.19

Molecularly Defined Renal Cell Carcinoma

Diagnosis	Molecular Alteration	Ancillary Tools
TFE3-rearranged renal cell carcinomas	*TFE3* (Xp11) rearrangement	TFE3 overexpression by IHC *TFE3* rearrangement by FISH or RNA-based fusion assay
TFEB-altered renal cell carcinomas	*TFEB* (6p21) rearrangement or amplification	TFEB overexpression by IHC *TFEB* alterations by FISH or RNA-based fusion assay
ELOC (formerly *TCEB1*)-mutated renal cell carcinoma	*ELOC* biallelic alterations	Next-generation sequencing
Fumarate hydratase (FH)-deficient renal cell carcinoma	*FH* germline or somatic alterations	FH loss by IHC 2-succino-cysteine (2SC) IHC
Succinate dehydrogenase (SDH)-deficient renal cell carcinoma	*SDHB* (most commonly)	SDHB loss by IHC
ALK-rearranged renal cell carcinomas	*ALK* rearrangement	ALK overexpression by IHC *ALK* rearrangement by FISH or RNA-based fusion assay
SMARCB1-deficient renal medullary carcinoma	*SMARCB1* deletion, rearrangement, or mutations	SMARCB1 loss by IHC

Source: adapted from ref. 31

benefit from therapy. Novel biological targets and mechanisms are still needed to improve the prognosis of patients with metastatic disease; directions currently under investigation include targeting HIF, metabolic pathways, cell cycle regulation, and novel immune mechanisms. Notably, belzutifan, a highly specific and well-tolerated HIF2α inhibitor, previously received FDA approval for the treatment of nonmetastatic RCC and various other tumors in patients with VHL disease (63).

Metastatic nccRCCs are less sensitive to the approved agents since these were mainly developed in ccRCC. Nevertheless, these agents have helped achieve better antitumor activity and improve outcomes in some patients. Combination TKI and ICI are now being evaluated and may further help patients. Enrolling nccRCC patients into clinical trials is an important treatment option currently. Meanwhile, advance in our understanding of each tumor type under the nccRCC umbrella will be essential for improving and optimizing patient outcomes in the future.

16.7 Penile Carcinoma

Penile carcinoma is a rare carcinoma, with an estimated 2,070 new cases and 470 deaths in 2022 (64). Most penile tumors are SCCs. SCC can be HPV (human papillomavirus) associated or HPV independent (31). High-risk HPV is present in 33% of HPV-associated penile SCC, with HPV 16 being the most common genotype from a list of prevalent subtypes. The average age for patients with HPV-associated penile SCC is younger than patients with HPV-independent SCC. HPV-independent SCC frequently involves the glans and occurs in older males. They are associated with long-standing inflammatory conditions such as lichen sclerosis and phimosis (31). The risk is threefold higher in men who are not circumcised.

16.7.1 Molecular Findings

The commonly altered genes in penile SCC include *TP53*, *CDKN2A*, and *PIK3CA*, followed by *MYC*, *HRAS*, and *SOX2* (65, 66). Although overall there is no correlation between specific mutations and HPV association, HPV-associated SCCs usually do not have *TP53* alterations or *EGFR* (epidermal growth factor receptor) amplifications (65). HPV-independent tumors and tumors with amplifications in *MYC* and *CCND1* may be associated with decreased disease-free survival. Data is still emerging on tumor mutation burden (TMB) and HPV association, with a large study by Nazha et al. noting a high TMB in a subset of HPV-associated SCC (66).

16.7.2 Current Treatment Including Targeted and Immuno-Therapeutic Agents

Treatment for penile carcinoma is usually through surgical resection and, when clinically indicated, inguinal lymph node dissection. Post-operative radiation therapy can be added depending on the lymph node status. Neo-adjuvant chemotherapy is recommended for patients with high tumor stage and/or confirmed inguinal nodal spread. First-line chemotherapy includes a combination of paclitaxel, ifosfamide, and cisplatin (TIP). Tumors with large size and local nodal spread are rarely controlled with one treatment modality (67). Recurrent or metastatic penile carcinoma is treated with first-line chemotherapy (TIP) (68). Subsequent-line systemic therapy includes the use of pembrolizumab, particularly in the setting of high TMB (> 10 mutations per Mb) or high microsatellite instability (MSI-High).

PD-L1 expression in penile carcinoma has been reported using variable PD-L1 clones. Variable scoring results (tumor score vs. tumor and infiltrating inflammatory cell score) and cutoff positive percentages were used (Table 16.20). Correlation studies between the expression of PD-L1 by IHC and clinical response to PD-L1 inhibitors are still accruing but initial data do not show a

TABLE 16.20

Summary of Available Reported Studies Investigating PD-L1 Expression in Penile Carcinoma

Study	#HPV Associated SCC	#HPV Independent SCC	PD-L1 Antibody Clone	PD-L1 Scoring Method	Positive Results	Clinical Response	Other Comments/ Prognosis
Cocks et al. 2017 (71)* $N = 53$	$N = 8$	$N = 45$	E1L3N, 1:100	Tumor and immune cells (> 0%)	21/53 total cases (40%) positive. No correlation with HPV status	N/A	Not predictive of tumor recurrence, progression, or cancer-related death
Davidsson et al. 2019 (72)* $N = 222$	$N = 75$	$N = 85$	Clone 28.8 1:400 Clone SP142 1:30	Tumor and Immune cells (separately scored) 1+ < 5%; 2+ > 5% to < 50%; 3+ > 50%	28.8 tumor $n = 70$ (32.1%) Immune cells $n = 99$ (45%) SP142: Tumor $n = 16$ (7.3%) Immune cells $n = 140$ (64.2%) No significant correlation with HPV status	N/A	SP142, independently associated with risk of poor clinical outcomes
Udager et al. 2016 (73) $N = 37$	$N = 5$	$N = 28$	Clone 5H1; 1:500	Tumor ≥ 5% tumor-infiltrating mononuclear cells ≥ 5%	23 (62.2%)	N/A	PD-L1 significantly expressed in lymph node metastases
Ottenhof et al. 2017 (74) $N = 210$	$N = 50$	$N = 150$	Clone E1L3N, 1:200	Tumor cells, ≥ 1%	HPV pos $n = 17$ (32.7%) HPV neg $n = 78$ (49.4%)	N/A	PD-L1 expression an independent predictor for survival
Deng et al. 2017 (75) $N = 116$	N/A	n/A	Clone E1L3N 1:100	Tumor cells and TILs ≥ 5%	Tumor cells $N = 62$ (53.4%) TILs $N = 91$ (79.8%)	N/A	High PD-L1 expression in tumor cells indicated a poor prognosis
Muller et al. 2022 (76) $N = 60$	$N = 31$	$N = 25$	Clone ZR3 1:200	TPS, staining (>0%) IC, positive immune reaction in immune cells (>0%)	TPS $N = 26$ (87%) IC $N = 25$ (83%)	N/A	PD-L1 expression was not associated with overall survival
Nazha et al. 2023 (66) $N = 108$	$N = 13$	$N = 16$#	SP142 dilution not provided	Tumor cells ≥ 1%	51%	N/A	N/A
El Zarif et al. 2023 (69) $N = 92$	$N = 17$	$N = 32$	N/A	Tumor proportion score (TPS)	$N = 17/26 = 65\%$	Combination or monotherapy ICI	ICI therapy benefited a small subset with overall ORR 13% and monotherapy 8.5% No correlation between PD-L1 positivity and response

Note: * Immunohistochemical staining for PD-L1 performed through Tissue microarray (TMA).

#only HPV 16 and 18 were performed and were negative; ICI, immune checkpoint inhibitors; TPS, tumor proportion score; IC, Immune cells; TIC, tumor infiltrating cells.

tangible correlation (69). Clinical trials on the efficacy of PD-L1 inhibitors in the setting of penile carcinoma are rare and limited by low numbers of enrolled patients. However, preliminary findings indicate a measurable response in a small percentage of patients (1 in 3 patients) (70). Future studies refining the PD-L1 IHC scoring method and correlation with anticipated therapy response could help determine the necessity for PD-L1 IHC staining in the setting of penile carcinoma.

Few studies report high level expression of PD-L1 correlates with poor prognosis and HPV negative status (74, 75), which is in keeping with what we know about PD-L1 and its role in helping tumor cells evade the immune system. Additional studies to further identify which subset of patients with penile SCC can benefit from immunotherapy are still needed.

16.8 Testicular Carcinoma

Testicular tumors represent around 1.5% of tumors that arise in males and are the most common tumor arising in young males between the ages of 15 and 40 years (31). The majority of testicular tumors are testicular germ cell tumors (TGCTs), with the remaining 5–10% consisting of sex cord stromal tumors and other less frequent tumors, including lymphoma and metastatic tumors from other primary sites.

TGCTs are broadly divided into seminomatous and non-seminomatous germ cell tumors and are thought to arise from a common precursor lesion, germ cell neoplasia *in situ* (GCNIS). Most patients present with a mixture of germ cell tumor subtypes with varying percentages and are diagnosed as "mixed germ cell tumor". Current surgical and chemotherapeutic treatment protocols result in over 95% cure rate of patients with testicular germ cell tumors (77). Discovery of additional biomarkers, including diagnostic, prognostic, and therapeutic biomarkers, would help clinicians better diagnose and treat these patients. This would prevent over-treatment when not needed and prompt neoadjuvant/adjuvant therapy when prognostically indicated.

16.8.1 Molecular Findings

GCNIS, believed to be the precursor lesion of TGCT, is thought to arise from incompletely differentiated primordial germ cells, possibly through non-disjunction resulting in tetraploid precursor cells (78). GCNIS then gains isochromosome 12p (i12p) as it gives rise to post-pubertal germ cell tumors (79). i12p was observed in most TGCT and absent only in a small subset of seminomas. i12p is also present in secondary somatic malignancies that rarely arise from TGCT (80).

Seminoma are currently genomically subcategorized into *KIT*-mutated and *KIT*-non-mutated tumors (81). The *KIT*-mutated seminoma seems to be associated with history of cryptorchidism and a higher level of accompanying immune response. *KIT* mutations were not observed in mixed germ cell tumors, despite the presence of seminoma in some of these tumors, suggesting that the occurrence of *KIT* mutations in seminoma may play a role in preventing further differentiation into other germ cell tumor subtypes. Other mutations, predominantly present in seminomas, involve *KRAS* and *NRAS* from the KIT-PI3K pathway.

In addition, global DNA methylation was differentially present in TGCT; seminoma generally lacks DNA methylation, while non-seminomatous germ cell tumors (NS-GCT) show varying levels of DNA methylation, suggesting that epigenetics may play a causative role in the development of the latter (81).

16.8.2 Treatment of Refractory Germ Cell Tumors

A small subset of patients develop recurrences that are refractory to first-line therapies and are subjected to salvage/high dose chemotherapy followed by bone marrow transplant (82, 83). The role of immune checkpoint inhibitors and specifically pembrolizumab is still under investigation and is currently used as a third-line therapy in patient with high tumor mutation burden or microsatellite unstable tumors (84, 85).

16.8.3 Additional Future Directions

In vitro response of refractory testicular cell lines to DNA methyltransferase inhibitors suggests a possible role for similar therapies in the future for the treatment of refractory NS-GCT (86). In addition, epigenetic silencing of homologous recombination (HR) DNA repair pathway genes in NS-GCT (*BRCA1* and *RAD51C*) raises the possibility of a therapeutic role for poly (ADP-ribose) polymerase (PARP) inhibitors (87).

16.9 Summary

The future of precision medicine and targeted therapy holds promise for optimization of treatment response and decreasing treatment side effect and toxicity. As these treatments are developed and refined, the role of the pathologists remains at the center of the multi-disciplinary care unit.

REFERENCES

1. SEER. SEER*Explorer: An interactive website for SEER cancer statistics [Internet]. Surveillance Research Program, National Cancer Institute; 2023 Apr 19. [updated: 2023 Jun 8; cited 2023 Sep 8]. Available from: https://seer.cancer.gov/statistics-network/explorer/. Data source(s): SEER Incidence Data, November 2022 Submission (1975–2020), SEER 22 registries. 2023.
2. Vellky JE, Ricke WA. Development and prevalence of castration-resistant prostate cancer subtypes. Neoplasia. 2020;22(11):566–75.
3. Zarrabi K, Paroya A, Wu S. Emerging therapeutic agents for genitourinary cancers. J Hematol Oncol. 2019;12(1):89.
4. Magers MJ, Iczkowski KA, Montironi R, et al. MYB-NFIB gene fusion in prostatic basal cell carcinoma: Clinicopathologic correlates and comparison with basal cell adenoma and florid basal cell hyperplasia. Mod Pathol. 2019;32(11):1666–1674.
5. Iczkowski KA, Montironi R. Adenoid cystic/basal cell carcinoma of the prostate strongly expresses HER-2/neu. J Clin Pathol. 2006;59(12):1327–1330.
6. Epstein JI, Egevad L, Amin MB, et al. The 2014 International Society of Urological Pathology (ISUP) consensus conference on gleason grading of prostatic carcinoma: Definition of grading patterns and proposal for a new grading system. Am J Surg Pathol. 2016;40(2):244–252.
7. Cancer Genome Atlas Research Network. The molecular taxonomy of primary prostate cancer. Cell. 2015;163(4):1011–1025.
8. He Y, Xu W, Xiao YT, Huang H, Gu D, Ren S. Targeting signaling pathways in prostate cancer: Mechanisms and clinical trials. Signal Transduct Target Ther. 2022;7(1):198.
9. Stopsack KH, Nandakumar S, Wibmer AG, et al. Oncogenic genomic alterations, clinical phenotypes, and outcomes in metastatic castration-sensitive prostate cancer. Clin Cancer Res. 2020;26(13):3230–3238.
10. Abida W, Cyrta J, Heller G, et al. Genomic correlates of clinical outcome in advanced prostate cancer. Proc Natl Acad Sci U S A. 2019;116(23):11428–31146.
11. Scher HI, Halabi S, Tannock I, et al. Design and end points of clinical trials for patients with progressive prostate cancer and castrate levels of testosterone: Recommendations of the Prostate Cancer Clinical Trials Working Group. J Clin Oncol. 2008;26(7):1148–1159.
12. Li Y, Yang R, Henzler CM, et al. Diverse AR gene rearrangements mediate resistance to androgen receptor inhibitors in metastatic prostate cancer. Clin Cancer Res. 2020;26(8):1965–1976.
13. Rickman DS, Beltran H, Demichelis F, Rubin MA. Biology and evolution of poorly differentiated neuroendocrine tumors. Nat Med. 2017;23(6):1–10.
14. Chung JH, Dewal N, Sokol E, et al. Prospective comprehensive genomic profiling of primary and metastatic prostate tumors. JCO Precis Oncol. 2019;3.
15. Jairath NK, Dal Pra A, Vince R, Jr., et al. A Systematic review of the evidence for the decipher genomic classifier in prostate cancer. Eur Urol. 2021;79(3):374–383.
16. Covas Moschovas M, Chew C, Bhat S, et al. Association between oncotype DX genomic prostate score and adverse tumor pathology after radical prostatectomy. Eur Urol Focus. 2022;8(2):418–424.

17. Sommariva S, Tarricone R, Lazzeri M, et al. Prognostic value of the cell cycle progression score in patients with prostate cancer: A systematic review and meta-analysis. Eur Urol. 2016;69(1):107–115.
18. Blume-Jensen P, Berman DM, Rimm DL, et al. Development and clinical validation of an in situ biopsy-based multimarker assay for risk stratification in prostate cancer. Clin Cancer Res. 2015;21(11):2591–2600.
19. Asif S, Teply BA. Biomarkers for treatment response in advanced prostate cancer. Cancers (Basel). 2021;13(22).
20. Armenia J, Wankowicz SAM, Liu D, et al. The long tail of oncogenic drivers in prostate cancer. Nat Genet. 2018;50(5):645–651.
21. Pritchard CC, Mateo J, Walsh MF, et al. Inherited DNA-repair gene mutations in men with metastatic prostate cancer. N Engl J Med. 2016;375(5):443–453.
22. NCCN-Prostate. Version 1.2023, National Comprehensive Cancer Network® (NCCN®), 2023. Available from: www.nccn.org/guidelines/guidelines-detail?category=1&id=1459.
23. Le DT, Durham JN, Smith KN, et al. Mismatch repair deficiency predicts response of solid tumors to PD-1 blockade. Science. 2017;357(6349):409–413.
24. Wu YM, Cieślik M, Lonigro RJ, et al. Inactivation of CDK12 delineates a distinct immunogenic class of advanced prostate cancer. Cell. 2018;173(7):1770–1782.e14.
25. Antonarakis ES, Isaacsson Velho P, Fu W, et al. CDK12-Altered prostate cancer: Clinical features and therapeutic outcomes to standard systemic therapies, poly (ADP-ribose) polymerase inhibitors, and PD-1 inhibitors. JCO Precis Oncol. 2020;4:370–381.
26. Sartor O, de Bono J, Chi KN, et al. Lutetium-177-PSMA-617 for metastatic castration-resistant prostate cancer. N Engl J Med. 2021;385(12):1091–1103.
27. Sweeney C, Bracarda S, Sternberg CN, et al. Ipatasertib plus abiraterone and prednisolone in metastatic castration-resistant prostate cancer (IPATential150): A multicentre, randomised, double-blind, phase 3 trial. Lancet. 2021;398(10295):131–142.
28. Jamaspishvili T, Berman DM, Ross AE, et al. Clinical implications of PTEN loss in prostate cancer. Nat Rev Urol. 2018;15(4):222–234.
29. Aggarwal R, Huang J, Alumkal JJ, et al. Clinical and genomic characterization of treatment-emergent small-cell neuroendocrine prostate cancer: A multi- institutional prospective study. J Clin Oncol. 2018;36(24):2492–2503.
30. Beltran H, Prandi D, Mosquera JM, et al. Divergent clonal evolution of castration-resistant neuroendocrine prostate cancer. Nat Med. 2016;22(3):298–305.
31. WHO. WHO Classification of Tumours Editorial Board. Urinary and Male Genital Tumours (WHO Classification of Tumours Series, 5th ed.; Vol. 8). Lyon: International Agency for Research on Cancer, 2022.
32. Beltran H, Rickman DS, Park K, et al. Molecular characterization of neuroendocrine prostate cancer and identification of new drug targets. Cancer Discov. 2011;1(6):487–495.
33. Robertson AG, Kim J, Al-Ahmadie H, et al. Comprehensive molecular characterization of muscle-invasive bladder cancer. Cell. 2017;171(3):540–556.e25.
34. Kamoun A, de Reyniès A, Allory Y, et al. A consensus molecular classification of muscle-invasive bladder cancer. Eur Urol. 2020;77(4):420–433.
35. Lindskrog SV, Prip F, Lamy P, et al. An integrated multi-omics analysis identifies prognostic molecular subtypes of non-muscle-invasive bladder cancer. Nat Commun. 2021;12(1):2301.
36. Knowles MA. Role of FGFR3 in urothelial cell carcinoma: Biomarker and potential therapeutic target. World J Urol. 2007;25(6):581–593.
37. Glaser AP, Fantini D, Shilatifard A, et al. The evolving genomic landscape of urothelial carcinoma. Nat Rev Urol. 2017;14(4):215–229.
38. Hoffman-Censits J, Choi W, Pal S, et al. Urothelial cancers with small cell variant histology have confirmed high tumor mutational burden, frequent TP53 and RB mutations, and a unique gene expression profile. Eur Urol Oncol. 2021;4(2):297–300.
39. Manzano RG, Catalan-Latorre A, Brugarolas A. RB1 and TP53 co-mutations correlate strongly with genomic biomarkers of response to immunity checkpoint inhibitors in urothelial bladder cancer. BMC Cancer. 2021;21(1):432.
40. NCCN, Bladder. 2023. Available from: www.nccn.org/guidelines/guidelines-detail?category=1&id=1417.
41. Jun T, Anker J, Galsky MD. Biomarkers for therapy selection in metastatic urothelial cancer. J Cancer Metastasis Treat. 2022;8:1.
42. Koshkin VS, O'Donnell P, Yu EY, Grivas P. Systematic review: Targeting HER2 in bladder cancer. Bladder Cancer. 2019;5:1–12.
43. Balar AV, Kamat AM, Kulkarni GS, et al. Pembrolizumab monotherapy for the treatment of high-risk non-muscle-invasive bladder cancer unresponsive to BCG (KEYNOTE-057): An open-label, single-arm, multicentre, phase 2 study. Lancet Oncol. 2021;22(7):919–930.
44. Harper HL, McKenney JK, Heald B, et al. Upper tract urothelial carcinomas: Frequency of association with mismatch repair protein loss and lynch syndrome. Mod Pathol. 2017;30(1):146–156.
45. Gayhart MG, Johnson N, Paul A, et al. Universal mismatch repair protein screening in upper tract urothelial carcinoma. Am J Clin Pathol. 2020;154(6):792–801.
46. Pires-Luis AS, Martinek P, Alaghehbandan R, et al. Molecular genetic features of primary nonurachal enteric-type adenocarcinoma, urachal adenocarcinoma, mucinous adenocarcinoma, and intestinal metaplasia/adenoma: Review of the literature and next-generation sequencing study. Adv Anat Pathol. 2020;27(5):303–310.
47. Maurer A, Ortiz-Bruechle N, Guricova K, et al. Comparative genomic profiling of glandular bladder tumours. Virchows Arch. 2020;477(3):445–454.
48. Sung H, Ferlay J, Siegel RL, et al. Global cancer statistics 2020: GLOBOCAN estimates of incidence and mortality worldwide for 36 cancers in 185 countries. CA Cancer J Clin. 2021;71(3):209–249.
49. Cai Q, Chen Y, Qi X, et al. Temporal trends of kidney cancer incidence and mortality from 1990 to 2016 and projections to 2030. Transl Androl Urol. 2020;9(2):166–181.
50. Siegel RL, Miller KD, Fuchs HE, Jemal A. Cancer statistics, 2022. CA Cancer J Clin. 2022;72(1):7–33.
51. Kotecha RR, Motzer RJ, Voss MH. Author correction: Towards individualized therapy for metastatic renal cell carcinoma. Nat Rev Clin Oncol. 2019;16(10):653.
52. Linehan WM, Srinivasan R, Schmidt LS. The genetic basis of kidney cancer: A metabolic disease. Nat Rev Urol. 2010;7(5):277–285.

53. Carlo MI, Hakimi AA, Stewart GD, et al. Familial kidney cancer: Implications of new syndromes and molecular insights. Eur Urol. 2019;76(6):754–764.
54. Cancer Genome Atlas Research Network. Comprehensive molecular characterization of clear cell renal cell carcinoma. Nature. 2013;499(7456):43–49.
55. Sato Y, Yoshizato T, Shiraishi Y, et al. Integrated molecular analysis of clear-cell renal cell carcinoma. Nat Genet. 2013;45(8):860–867.
56. Mitchell TJ, Turajlic S, Rowan A, et al. Timing the landmark events in the evolution of clear cell renal cell cancer: TRACERx renal. Cell. 2018;173(3):611–623.e17.
57. Turajlic S, Xu H, Litchfield K, et al. Deterministic evolutionary trajectories influence primary tumor growth: TRACERx renal. Cell. 2018;173(3):595–610.e11.
58. Turajlic S, Xu H, Litchfield K, et al. Tracking cancer evolution reveals constrained routes to metastases: TRACERx renal. Cell. 2018;173(3):581–594.e12.
59. Linehan WM, Spellman PT, Ricketts CJ, et al. Comprehensive molecular characterization of papillary renal-cell carcinoma. N Engl J Med. 2016;374(2):135–145.
60. Davis CF, Ricketts CJ, Wang M, et al. The somatic genomic landscape of chromophobe renal cell carcinoma. Cancer Cell. 2014;26(3):319–330.
61. Casuscelli J, Weinhold N, Gundem G, et al. Genomic landscape and evolution of metastatic chromophobe renal cell carcinoma. JCI Insight. 2017;2(12).
62. Motzer RJ, Jonasch E, Agarwal N, et al. Kidney cancer, version 3.2022, NCCN clinical practice guidelines in oncology. J Natl Compr Canc Netw. 2022;20(1):71–90.
63. Jonasch E, Donskov F, Iliopoulos O, et al. Belzutifan for renal cell carcinoma in von Hippel-Lindau disease. N Engl J Med. 2021;385(22):2036–2046.
64. Siegel RL, Miller KD, Jemal A. Cancer statistics, 2019. CA Cancer J Clin. 2019;69(1):7–34.
65. McDaniel AS, Hovelson DH, Cani AK, et al. Genomic profiling of penile squamous cell carcinoma reveals new opportunities for targeted therapy. Cancer Res. 2015;75(24):5219–5227.
66. Nazha B, Zhuang T, Wu S, et al. Comprehensive genomic profiling of penile squamous cell carcinoma and the impact of human papillomavirus status on immune-checkpoint inhibitor-related biomarkers. Cancer. 2023;129(24):3884–3893.
67. Pagliaro LC, Crook J. Multimodality therapy in penile cancer: When and which treatments? World J Urol. 2009;27(2):221–225.
68. NCCN-Penile. Version 1.2023, ©2022 National Comprehensive Cancer Network® 2023. Available from: https://www.nccn.org/guidelines/guidelines-detail?category=1&id=1456.
69. El Zarif T, Nassar AH, Pond GR, et al. Safety and efficacy of immune checkpoint inhibitors in advanced penile cancer: Report from the Global Society of Rare Genitourinary Tumors. J Natl Cancer Inst. 2023.
70. Naing A, Meric-Bernstam F, Stephen B, et al. Phase 2 study of pembrolizumab in patients with advanced rare cancers. J Immunother Cancer. 2020;8(1).
71. Cocks M, Taheri D, Ball MW, et al. Immune-checkpoint status in penile squamous cell carcinoma: A North American cohort. Hum Pathol. 2017;59:55–61.
72. Davidsson S, Carlsson J, Giunchi F, et al. PD-L1 expression in men with penile cancer and its association with clinical outcomes. Eur Urol Oncol. 2019;2(2):214–221.
73. Udager AM, Liu TY, Skala SL, et al. Frequent PD-L1 expression in primary and metastatic penile squamous cell carcinoma: Potential opportunities for immunotherapeutic approaches. Ann Oncol. 2016;27(9):1706–1712.
74. Ottenhof SR, Djajadiningrat RS, de Jong J, Thygesen HH, Horenblas S, Jordanova ES. Expression of programmed death ligand 1 in penile cancer is of prognostic value and associated with HPV status. J Urol. 2017;197(3 Pt 1):690–697.
75. Deng C, Li Z, Guo S, et al. Tumor PD-L1 expression is correlated with increased TILs and poor prognosis in penile squamous cell carcinoma. Oncoimmunology. 2017;6(2):e1269047.
76. Müller T, Demes M, Lehn A, et al. The peri- and intratumoral immune cell infiltrate and PD-L1 status in invasive squamous cell carcinomas of the penis. Clin Transl Oncol. 2022;24(2):331–341.
77. Stang A, Jansen L, Trabert B, et al. Survival after a diagnosis of testicular germ cell cancers in Germany and the United States, 2002–2006: A high resolution study by histology and age. Cancer Epidemiol. 2013;37(4):492–497.
78. Frigyesi A, Gisselsson D, Hansen GB, et al. A model for karyotypic evolution in testicular germ cell tumors. Gene Chromosome Canc. 2004;40(3):172–178.
79. Ottesen AM, Skakkebaek NE, Lundsteen C, et al. High-resolution comparative genomic hybridization detects extra chromosome arm 12p material in most cases of carcinoma in situ adjacent to overt germ cell tumors, but not before the invasive tumor development. Gene Chromosome Canc. 2003;38(2):117–125.
80. Kum JB, Ulbright TM, Williamson SR, et al. Molecular genetic evidence supporting the origin of somatic-type malignancy and teratoma from the same progenitor cell. Am J Surg Pathol. 2012;36(12):1849–1856.
81. Shen H, Shih J, Hollern DP, et al. Integrated molecular characterization of testicular germ cell tumors. Cell Rep. 2018;23(11):3392–3406.
82. Sheridan WP, Boyd AW, Green MD, et al. High-dose chemotherapy with busulphan and cyclophosphamide and bone-marrow transplantation for drug- sensitive malignancies in adults: A preliminary report. Med J Aust. 1989;151(7):379–386.
83. Allen JC, Kirschner A, Scarpato KR, Morgans AK. Current management of refractory germ cell tumors and future directions. Curr Oncol Rep. 2017;19(2):8.
84. Marabelle A, Fakih M, Lopez J, et al. Association of tumour mutational burden with outcomes in patients with advanced solid tumours treated with pembrolizumab: Prospective biomarker analysis of the multicohort, open-label, phase 2 KEYNOTE-158 study. Lancet Oncol. 2020;21(10):1353–1365.
85. Le DT, Uram JN, Wang H, et al. PD-1 Blockade in tumors with mismatch-repair deficiency. N Engl J Med. 2015;372(26):2509–2520.
86. Albany C, Hever-Jardine MP, von Herrmann KM, et al. Refractory testicular germ cell tumors are highly sensitive to the second generation DNA methylation inhibitor guadecitabine. Oncotarget. 2017;8(2):2949–2959.
87. Cavallo F, Graziani G, Antinozzi C, et al. Reduced proficiency in homologous recombination underlies the high sensitivity of embryonal carcinoma testicular germ cell tumors to Cisplatin and poly (adp-ribose) polymerase inhibition. PLoS ONE. 2012;7(12):e51563.

17

Female Genital Tract Tumors

Krisztina Hanley, Jane L. Meisel, Sarah J. Wood, and Gulisa Turashvili

17.1 Introduction

Gynecological cancers involve all parts of the female genital tract, with endometrial cancer being the most common (1). Many factors, including viruses, estrogen, tobacco smoking, and exposure to other carcinogens and radiation, all play a role in the development of cancers of the female genital tract. This chapter will summarize the most recent advances in precision pathology of gynecologic tumors in the era of precision medicine.

17.2 Uterine Epithelial Tumors

Endometrial carcinomas (ECs) represent the most common gynecologic malignancy in developed countries and are clinically managed based on pathologic and molecular findings (2).

17.2.1 Histologic Classification

ECs include endometrioid and non-endometrioid subtypes (Table 17.1). Endometrioid adenocarcinoma (EA), the only subtype graded based on the proportion of nonsquamous solid growth, is composed of neoplastic glands with smooth luminal outlines and frequent squamous, mucinous, or secretory differentiation, lined by columnar cells with low-grade atypia and variable mitoses (Figure 17.1A-B).

All non-endometrioid ECs (NECs) are high-grade by convention. Serous carcinoma (SC) exhibits papillary, glandular and/or solid architecture and high-grade atypia (Figure 17.1C). Clear cell carcinoma (CCC) is characterized by tubulocystic, papillary, and/or solid architecture with low-to-intermediate grade atypia (Figure 17.1D). Undifferentiated carcinoma (UC) shows solid sheets of monomorphic, discohesive cells, while dedifferentiated carcinoma (DC) displays a second component of low-grade EA (Figure 17.1E) (3). Carcinosarcoma (CS) is composed of sharply

TABLE 17.1

Morphology and Immunophenotype of Endometrial Carcinomas

Histotype	Morphology	IHC
Endometrioid adenocarcinoma, low-grade	< 50% nonsquamous solid growth (< 5% in FIGO grade 1, 6–50% in FIGO grade 2); oval or round glands with smooth outlines lined by columnar to cuboidal cells with low-grade oval to round nuclei, ±squamous, secretory or mucinous differentiation, ±background EIN	WT p53, ER/PR(+), PTEN(∓), ARID1A(∓), p16(-), MMR(∓)
Endometrioid adenocarcinoma, high-grade	> 50% nonsquamous solid growth or, rarely, 6–50% solid growth with diffuse marked nuclear atypia	Abn p53 (25-30%), ER/PR(+), PTEN(∓), ARID1A(∓), MMR(∓)
Serous carcinoma	Papillary, glandular or solid growth, marked diffuse cytologic atypia with brisk mitoses, apoptotic bodies, tumor cell budding and tufting, ±psammoma bodies, ±background atrophic endometrium or polyp	Abn p53, p16(+), PTEN(+), ARID1A(+), MMR(+)
Clear cell carcinoma	Tubulocystic, papillary or solid growth, cuboidal to polygonal cells with variable nuclear pleomorphism and mitotic rate, ±hobnailing, cytoplasmic clearing	Abn p53 (30%), ER/PR(-), PTEN(-), ARID1A(-), p16(-)
Un/dedifferentiated carcinoma	Diffuse sheets of monomorphic discohesive cells (undifferentiated), associated with low-grade endometrioid adenocarcinoma (dedifferentiated), ±alveolar, nested, corded or trabecular growth, rhabdoid/plasmacytoid morphology, focal marked atypia, multinucleation, spindling, and "abrupt" keratinization	WT p53 (most), PanCK(∓), E-cadherin(∓), MMR(∓), p16(-)
Mesonephris and Mesonephric-like carcinomas	Admixture of papillary, ductal, retiform, solid or spindled growth, small glands and tubules with luminal eosinophilic colloid-like material, moderately atypical vesicular nuclei, often angulated or overlapping	WT p53, GATA3(±), TTF1(±), p16(-), MMR(+)
Gastric (gastrointestinal)-type carcinoma	Glands formed by mucin-containing epithelial cells with low-grade nuclei, ±goblet cells	WT p53, ER/PR(-), p16(-), MMR(+)
Squamous cell carcinoma	Morphology similar to squamous cell carcinomas of other sites; may appear deceptively bland, invading along a broad front	WT p53, p63(+), p40(+), p16(±), MMR(+)

(Continued)

DOI: 10.1201/9781003513469-17

TABLE 17.1 (Continued)

Histotype	Morphology	IHC
Carcinosarcoma	Biphasic tumor composed of malignant high-grade epithelial and mesenchymal and sarcomatous elements, the latter with or without heterologous differentiation	Abn p53 (most), p16(+), MMR(±)

Notes: [a]For p16 staining, (+) denotes diffuse, block-like expression, (-) denotes negative, focal, or patchy staining; Abn, abnormal; EIN, endometrioid intraepithelial neoplasia; ER/PR, estrogen and progesterone receptors; FIGO, The International Federation of Gynecology and Obstetrics; MMR, mismatch repair; PanCK, pan-cytokeratin; WT, wild-type

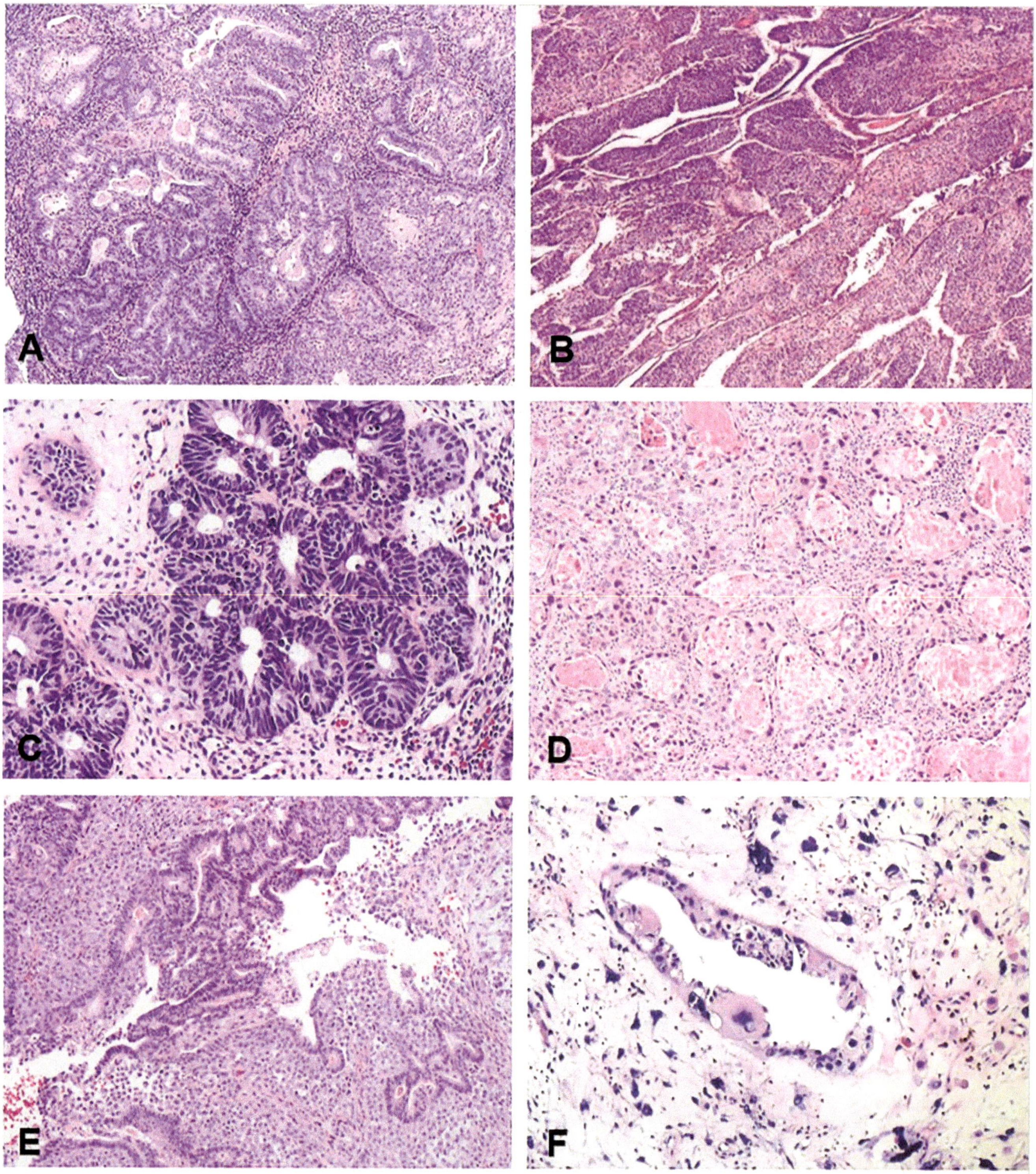

FIGURE 17.1 Uterine epithelial tumors. (A) Low-grade (FIGO grade 1-2) endometrioid adenocarcinoma (H&E, ×100). (B) High-grade (FIGO grade 3) endometrioid adenocarcinoma (H&E, ×40). (C) Serous carcinoma (H&E, ×100). (D) Clear cell carcinoma (H&E, ×40). (E) Dedifferentiated carcinoma (H&E, ×40). (F) Carcinosarcoma with heterologous (rhabdomyosarcomatous) differentiation (H&E, ×100).

demarcated malignant epithelial and sarcomatous components (Figure 17.1F). Mixed carcinoma exhibits ≥ 2 distinct components, with ≥ 1 being SC or CCC. Rare NECs include mesonephric, mesonephric-like, squamous cell and gastric (gastrointestinal)-type mucinous carcinomas (4).

17.2.2 Molecular Classification and Genetic Alterations

Over the past decade, the EC classification has undergone a paradigm shift due to an emerging molecular classification system. In 2013, an integrated genomic analysis by the Cancer Genome Atlas (TCGA) Research Network (5) identified four subtypes (Table 17.2):

1) *POLE*-mutated/ultramutated EC, defined by mutations in the exonuclease domain of the DNA polymerase epsilon (POLE), an enzyme involved in DNA replication and repair, and ultra-high tumor mutation burden (TMB) (6). Characteristic features include EA or serous-like morphology with tumor giant cells, abundant tumor infiltrating lymphocytes (TILs), and favorable prognosis (progression-free survival [PFS]) (7, 8).
2) Copy number high (CNH) EC exhibits *TP53* mutations, high copy number alterations and SC or serous-like morphology in 93% of cases, followed by CS and CCC (9). This subtype is associated with poor prognosis, increased rates (~20–25%) of human epidermal growth factor 2 (*HER2*) amplification, and homologous recombination deficiency (HRD) (10, 11).
3) Microsatellite instability high (MSI-H) EC shows defects in DNA mismatch repair (MMR) genes, high TMB, EA morphology, abundant TILs, and intermediate prognosis.
4) Copy number-low EC (so-called no specific molecular profile [NSMP]) is genomically stable, MMR-proficient EA with moderate TMB, common mutations in the PI3K/Akt and Wnt/CTNNB1 signaling pathways, and intermediate to favorable prognosis.

Both the histologic and molecular subtypes of EC are characterized by certain gene mutations. Genes frequently mutated in EA include *PTEN* (77%), *PIK3CA* (53%), *PIK3R1* (37%), *CTNNB1* (36%), *ARID1A* (35%), and *KRAS* (24%). Almost all SCs show *TP53* mutations, less commonly *PIK3CA* (41.9%), *FBXW7* (30.2%), and *PPP2R1A* (36.6%) (12). However, *TP53* mutations may be seen in ~30% of high-grade EA and CCC (13). CCC may show *ARID1A* and rarely *PTEN* mutations. MMR deficiency has been reported in ~50% of UC/DC and ~30% of EA and CCC but only 10% of SC (14, 15).

17.2.3 Testing Strategies

17.2.3.1 Molecular Classification

The World Health Organization (WHO) recommends molecular subtyping of EC when resources are available. However, given the limited availability of *POLE* sequencing, no universal or standardized approach currently exists for routine application of the TCGA classification in practice (4). A combined approach with *POLE* sequencing and immunohistochemistry (IHC) for p53 and MMR proteins has been proposed as a surrogate assay including the ProMisE (Proactive Molecular Risk Classifier for Endometrial Cancer) recommending MMR IHC first, followed by *POLE* sequencing and p53 IHC (16, 17), although *POLE*-mutated ECs will be missed (18). Another approach using *POLE* sequencing and IHC for p53 and 2 MMR proteins (PMS2, MSH6) has been validated in three independent studies (16, 17, 19). If *POLE* sequencing is unavailable, MSI-H and CNH groups can still be identified using MMR and p53 IHC (20).

MMR IHC has a dual purpose of molecular subtyping and Lynch syndrome screening. When interpreting MMR IHC, an absence of nuclear staining should be noted for MMR proteins, which function in dimers (MLH1/PMS2 and MSH2/MSH6) (Figure 17.2A). MMR deficiency may be due to germline or somatic mutations (21). In most tumors, MLH1 deficiency is sporadic due to epigenetic silencing of the *MLH1* gene via *MLH1* promoter methylation. Reflex *MLH1* promoter methylation testing is therefore performed in MLH1/PMS2-deficient tumors. Patients with non-methylated EC should undergo germline testing (22).

Three abnormal or mutation-type IHC patterns of p53 expression include nuclear overexpression in 80–100% of cells (non-synonymous missense mutations) (Figure 17.2B), complete absence (null-pattern, loss of function mutations) (Figure 17.2C) or, rarely, cytoplasmic expression (loss of function mutation disrupting nuclear localization domain) (Figure 17.2D) (23).

17.2.3.2 HER2 Testing

Approximately 30% of SCs are positive for HER2, a tyrosine kinase receptor critical in key oncogenic signaling pathways (24, 25). A subset of carcinosarcomas and clear carcinomas also express HER2,

TABLE 17.2

Genomic Subtypes of Endometrial Carcinoma

	Definition	Other Molecular Features	Morphology
POLE-mutated/ultramutated	*POLE* mutations Ultra-high TMB	*POLE, PTEN, PIK3CA, FBXW7, ARID1A*	High-grade ("serous-like"), giant cells, TILs
MSI-H/hypermutated	MMR-deficient High TMB	*POLE* wild-type, *KRAS, PTEN*	May be high-grade, endometrioid, TILs
Copy number high/p53-abnormal	*TP53* mutations High copy number alterations	*POLE* wild-type, MMR(+)	Typically high-grade, mostly serous
Copy number low	Low number of copy number alterations	NSMP, *POLE* and *TP53* wild-type, MMR(+), *PTEN, KRAS, ARID1A, CTNBB1*	Endometrioid (any grade, mostly low)

Abbreviations: MMR, mismatch repair; MSI-H, microsatellite instability high; NSMP, no specific molecular profile; *POLE*, polymerase epsilon; TILs, tumor infiltrating lymphocytes; TMB, tumor mutation burden

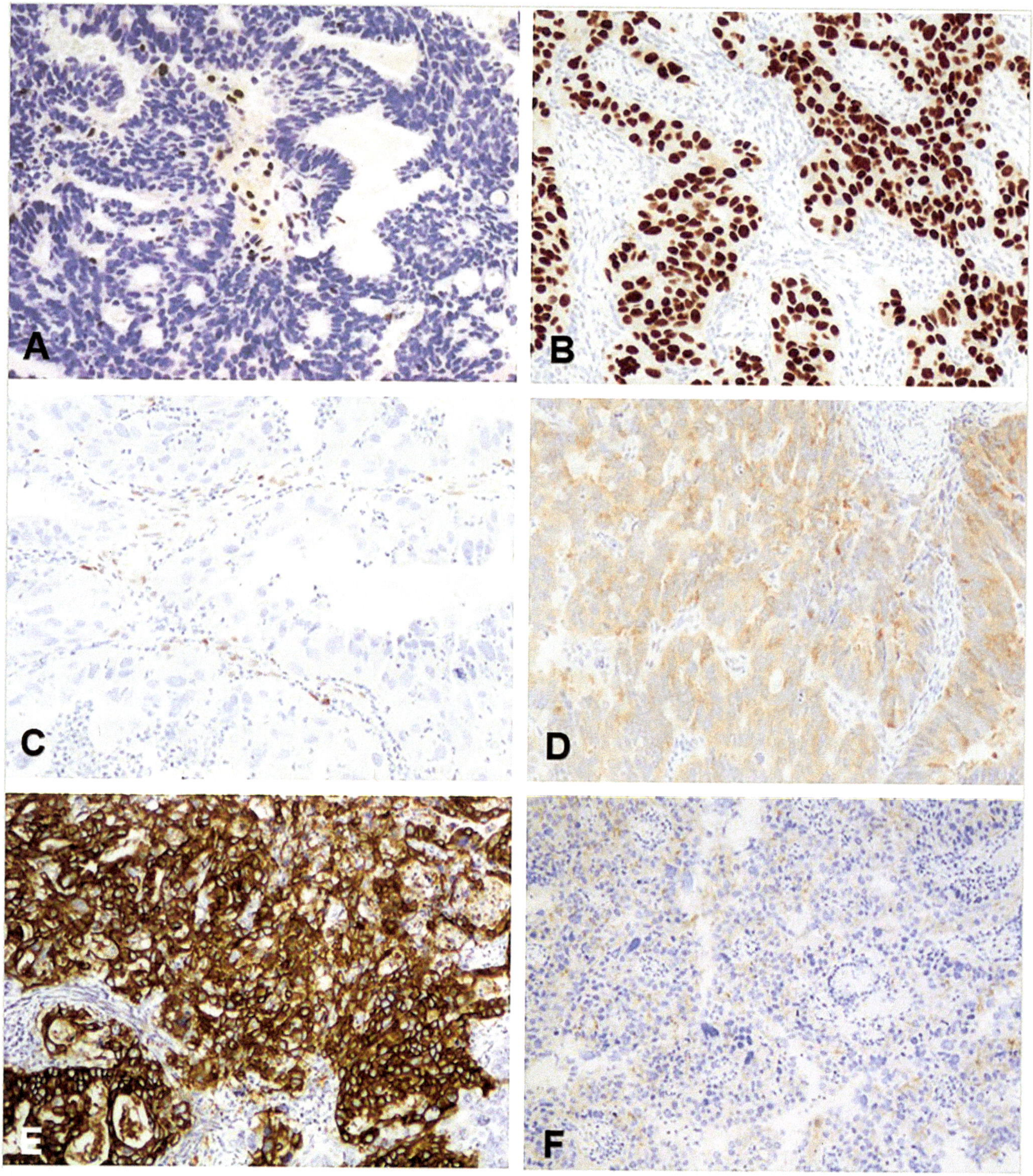

FIGURE 17.2 Interpretation of immunohistochemical stains. (A) Loss of MSH6 expression with positive internal control. (B) Abnormal p53 expression (strong diffuse staining). (C) Abnormal complete absence of p53 expression (null pattern). (D) Abnormal cytoplasmic expression of p53. (E) Positive HER2 protein over expression (score 3+). (F) Negative HER2 protein over expression (score 1+). All figures at ×100.

and HER2 positivity is associated with abnormal p53 expression. HER2 positivity is defined by IHC based on protein overexpression with > 30% of tumor cells showing strong complete or lateral/basolateral membranous staining (score 3+) (Figure 17.2E–F), or gene amplification by fluorescent in situ hybridization (FISH) based on a *HER2/CEP17* ratio of ≥ 2.0 or a *HER2/CEP17* ratio of < 2.0 and average *HER2* copy number of ≥ 6.0/nucleus (26).

17.2.3.3 Ongoing Clinical Trials and Therapeutics

Discovery and integration of the TCGA subtypes has changed the landscape of EC treatment. NSMP EAs are generally hormone receptor positive and respond to hormonal therapy. In a meta-analysis of *POLE*-mutated ECs, adjuvant therapy was not associated with improved outcomes suggesting possible overtreatment (27). This has led to trials assessing the safety of de-escalation adjuvant treatment, including PORTEC-4a (*POLE*-mutated EC) and TAPER (tailored adjuvant therapy in *POLE*-mutated and NSMP EC). The outcomes of these trials will shape future guidelines on the role of adjuvant therapies.

The US Food and Drug Administration (FDA) has approved immune checkpoint inhibitors for treatment of metastatic or recurrent MSI-H EC (28). Keynote-775, a phase III open-label randomized trial for metastatic EC progressed following ≥ 1 platinum-based chemotherapy regimen was published in early 2022 (29). In the study, patients received oral lenvatinib plus intravenous pembrolizumab vs. physician's choice chemotherapy (paclitaxel or doxorubicin). Among 697 patients with MMR-proficient EA, PFS was 6.6 months vs. 3.8 months for standard chemotherapy (HR = 0.60, 95% CI: 0.50–0.72, $p < 0.001$). Median overall survival (OS) was also significantly improved with lenvatinib plus pembrolizumab vs. chemotherapy (17.4 vs. 12 months; HR = 0.68, 95% CI: 0.56–0.84, $p < 0.001$). Similar improved PFS and OS were reported in the entire study population of 827 patients. Following this trial, the FDA approved pembrolizumab in combination with lenvatinib for patients with advanced MMR-proficient EC.

17.2.3.4 HER2-Positive SC and Other Gynecologic Neoplasms

Trastuzumab is a monoclonal antibody that binds to the extracellular domain of HER2, thus inhibiting proliferation of HER2-overexpressing cells. In a randomized phase II trial involving 61 subjects, patients with stage III–IV or recurrent HER2-positive SC were randomized to receive trastuzumab with standard platinum-based chemotherapy (carboplatin/paclitaxel) vs. platinum-based chemotherapy alone (30). Compared with the control arm, the trastuzumab arm showed higher median PFS (12.9 vs. 8 months; HR = 0.46, 95% CI: 0.28–0.76, $p = 0.005$) and OS (29.6 vs. 24.4 months; HR 0.58, 95% CI: 0.34–0.99, $p = 0.046$). Following this trial, trastuzumab was approved by the FDA for HER2-overexpressing metastatic or recurrent SC. Trastuzumab can be added to front-line chemotherapy and continued until disease progression. In the recent DESTINY-PanTumor02 trial (NCT04482309), an antibody-drug conjugate trastuzumab-deruxtecan (T-DXd) improved PFS and OS in multiple tumor types, including gynecologic carcinomas (objective response rates: 57.5% for endometrial, 50.0% for cervical, 45.0% for ovarian (31). This led to accelerated approval of T-DXd for unresectable or metastatic HER2-positive (IHC 3+) solid tumors who have received prior systemic treatment and have no satisfactory alternative treatment options.

17.3 Uterine Mesenchymal Neoplasms

Uterine mesenchymal tumors are largely categorized as smooth muscle, endometrial stromal and miscellaneous neoplasms, while mesenchymal tumors of the lower genital tract are heterogeneous and include a *NTRK*-rearranged spindle cell neoplasm/sarcoma (Table 17.3).

TABLE 17.3

Morphology, Immunophenotype, and Genomic Alterations in Targetable Mesenchymal Tumors

	Morphology	IHC
IMT	– Three morphologic patterns: 1) Loose myxoid—hypocellular areas with scattered cells in an abundant myxoid matrix (fasciitis-like or tissue culture-like appearance). 2) Fascicular/compact—cellular composed of intersecting fascicles or storiform growth pattern 3) Hyalinized pattern—dense collagenous matrix with scattered bland tumor cells • Spindled tumor cells with wispy eosinophilic cytoplasm and bland elongated nuclei, ±ganglion-like cells, epithelioid cells, Touton giant cells; ∓severe atypia, mitoses • Lymphoplasmacytic inflammatory infiltrate, rarely mixed • Stromal decidualization in pregnancy	ALK(+) in 95%, muscle markers (SMA, desmin, h-caldesmon) (+), CD10(±), keratin(∓), S100(∓), CD34(∓), CD117(∓), WT p53
PEComa	• Discohesive nests, sheets and/or fascicles of epithelioid and/or spindled cells with clear to eosinophilic granular cytoplasm surrounded by delicate thin-walled vessels, radial/perivascular distribution of tumor cells, multinucleated cells, cells with lipid-rich or rhabdoid cytoplasm, stromal hyalinization • Expansile, permeative or infiltrative growth • *TFE3* translocation-associated PEComas: uniform epithelioid cells with clear or clear to eosinophilic cytoplasm and nested, alveolar, or solid architecture • Variable cytologic atypia, mitoses, and melanin pigment	HMB45(±): more sensitive, melan-A(±): more specific), muscle markers (SMA, desmin, h-caldesmon) (+), cathepsin K(+), S100(∓), MITF(∓), tyrosinase(∓), keratins(∓), ER/PR(∓) *TFE3* translocation-associated PEComas: TFE3(+), HMB45(+), cathepsin K(+), melan-A(∓), muscle markers (∓)
NTRK-sarcoma	• Uniform spindle cells with mild to moderate cytologic atypia and variable mitoses • Scattered atypical symplastic-like cells, staghorn vascular pattern, and necrosis	S100(+), CD34(+), TRK(+), cyclin D1(+), CD10(-), muscle markers(-), BCOR(-), ER/PR(-)

Abbreviations: IHC, immunohistochemistry; IMT, inflammatory myofibroblastic tumor; PEComa, perivascular epithelioid cell tumor; ER, estrogen receptor; PR, progesterone receptor; SMA, smooth muscle actin; WT, wild-type

17.3.1 Inflammatory Myofibroblastic Tumors

17.3.1.1 Etiopathogenesis and Pathologic Diagnosis

Inflammatory myofibroblastic tumor (IMT) is a miscellaneous uterine neoplasm that may involve the corpus or cervix. Most IMTs exhibit rearrangements of the anaplastic lymphoma kinase gene (*ALK*) with partners such as *IGFBP5*, *THBS1*, and *TIMP3* (32, 33). Rare alterations include *ETV6::NTRK3, ROS* or *RET* fusions (34, 35).

IMTs are usually well circumscribed. Morphologic patterns include loose myxoid, fascicular/compact, and hyalinized architecture (33, 35, 37). Tumor cells are spindled with wispy eosinophilic cytoplasm and bland elongated nuclei (Figure 17.3A–B), usually associated with a variable lymphoplasmacytic inflammatory infiltrate (Figure 17.3C). Stromal decidualization can be seen during pregnancy (33).

Although most uterine IMTs are benign, extrauterine spread and/or recurrences may occur (33, 36). Necrosis, tumor size > 7 cm, moderate to marked atypia, high mitotic count, and lymphovascular space invasion (LVSI) have been associated with aggressive behavior (33).

17.3.1.2 Testing Strategy

Most (~95%) IMTs can be diagnosed based on the expression of the ALK protein by IHC (Figure 17.3D), usually correlating with *ALK* gene rearrangements and resulting in constitutive activation of tyrosine kinase activity (33, 38). Muscle markers (smooth muscle actin [SMA], desmin, h-caldesmon) and CD10 may be expressed. *ALK* rearrangements (2p23.2-p23.1) are detected by FISH in 75% of cases (39).

17.3.1.3 Ongoing Clinical Trials and Therapeutics

On 07/14/2022, the FDA approved crizotinib, a first-generation tyrosine kinase inhibitor (TKI), which subsequently inhibits ALK, for patients with unresectable, recurrent or refractory ALK-positive IMTs, regardless of tumor site (tissue-agnostic). Currently,

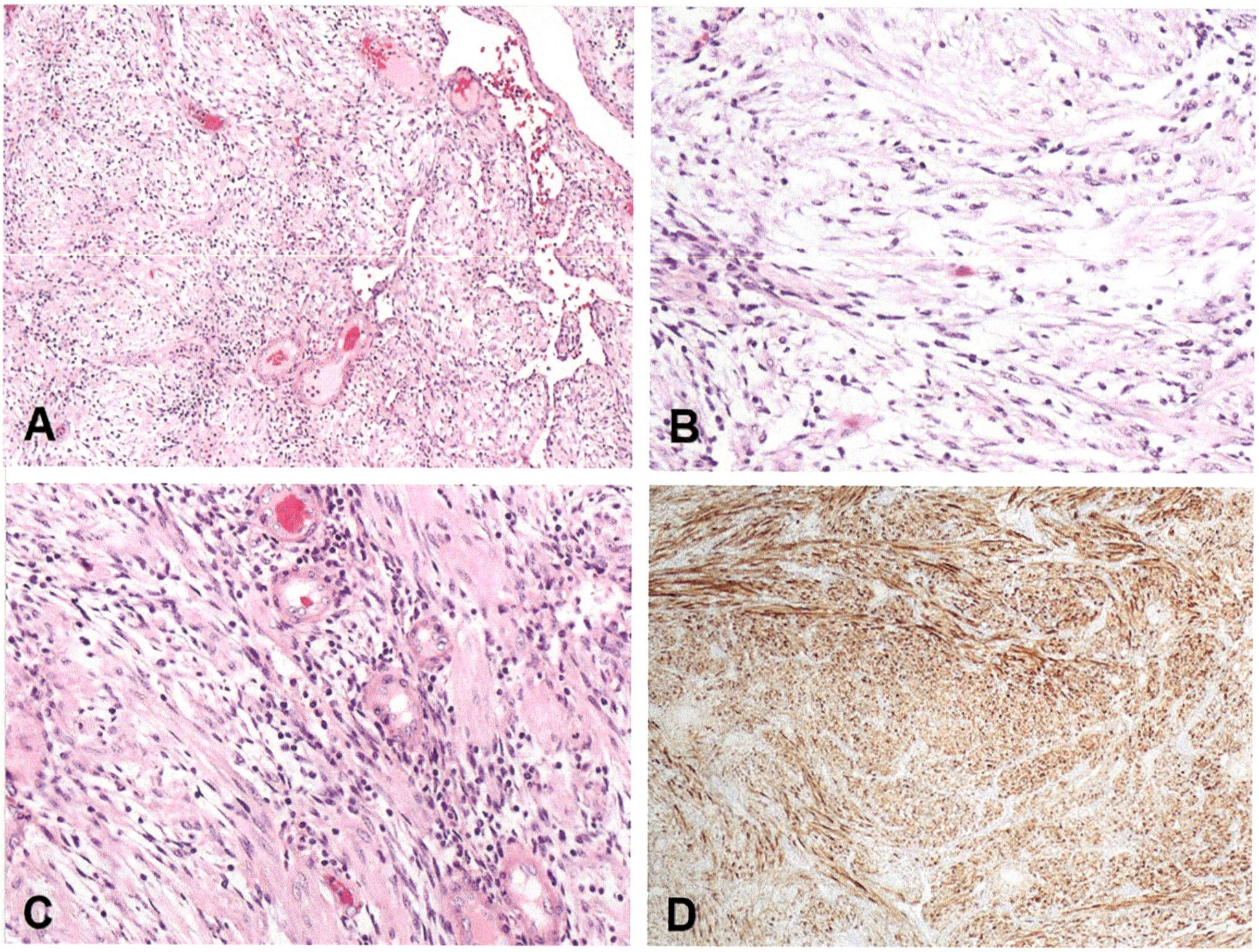

FIGURE 17.3 Inflammatory myofibroblastic tumor. (A) Fascicular growth pattern (H&E, ×40); (B) Spindled cells with mild cytologic atypia and myxoid background (H&E, ×100); (C) Associated lymphoplasmacytic infiltrate (H&E, ×100); (D) Granular cytoplasmic positivity for ALK protein (IHC, ×40).

crizotinib is the only targeted therapy approved for IMTs, although newer-generation TKIs, such as alectinib, appear promising.

17.3.2 Perivascular Epitheliod Cell Tumors

17.3.2.1 Etiopathogenesis and Pathologic Diagnosis

Perivascular epitheliod cell tumor (PEComa) is a miscellaneous mesenchymal neoplasm with myomelanocytic differentiation, usually involving the corpus or, rarely, the lower genital tract, ovary, and broad ligament. Most cases are sporadic, but 10% are associated with tuberous sclerosis (40, 41). PEComas exhibit inactivating mutations of *TSC1/TSC2* resulting in upregulation of mTOR signaling as well as *TFE3*, *RAD51B*, or *HTR4::ST3GAL1* fusions (40, 42, 43). *TSC* mutations and *TFE3* fusions appear mutually exclusive (44). Most malignant PEComas harbor alterations in *TP53*, *ATRX*, or *RB1* (45).

PEComas may have well-circumscribed or infiltrative borders (40). Microscopic features include discohesive nests, sheets, and/or fascicles of epithelioid and/or spindled cells with clear to eosinophilic granular cytoplasm surrounded by delicate thin-walled vessels, perivascular distribution of tumor cells, multinucleated cells (Figure 17.4A–B), lipid-rich or rhabdoid morphology, and stromal hyalinization. Expansile, permeative, or infiltrative growth may be seen (40, 41). *TFE3* translocation associated PEComas tend to exhibit uniform epithelioid cells with clear to eosinophilic cytoplasm and nested, alveolar, or solid architecture. Variable cytologic atypia, mitoses, and melanin pigment are identified (42).

Three algorithms have been proposed for stratifying PEComas as benign uncertain malignant potential and malignant subtypes (40, 41, 46). The largest series indicated that gynecologic-specific criteria should include ≥ 3 features for malignancy: size ≥ 5 cm, high-grade atypia, mitoses > 1/50 high-power fields, necrosis, and LVSI (39). Limited data suggest the association of *RAD51B* fusions with unfavorable outcomes (40).

17.3.2.2 Testing Strategy

PEComas are positive for melanocytic (HMB45: more sensitive, melan-A: more specific) and muscle markers

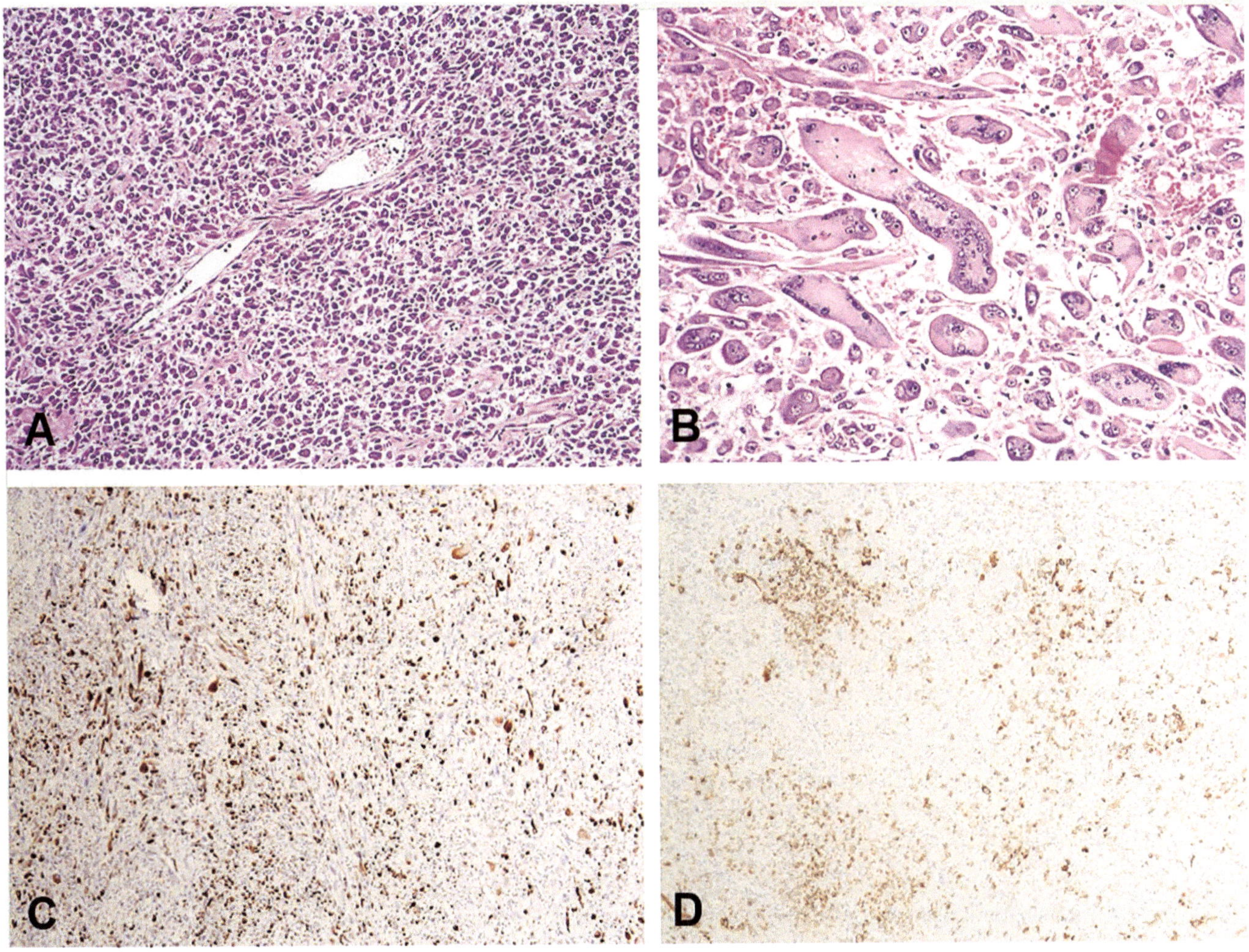

FIGURE 17.4 Malignant perivascular epithelioid cell tumor. (A) Sheets of epithelioid to spindled cells (H&E, ×100); (B) High-grade cytologic atypia and multinucleated forms (H&E, ×200); (C) Patchy staining for desmin (IHC, ×100); (D) Patchy staining for HMB-45 (IHC, ×100).

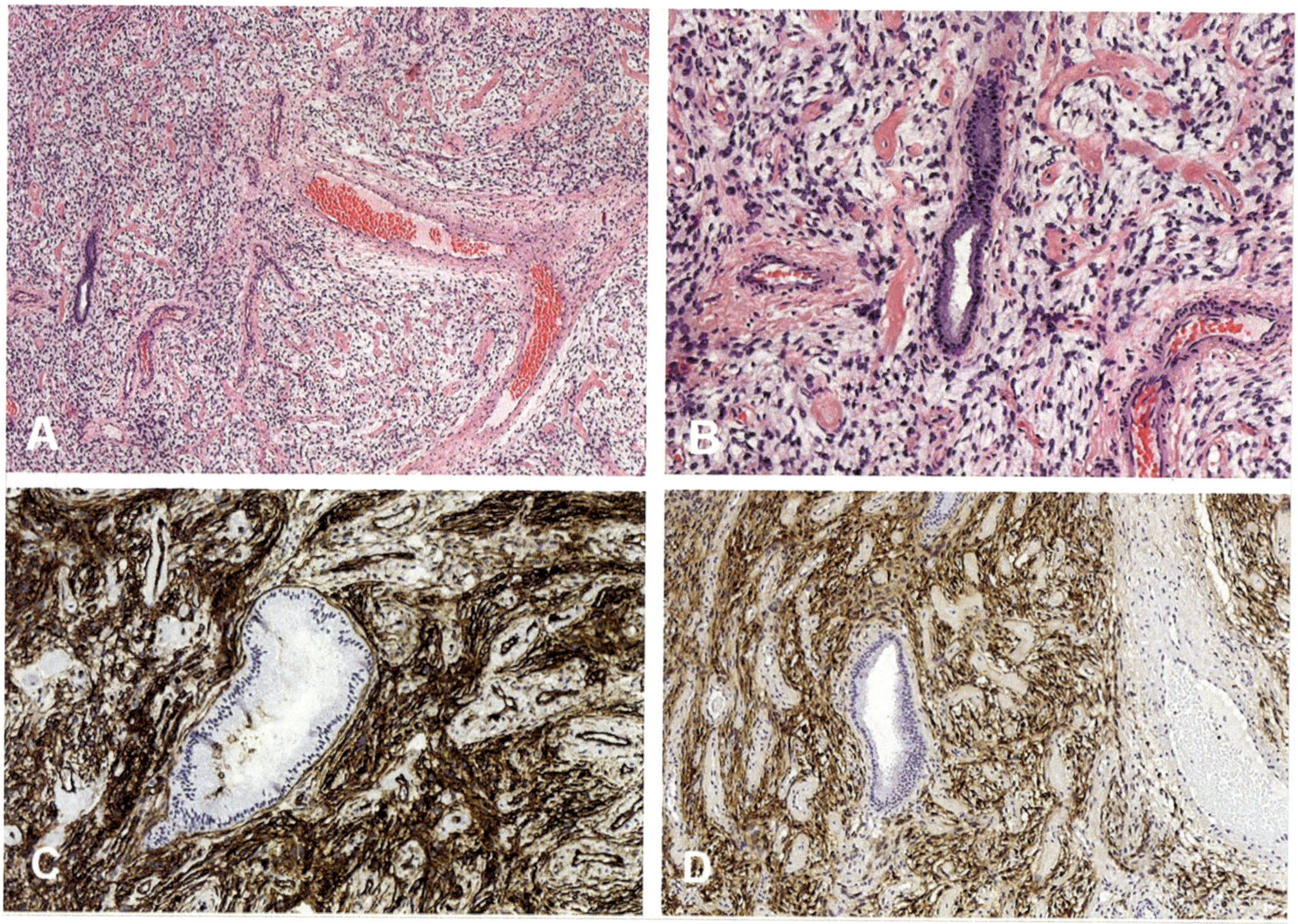

FIGURE 17.5 *NTRK*-rearranged spindle cell sarcoma. (A) Uniform spindled cells (H&E, ×40); (B) Mild cytologic atypia (H&E, ×200). Diffuse staining for S100 (C) and CD34 (D) (IHC, ×200).

(Figure 17.4C-D). Diagnosis requires expression of HMB45 or melan-A and ≥ 1 muscle marker. Expression of cathepsin-K, S100, MITF, tyrosinase, keratins, and hormone receptors is variable (40, 41). *TFE3* translocation-associated PEComas are diffusely positive for TFE3, HMB45, and cathepsin-K, with focal to absent melan-A and muscle markers (42). *TFE3* rearrangement or fusion may be confirmed by FISH.

17.3.2.3 Ongoing Clinical Trials and Therapeutics

Metastatic or recurrent PEComas may be treated with chemotherapy and radiation. mTOR inhibitors, such as sirolimus, everolimus, and temsirolimus, have shown variable results in tumors with *TSC1/TSC2* mutations (47). In the only prospective trial involving 31 patients, the overall response rate (ORR) to nab-Sirolimus was 38.7%, including 92% complete response (CR) and 8% partial response (PR); 51.6% had stable disease, and 9.7% progressed (48). Tumors with *TFE3* fusions are unresponsive to mTOR inhibitors (41).

17.3.3 *NTRK*-Rearranged Spindle Cell Neoplasm

17.3.3.1 Etiopathogenesis and Pathologic Diagnosis

NTRK-rearranged spindle cell neoplasm is a low-grade spindle cell sarcoma involving the lower uterine segment or cervix (48). *NTRK1/2/3* genes are neurotrophic tyrosine kinase receptors encoding the TRK family of TRK A/B/C proteins. *NTRK* fusions with gene partners such as *SPECC1L*, *RBPMS*, *LMNA*, *TPR*, and *TPM3* activate the downstream signaling cascades via PI3K, RAS/MAPK/ERK, and PLCgamma (49, 50).

Microscopically, *NTRK*-rearranged spindle cell neoplasm is composed of uniform spindle cells with mild-to-moderate cytologic atypia and variable mitoses (Figure 17.5A–B) (50). Scattered atypical symplastic-like cells, staghorn vessels, and necrosis may be present.

17.3.3.2 Testing Strategy

By IHC, the tumor cells are positive for S100, CD34 (Figure 17.5C–D), Trk, and cyclin D1 and negative for CD10, muscle markers, BCOR, and hormone receptors (51). Demonstration of *NTRK* fusion by RNA sequencing or FISH is diagnostic.

17.3.3.3 Ongoing Clinical Trials and Therapeutics

NTRK fusion-positive neoplasms can be targeted with either larotrectinib or entrectinib. In November 2018, the FDA granted accelerated approval for larotrectinib, a highly selective NTRK inhibitor, for patients with metastatic or inoperable solid tumors harboring an *NTRK* fusion based on data from three multicenter, tissue-agnostic, single-arm clinical trials:

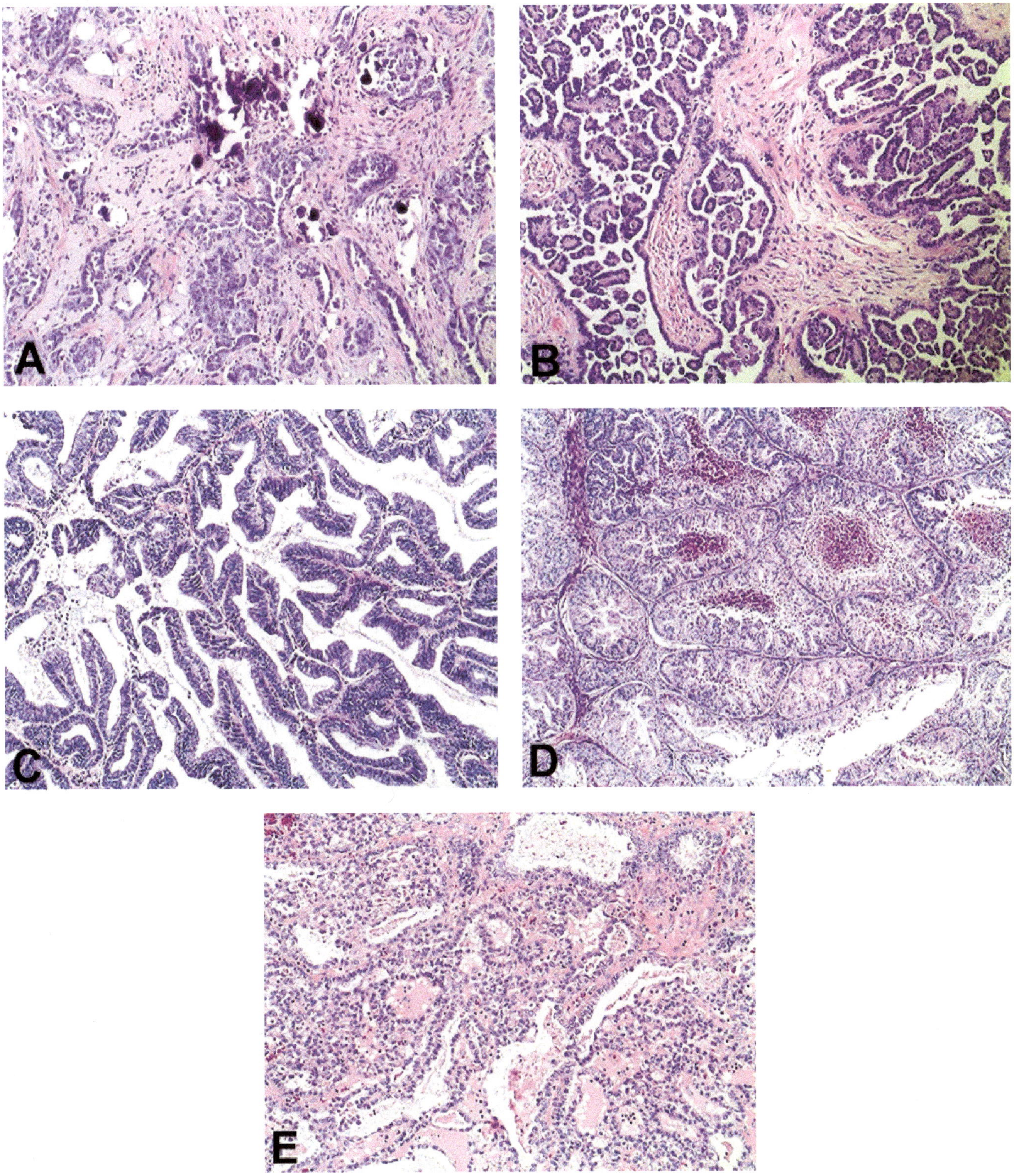

FIGURE 17.6 Five major histologic subtypes of ovarian carcinoma (H&E). (A) High-grade serous (×100); (B) Low-grade serous (×100); (C) Endometrioid (×200); (D) Mucinous (×100); and (E) Clear cell (×100).

LOXO-TRK-14001, SCOUT, and NAVIGATE. In these trials, patients with unresectable or metastatic solid tumors with *NTRK* fusion who had progressed following standard systemic therapy were treated with larotrectinib. ORR was 75%, including 22% CR and 53% PR. Subsequently, on 08/15/2019, the FDA granted accelerated approval for the second NTRK inhibitor, entrectinib, for the same indication based on multicenter, single-arm clinical trials: ALKA, STARTRK-1, and STARTRK-2.

17.4 Ovarian Epithelial Tumors

Ovarian cancer (OC) is the most lethal gynecologic cancer. The standard treatment for newly diagnosed advanced OC is cytoreductive surgery and platinum-based chemotherapy (52, 53). Although most patients respond well to front-line therapy, ~70% recur within 3 years, and recurrences are generally deemed incurable (53, 54). Additional strategies, particularly molecularly targeted treatment options, are needed to improve outcomes in front-line and recurrent-disease settings.

17.4.1 Histologic Classification

OC includes five major histologic subtypes: high-grade serous carcinoma (HGSC), low-grade serous carcinoma (LGSC), endometrioid adeno carcinoma (EA), mucinous carcinoma (MC), and clear cell carcinoma (CCC) (Figure 17.6A–E), characterized by different etiology, syndromic associations, hallmark precursor lesions, and mutated genes/pathways (Table 17.4).

17.4.2 Systemic Therapy

17.4.2.1 Anti-Angiogenesis Treatment

OC cell lines frequently express vascular endothelial growth factor (VEGF) (55). Bevacizumab is a monoclonal antibody that binds to all isoforms of the VEGF-receptor ligand, and decreased VEGF expression is associated with reduced tumor vascularization and angiogenesis (56). A phase III trial ICON7 examined the effect of adding intravenous bevacizumab to front-line platinum-based chemotherapy, followed by bevacizumab alone for 12 cycles or until disease progression (57). The addition of bevacizumab resulted in slightly improved PFS at 21.8 vs. 20.3 months with standard therapy alone (HR = 0.81, 95% CI: 0.70–0.95, p = 0.004) (57), without OS benefit (45.5 vs. 44.6 months, 95% CI: 44.2–46.7, p = 0.85) (58). Similarly, GOG218, a double-blind placebo-controlled phase III trial, examined bevacizumab in the front-line setting among 1873 patients with stage III-IV OC post-surgery, all treated with platinum-based chemotherapy with paclitaxel at standard dosages for six cycles (59). Median PFS was 10.3 months in control arm, 11.2 months in bevacizumab-initiation arm with bevacizumab in cycles 2–6 (HR = 0.908, 95% CI: 0.75–1.04), and 14.1 months in bevacizumab-throughout group with bevacizumab in cycles 2–6 and an additional 16 cycles of maintenance bevacizumab (HR = 0.717, 95% CI: 0.625–0.824, p < 0.001) (59). No OS difference was identified after extended follow-up (59, 60).

The OCEANS trial, a double-blind placebo-controlled phase III trial, randomized 484 patients with recurrent platinum-sensitive OC to gemcitabine and carboplatin (GC) plus bevacizumab vs. GC plus placebo for six to ten cycles, followed by bevacizumab or placebo until disease progression (61). PFS was better in the bevacizumab arm compared to placebo arm (12.4 vs. 8.4 months; HR = 0.484, 95% CI: 0.388–0.605, p < 0.001). Objective response rate (78.5 vs. 57.4 months, p < 0.001) and duration of response (10.4 vs. 7.4 months, HR = 0.534, 95% CI: 9.408–0.698) were also better. At the last follow-up, 72.9% of the patients were deceased, and median OS was similar between the two cohorts (33.6 vs. 32.9 months; HR = 0.95, p = 0.65).

Thus, while the addition of anti-angiogenics improves PFS in both the frontline and recurrent disease setting, there is no OS benefit. Additionally, there is currently no biomarker testing to quantitate VEGF expression.

17.4.2.2 PARP Inhibition

Poly(adenosine diphosphate-ribose) polymerases (PARPs) are nuclear proteins binding to damaged DNA and activating repair of single-strand DNA breaks (SSDB) (62). If the SSDB

TABLE 17.4

Subtypes of Ovarian Carcinoma

	HGSC	LGSC	CCC	EA	MC
Incidence	70%	10%	5%	10%	2%
Syndromic association	Hereditary breast and ovarian cancer syndrome	-	Lynch syndrome	Lynch syndrome	-
Hallmark precursor lesion	Serous tubal intraepithelial carcinoma	Serous borderline tumor	Endometriosis	Endometriosis	Mucinous borderline tumor
Mutated genes/pathways	*BRCA1/2* (14–18%), *TP53*, homologous recombinant deficiency	*BRAF* (38%), *KRAS* (19%), activated *MAPK* pathway	*ARID1A* (40–67%), *PIK3CA* (33%), *PTEN* (37%), *TERT* promoter (16%), *KRAS* (10%), *TP53* (< 10%), MMR genes: *MLH1*, *PMS2*, *MSH2*, *MSH6* (6%)	*CTNNB1* (50%), *PIK3CA* (40%), *ARID1A* (30%), *KRAS* (30%), *PTEN* (16%), *PPP2R1A* (16%)	*KRAS* (30–75%), *CDKN2A* (76%) *HER2* (15–26%), *TP53* (64%)

Abbreviations: CCC, clear cell carcinoma; EA, endometrioid carcinoma; HGSC, high-grade serous carcinoma; LGSC, low-grade serous carcinoma; MC, mucinous carcinoma; MMR, mismatch repair is unrepaired, upon reaching the DNA replication fork, a double-strand DNA break (DSDB) is generated, requiring homologous recombination (HR) for high fidelity repair (62, 63). PARP inhibitors (PARPi), such as olaparib, trap PARPs on DNA sites, thereby preventing their ability to repair the SSDB. In HRD-positive tumors, such as tumors with *BRCA1/2* mutations, PARPi leads to accumulation of DNA damage and genomic instability resulting in tumor cell death (64, 65).

Olaparib has been approved as maintenance therapy for relapsed, platinum-sensitive OC regardless of *BRCA* mutation status (66). Several pivotal trials recently evaluated PARPi in the front-line setting as maintenance therapy. In 2018, the FDA approved olaparib as maintenance treatment for adult patients with advanced epithelial ovarian, fallopian tube, or primary peritoneal cancer who achieved complete response (CR) or partial response (PR) to first-line platinum-based chemotherapy with deleterious or suspected deleterious germline or somatic *BRCA* mutation. Approval was based on the SOLO-1 study, a phase III randomized double-blinded, placebo-controlled trial comparing efficacy of olaparib vs. placebo in *BRCA 1/2* mutated advanced tumors following first-line platinum-based chemotherapy. PFS was 13.8 months in placebo arm and was not reached in the olaparib arm with an unprecedented 70% reduction in the hazard for progression or death (HR = 0.30, 95% CI: 0.23–0.41, $p <$ 0.01). Additionally, at 3 years, 60% of olaparib-treated patients, compared to 27% of placebo arm, remained progression-free, suggesting benefit of PARPi may extend beyond the 2 years of therapy (62, 66).

Following SOLO-1, the PRIMA study evaluated the PARPi niraparib in the frontline maintenance setting in a broader population of advanced ovarian cancer (67). In this randomized, double-blinded, placebo-controlled phase III trial, niraparib vs. placebo was given following PR or CR to front-line platinum-based chemotherapy for a duration of 3 years. There was no exclusion for biomarker status, though patients were stratified by HRD status defined as deleterious *BRCA1/2* mutation or HRD score ≥ 42. In the HRD cohort, median PFS was 22.1 vs. 10.9 months in the niraparib group compared to placebo (HR = 0.40, 95% CI: 0.27–0.62, $p < 0.001$). In HR-proficient group, the PFS was 8.1 vs. 5.4 months (HR = 0.68, 95% CI: 0.49–0.94). Following the PRIMA study, on 4/29/2020, niraparib gained FDA approval as maintenance treatment in patients with advanced ovarian, fallopian tube, or primary peritoneal cancer who are in CR or PR following first-line platinum-based therapy, regardless of biomarker status.

Most recently, the ATHENA was a randomized phase III trial evaluating rucaparib monotherapy as maintenance treatment in patients with newly diagnosed OC, regardless of biomarker status (68). Patients with stage III–IV high-grade ovarian cancer undergoing surgical cytoreduction and responding to first-line platinum-based chemotherapy were assigned to oral rucaparib vs. placebo. Median PFS was 28.7 months with rucaparib vs. 11.1 months with placebo in the HRD-positive population (HR = 47, 95% CI: 0.31–0.72, $p = 0.0004$) and 12.1 months vs. 9.2 months in the HRD-negative population (HR = 0.65; 95% CI: 0.45–0.95). The ATHENA trial showed benefit of rucaparib as maintenance therapy in the first-line setting but with greater impact in HRD-positive tumors.

In summary, PARPi have established a key role in the treatment of OC both in the frontline and recurrent disease setting. The degree of benefit of PARPi in the maintenance setting is consistently greater among *BRCA*-mutated or HRD-positive patients, which highlights the importance of universal germline and tumor *BRCA* testing in all OC patients. In the recurrent disease setting, PARPi are approved as maintenance therapy if a response to the most recent platinum-based therapy is achieved, regardless of *BRCA* mutation status. Ongoing studies are needed to answer clinical questions such as choice and duration of PARPi, the role of PARPi after progression while on PARPi, and potential synergy between PARPi and immunotherapy.

17.5 Epithelial Tumors of the Female Lower Genital Tract

17.5.1 Cervical and Vulvar Squamous Cell Carcinoma

Squamous cell carcinoma (SCC) is the most common malignancy of the cervix, usually associated with high-risk human papillomavirus (HR-HPV) (Figure 17.7A). Most vulvar cancers are SCCs, which are divided into HPV-associated and HPV-independent categories (Figure 17.7C, D). Vulvar SCC is usually treated with surgical resection followed by adjuvant therapy, typically platinum-based chemotherapy and concurrent radiation therapy (69, 70). In patients with recurrent or metastatic SCC, treatment options are limited.

17.5.2 Immune Checkpoint Inhibitors

Checkpoint inhibitor therapy blocks the immunosuppressive interaction by targeting either the checkpoint (PD-1) or its ligand (PD-L1), resulting in cytotoxic T-cell activation against the tumor cells. PD-L1 expression is assessed by IHC as a combined positive score (CPS) using the 22C3 parmaDx kit (Agilent) (Figure 17.7B, Table 17.5). CPS is determined based on PD-L1 expression in the tumor cells, tumor-associated lymphocytes, and macrophages and is calculated by the following formula:

$$CPS = \frac{\text{Total Number of PD} - \text{L1} - \text{positive tumor cells, lymphocytes, macrophages}}{\text{Total number of viable tumor cells}} \times 100$$

$$\text{CPS} = 1 - 100 \text{ is considered positive } (< 1 \text{ negative}, \geq 1 \text{ positive})$$

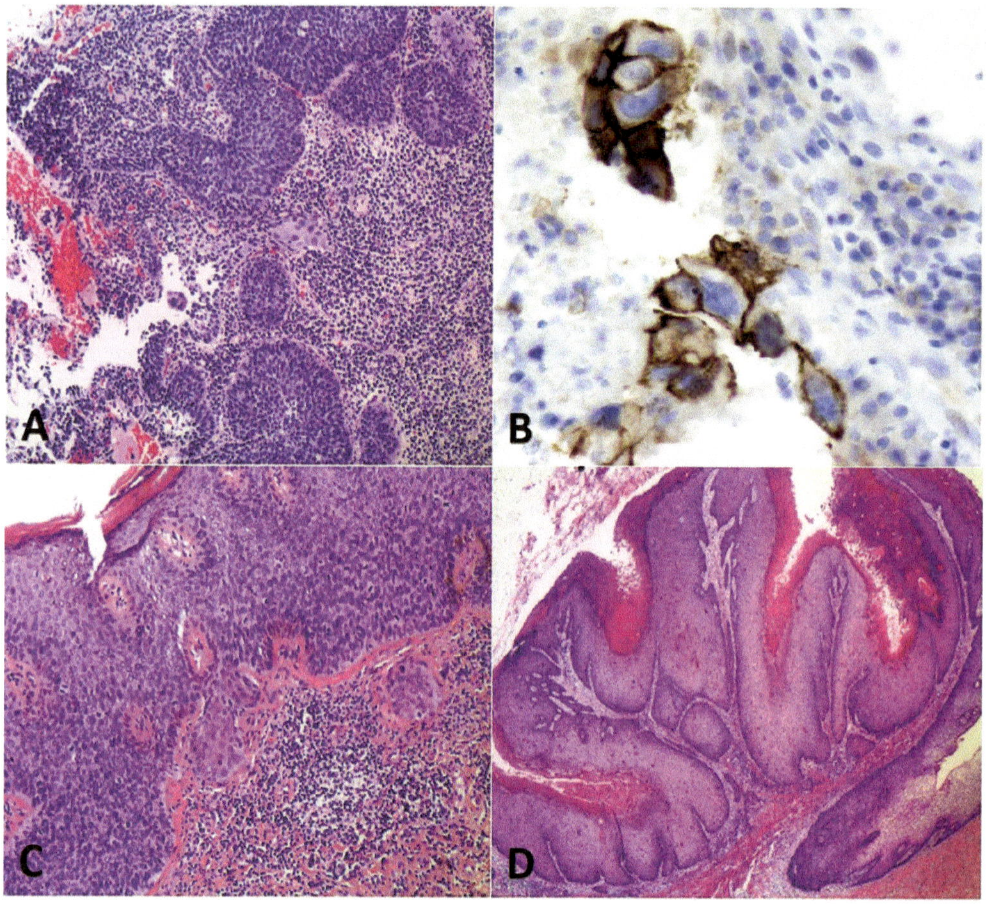

FIGURE 17.7 Invasive squamous cell carcinoma. (A) Cervical, HPV-associated (H&E ×100); (B) Cervical with PDL-1 expression (IHC, ×400); (C) Vulva, HPV-associated (H&E, ×100); (D) Vulva, HPV-independent (H&E, ×40).

TABLE 17.5

Assessment of PD-L1 Expression by Immunohistochemistry

Key Points for Interpretation of PD-L1 IHC Staining Results	Limitations and Challenges
Averaged across the entire tumor, peritumoral and intratumoral lymphocytes and macrophages	Low positive predictive value of immunohistochemistry on treatment response
Assessed at 200× magnification	FDA approval is specific for 22C3 pharmaDX kit (Dako autostainer)
Positive staining is membranous in tumor cells and membranous or cytoplasmic in immune cells	Requires internal quality control and validation protocols
Non-specific weak positivity of plasma cells should be ignored	Impact of delayed fixation on results

Abbreviations: FDA, Food and Drug Administration; IHC, immunohistochemistry

In patients with *de novo* metastatic disease, pembrolizumab is recommended with chemotherapy plus bevacizumab based on data from a phase III double-blinded randomized control trial where patients with persistent, recurrent, or *de novo* metastatic cervical cancer received pembrolizumab vs. placebo plus platinum-based chemotherapy with or without bevacizumab (at physician's discretion) (71). Those in the pembrolizumab arm had improvement in PFS compared to placebo (10.4 vs. 8.2 months; HR = 0.65; 95% CI: 0.53–0.79; $p = 0.001$). Benefits were similar between the overall population and those with PD-L1 CPS of ≥ 1 and ≥ 10, though only 69/617 patients had CPS < 1%, and there is less certainty about the degree of benefit in this group (HR = 0.94, 95% CI: 0.52–1.70). For women with disease progression after first-line therapy, pembrolizumab can reasonably be given prior to additional cytotoxic chemotherapy if tumors display PD-L1 expression ≥1%, per KEYNOTE-028 (assuming pembrolizumab was not given in the first-line setting) (72). Following this study, the FDA granted accelerated approval for pembrolizumab in patients with advanced, PD-L1-positive progressive cervical cancer on or after chemotherapy.

17.5.3 EGFR Inhibitors

Increased expression of the epidermal growth factor receptor (EGFR) occurs in 40–67% of cases (73) and leads to tumor angiogenesis, metastasis, and inhibition of apoptosis (74). Erlotinib

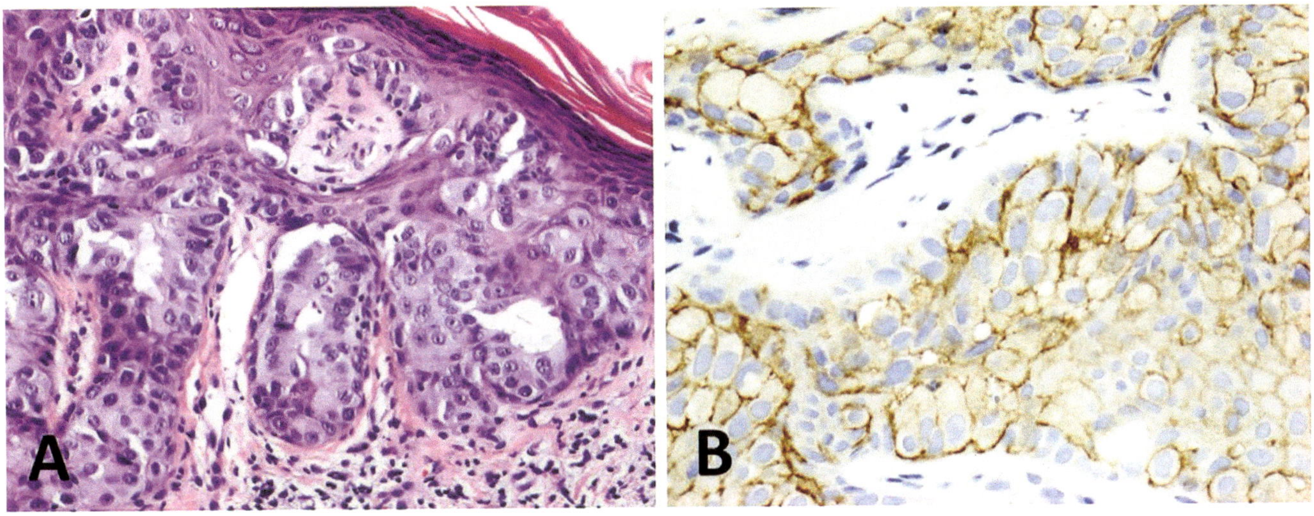

FIGURE 17.8 Vulvar Paget disease. (A) Morphology (H&E, ×200); (B) HER2 overexpression (IHC, ×400).

is an EGFR inhibitor and selectively blocks EGFR-TK activity, resulting in inhibition of intracellular phosphorylation, further downstream signaling, and cell death. In a prospective phase II trial including 41 patients with SCC who received oral erlotinib, overall clinical benefit rate was 67.5% (27.5% PR, 40% stable disease, 17.5% progressive disease), although duration of response was short-lived, with a median of 3 months (75, 76). Given the poor prognosis and limited treatment options in recurrent or metastatic SCC, inhibition of EGFR-signaling with erlotinib may be beneficial and further research is ongoing.

17.5.4 HER2-Positive Vulvar Paget Disease

Vulvar Paget disease (VPD) is a rare intraepidermal adenocarcinoma affecting postmenopausal patients (Figure 17.8A) (77, 78). The standard treatment is surgical excision, although recurrence is common and multiple excisions are often required regardless of margin status. Advanced VPD has no standard therapy options. Approximately 25% of VPD overexpresses HER2 (Figure 17.8B) (6). To date, there have been five case reports of advanced HER2-positive VPD in which trastuzumab was effective (69, 70, 73, 79). In a retrospective case series, CR or PR was observed in all four patients with advanced HER2-positive VPD treated with trastuzumab and paclitaxel followed by trastuzumab maintenance (79).

17.6 Summary

Various tumors arise from the female genital tract and harbor numerous genetic aberrations, affecting many signal transduction and metabolic pathways. Some genetic abnormalities are unique for the female genital tract, whereas others are shared with tumors in the other organs and systems. To achieve optimal clinical outcomes, precision pathologists need to employ various testing strategies to identify as many therapeutic targets as possible for FDA-approved targeting drugs and each patient's metabolic biomarkers. This information is critically important for oncologists to manage patients with the best clinical results.

REFERENCES

1. Centers for Disease Control and Prevention. Basic information about gynecologic cancers. June 13, 2023. Accessed November 1, 2023. Available at: https://www.cdc.gov/gynecologic-cancer/about/?CDC_AAref_Val=https://www.cdc.gov/cancer/gynecologic/basic_info/index.htm.
2. Bray F, Ferlay J, Soerjomataram I, et al. Global cancer statistics 2018: GLOBOCAN estimates of incidence and mortality worldwide for 36 cancers in 185 countries. CA Cancer J Clin. 2018;68(6):394–424.
3. Stewart CJ, Crook ML. SWI/SNF complex deficiency and mismatch repair protein expression in undifferentiated and dedifferentiated endometrial carcinoma. Pathology. 2015;47(5):439–445.
4. Buza N. Immunohistochemistry in gynecologic carcinomas: Practical update with diagnostic and clinical considerations based on the 2020 WHO classification of tumors. Semin Diagn Pathol. 2022;39(1):58–77.
5. Cancer Genome Atlas Research Network, Kandoth C, Schultz N, et al. Integrated genomic characterization of endometrial carcinoma. Nature. 2013;497(7447):67–73.
6. Church DN, Stelloo E, Nout RA, et al. Prognostic significance of POLE proofreading mutations in endometrial cancer. J Natl Cancer Inst. 2015;107(1):402.
7. van Gool IC, Eggink FA, Freeman-Mills L, et al. POLE proofreading mutations elicit an antitumor immune response in endometrial cancer. Clin Cancer Res. 2015;21(14):3347–3355.
8. McConechy MK, Talhouk A, Leung S, et al. Endometrial carcinomas with POLE exonuclease domain mutations have a favorable prognosis. Clin Cancer Res. 2016;22(12):2865–2873.
9. Jamieson A, Thompson EF, Huvila J, et al. p53abn endometrial cancer: Understanding the most aggressive endometrial cancers in the era of molecular classification. Int J Gynecol Cancer. 2021;31(6):907–913.
10. Ashley CW, Da Cruz Paula A, Kumar R, et al. Analysis of mutational signatures in primary and metastatic endometrial cancer reveals distinct patterns of DNA repair defects and shifts during tumor progression. Gynecol Oncol. 2019;152(1):11–19.
11. de Jonge MM, Auguste A, van Wijk LM, et al. Frequent homologous recombination deficiency in high-grade endometrial carcinomas. Clin Cancer Res. 2019;25(3):1087–1097.

12. Yeramian A, Moreno-Bueno G, Dolcet X, et al. Endometrial carcinoma: Molecular alterations involved in tumor development and progression. Oncogene. 2013;32(4):403–413.
13. Bosse T, Nout RA, McAlpine JN, et al. Molecular classification of grade 3 endometrioid endometrial cancers identifies distinct prognostic subgroups. Am J Surg Pathol. 2018;42(5):561–568.
14. Murali R, Davidson B, Fadare O, et al. High-grade endometrial carcinomas: morphologic and immunohistochemical features, diagnostic challenges and recommendations. Int J Gynecol Pathol. 2019;38 Suppl 1:S40–S63.
15. DeLair DF, Burke KA, Selenica P, et al. The genetic landscape of endometrial clear cell carcinomas. J Pathol. 2017;243(2):230–241.
16. Talhouk A, McConechy MK, Leung S, et al. Confirmation of ProMisE: a simple, genomics-based clinical classifier for endometrial cancer. Cancer. 2017;123(5):802–813.
17. Stelloo E, Nout RA, Osse EM, et al. Improved risk assessment by integrating molecular and clinicopathological factors in Early-stage Endometrial Cancer-Combined Analysis of the PORTEC Cohorts. Clin Cancer Res. 2016;22(16):4215–4224.
18. Cho KR, Cooper K, Croce S, et al. International Society of Gynecological Pathologists (ISGyP) endometrial cancer project: Guidelines from the special techniques and ancillary studies group. Int J Gynecol Pathol. 2019;38 Suppl 1:S114–S122.
19. Talhouk A, McConechy MK, Leung S, et al. A clinically applicable molecular-based classification for endometrial cancers. Br J Cancer. 2015;113(2):299–310.
20. Soslow RA, Tornos C, Park KJ, et al. Endometrial carcinoma diagnosis: use of FIGO grading and genomic subcategories in clinical practice: recommendations of the International Society of Gynecological Pathologists. Int J Gynecol Pathol. 2019;38 Suppl 1:S64–S74.
21. Geurts-Giele WR, Leenen CH, Dubbink HJ, et al. Somatic aberrations of mismatch repair genes as a cause of microsatellite-unstable cancers. J Pathol. 2014;234(4):548–559.
22. Buchanan DD, Tan YY, Walsh MD, et al. Tumor mismatch repair immunohistochemistry and DNA MLH1 methylation testing of patients with endometrial cancer diagnosed at age younger than 60 years optimizes triage for population-level germline mismatch repair gene mutation testing. J Clin Oncol. 2014;32(2):90–100.
23. Kobel M, Piskorz AM, Lee S, et al. Optimized p53 immunohistochemistry is an accurate predictor of TP53 mutation in ovarian carcinoma. J Pathol Clin Res. 2016;2(4):247–258.
24. Buza N, English DP, Santin AD, Hui P. Toward standard HER2 testing of endometrial serous carcinoma: 4-year experience at a large academic center and recommendations for clinical practice. Mod Pathol. 2013;26(12):1605–1612.
25. Buza N, Hui P. Marked heterogeneity of HER2/NEU gene amplification in endometrial serous carcinoma. Gene Chromosome Canc. 2013;52(12):1178–1186.
26. Buza N. HER2 testing and reporting in endometrial serous carcinoma: practical recommendations for HER2 immunohistochemistry and fluorescent in situ hybridization: proceedings of the ISGyP Companion Society Session at the 2020 USCAP Annual Meeting. Int J Gynecol Pathol. 2021;40(1):17–23.
27. McAlpine JN, Chiu DS, Nout RA, et al. Evaluation of treatment effects in patients with endometrial cancer and POLE mutations: an individual patient data meta-analysis. Cancer. 2021;127(14):2409–2422.
28. Le DT, Uram JN, Wang H, et al. PD-1 blockade in tumors with mismatch-repair deficiency. N Engl J Med. 2015; 372(26):2509–2520.
29. Makker V, Rasco D, Vogelzang NJ, et al. Lenvatinib plus pembrolizumab in patients with advanced endometrial cancer: An interim analysis of a multicentre, open-label, single-arm, phase 2 trial. Lancet Oncol. 2019;20(5):711–718.
30. Fader AN, Roque DM, Siegel E, et al. Randomized phase II trial of carboplatin-paclitaxel compared with carboplatin-paclitaxel-trastuzumab in advanced (stage III-IV) or recurrent uterine serous carcinomas that overexpress Her2/Neu (NCT01367002): updated overall survival analysis. Clin Cancer Res. 2020;26(15):3928–3935.
31. Meric-Bernstam F, Makker V, Oaknin A, et al. Efficacy and safety of trastuzumab deruxtecan in patients with HER2-expressing solid tumors: Primary results from the DESTINY-PanTumor02 phase II trial. J Clin Oncol. 2024;42(1):47-58.
32. Haimes JD, Stewart CJR, Kudlow BA, et al. Uterine inflammatory myofibroblastic tumors frequently harbor ALK fusions with IGFBP5 and THBS1. Am J Surg Pathol. 2017;41(6):773–780.
33. Bennett JA, Nardi V, Rouzbahman M, et al. Inflammatory myofibroblastic tumor of the uterus: A clinicopathological, immunohistochemical, and molecular analysis of 13 cases highlighting their broad morphologic spectrum. Mod Pathol. 2017;30(10):1489–1503.
34. Takahashi A, Kurosawa M, Uemura M, et al. Anaplastic lymphoma kinase-negative uterine inflammatory myofibroblastic tumor containing the ETV6-NTRK3 fusion gene: A case report. J Int Med Res. 2018;46(8):3498–3503.
35. Cheek EH, Fadra N, Jackson RA, et al. Uterine inflammatory myofibroblastic tumors in pregnant women with and without involvement of the placenta: A study of 6 cases with identification of a novel TIMP3-RET fusion. Hum Pathol. 2020;97:29–39.
36. Parra-Herran C, Quick CM, Howitt BE, et al. Inflammatory myofibroblastic tumor of the uterus: Clinical and pathologic review of 10 cases including a subset with aggressive clinical course. Am J Surg Pathol. 2015;39(2):157–168.
37. Mohammad N, Haimes JD, Mishkin S, et al. ALK is a specific diagnostic marker for inflammatory myofibroblastic tumor of the uterus. Am J Surg Pathol. 2018;42(10):1353–1359.
38. Fuehrer NE, Keeney GL, Ketterling RP, et al. ALK-1 protein expression and ALK gene rearrangements aid in the diagnosis of inflammatory myofibroblastic tumors of the female genital tract. Arch Pathol Lab Med. 2012;136(6):623–626.
39. Zarei S, Abdul-Karim FW, Chase DM, et al. Uterine inflammatory myofibroblastic tumor showing an atypical ALK signal pattern by FISH and DES-ALK fusion by RNA sequencing: a case report. Int J Gynecol Pathol. 2020;39(2):152–156.
40. Bennett JA, Braga AC, Pinto A, et al. Uterine PEComas: a morphologic, immunohistochemical, and molecular analysis of 32 tumors. Am J Surg Pathol. 2018;42(10):1370–1383.
41. Schoolmeester JK, Howitt BE, Hirsch MS, et al. Perivascular epithelioid cell neoplasm (PEComa) of the gynecologic tract: Clinicopathologic and immunohistochemical characterization of 16 cases. Am J Surg Pathol. 2014;38(2):176–188.

42. Schoolmeester JK, Dao LN, Sukov WR, et al. TFE3 translocation-associated perivascular epithelioid cell neoplasm (PEComa) of the gynecologic tract: Morphology, immunophenotype, differential diagnosis. Am J Surg Pathol. 2015;39(3):394–404.
43. Agaram NP, Sung YS, Zhang L, et al. Dichotomy of genetic abnormalities in PEComas with therapeutic implications. Am J Surg Pathol. 2015;39(6):813–825.
44. Malinowska I, Kwiatkowski DJ, Weiss S, et al. Perivascular epithelioid cell tumors (PEComas) harboring TFE3 gene rearrangements lack the TSC2 alterations characteristic of conventional PEComas: Further evidence for a biological distinction. Am J Surg Pathol. 2012;36(5):783–784.
45. Bennett JA, Ordulu Z, Pinto A, et al. Uterine PEComas: Correlation between melanocytic marker expression and TSC alterations/TFE3 fusions. Mod Pathol. 2022;35(4):515–523.
46. Folpe AL, Mentzel T, Lehr HA, et al. Perivascular epithelioid cell neoplasms of soft tissue and gynecologic origin: A clinicopathologic study of 26 cases and review of the literature. Am J Surg Pathol. 2005;29(12):1558–1575.
47. Benson C, Vitfell-Rasmussen J, Maruzzo M, et al. A retrospective study of patients with malignant PEComa receiving treatment with sirolimus or temsirolimus: The Royal Marsden Hospital experience. Anticancer Res. 2014; 34(7):3663–3668.
48. Wagner AJ, Ravi V, Riedel RF, et al. nab-sirolimus for patients with malignant perivascular epithelioid cell tumors. J Clin Oncol. 2021;39(33):3660–3670.
49. Chiang S, Cotzia P, Hyman DM, et al. NTRK fusions define a novel uterine sarcoma subtype with features of fibrosarcoma. Am J Surg Pathol. 2018;42(6):791–798.
50. Hodgson A, Pun C, Djordjevic B, Turashvili G. NTRK-rearranged cervical sarcoma: expanding the clinicopathologic spectrum. Int J Gynecol Pathol. 2021;40(1):73–77.
51. Croce S, Hostein I, Longacre TA, et al. Uterine and vaginal sarcomas resembling fibrosarcoma: A clinicopathological and molecular analysis of 13 cases showing common NTRK-rearrangements and the description of a COL1A1-PDGFB fusion novel to uterine neoplasms. Mod Pathol. 2019;32(7):1008–1022.
52. Ledermann JA, Raja FA, Fotopoulou C, et al. Newly diagnosed and relapsed epithelial ovarian carcinoma: ESMO Clinical Practice Guidelines for diagnosis, treatment and follow-up. Ann Oncol. 2013;24 Suppl 6:vi24–vi32.
53. NCCN clinical practice guidelines in oncology: ovarian cancer version 2.2024. Accessed 5/28/2024. Availabe at: www.nccn.org/professionals/physiain_gls/pdf/ovarian.pdg
54. Giornelli GH. Management of relapsed ovarian cancer: A review. Springerplus. 2016;5(1):1197.
55. Hoskins P, Vergote I, Cervantes A, et al. Advanced ovarian cancer: Phase III randomized study of sequential cisplatin-topotecan and carboplatin-paclitaxel vs carboplatin-paclitaxel. J Natl Cancer Inst. 2010;102(20):1547–1556.
56. Armstrong DK, Bundy B, Wenzel L, et al. Intraperitoneal cisplatin and paclitaxel in ovarian cancer. N Engl J Med. 2006;354(1):34–43.
57. Perren TJ, Swart AM, Pfisterer J, et al. A phase 3 trial of bevacizumab in ovarian cancer. N Engl J Med. 2011; 365(26):2484–2496.
58. Oza AM, Cook AD, Pfisterer J, et al. Standard chemotherapy with or without bevacizumab for women with newly diagnosed ovarian cancer (ICON7): Overall survival results of a phase 3 randomised trial. Lancet Oncol. 2015;16(8):928–936.
59. Burger RA, Brady MF, Bookman MA, et al. Incorporation of bevacizumab in the primary treatment of ovarian cancer. N Engl J Med. 2011;365(26):2473–2483.
60. Burger RA, Enserro D, Tewari KS, et al. Final overall survival (OS) analysis of an international randomized trial evaluating bevacizumab (BEV) in the primary treatment of advanced ovarian cancer: a NRG oncology/Gynecologic Oncology Group (GOG) study. J Clin Oncol. 2018;36(15_suppl):5517–5517.
61. Aghajanian C, Blank SV, Goff BA, et al. OCEANS: A randomized, double-blind, placebo-controlled phase III trial of chemotherapy with or without bevacizumab in patients with platinum-sensitive recurrent epithelial ovarian, primary peritoneal, or fallopian tube cancer. J Clin Oncol. 2012;30(17):2039–2045.
62. Pothuri B, O'Cearbhaill R, Eskander R, Armstrong D. Frontline PARP inhibitor maintenance therapy in ovarian cancer: A Society of Gynecologic Oncology practice statement. Gynecol Oncol. 2020;159(1):8–12.
63. Murai J, Huang SY, Das BB, et al. Trapping of PARP1 and PARP2 by clinical PARP inhibitors. Cancer Res. 2012;72(21):5588–5599.
64. O'Connor MJ. Targeting the DNA damage response in cancer. Mol Cell. 2015;60(4):547–560.
65. Kaufman B, Shapira-Frommer R, Schmutzler RK, et al. Olaparib monotherapy in patients with advanced cancer and a germline BRCA1/2 mutation. J Clin Oncol. 2015;33(3):244–250.
66. Moore K, Colombo N, Scambia G, et al. Maintenance olaparib in patients with newly diagnosed advanced ovarian cancer. N Engl J Med. 2018;379(26):2495–2505.
67. Gonzalez-Martin A, Pothuri B, Vergote I, et al. Niraparib in patients with newly diagnosed advanced ovarian cancer. N Engl J Med. 2019;381(25):2391–2402.
68. Monk BJ, Parkinson C, Lim MC, et al. A randomized, phase III trial to evaluate rucaparib monotherapy as maintenance treatment in patients with newly diagnosed ovarian cancer (ATHENA-MONO/GOG-3020/ENGOT-ov45). J Clin Oncol. 2022;40(34):3952–3964.
69. Siegel RL, Miller KD, Fuchs HE, Jemal A. Cancer statistics, 2022. CA Cancer J Clin. 2022;72(1):7–33.
70. Gill BS, Bernard ME, Lin JF, et al. Impact of adjuvant chemotherapy with radiation for node-positive vulvar cancer: A National Cancer Data Base (NCDB) analysis. Gynecol Oncol. 2015;137(3):365–372.
71. Colombo N, Dubot C, Lorusso D, et al. Pembrolizumab for persistent, recurrent, or metastatic cervical cancer. N Engl J Med. 2021;385(20):1856–1867.
72. Chung HC, Ros W, Delord JP, et al. Efficacy and safety of pembrolizumab in previously treated advanced cervical cancer: results from the phase II KEYNOTE-158 study. J Clin Oncol. 2019;37(17):1470–1478.
73. Johnson GA, Mannel R, Khalifa M, et al. Epidermal growth factor receptor in vulvar malignancies and its relationship to metastasis and patient survival. Gynecol Oncol. 1997;65(3):425–429.
74. Olawaiye A, Lee LM, Krasner C, Horowitz N. Treatment of squamous cell vulvar cancer with the anti-EGFR tyrosine kinase inhibitor Tarceva. Gynecol Oncol. 2007;106(3):628–630.

75. Woelber L, Mathey S, Prieske K, et al. Targeted therapeutic approaches in vulvar squamous cell cancer (VSCC): case series and review of the literature. Oncol Res. 2021;28(6):645–659.
76. Horowitz NS, Olawaiye AB, Borger DR, et al. Phase II trial of erlotinib in women with squamous cell carcinoma of the vulva. Gynecol Oncol. 2012;127(1):141–146.
77. Karam A, Berek JS, Stenson A, et al. HER-2/neu targeting for recurrent vulvar Paget's disease A case report and literature review. Gynecol Oncol. 2008;111(3):568–571.
78. Parker LP, Parker JR, Bodurka-Bevers D, et al. Paget's disease of the vulva: Pathology, pattern of involvement, and prognosis. Gynecol Oncol. 2000;77(1):183–189.
79. Bartoletti M, Mazzeo R, De Scordilli M, et al. Human epidermal growth factor receptor-2 (HER2) is a potential therapeutic target in extramammary Paget's disease of the vulva. Int J Gynecol Cancer. 2020;30(11):1672–1677.

18

Neuroendocrine Neoplasms

Xianfeng F. Zhao

18.1 Introduction

Compared to the other organs, the neuroendocrine organs are relatively small yet critical for the homeostasis of human bodies. These organs include the hypothalamus, pituitary, pineal bodies, thyroids, parathyroids, adrenals, endocrine pancreas, ovaries, testes, and organs with tissues that carry endocrine functions. The American Society of Clinical Oncology estimated that over 12,000 people in the United States are diagnosed with neuroendocrine tumors each year, and approximately 175,000 people are living with these diagnosed tumors (1). Since endocrine cancers in ovaries and testes are discussed in the male and female reproductive systems, this chapter will focus on pituitary, thyroid, parathyroid, adrenal, and pancreatic endocrine cancers (Table 18.1) (2, 3).

18.2 Pituitary Tumors

The pituitary gland is the largest neuroendocrine organ in the brain. Most pituitary tumors are benign adenomas, but due to the limited space of the skull, they can have a malignant potential. Craniopharyngioma (CP) is a benign brain tumor which has a malignant clinical course. It is routinely treated with surgery, but complete removal is neither feasible nor curative. Recent genetic findings that majority of papillary CP harbors a hotspot *BRAF* (V600E) mutation opened the door to targeted therapy with FDA-approved agents that target BRAF and MEK (4). *CTNNB1* and *EGFR* are often overexpressed in adamantinomatous CP (aCP), and *VEGF* is overexpressed in aCP and recurrent CP. Therefore, molecular analysis of *BRAF*, *CTNNB1*, *EGFR*, and *VEGF* and the genes of the WNT, PI3K/AKT/mTOR, and RAS-MEK-ERK pathways should be routinely performed whenever enough specimen is obtained.

Encased in sellar turcica, pituitary tumors were evaluated by World Health Organization (WHO) classification for aggressiveness by emphasizing tumor proliferation and invasion (5). Causing mass effect symptoms, high Ki-67 proliferation index (11.9 ± 3.4%), and failure to respond to standard, multiple treatment steps also contribute to its aggressiveness. Therefore, the ultimate therapeutic goal is to manage mass effect and excess hormonal syndromes and limit damage to the normal pituitary gland (Figure 18.1). Currently, peptide receptor radionuclide therapy (PRRT) (a radionuclide linked by a chelator to a somatostatin receptor ligand (SRL) that binds cell surface somatostatin receptors (SSTRs)) is the preferred therapy for aggressive pituitary carcinomas (Figure 18.2). Novel targeted therapies are under investigation (Figure 18.3). Due to its rarity, there are no documented large-scale clinical trials for aggressive pituitary adenomas or carcinomas.

18.3 Thyroid Cancers

Thyroid cancer is the most common endocrine cancer, accounting for approximately 33,500 cases per year in the United States (6) and ranging from indolent, well-differentiated tumors to extremely aggressive, poorly differentiated, or anaplastic cancers. Its incidence is rapidly increasing in the last decade. Most thyroid cancers are differentiated thyroid cancers (DTCs) (approximately 85%), which include papillary thyroid cancer (PTC), follicular thyroid cancer (FTC), Hürthle cell cancer (HCC), and poorly differentiated thyroid cancer (PDTC). Medullary thyroid cancer arising from the parafollicular C cells accounts for approximately 1–2% of thyroid cancers. Anaplastic thyroid cancer (ATC) is a rapidly fatal form of thyroid cancer, which accounts for approximately 1–2% of all thyroid cancers but 50% of the thyroid cancer deaths. It can arise in the normal thyroid gland or in ectopic thyroid tissue.

18.3.1 Differentiated Thyroid Cancers

DTCs are further classified by WHO classification into papillary, follicular, medullary, and anaplastic/undifferentiated carcinoma, based on morphology and clinical features (Figure 18.4). They are distinct entities as supported by the involved genes in these malignancies (Table 18.2). The mainstay therapy of DTC remains radical surgery followed by radioactive iodine ablative treatment (RAI), with an 80% cure rate (7). Once refractory to RAI (in ~5% of the cases), the DTC carries a grave prognosis. Chemotherapy plays no role in treating RAI-refractory DTC, which can be managed with targeted agents.

18.3.1.1 Papillary Thyroid Cancer

PTC is well-differentiated thyroid cancer with distinctive nuclear features. It is often first diagnosed by cytology of fine needle–aspirated (FNA) thyroid nodules. The nuclei of PTC are often larger than their normal counterparts and tend to be elongated with irregular nuclear contour, grooves, and pseudo-inclusions

DOI: 10.1201/9781003513469-18

TABLE 18.1

Common Endocrine Neoplasms

Organs		Tumors	Features
Pituitary		Pituitary adenoma	10~15% of primary brain tumors, benign with malignant potential
		Pituitary carcinoma	0.2% of all pituitary tumors, local craniospinal metastases or systemic metastases to lung, liver, lymph nodes and bone
		Pituitary blastoma	Rare, lethal tumor in children and young adults, often with germline *DICER1* mutations (DICER1 syndrome)
		Craniopharyngioma	0.17~0.2/100,000 in the U.S., benign epithelial tumor with mass effects
		Neuronal and paraneuronal tumors	Rare low-grade tumor with minimal risk for an aggressive clinical course
Thyroid		Differentiated carcinoma	Most common endocrine neoplasia (2.9% of all cancers, > 90% of thyroid cancers), originating from thyroid follicular cells with four major subtypes: papillary, follicular, Hurthle cell, and poorly differentiated
		Medullary carcinoma	2–4% of all thyroid cancers, originating from neural crest C cells
		Anaplastic/undifferentiated carcinoma	Approximately 1–2% of thyroid cancers, also the most aggressive form of thyroid cancers
Parathyroid		Parathyroid adenoma	~6/100,000 in the U.S., derived from the parenchymal cells of the parathyroids with primary hyperparathyroidism (PHPT)
		Parathyroid carcinoma	~0.06/100,000 in the U.S., histologically similar to adenoma with invasion, metastasis, and severe PHPT
Adrenal	Cortex	Adrenal cortical carcinoma	0.05~0.2/100,000, 50–60% with Cushing syndrome, 20–30% of female having hyperandrogenism
		Adrenal cortical adenoma	1–10%, endocrine-inactive, majority non-functioning and asymptomatic, most found by autopsy
	Medulla	Pheochromocytoma/ paraganglioma (PPGL)	1–2/100,000, ~5–10% metastasize, increased release of catecholamines leads to either constant or episodic hypertension in patients
Pancreas		Islet-cell carcinomas	Low-grade tumors with metastatic potential, a.k.a. insulinoma, glucagonoma, somatostatinoma, gastrinoma, VIPoma, based on the produced hormones
Other		Inherited tumor syndromes	Autosomal dominant inheritance, including MEN1 (*MENIN*), MEN2a (*RET*), and MEN2b (*RET*)

Source: from ref. 2-5, 7, 16 and 18

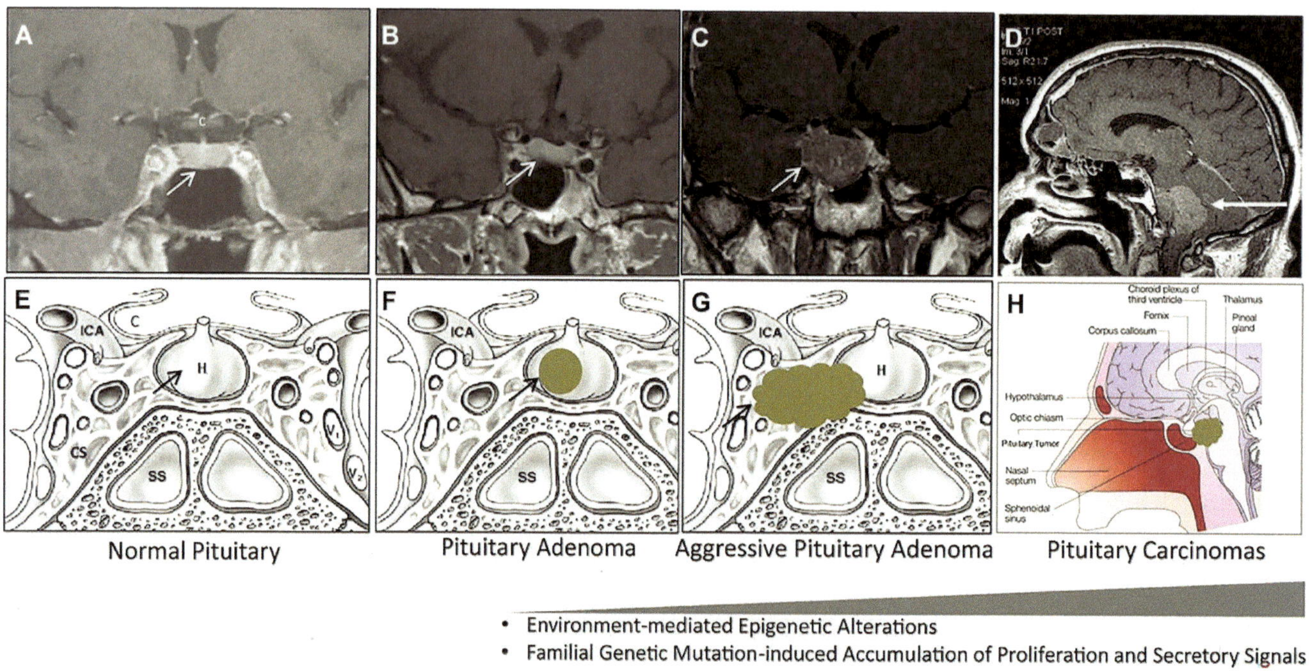

FIGURE 18.1 A model of pituitary tumor pathogenesis from normal pituitary cell to adenoma to "aggressive" locally invasive recurrent tumor to carcinoma (adapted from ref. 5). Accumulation of aberrant cellular proliferative and secretory signals is caused by environmentally induced epigenetic changes in some cases on a back-drop of inherited genetic mutations. Top panel (from left to right): coronal images of pituitary region showing normal gland (A), pituitary microadenoma (B), locally invasive pituitary macroadenoma growing despite maximal standard therapy (aggressive tumor, (C) and pituitary carcinoma (D). Lower panel: cartoon depicting schematically the changes seen on MRI series (E-H). C, optic chiasm; CS, cavernous sinus; ICA, internal carotid artery; H, hypophysis; SS, sphenoid sinus.

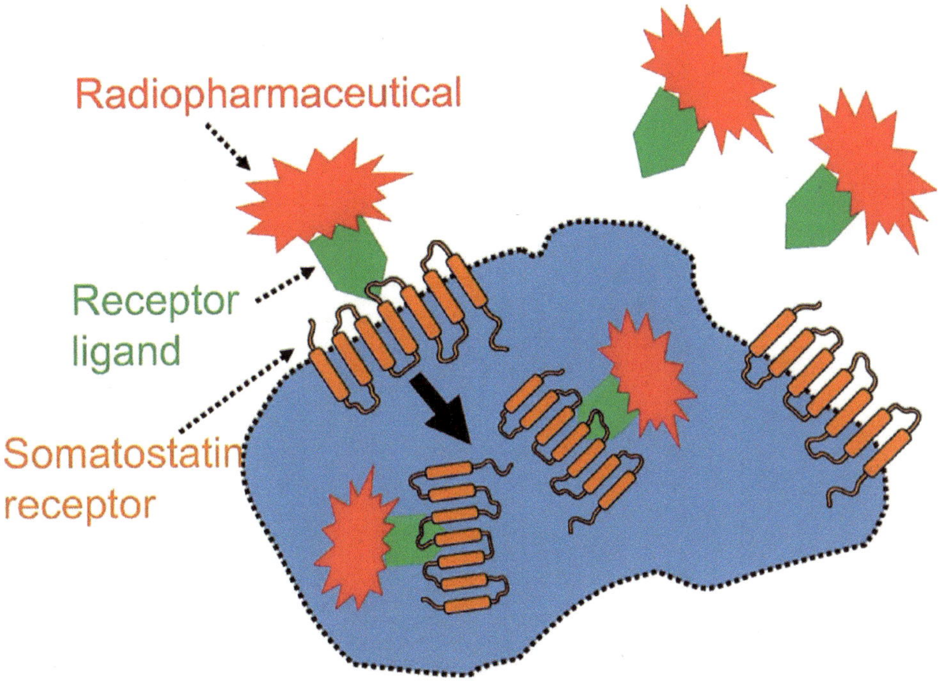

FIGURE 18.2 Principles of peptide receptor radionuclide therapy (PRRT) (adapted from ref. 5): Radiopharmaceuticals are linked to the receptor ligand, which binds to its specific receptor at the surface of the tumor cell. The complex is subsequently internalized. Radioactivity is thereby specifically transported into target cells.

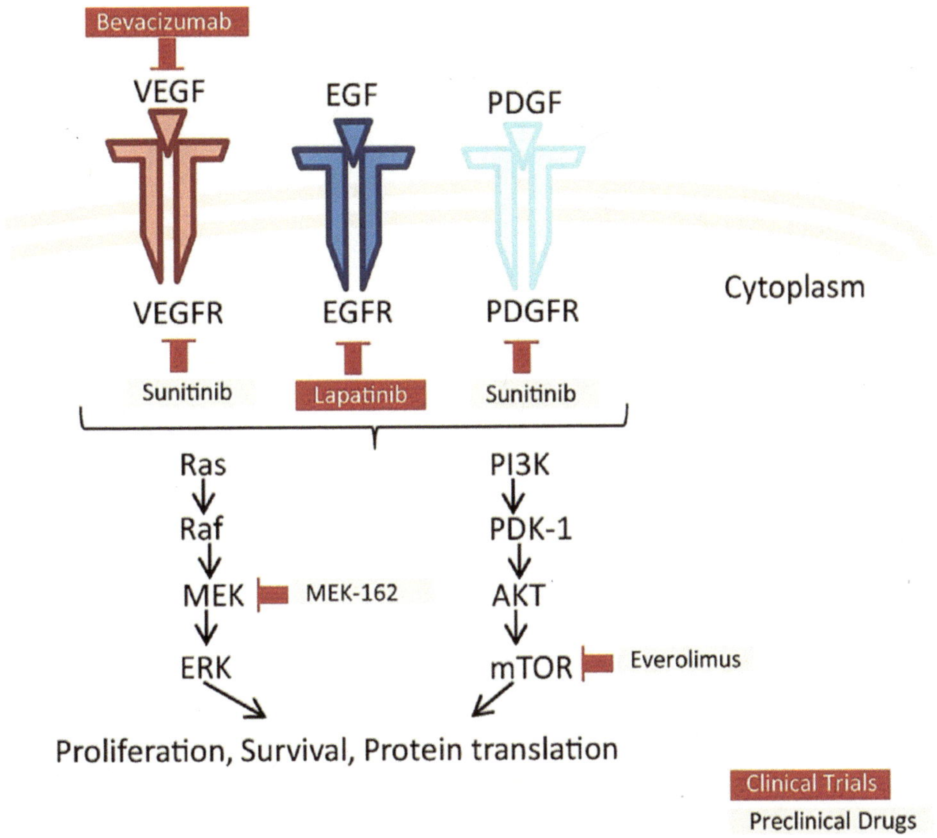

FIGURE 18.3 Novel targeted therapies for pituitary cancer (adapted from ref. 5). Immunotherapy (bevacizumab) and small molecule kinase inhibitors (such as sunitinib, lapatinib, and everolimus) targeting different signal transduction pathways at various levels.

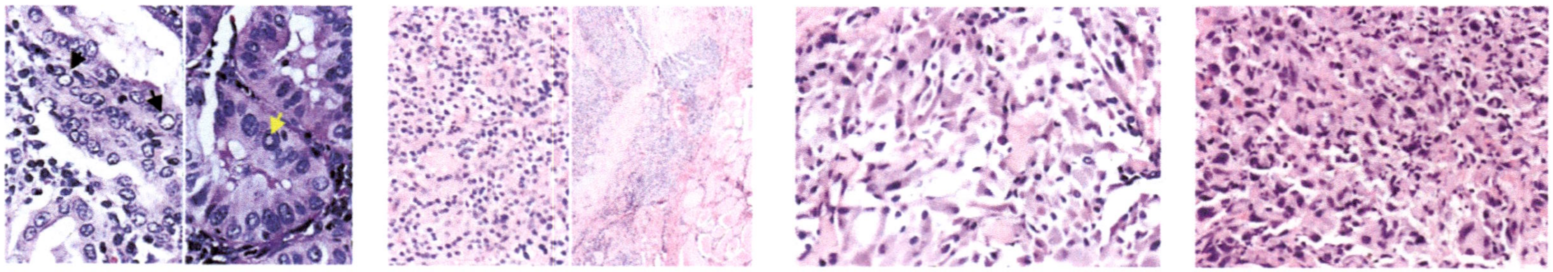

	A	B	C	D
Cytology	Papillary architecture with psammoma bodies, intranuclear pseudo-inclusions, nuclear grooves and pale finely chromatin	Microfollicles (6 - 12 nuclei) with nuclear enlargement, overlapping and crowding	Plasmacytoid cells with eccentric nuclei with granular chromatin ("salt and pepper") and abundant cytoplasm	Pleomorphic cells, neoplastic giant cells, spindle cells or squamoid cells in a background of tumor diathesis and inflammation
Histology	True papillae with nuclear grooves and inclusions, and Orphan Annie nuclei	Trabecular or solid pattern of follicles, no nuclear features of papillary thyroid carcinoma, capsular invasion seen	Plasmacytoid cells in nests, cords or follicles, and with finely stippled chromatin and indistinct nucleoli, granular cytoplasm. Amyloid deposits seen	Pleomorphic cells with widely invasive growth, extensive tumor necrosis, marked nuclear pleomorphism and high mitotic activity
Calcitonin	-	-	+	-
CK7	+	+	+	+
CK20	-	-	-	-
TTF1	+	+	+ (weak to moderate)	-
Thyroglobulin	+	+	-	-
PAX8	+	+	+ (variable)	+
BRAF V600E	**+**	-	-	**-/+**
NRAS Q61R	**+**	**-/+**	-	**-/+**

FIGURE 18.4 Pathological characteristics of major thyroid cancers. (A) Papillary thyroid cancer (by courtesy of Dr. Twisha Oza, from University of Tennessee Health Science Center (UTHSC)). (B) Follicular thyroid cancer with microfollicles and capsular invasion (by courtesy of Dr. Leslie Lopez-Calderon, from UTHSC). (C) Medullary thyroid cancer with plasmacytoid cells and focal amyloid-like deposition (by courtesy of Leslie Lopez-Calderon, from UTHSC). (D) Undifferentiated thyroid cancer (by courtesy of Pathology Outlines, contributed by Dr. Ayana Suzuki, Kameda Medical Center, and Dr. Shuanzeng Wei, Fox Chase Cancer Center). The potential targetable biomarkers are in bold.

TABLE 18.2

Genetic alterations and therapeutic targets of thyroid cancers

Cancer	Altered Oncogene	Altered Tumor Suppressor	Drug
Differentiated			
Papillary	*BRAF, HRAS, KRAS, NRAS, RET, EIF1AX, PAR-γ, NTRK1/3,* and *THADA; TERT*		vandetanib, cabozantinib, sorafenib, lenvatinib
Follicular	*RAS, TERT*	*PTEN, TP53, RB1,* and *MEN1*	
Hürthle cell	*NRAS, TERT, DAXX, ATRX, EIF1AX*		
Poorly differentiated	*EIF1AX, TERT*		
Undifferentiated/anaplastic	*BRAF*	*EIF1AX, ATM, RB1, NF2,* and *MEN1*	dabrafenib, trametinib
Medullary	*RET, RAS*		vandetanib, cabozantinib, sorafenib, lenvatinib

Source: compiled from ref. 2

(Figure 18.4A). Histologically it can be divided into classical variant, follicular variant, and tall cell variant. Molecular studies can be performed on the FNA specimens. The Cancer Genome Atlas (TGCA) project revealed genetic alterations that commonly occur in PTC (8). The most common genetic alterations are *BRAF* V600E and *RAS* (*HRAS*, *KRAS*, and *NRAS*) mutations that comprise approximately 75% of oncogenic drivers in PTC. This study extended the set of known PTC driver alterations to include *EIF1AX*, *PPM1D*, and *CHEK2* and diverse gene fusions, which enable us to identify at least one oncogenic driver for 96.5% of the PTC (8). The occurrence of *BRAF* and *RAS* mutations are mutually exclusive, and additional mutations do not seem to have a clonal advantage. However, *BRAF* mutations preferably activate the MAPK pathway, whereas *RAS* mutations drive the oncogenic process down both MAPK and PI3K signal transduction pathways. Multiple kinases have been identified in the development of PTC and can serve as molecular targets for therapy (Table 18.3). Detection of these genes and components of these related pathways should be routinely performed in pathology labs.

Although the FDA has approved many targeting agents, a recent genomic analysis of the 128 targetable genes with the FDA-approved 129 targeting agents indicated that PTC only showed predictive sensitivity to the selective and non-selective BRAF inhibitors (9), suggesting that the treatment strategy needs to focus on overcoming the drug resistance to BRAF inhibitors and searching for mechanisms other than the current genetic alterations.

18.3.1.2 Follicular Thyroid Cancer

As the second most common thyroid cancer of follicular cell origin, FTC is featured by the microfollicular formation on cytology and vascular and capsular invasion on histology. The oncocytic variant (a.k.a. Hürthle cell carcinoma) represents over 75% of FTC (Figure 18.4B). Two predominant genetic alterations drive FTC development; *RAS* single nucleotide mutations occur in 40–50% of FTC, whereas *PAX8::PPRAγ* rearrangements are found in 30–40% of FTC cases (10). *RAS* mutations and *PAX8::PPARγ* rearrangements are mutually exclusive, suggesting one of these two oncogenic drivers is sufficient for the cancer development. Interestingly, these two genetic alterations are common in FTC and the follicular variant of PTC, but not in classical PTC, suggesting the follicular variant of PTC is akin to FTC. Besides *RAS* mutations and *PAX8::PPRAγ* genetic alterations, mutations and/or gene copy number variations of the PI3K/AKT pathway have been identified in FTC (11). For example, *PIK3A* gene amplification has been found in approximately 24% of the FTCs (12). All these provide effective therapeutic targets for the therapy of FTC.

18.3.1.3 Hürthle Cell Carcinoma

Although the exact origin of Hürthle cells remains controversial, HCC is believed to also derive from follicular cells and thus is currently considered an oncocytic variant of FTC (~5% of all thyroid cancers) by the most recent edition of WHO classification of endocrine neoplasms (13). However, HCC is a morphologically, clinically, and genetically distinct entity (12). In contrast to FTC that prefers tedious hematogenous metastasis and PTC that favors localized invasion and lymphatic metastasis, HCC loves both. The mutational profiles are quite different from PTC and FTC; no *BRAF* mutations were detected, and the frequency of *NRAS* mutation was quite low per at least one study (14). Most common mutated genes are *MADCAM1* (20%), *EIF1AX* (11%), *UBXN11* (9%), *NRAS* (9%), and *SIRPA* (7%). Co-occurrence of *EIF1AX* and *NRAS* mutations was not identified. Furthermore, gene mutations important in PDTCs and ATCs (*TP53*, *TERT* promoter, *PTEN*, *PIK3CA*, and *ATM*) were detected, but in low frequencies.

18.3.1.4 Poorly Differentiated Thyroid Cancer

PDTC is a neoplasm of follicular cell origin with intermediate features between the well-differentiated thyroid cancers (PTC and FTC) and undifferentiated/anaplastic thyroid cancers. It is characterized by the lack of classic PTC nuclear features, high mitotic rate, and tumor necrosis (11). Vascular and local invasion and lymph node and distant metastasis are common in PDTC. The frequent coexistence of other types of DTC with PDTC suggests PDTC may represent transformed PTCs or FTCs or underwent dedifferentiation. As in other DTCs, *RAS* and *BRAF* mutations are the major oncogenic drivers in PDTC; *RAS* mutations occur in 20–50% of the PDTCs, whereas *BRAF* mutations are present in approximately 35% of the PDTCs, and they are

TABLE 18.3

Frequency of Thyroid Cancer Genetic Alterations

Histologic Type	Mutations (~75%)	Gene Fusions (~15%)	Other Alterations	Reference
Differentiated				
Papillary	*BRAF*V600 (59%)	*RET* (8%)	*TERT* promoter mutation	8, 9
	*NRAS*Q61 (8%)	*NTRK* (3%)	*TP53* promoter mutation	
	HRAS (3.5%)	*BRAF*		
	KRAS (0.8%)	*ALK*		
	*TOP2A*K1199 (0.5%)	*THADA*		
	*EIF1AX*G9 (0.8%)			
Follicular	*RAS* (40–50%)	*PAX8::PPARγ* (30–40%)	*PI3CA* amplification (24%)	9, 10
	PTEN		*PTEN* epigenetic silencing	11
Hürthle cell	*EIF1AX* (11%)			13, 14
	NRAS (9%)			
	TERT, DAXX, ATRX	*RET*		
Poorly differentiated	*RAS* (20–50%)	*ALK*	*TERT* promoter mutation	10, 15, 17
	BRAF (35%)	*RET*	+1q, -1p, -13q, -15q, -22q	
	TP53 (10–35%)	*PAX8::PPARγ*		
	CTNNB1			
	EIF1AX (11%)			
Undifferentiated/anaplastic	*BRAF*V600E (26–45%)	*RET, ALK*, and *NTRK*	*TERT* promoter mutation	15, 16
	RAS (22–24%)			
	PIK3CA (17–18%)			
	PTEN (12–15%)			
	CTNNB1 (38–60%)			
	Axin (82%)			
	EIF1AX (9%)			
	TP53 (55–73%)			
	SWI/SNF (36%)			
Medullary				
Hereditary	*RET* (95%-100%)			17, 18
Sporadic	*RET* (40–50%)			
	RAS (17–40%)			

mutually exclusive (15). Ninety-two percent of *RAS* mutations were found in PDTC-Turin, whereas 81% of *BRAF* mutations were detected in PDTC-MSK. In contrast to well-differentiated thyroid cancers, PDTC and undifferentiated thyroid cancers often show co-occurrence of *EIF1AX* and *RAS* mutations (15). When *TERT* promoter mutations and *TP53* mutations are present with either *RAS* or *BRAF* mutations, PDTC becomes more aggressive. Other genetic alterations include *ALK* rearrangements and *CTNNB1* and *EIF1AX* mutations (Table 18.3). Targeted therapies employ the FDA-approved inhibitors for RAS, BRAF, and ALK and multikinase inhibitors.

18.3.2 Undifferentiated/Anaplastic Thyroid Cancer

Undifferentiated or anaplastic thyroid cancer (ATC) is an extremely rare and aggressive thyroid cancer (Figure 18.4D). It comprises 1.3% to 9.8% of all thyroid cancers globally, 1.7% in the U.S. (16). Compatible with its aggressive clinical behavior, ATCs are dedifferentiated PTCs, FTCs, HCCs, and PDTCs with multiple genetic mutations (Table 18.3). *BRAF*V600E mutation was present in 45% of ATCs, whereas mutations in *NRAS, HRAS*, or *KRAS* occurred in 24% of ATCs, respectively, and they were mutually exclusive with *BRAF* and gene fusions (15). Co-occurrence of *EIF1AX* and *RAS* mutations, *PIK3CA* and *PTEN* mutations, and *PIK3CA* and *BRAF* mutations were found in ATCs (15). In addition, ATCs also had a greater mutation burden than PDTCs, including a higher frequency of mutations in *TP53, TERT* promoter, PI3K/AKT/mTOR pathway effectors, SWI/SNF subunits, and histone methyltransferases.

18.3.3 Medullary Thyroid Cancer

MTC is the only thyroid cancer arising from the parafollicular C cells that normally produce calcitonin and constitutes approximately 1–2% of the thyroid cancers (2). MTC shows all the immunophenotypes of a neuroendocrine tumor (Figure 18.4C).

Almost all the inherited (as part of the MEN II syndrome) and half of the sporadic MTCs are driven by *RET* inactivating point mutations, in 95% of hereditary MTC and 45% of the sporadic MTC (11). The only other oncogenic driver in sporadic MTC is *RAS* mutations (*HRAS* or *KRAS*), which are found in 17% of the RET-negative cases. Some studies reported even higher prevalence (40%) of *RAS* mutations in RET-negative cases (17). These two genetic alterations are also mutually exclusive. Several RET inhibitors have been approved by FDA for the treatment of MTC (18). Earlier multi-target tyrosine kinase inhibitors are relatively nonspecific, and their modest activities and significant side effects limited their use in MTC therapies (19). Recently approved tyrosine kinase inhibitors specifically targeting RET yielded much better clinical responses; however, new mutations emerging in RET led to drug resistance to these inhibitors (20) (Figure 18.5). *MET* amplification was also identified as one of the mechanisms in drug resistance to selpercatinib, a RET-specific inhibitor; however, this drug resistance can be reversed by addition of the MET/ALK/ROS1 inhibitor crizotinib to the combined regimen (21). In contrast to targeting RET, clinical trials with RAS inhibitors yielded less promising clinical outcomes. New strategies to target the components of the pathways downstream of RET are being explored for MTC, but intolerance due to toxicities limited their use in combination therapies (22).

18.4 Parathyroid Tumors

Parathyroid carcinoma (PCA) is a rare indolent malignancy occurring in approximately 6 in 10 million people (23) and originating from the parenchymal cells of parathyroid glands. Patients with PCA are often associated with hyperparathyroidism with

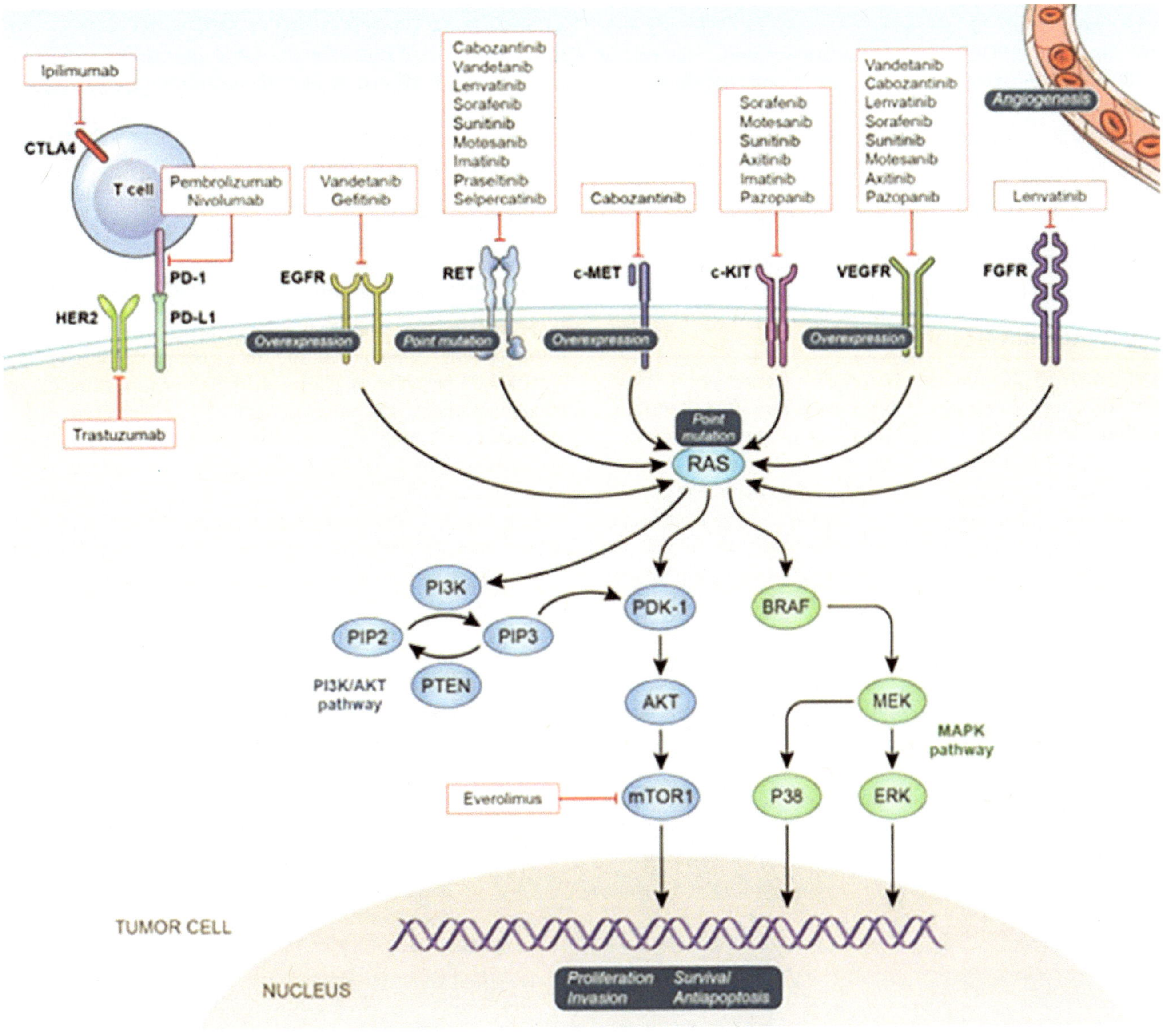

FIGURE 18.5 Oncogenic signaling pathways in MTC. Potential and confirmed therapeutic targets in MTC are depicted with currently available targeted agents (adapted from ref. 20). RAS plays the critical role in the signal transduction of MTC oncogenesis and is considered the key functional "node".

hypercalcemia and thus often misdiagnosed as primary hyperparathyroidism (PHPT) (24). Generally, PCA is treated with *en bloc* surgical resection, while biopsy should be avoided due to the risk of potential tumor implantation (25). Pathological diagnosis of PCA remains a challenge due to lack of differentiating markers between PCA and parathyroid adenoma. Various criteria have been proposed for the differential diagnosis, but their reliability remains controversial (26). The most reliable histological features may include local infiltration beyond the capsule, lymph node, vascular and distant metastasis. Lack of nuclear staining for parafibromin resulting from *HRPT2* mutations has been the surrogate for the diagnosis of PCA based on the high incidence of *HRPT2* mutations in 70% of sporadic PCA and only rarely in benign PHPT (27). Expression of PGP9.5 can also be used to assist parafibromin in diagnosing PCA. Oncogenic drivers of PCA have not been well defined. Some studies identified the loss of *RB* and *TP53* genes and *CCND1* overexpression as major potential oncogenic drivers in addition to *HRPT2* mutations (28). Microarray analysis of PCA as compared with normal parathyroid tissues identified overexpression of *UCHL1*, a gene that encodes the PGP9.5 protein, further supporting the role of PGP9.5 as a diagnostic biomarker and a potential therapeutic target for PCA. Due to its rarity, PCA drew much less attention from both investigators and pharmaceutical companies, and as a result, to date, there is no FDA-approved targeting agent available for PCA treatment.

18.5 Tumors of the Adrenal Gland

18.5.1 Adrenocortical Carcinoma

Compared to benign adrenocortical adenomas (1–10%), adrenocortical carcinoma (ACC) is a rare (0.5–2/million) malignancy (29), with more than half of the patients being associated with Cushing syndrome, approximately 20–30% of the female patients having hyperandrogenism, and a small number of patients with estrogen and/or mineralocorticoid excess. Although localized disease can be potentially cured by complete surgical resection, recurrent or metastatic diseases occur in over half of the patients who have undergone complete resection. Mitotane, a derivative of insecticide DDT, is the only FDA-approved drug for ACC (29), which has a low response rate and a high systemic toxicity. A combination of mitotane with cytotoxic chemotherapy yielded only limited clinical outcomes.

Genetic alterations in ACC were comprehensively analyzed by two major studies from the European Network for the Study of Adrenal Tumors (ENSAT) and TCGA projects, which identified multiple ACC driver genes (30, 31). Alterations of the *IGF2* gene were identified as major genetic abnormalities; either loss of heterozygosity in *IGF2* locus or *IGF2* expression is detected in 80–90% of the tumors analyzed (30). Among the nine genes (*ZNRF3*, *CTNNB1*, *TP53*, *CDKN2A*, *RB1*, *MEN1*, *DAXX*, *MED12*, and *TERT*) that displayed damaging mutations, homozygous deletions, or high-level amplifications in ≥ 5% of ACCs, *ZNRF3* was the most frequently altered tumor suppressor gene (21%), which is related to the β-catenin pathway (30, 31) (Table 18.4). *CTNNB1* and *ZNRF3* alterations were mutually exclusive in this study (30). Collectively the genes altered most frequently by somatic mutations, DNA copy number alterations, and epigenetic silencing were *TP53* (21%), *ZNRF3* (19%), *CDKN2A* (15%), *CTNNB1* (16%), *TERT* (14%), and *PRKAR1A* (11%) (31). These driver genes are candidates for future targeted therapies.

18.5.2 Pheochromocytoma/paraganglioma

Pheochromocytoma is a rare tumor that develops in the medulla of the adrenal gland, and the incidence is approximately 1–2/100,000 per year. When the same tumor forms outside of the adrenal gland, it is called paraganglioma. Therefore, these two tumors are often mentioned together as pheochromocytoma/paraganglioma (PPGL). Increased release of catecholamines (epinephrine and norepinephrine) by PPGL leads to either constant or episodic hypertension in the patients. Radical

TABLE 18.4

Genetic Abnormalities of Adrenocortical Carcinoma

Genetic Alterations	Chromosome	Chromosomal Remodeling	Wnt/β-Catenin Pathway (39%)	P53-Rb Pathway (33%)	Other Pathways
Gains	4, 5, 7, 8, 12, 16, 19, 20				
Homozygous deletions	1p, 22		*ZNRF3* (22q12.1) (16–21%)	*CDKN2A* (9p21.3) (11%) *RB1* (13q14) (7%)	
Loss of heterozygosity	16 autosomes (>30%);				*IGF2* (11p15) (82%)
Amplification		*TERT* (5p15.33) (6–15%) *TERF2* (16q22.1) (7%)		*CDK4* (12q14) (2%) *MDM2* (2%)	
Activating mutations			*CTNNB1* (16%)	*CCNE1* (19q12) (6%)	
Inactivating mutations		*DAXX* (6%) *MEN1* (7%) *ATRX* (4%)	*MED12* (5%) *APC* (2%)	*TP53* (16%) *RPL22* (7%)	*PRKAR1A* (8%)

Source: adapted from ref. 30 and 31

surgery, radiation, and chemotherapy are the current mainstays of treatment. Recent comprehensive molecular analysis identified three major pathways in PPGL: pseudohypoxic, kinase, and WNT signaling (32).

Mutations in genes encoding the Krebs cycle enzymes lead to upregulation of the hypoxia-inducible factor (HIF) signaling pathway. Tumors with these pseudohypoxic mutations are aggressive and often metastatic noradrenergic phenotypes. Tumors with dysregulated kinase pathways harbor mutations of the components of PI3K/AKT/mTOR and RAS/MAPK signal transduction pathways. These tumors originate from the adrenal gland with an adrenergic phenotype. Activation of WNT and Hedgehog pathways can also be present in pheochromocytomas with numerous mutations in the components of these signaling pathways, and MYC and cyclin D1 as their downstream targets. Activation of these three major pathways plays a critical role in the oncogenesis of PPGL (32).

As a rare cancer, PPGL lagged other tumors on targeted therapy. Some off-label tyrosine kinase inhibitors (sunitinib, cabozantinib) are in clinical use for the treatment of PPGLs (33). So far sunitinib is the only targeted drug that has been investigated in a randomized placebo-controlled clinical trial. It is clinically used for the treatment of recurrent and metastatic PPGLs. Molecular therapeutic agents mainly targeting the pseudohypoxic and kinase signaling pathways are being investigated in clinical trials. These include HIF2α inhibitor belzutifan, temozolomide, olaparib, talazoparib, cabozantinib, and atezolizumab (33).

18.6 Pancreatic Endocrine Cancers

Neuroendocrine carcinomas of the pancreas include carcinoid and islet cell carcinoma, generally occurring as part of hereditary cancer syndromes, which affect several other organs as well (Table 18.5) (34). Multiple genetic abnormalities and aberrant expression of oncoproteins form the basis for targeted therapy (34). These include the roles of MENIN, TSC2, NF-1, vHL, p53, BCL2, BAX, VEGF, IGF, PDGF, EGFR, and mTOR. Due to the rarity of these tumors, the current approach is to identify the therapeutic targets with available FDA-approved targeted molecules for the treatment of other tumors. See Chapter 15 for further details.

18.7 Pharmacomics

Since almost all the targeted drugs for endocrine tumors are also being used in precision therapy for other cancers, pharmacogenomics, pharmacoproteomics, and pharmacometabolomics have been extensively discussed in other chapters (such as Chapters 4 and 11) and thus will not be reiterated here.

18.8 Precision Diagnosis of Neuroendocrine Tumors

Excisional biopsies of the pituitary, thyroid, and parathyroid glands provide plenty of tumor cells for diagnosis and molecular studies for therapeutic targets. However, since the adrenal gland and pancreas are deeply located in the abdomen, FNA and core needle biopsy may be the major procedures for specimen acquisition. With limited amount of tissues and cells, the specimen should be prioritized to diagnosis and identification of therapeutic targets. Precision pathology testing strategies are depicted in Figure 18.6. Immunohistochemistry will be performed for the pathological diagnosis and identification of the overexpressed oncoproteins, and NGS with tumor-specific panels will also be performed to detect mutated oncogenic drivers for targeted therapy. While NGS is used for the detection of oncogene driver mutations, a highly sensitive and high-throughput protein assay is needed for the evaluation of activated kinases that can be targeted by FDA-approved or commercially available off-label TKIs and other kinase inhibitors.

18.9 Summary

Neuroendocrine neoplasms originate from the specialized endocrine organs and tissues that produce hormones for the homeostasis of the body. Most of the molecular genomic/genetic work has been done in the thyroid, parathyroid, and adrenal gland due to organ accessibility and tissue availability. Many target agents are either already in clinical use or still in clinical trials. Some dismal results of clinical trials might be due to the traditional stratification of patients and lack of consideration of the subjects' pharmacomics. A well-crafted strategy with combined effective therapeutic targets and individualized pharmacomics will likely lead to optimal clinical outcomes.

TABLE 18.5

Genetic Syndromes Associated with the Development of Low-Grade Neuroendocrine Tumors

Syndrome	Gene (Location)	Tumor Location	Molecular Mechanism
MEN1	*MENIN*	Pancreas, lung, thymus	Menin as part of a histone methyltransferase complex regulates gene transcription
Tuberous sclerosis 2	*TSC2* (16p13.3)	Pancreas	Loss leads to constitutive mTOR activation
Neurofibromatosis	*NF-1* (17q11.2)	Ampulla of Vater, duodenum, mediastinum	Loss leads to constitutive mTOR activation
von Hippel-Lindau	*VHL* (3p26–p25)	Pancreas	Loss lead to increase HIF activity

Source: modified from ref. 34

Abbreviations: MEN1, multiple endocrine neoplasia type 1 syndrome; HIF, hypoxia-induced factor.

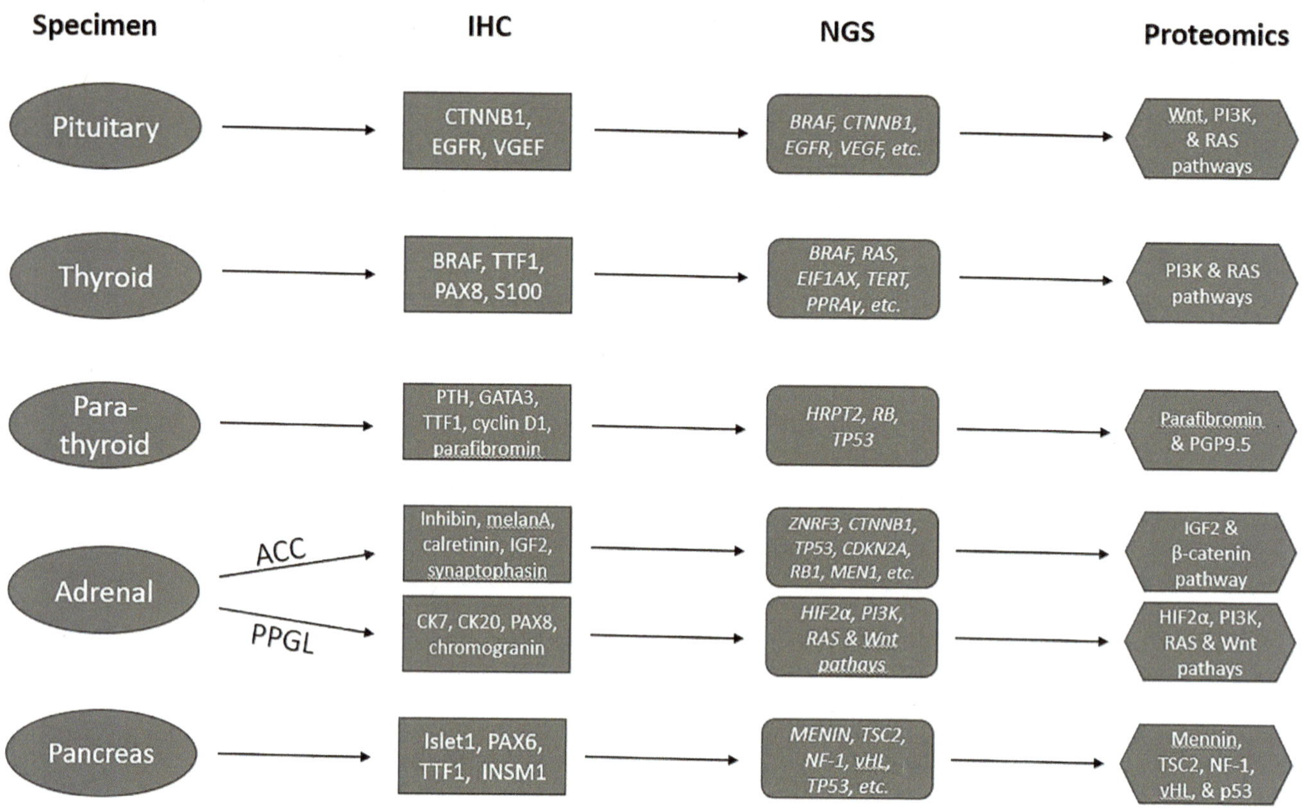

FIGURE 18.6 Precision testing strategies for neuroendocrine tumors. For pituitary tumors, the first step is to use IHC to evaluate the overexpressed CTNNB1, EGFR, and VGEF on the tissue sections. Then the tissue will be tested for the mutations in the *BRAF*, *CTNNB1*, *EGFR*, and *VEGF* and the genes of the WNT, PI3K/AKT/mTOR, and RAS-MEK-ERK pathways. Finally, the kinase activities of the WNT, PI3K/AKT/mTOR, and RAS-MEK-ERK pathways will be analyzed for precision therapy. For thyroid cancers, parathyroid cancers, adrenocorticoid carcinoma, adrenal medullary carcinoma, and pancreatic islet cell carcinomas, the testing will proceed similarly to pituitary tumors except for the different oncogenic drivers being tested.

REFERENCES

1. ASCO. Neuroendocrine Tumors: Statistics. Cancer.Net. 02/2022. Retrieved 3 January 2023 www.cancer.net/cancer-types/neuroendocrine-tumors/statistics#:~:text=Overall%2C%20it%20is%20estimated%20that,has%20been%20increasing%20for%20years.
2. Asban A, Patel AJ, Reddy S, et al. Cancer of the endocrine system. In: Niederhuber JE, Armitage JA, Kastan MB et al., eds., Abeloff's Clinical Oncology (6th Edition), 2020;1074–1107.
3. de Kock L, Sabbaghian N, Plourde F, et al. Pituitary blastoma: A pathognomonic feature of germ-line DICER1 mutations. Acta Neuropathol. 2014; 128(1): 111–122.
4. Reyes M, Taghvaei M, Yu S, et al. Targeted therapy in the management of modern craniopharyngiomas. Front Biosci (Landmark Ed). 2022; 27(4): 136.
5. Petersenn S, Heaney AP. Targeted systemic and peptide radioligand therapy for aggressive pituitary tumors and carcinomas. Rev Endocr Metab Disord. 2020; 21(2): 277–286.
6. Cabanillas ME, Ryder M, Jimenez C. Targeted therapy for advanced thyroid cancer: Kinase inhibitors and beyond. Endocr Rev. 2019; 40(6): 1573–1604.
7. Lorusso L, Cappagli V, Valerio L, et al. Thyroid cancers: from surgery to current and future systemic therapies through their molecular identities. Int J Mol Sci. 2021; 22(6): 3117.
8. Cancer Genome Atlas Research Network. Integrated genomic characterization of papillary thyroid carcinoma. Cell. 2014; 159(3): 676–690.
9. Hescheler DA, Riemann B, Hartmann MJM, et al. Targeted therapy of papillary thyroid cancer: a comprehensive genomic analysis. Front Endocrinol (Lausanne). 2021; 12: 748941.
10. Laha D, Nilubol N, Boufraqech M. New therapies for advanced thyroid cancer. Front Endocrinol (Lausanne). 2020; 11: 82.
11. Valerio L, Pieruzzi L, Giani C, et al. Targeted therapy in thyroid cancer: state of the art. Clin Oncol (R Coll Radiol). 2017; 29(5): 316–324.
12. McFadden DG, Sadow PM. Genetics, diagnosis, and management of Hürthle cell thyroid neoplasms. Front Endocrinol (Lausanne). 2021; 12: 696386.
13. DeLellis RA, Lloyd RV, Heitz PU, Eng C (Eds.): World Health Organization Classification of Tumours: Pathology and Genetics of Tumors of Endocrine Organs. IARC Press: Lyon, 2004;69–70.
14. Ganly I, Makarov V, Deraje S, et al. Integrated genomic analysis of Hürthle cell cancer reveals oncogenic drivers, recurrent mitochondrial mutations, and unique chromosomal landscapes. Cancer Cell. 2018; 34(2): 256–270.
15. Landa I, Ibrahimpasic T, Boucai L, et al. Genomic and transcriptomic hallmarks of poorly differentiated and anaplastic thyroid cancers. J Clin Invest. 2016; 126(3): 1052–1066.

16. Smallridge RC, Copland JA. Anaplastic thyroid carcinoma: Pathogenesis and emerging therapies. Clin Oncol. 2010; 22(6): 486–497.
17. Raue F, Frank-Raue K. Thyroid Cancer: risk-stratified management and individualized therapy. Clin Cancer Res. 2016; 22(20): 5012–5021.
18. Miller KC, Chintakuntlawar AV. Molecular-driven therapy in advanced thyroid cancer. Curr Treat Options Oncol. 2021; 22(3): 24.
19. Ancker OV, Krüger M, Wehland M, et al. Multikinase inhibitor treatment in thyroid cancer. Int J Mol Sci. 2019; 21(1): 10.
20. Okafor C, Hogan J, Raygada M, et al. Update on targeted therapy in medullary thyroid cancer. Front Endocrinol (Lausanne). 2021; 12: 708949.
21. Rosen EY, Johnson ML, Clifford SE, et al. Overcoming MET-dependent resistance to selective RET inhibition in patients with RET fusion-positive lung cancer by combining Selpercatinib with Crizotinib. Clin Cancer Res. 2021; 27(1): 34–42.
22. Bardia A, Gounder M, Rodon J, et al. Phase Ib study of combination therapy with MEK inhibitor Binimetinib and phosphatidylinositol 3-kinase inhibitor buparlisib in patients with advanced solid tumors with RAS/RAF alterations. Oncologist. 2020; 25(1): e160–e169.
23. Lee PK, Jarosek SL, Virnig BA, et al. Trends in the incidence and treatment of parathyroid cancer in the United States. Cancer. 2007; 109(9): 1736–1741.
24. Schoretsanitis G, Daskalakis M, Melissas J, et al. Parathyroid carcinoma: clinical presentation and management. Am J Otolaryngol. 2009; 30(4): 277–280.
25. Agarwal G, Dhingra S, Mishra SK, et al. Implantation of parathyroid carcinoma along fine needle aspiration track. Langenbecks Arch Surg. 2006; 391(6): 623–626.
26. Sandelin K, Tullgren O, Farnebo LO. Clinical course of metastatic parathyroid cancer. World J Surg. 1994; 18(4): 594–598.
27. Howell VM, Gill A, Clarkson A, et al. Accuracy of combined protein gene product 9.5 and parafibromin markers for immunohistochemical diagnosis of parathyroid carcinoma. J Clin Endocrinol Metab. 2009; 94(2): 434–441.
28. Adam MA, Untch BR, Olson JA Jr. Parathyroid carcinoma: Current understanding and new insights into gene expression and intraoperative parathyroid hormone kinetics. Oncologist. 2010; 15(1): 61–72.
29. Alyateem G, Nilubol N. Current status and future targeted therapy in adrenocortical cancer. Front Endocrinol (Lausanne). 2021; 12: 613248.
30. Assie G, Letouze E, Fassnacht M, et al. Integrated genomic characterization of adrenocortical carcinoma. Nat Genet. 2014; 46(6): 607–612.
31. Zheng S, Cherniack AD, Dewal N, et al. Comprehensive pan-genomic characterization of adrenocortical carcinoma. Cancer Cell. 2016; 29(5): 723–736.
32. Jochmanova I, Pacak K. Genomic landscape of pheochromocytoma and paraganglioma. Trends Cancer. 2018; 4(1): 6–9.
33. Wang K, Crona J, Beuschlein F, et al. Targeted therapies in pheochromocytoma and paraganglioma. J Clin Endocrinol Metab. 2022; 107(11): 2963–2972.
34. Yao JC. Neuroendocrine tumors. Molecular targeted therapy for carcinoid and islet-cell carcinoma. Best Pract Res Clin Endocrinol Metab. 2007; 21(1): 163–172.

19

Myeloid Neoplasms

George Deeb and Shiyong Li

19.1 Introduction

Myeloid neoplasms consist of a heterogeneous group of hematopoietic disorders derived from bone marrow progenitor cells. The signs and symptoms of patients with myeloid neoplasms range from asymptomatic to chronic and acute leukemias with or without extramedullary tissue involvement. According to the NCI Cancer Statistics, myeloid together with lymphoid neoplasms affect approximately 60,000 patients per year in the United States (Leukemia—Cancer Stat Facts) and is the 11th leading cause of death with acute myeloid leukemia attributing to almost half of the death. Tremendous progress has been made in our understanding of the normal hematopoiesis and the underlying pathobiology of myeloid neoplasms owing to technological advances in the last several decades. As a result, the diagnosis and classification of myeloid neoplasms have evolved from simple morphological examination to an integrated approach that includes not only morphologic examination but also immunophenotyping, cytogenetics, and molecular genetics testing (Table 19.1) (1-3). Despite the early success in the treatment of acute promyelocytic leukemia and chronic myeloid leukemia with small molecule-targeted therapies, chemotherapy with or without bone marrow transplantation remains the mainstay standard treatment for patients with myeloid neoplasms. In recent years, new targets have been discovered, and novel therapies against these new biomarkers have been developed and become part of the treatment armamentarium for patients with myeloid neoplasms (Table 19.2) (4-6). This chapter will focus on how precision pathology can aid in

TABLE 19.1

Overview of the Current Classifications of Myeloid Neoplasms

WHO HAEM5	ICC
Clonal hematopoiesis	**Premalignant clonal cytopenias and/or monocytosis**
Clonal hematopoiesis of indeterminate potential	Clonal hematopoiesis
Clonal cytopenia of undetermined significance	Clonal cytopenia of undetermined significance
	Clonal cytopenia with monocytosis of undetermined significance
	Clonal monocytosis of undetermined significance
Myeloproliferative neoplasms	**Myeloproliferative neoplasms**
Chronic myeloid leukemia	Chronic myeloid leukemia
Polycythaemia vera	Polycythemia vera
Essential thrombocythemia	Essential thrombocythemia
Primary myelofibrosis	Primary myelofibrosis
Chronic neutrophilic leukemia	Chronic neutrophilic leukemia
Chronic eosinophilic leukemia	Chronic eosinophilic leukemia, NOS
Myeloproliferative neoplasm, NOS	Myeloproliferative neoplasm, unclassifiable
Juvenile myelomonocytic leukemia	
Mastocytosis	**Mastocytosis**
Cutaneous mastocytosis	Cutaneous mastocytosis
Systemic mastocytosis	Systemic mastocytosis
Mast cell sarcoma	Mast cell sarcoma

(Continued)

DOI: 10.1201/9781003513469-19

TABLE 19.1 (Continued)

WHO HAEM5	ICC
Myelodysplastic neoplasms (MDS)	**Myelodysplastic syndromes (MDS)**
MDS with defining genetic abnormalities	
MDS with low blasts and isolated 5q deletion	MDS with del(5q)
MDS with low blasts and *SF3B1* mutation	MDS with mutated *SF3B1*
MDS with biallelic *TP53* inactivation	MDS with mutated *TP53*
MDS, morphologically defined	
MDS with low blasts	MDS, NOS
	MDS, NOS without dysplasia
	MDS, NOS with single lineage dysplasia
	MDS, NOS with multilineage dysplasia
MDS, hypoplastic	
MDS with increased blasts (MDS-IB)	
MDS-IB1	MDS with excess blasts
MDS-IB2	MDS/AML
	MDS/AML with mutated *TP53*
	MDS/AML with MDS-related gene mutations
	MDS/AML with MDS-related cytogenetic abnormalities
	MDS/AML, NOS specified
MDS with fibrosis	
MDS of childhood	
Childhood MDS with low blasts	
Childhood MDS with increased blasts	
	Pediatric and/or germline mutation-associated disorders
	Refractory cytopenia of childhood
	Refractory cytopenia of childhood
	Juvenile myelomonocytic leukemia
	Juvenile myelomonocytic leukemia-like neoplasms
	Noonan syndrome-associated myeloproliferative disorder
	Hematologic neoplasms with germline predisposition
Myelodysplastic/myeloproliferative neoplasms (MDS/MPN)	**Myelodysplastic/myeloproliferative neoplasms (MDS/MPN)**
Chronic myelomonocytic leukemia	Chronic myelomonocytic leukemia
MDS/MPN with neutrophilia	Atypical chronic myeloid leukemia
MDS/MPN with *SF3B1* mutation and thrombocytosis	MDS/MPN with thrombocytosis and *SF3B1* mutation
MDS/MPN with ring sideroblasts and thrombocytosis	MDS/MPN with ring sideroblasts and thrombocytosis, NOS
MDS/MPN, NOS	MDS/MPN, NOS
Myeloid/lymphoid neoplasms with eosinophilia and tyrosine kinase gene fusions	**Myeloid/lymphoid neoplasms with eosinophilia and tyrosine kinase gene fusions**
Myeloid/lymphoid neoplasm with *PDGFRA* rearrangement	Myeloid/lymphoid neoplasm with *PDGFRA* rearrangement
Myeloid/lymphoid neoplasm with *PDGFRB* rearrangement	Myeloid/lymphoid neoplasm with *PDGFRB* rearrangement
Myeloid/lymphoid neoplasm with *FGFR1* rearrangement	Myeloid/lymphoid neoplasm with *FGFR1* rearrangement
Myeloid/lymphoid neoplasm with *JAK2* rearrangement	Myeloid/lymphoid neoplasm with *JAK2* rearrangement
Myeloid/lymphoid neoplasm with *FLT3* rearrangement	Myeloid/lymphoid neoplasm with *FLT3* rearrangement
Myeloid/lymphoid neoplasm with *ETV6::ABL1* fusion	Myeloid/lymphoid neoplasm with *ETV6::ABL1* fusion
Myeloid/lymphoid neoplasm with other gene fusions	
	Blastic plasmacytoid dendritic cell neoplasm
Acute myeloid leukemias (AML)	**Acute myeloid leukemias (AML)**
AML with defining genetic abnormalities	
APL with *PML::RARA* fusion	APL with t(15;17)(q24.1;q21.2)/*PML::RARA*

(Continued)

TABLE 19.1 (Continued)

WHO HAEM5	ICC
	APL with other *RARA* rearrangements
AML with *RUNX1::RUNX1T1* fusion	AML with t(8;21)(q22;q22.1)/*RUNX1:: RUNX1T1*
Acute myeloid leukemia with *CBFB::MYH11* fusion	AML with inv(16)(p13.1q22) or t(16;16)(p13.1;q22)/ *CBFB::MYH11*
AML with *DEK::NUP214* fusion	AML with t(6;9)(p22.3;q34.1)/*DEK::NUP214*
AML with *RBM1::MRTFA* fusion	
AML with *BCR::ABL1* fusion	AML with t(9;22)(q34.1;q11.2)/*BCR::ABL1*
AML with *KMT2A* rearrangement	AML with t(9;11)(p21.3;q23.3)/*MLLT3::KMT2A*
	AML with other *KMT2A* rearrangements
AML with *MECOM* rearrangement	AML with inv3(q21.3q26.2) or t(3;3)(q21.3/q26.2)/ *GATA2; MECOM*
	AML with other *MECOM* rearrangements
AML with *NUP98* rearrangement	
AML with *NPM1* mutation	AML with mutated *NPM1*
AML with *CEBPA* mutation	AML with in-frame bZIP *CEBPA* mutations
	AML with mutated *TP53*
AML, myelodysplasia-related	AML with myelodysplasia-related gene mutations
	AML with myelodysplasia-related cytogenetic abnormalities
AML with other defined genetic abnormalities	AML with other rare recurring translocations
AML, defined by differentiation	AML, NOS
AML with minimal differentiation	
AML without maturation	
AML with maturation	
Acute basophilic leukemia	
Acute myelomonocytic leukemia	
Acute monocytic leukemia	
Acute erythroid leukemia	
Acute megakaryoblastic leukemia	
Myeloid sarcoma	Myeloid sarcoma
Acute leukemia of mixed or ambiguous lineage (ALAL/ MPAL)	**Acute leukemia of ambiguous lineage**
ALAL/MPAL with defining genetic abnormalities	
MPAL with *BCR::ABL1* fusion	MPAL with t(9;22)(q34.1;q11.2)/*BCR::ABL1*
MPAL with *KMT2A* rearrangement	MPAL with t(v;11q23.3)/*KMT2A* rearranged
ALAL with other defined genetic alterations	
With *ZNF384* rearrangement	
With *BCL11B* rearrangement	
ALAL/MPAL, immunophenotypically defined	
MPAL, B/myeloid	MPAL, B/myeloid, NOS
MPAL, T/myeloid	MPAL, T/myeloid, NOS
MPAL, rare types	
ALAL, NOS	
Acute undifferentiated leukemia	Acute undifferentiated leukemia
Secondary myeloid neoplasms	
Myeloid neoplasms post cytotoxic therapy	Qualifier for MDS or AML
Myeloid neoplasms associated with germline predisposition	
Without a preexisting platelet disorder or organ dysfunction	
With pre-existing platelet disorder	

(Continued)

TABLE 19.1 (Continued)

WHO HAEM5	ICC
With potential organ dysfunction	
Myeloid proliferations associated with Down syndrome	
	Myeloid proliferations associated with Down syndrome
Histiocytic/dendritic cell neoplasms	**Histiocytic/dendritic cell neoplasms**
Plasmacytoid dendritic cell neoplasms	
Mature plasmacytoid dendritic cell proliferation	
Blastic plasmacytoid dendritic cell neoplasm	
Langerhans cell neoplasms	
Langerhans cell histiocytosis	Langerhans cell histiocytosis
Langerhans cell sarcoma	Langerhans cell sarcoma
Other dendritic cell neoplasm	
Indeterminate dendritic cell neoplasm	indeterminate dendritic cell neoplasm
Interdigitating dendritic cell neoplasm	interdigitating dendritic cell neoplasm
Histiocytic neoplasms	
Juvenile xanthogranuloma	Xanthogranuloma
Erdheim-Chester disease	Erdheim-Chester disease
Rosai-Dorfman disease	Rosai-Dorfman-Destombes disease
ALK-positive histiocytosis	ALK-positive histiocytosis
Histiocytic sarcoma	Histiocytic sarcoma

Source: ref. 2-3 WHO HAEM5, 5th Edition of World Health Organization Classification of Hematolymphoid Neoplasms; ICC, International Consensus Classification;

Abbreviations: AML, acute myeloid leukemia; APL, acute promyelocytic leukemia; MDS, myelodysplastic syndrome/neoplasm; MDS/MPN, myelodysplastic/myeloproliferative neoplasm; ALAL/MPAL, acute leukemia of ambiguous lineage/mixed phenotype acute leukemia; bZIP, basic leucine zipper domain; NOS, not otherwise specified.

TABLE 19.2

Summary of Targeted Therapy for Myeloid Neoplasms (ref. 4-6)

Targets	Drugs	Disease Categories	Current Status
BCR-ABL1	Imatinib	CML	FDA approved
	Nilotinib	CML	FDA approved
	Dasatinib	CML	FDA approved
	Bosutinib	CML	FDA approved
	Ponatinib	CML	FDA approved
	Padotinib	CML	Investigational
PML-RARA	Arsonic trioxide	APL	FDA approved
	ATRA	APL	FDA approved
PDGFRA/B	Imatinib	MLN-TK	FDA approved
FGFR1	Pemigatinib	MLN-TK	FDA approved
KIT	Avapritinib	SM	FDA approved
IDH1	Ivosidenib	MDS/AML	FDA approved
	Olutasidenib	MDS/AML	FDA approved
	ACC1 inhibitors	MDS/AML	Investigational
BCL2	Venetoclax	MDS/AML	FDA approved
IDH2	Enasidenib	MDS/AML	FDA approved
FLT3	Midostrurin	AML	FDA approved
	Gilteritinib	AML	FDA approved
	Sorafenib	AML	FDA approved
	Quizartinib	AML	Investigational
JAK2	Ruxolitnib	MPN	FDA approved
	Pacritinib	MPN	FDA approved
	Fedratinib	MPN	Investigational
	NS-018	MPN	Investigational

(Continued)

TABLE 19.2 (Continued)

Targets	Drugs	Disease Categories	Current Status
NPM1	Actinomycin D	AML/MDS	Investigational
	PARP inhibitors	AML/MDS	Investigational
	DOT1L inhibitors	AML/MDS	Investigational
	XPO inhibitors	AML/MDS	Investigational
DNMT	Azacitidine	MDS	FDA approved
	Decitabine	MDS	FDA approved
	SETD1B inhibitors	AML	Investigational
RARA	Tamibarotene	AML	Investigational
RAS	Tipifarnib	MDS	Investigational
	Rigosertib	MDS	Investigational
	Trametinib	MDS	Investigational
FLT3	Midostaurin	AML	FDA approved
	Gilteritinib	AML	FDA approved
	Quizrtinib	AML	Investigational
	Crenolanib	AML	Investigational
TP53	Nutlin analogs	AML	Investigational
	Eprenetapopt	AML	Investigational
ZRSR2	RBM39 inhibitors	AML	Investigational
	H3B-8800	AML	Investigational
SF3B1	Vitamin B5	MDS or MDS/MPN	Investigational
	RBM39 inhibitors	MDS or MDS/MPN	Investigational
	H3B-8800	MDS or MDS/MPN	Investigational
U2AF1	RBM39 inhibitors	AML/MDS	Investigational
	H3B-8800	AML/MDS	Investigational
SRSF2	RBM39 inhibitors	AML/MDS	Investigational
	H3B-8800	AML/MDS	Investigational
TET2	XPO inhibitors	AML/MDS	Investigational
	Ascorbic acid	AML/MDS	Investigational
RAD21	XPO inhibitors	AML/MDS	Investigational
	PARP inhibitors	AML/MDS	Investigational
	DOT1L inhibitors	AML/MDS	Investigational
SMC1A	XPO inhibitors	AML/MDS	Investigational
	PARP inhibitors	AML/MDS	Investigational
	DOT1L inhibitors	AML/MDS	Investigational
STAG2	XPO inhibitors	AML/MDS	Investigational
	PARP inhibitors	AML/MDS	Investigational
	DOT1L inhibitors	AML/MDS	Investigational
SMC3	XPO inhibitors	AML/MDS	Investigational
	PARP inhibitors	AML/MDS	Investigational
	DOT1L inhibitors	AML/MDS	Investigational
KMT2A/MLL	SNDX-5613	AML/MDS	Investigational
	DOT1L inhibitors	AML/MDS	Investigational
	Menin-MLL inhibitors	AML/MDS	Investigational
GDF-11	Luspatercept	MDS or MDS/MPN	FDA approved
SMO	Glasdegib	AML	FDA approved
PD1	Pembrolizumab	AML/MDS	Investigational
	Nivolumab	AML/MDS	Investigational
PD-L1	Atezolizumab	AML/MDS	Investigational
CTLA-4	Ipilimumab	AML/MDS	Investigational
CD43	Magrolimab	AML/MDS	Investigational
CD33	Gemtuzumab Ozogamicin	AML	FDA approved
CD123	CAR-T	AML	Investigational

Abbreviations: AML, acute myeloid leukemia; APL, acute promyelocytic leukemia; ATRA, all-trans retinoic acid; MDS, myelodysplastic syndrome/neoplasm; MDS/MPN, myelodysplastic/myeloproliferative neoplasm; SM, systemic mastocytosis; MLN-TK, myeloid/lymphoid neoplasms with eosinophilia and tyrosine kinase gene fusion; FDA, Food and Drug Administration.

the diagnosis, classification, and personalized management of patients with common myeloid neoplasms.

19.2 Myelodysplastic Syndromes/Neoplasms

Myelodysplastic syndrome/neoplasm (MDS) is a heterogeneous group of clonal hematopoietic stem cell disorder characterized by morphologic dysplasia affecting one or more of the myeloid lineages, ineffective hematopoiesis resulting in peripheral cytopenia, and an increased risk of transformation to acute myeloid leukemia (7, 8). The estimated overall incidence of MDS is approximately 4 per 100,000 in the United States and continues to increase with aging and accumulation of driver gene mutations (9). It is mainly a disease of the elderly. At the time of the MDS diagnosis, more than 80% of patients are 60 years or older (median age, 76) with a slight male predominance.

Morphological examination to assess the presence of dysplasia and to enumerate blasts remains an essential step in the diagnostic evaluation of MDS (Figures 19.1A, 19.2A–C, and 19.3). Dysplasia affecting at least 10% of one or more of the myeloid lineage (granulocytic, erythroid, and megakaryocytic) cells is required by the current World Health Organization 5th edition and International Consensus Classification (ICC) systems (2, 3). It is also a major diagnostic criterion proposed by the International Working Group for MDS (10). In regard to the latter, the presence of more than 15% ring sideroblasts is considered sufficient to fulfill the 10% dysplasia criterion affecting the erythroid lineage. The blast cutoff for MDS diagnosis is different between two classification systems (Table 19.3). The WHO classification defines MDS as having less than 20% blasts in the blood or bone marrow and without AML-defining genetic abnormalities. In contrast, the ICC redefines cases with 10–19% blasts as MDS/AML, emphasizing the biological continuum between MDS and AML. The demonstration of aberrant immunophenotypic profiles by multiparameter flow cytometry may help support the diagnosis of MDS (11). When blasts are not increased and morphological dysplasia is equivocal, detection of clonal cytogenetic and/or molecular genetic abnormalities is required to diagnose MDS. The cytogenetic abnormalities frequently involve chromosomes 5, 7, 8, 11, 13, 17, and 20 with either gain or loss. The molecular genetic aberrations include disease-defining mutations of *SF3B1* and *TP53* genes or other clonal hematopoiesis driver gene mutations (Figures 19.1B and C; Figures 19.2D and E; Table 19.4).Both the WHO 5th edition and ICC classification systems recognize subtypes of MDS that are genetically defined (Tables 19.1 and 19.3). The genetically defined MDS strata are based on detection of clonal copy number changes (loss of genetic material affecting mainly chromosomes 5q and 17p/*TP53*), copy neutral loss of heterozygosity of 17p/*TP53*, and mutated genes (*SF3B1* and *TP53*). The genomic landscape of MDS is not limited to the genetic abnormalities that diagnose the disease and define certain disease subtypes. There are numerous additional pathogenic variants of mutated genes that are also detected in MDS and implicated in the disease pathogenesis, prognosis, and progression to AML. In this regard, the somatic mutations affecting the following genes *TP53*, *EZH2*, *ETV6*, *RUNX1*, and *ASXL1*

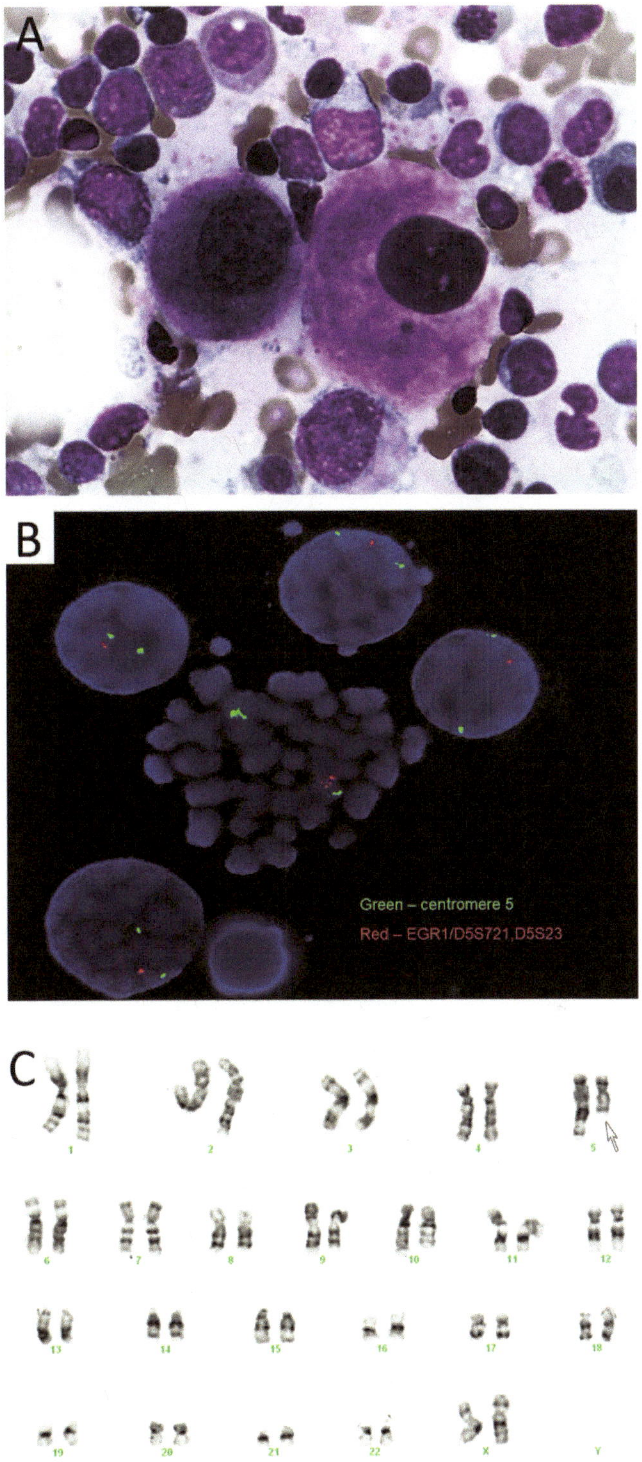

FIGURE 19.1 MDS with del(5q). (A) Wright-Giemsa-stained bone marrow aspirate smear shows dysplastic hypolobated megakaryocytes. (B) FISH analysis shows loss of 5q signal (red). (C) Chromosome analysis shows loss of 5q31 (arrow).

have been shown to predict poor outcome of patients with MDS in multivariant analysis (12). In this study, approximately 45% of the tested patients had at least one mutation. The frequency of patients with at least one oncogenic mutation increased to 74–90% when larger cohorts were tested (12-17). Currently, molecular genetic testing of patients with MDS, via targeted

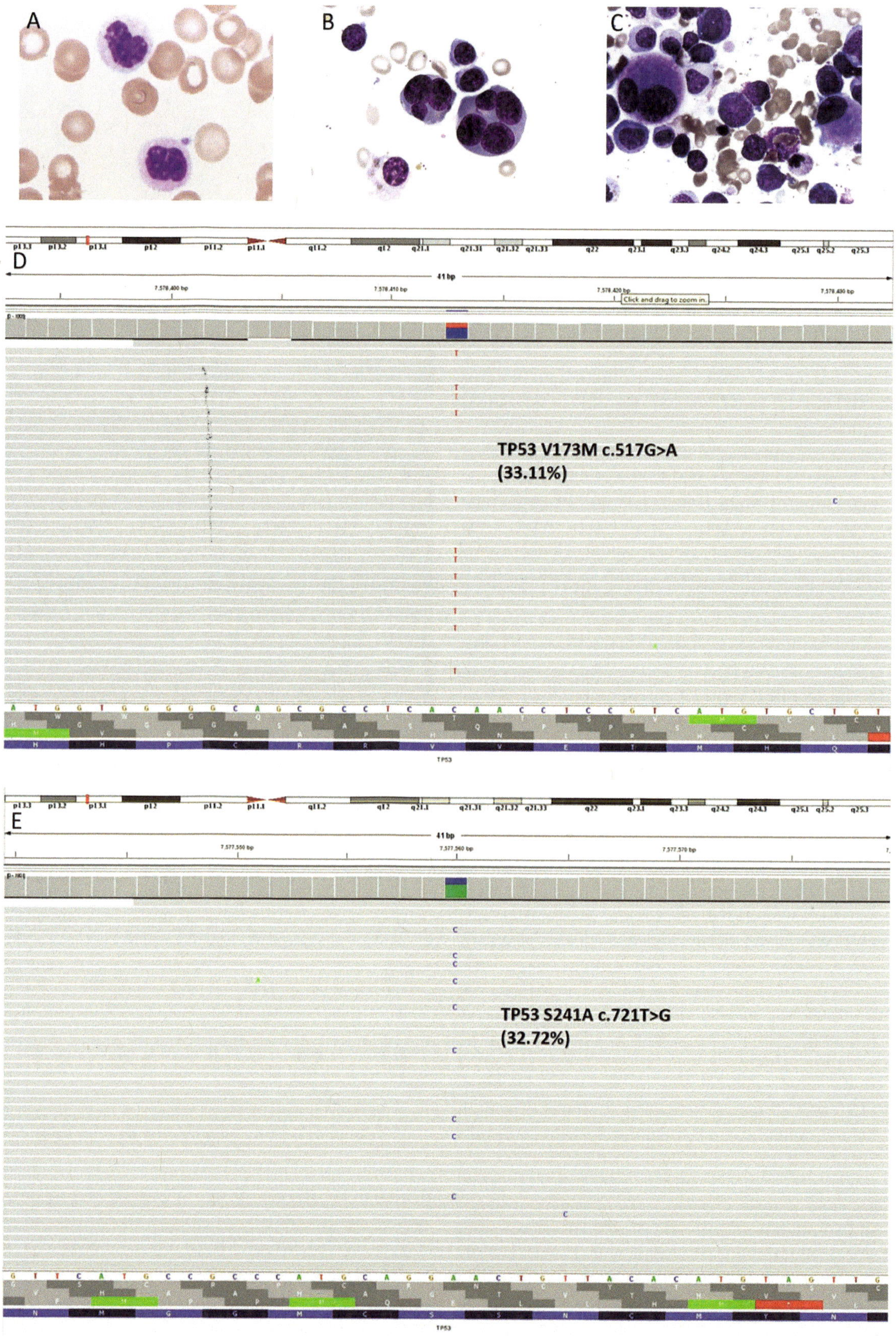

FIGURE 19.2 MDS with biallelic *TP53* inactivation or mutated *TP53*. (A) Wright-Giemsa-stained blood smear shows dysplastic neutrophils. (B and C) Wright-Giemsa-stained bone marrow aspirate shows dysplastic erythroid precursor cells and megakaryocytes. (D and E) Next-generation sequencing (NGS) analysis shows the presence double *TP53* mutations.

TABLE 19.3

Classification of Myelodysplastic Syndrome/Neoplasms

	Blast Count and Other Cyto-/ Histo-Morphologic Features	Genetic Abnormalities
MDS, genetically defined (with defining genetic abnormalities)		
MDS with low blasts and isolated 5q deletion (MDS-5q)	< 5% blasts in BM and < 2% blasts in PB	5q deletion alone, or with 1 other abnormality other than monosomy 7 or 7q deletion
MDS with low blasts and *SF3B1* mutation (MDS-*SF3B1*) *,**	< 5% blasts in BM and < 2% blasts in PB	Absence of 5q deletion, monosomy 7, or complex karyotype
MDS with biallelic (or multi-hit) *TP53* inactivation (MDS-bi*TP53*) (**ICC)	< 20% blasts in BM and PB and < 30% erythroblasts in BM (**ICC)	Usually complex karyotype. Two or more *TP53* mutations, or 1 mutation with evidence of *TP53* copy number loss or copy neutral loss of heterozygosity (LOH)
MDS, morphologically defined (not meeting criteria for MDS with defining genetic abnormalities)		
MDS with low blasts (MDS-LB) ***	< 5% blasts in BM and < 2% blasts in PB	No defining genetic abnormalities
MDS, hypoplastic (MDS-h) (≤ 25% bone marrow cellularity, age adjusted) (**ICC)	< 5% blasts in BM and < 2% blasts in PB	No defining genetic abnormalities or increased blasts
MDS with increased blasts (MDS-IB)		No diagnostic criteria of MDS with biallelic *TP53* inactivation or AML
MDS-IB: MDS-IB1 (**ICC)	5–9% blasts in BM or 2–4% blasts in PB	
MDS-IB: MDS-IB2 (**ICC)	10–19% blasts in BM or 5–19% blasts in PB or Auer rods. No significant reticulin fibrosis	
MDS-IB: MDS with fibrosis (MDS-f) (**ICC)	5–19% blasts in BM or 2–19% blasts in PB, with significant reticulin fibrosis (grade 2 or 3)	

Note: BM = Bone marrow, PB = Peripheral blood.

* = MDS with low blasts and ring sideroblasts: < 5% blasts in BM, < 2% blasts in PB, ≥ 15% ring sideroblasts and wild-type *SF3B1* and No other defining genetic abnormalities. According to WHO classification, this entity cannot be rendered if the *SF3B1* variant is at a variant allele frequency (VAF) of < 5%.

**ICC, International Consensus Classification. The following are some differences from the WHO classification addressed or specified by ICC. *SF3B1* mutation should be detected with VAF >= 10% and without multi-hit *TP53* or *RUNX1*. *TP53* mutations should be encountered with VAF > 10%. MDS-h and MDS-f are not recognized. MDS-IB1 is designated "MDS with excess blasts". Although 2% PB blasts mandates classification of an MDS case as MDS-EB, 1% blasts in PB on 2 separate occasions qualifies for MDS-EB too. MDS-IB2 is designated as "MDS/acute myeloid leukemia (AML) (10–19% blasts in BM or PB in adult patients ≥18 year old)". MDS not otherwise specified (NOS) without dysplasia, or with single lineage or multilineage dysplasia is recognized by ICC.

*** = MDS-LB could be optionally divided into MDS-LB with single or multilineage (two or more lineages) dysplasia.

next-generation sequencing (NGS), has been a routine laboratory practice that is critical for the diagnosis, classification, prognosis, and defining germline predisposition of MDS.

A battery of genes shown to be mutated in association with MDS has been recommended for testing by the ICC and the International MDS group (Molecular International Prognostic Scoring System, IPSS-M) (6, 18-23). These genes collectively included *ASXL1, BCOR, BCORL1, CBL, CEBPA, CSF3R, DDX41, DNMT3A, ETV6, ETNK1, EZH2, FLT3*-ITD, *FLT3*-TKD, *GATA2, GNB1, IDH1, IDH2, JAK2, KIT, KRAS, KMT2A*-PTD, *NF1, NPM1, NRAS, PHF6, PPM1D, PRPF8, PTPN11, RAD21, RUNX1, SAMD9, SAMD9L, SETBP1, SF3B1, SRSF2, STAG2, TET2, TP53, U2AF1, UBA1, WT1*, and *ZRSR2* (Table 19.4). Incorporation of molecular genetic markers (mutated oncogenes) in the IPSS for MDS, though needing more future validation, may further enhance the predictive power of the IPSS especially within the group of patients with low-grade disease or those who may benefit from allogeneic transplant (19-21, 24). Regarding the latter, a practical IPPS-M Risk Calculator has been available for healthcare providers to stratify the risk of patients with MDS and predict clinical outcomes. The input information includes clinical, cytogenetic, and molecular data (https://mds-risk-model.com).

Deciphering the genetic code of MDS has been shown to be promising in developing potential targeted therapy (25-28). Patients with low-risk MDS are typically managed with either supportive treatment such as blood transfusion or chemotherapy with hypomethylating agents, such as azacitidine (Vidaza) or decitabine (Dacogen) (25). Standard chemotherapy such as cytarabine (ara-C) with or without idarubicin or daunorubicin may be used for patients with high-risk MDS to prevent transformation to acute myeloid leukemia. Immunomodulating agents such as lenalidomide (Revlimid) have been shown to eliminate the need for blood transfusions in low-grade MDS, particularly MDS with del5q (29, 30). Recently, the Food and Drug Administration (FDA) approved luspatercept for the treatment of anemia in patients with low to intermediate-risk MDS with ring sideroblasts (RS) (www.fda.gov/drugs/resources-information-approved-drugs/fda-approves-luspatercept-aamt-anemia-adults-mds). Targeted therapy against driver gene mutations for MDS

TABLE 19.4

Summary of Driver Gene Mutations and Their Prognostic Significance in MDS

Genes	Frequency in MDS (%)	Implicated Biological Pathways	Prognostic Significance
ASXL1 *,**	10–20	Chromatin modification (epigenetics)(epigenetic modifiers)epigenetic regulators and chromatin-remodeling factors	Poor
BCOR *,**	< 5	Epigenetic modifiers	Poor
BCORL1 *,**		Epigenetic modifiers	
CBL *[a]	2–5	Signal transduction (RAS pathway) (signaling molecule) Receptor tyrosine kinases/signaling	Poor
CEBPA *,** [a]		Transcription factor (Transcriptional regulation)	
CSF3R **		Receptors	
DDX41 [a]		Currently unclear	
DNMT3A *,**	10–15	DNA methylation (epigenetics)(epigenetic modifiers) epigenetic regulators and chromatin-remodeling factors	Poor
ETV6 *,** [a]	2–5	Transcription factor (Transcriptional regulation)	Poor
ETNK1 * [b]	N/A	Phosphatidylethanolamine synthesis pathway [c]	N/A
EZH2 *,**	5–10	Chromatin modification (epigenetics)	Poor
FLT3-ITD *		Signal transduction (signaling molecule) Receptor tyrosine kinases/signaling	Poor
FLT3-TKD *		Signal transduction (signaling molecule) Receptor tyrosine kinases/signaling	Poor
GATA2 *,**[a]	< 5	Transcriptional regulation	Poor
GNB1 *,**		Signal transduction (signaling molecule)	
IDH1 *,**	1–2	DNA methylation (epigenetics)(epigenetic modifiers) epigenetic regulators and chromatin-remodeling factors	Poor
IDH2 *,**	2–5	DNA methylation (epigenetics)(epigenetic modifiers)	Poor
JAK2 **	3–5	Signal transduction (signaling molecule) Receptor tyrosine kinases/signaling	N/A (unclear)
KIT **	1–5	Signal transduction (signaling molecule) Receptor tyrosine kinases/signaling	N/A (unclear)
KRAS *,** [a]	1–5	Signal transduction (RAS pathway) (signaling molecule)	Poor
KMT2A-PTD *,**		Transcriptional coactivator [d]	Poor
NF1 *[a]		Signal transduction (RAS pathway) (signaling molecule)	Poor
NPM1 *	1–2	(Signaling molecule)	
NRAS *,**[a]	3–5	Signal transduction (RAS pathway) (signaling molecule)	Poor
PHF6 *,**	5	Transcription factors	Poor
PPM1D *,**		TP53 related	
PRPF8 *	< 1	RNA splicing [e]	
PTPN11 *,** [a]	< 5	Signal transduction (signaling molecule) Receptor tyrosine kinases/signaling	Poor
RAD21 **	< 5	Cohesin complex	N/A (unclear)
RUNX1 *,**[a]	8–10	Transcription factor (transcriptional regulation)	Poor
SAMD9 ***[a]		Cellular proliferation pathway	
SAMD9L ***[a]		Cellular proliferation pathway	
SETBP1 *,**		DNA replication [f]	
SF3B1 *,**	14–30	RNA splicing	Good (unfavorable if combined with del5q)
SRSF2 *,**		RNA splicing	Poor
STAG2 *,**	5–10	Cohesion complex	Poor
TET2 **	19–30	DNA methylation (epigenetics) (epigenetic modifiers) (epigenetic regulators and chromatin-remodeling factors)	Poor

(Continued)

TABLE 19.4 (Continued)

Genes	Frequency in MDS (%)	Implicated Biological Pathways	Prognostic Significance
TP53 *,** [a]	7–10, and 50 in complex karyotype	DNA repair and gene expression control	Poor
U2AF1 *,**	8	RNA splicing	Poor
UBA1 [g]	N/A	Ubiquitylation	N/A
WT1 *,**	< 1	Transcription factor (transcriptional regulation)	Poor
ZRSR2 **	5–10	RNA splicing	N/A

Notes: Px = Prognosis.

[a]These genes are associated with germline predisposition to hematologic neoplasms. *KRAS*, *NRAS*, and *PTPN11* are associated with Noonan syndrome and *CBL* is associated with CBL syndrome (both are inherited as autosomal dominant traits).
[b] Ref. 16.
[c] www.ncbi.nlm.nih.gov/gene/55500.
[d] www.ncbi.nlm.nih.gov/gene/4297.
[e] www.ncbi.nlm.nih.gov/gene/10594.
[f] www.ncbi.nlm.nih.gov/gene/26040.
[g] Ref. 15.
* List of genes incorporated in the International Prognostic Scoring System (IPSS-M) for MDS. Website (IPSS-M Risk Calculator): https://mds-risk-model.com and citation: Bernard, E et al. NEJM Evid 2022; 1 (7), DOI: 10.1056/EVIDoa2200008.
** Clonal hematopoiesis driver mutations associated with clonal cytopenia of undetermined significance by the WHO 5th edition. Additional genes that are not mentioned previously included *CTCF* and *BRCC3*, and those labeled as "other", including *BRAF, CALR, CUX1, JAK3, KDM6A, MPL, MYD88, NOTCH1, PIGA, PRPF40B, PTEN, SF1, SF3A1, SMC1A, SMC3,* and *STAT3.* Of note, *GNAS* (less than 1% of tested MDS patients) was not mentioned by ICC or IPSS-M but mentioned by Bejar et al. (ref. 12) and the aforementioned gene list.
*** Testing for *SAMD9* and *SAMD9L* genes is recommended for pediatric patients.

is limited. MDS with *IDH1* mutation may be treated with IDH1 inhibitors such as ivosidenib. Other small molecules or immunomodulating drugs have also been under active experimental investigation as potential therapeutic modalities for patients with MDS (Table 19.2) (31). Given the complexity of MDS oncogenesis, immune response, and microenvironment, the ultimate therapeutic approaches may target the genetic make-up and genome instability, the imbalanced apoptosis and blocking of differentiation, immune dysregulation, and immune evasion (escape), and/or tumor-promoting inflammation.

19.3 Myeloproliferative Neoplasms

Myeloproliferative neoplasm (MPN) is a group of hematopoietic stem cell disorders characterized by uncontrolled proliferation of one or more myeloid lineage cells (32). The hallmark of MPN is peripheral cytosis without morphologic dysplasia or increased blasts at initial diagnosis. The underlying pathogenesis of MPN invariably involves oncogenic gene fusions or driver gene mutations that mainly affect the tyrosine kinase receptor-ligand pathways and therefore are amenable to targeted therapy with small molecule inhibitors or antagonists (Table 19.2). The natural history of MPN, if untreated, is progression from asymptomatic to more aggressive disease, including bone marrow failure and acute myeloid leukemia.

The prototypical MPN is *BCR::ABL1*-positive chronic myeloid leukemia (CML). It is the most common MPN, with an estimated annual incidence of 1–2 per 100,000 in the United States (32-34). CML usually has a chronic phase and inevitably progresses to accelerated and/or blast phase if left untreated. In chronic phase, the peripheral blood always has high white blood cell counts with left shift and frequent basophilia. Dysplasia is absent or minimal. The bone marrow is hypercellular with myeloid lineage cell predominance and frequent small megakaryocytes. In blast phase, blasts are increased resembling acute leukemia.

The *BCR::ABL1* gene fusion plays an essential role in the CML pathogenesis and is diagnostic of CML in the appropriate clinical and hematologic settings. It also offers a clinically effective targeted therapy using ABL-specific tyrosine kinase inhibitors (TKIs) (Table 19.2). With the advent of TKIs, the prognosis of CML has significantly improved with a high rate of complete molecular response, prolonged survival, and treatment-free remission in a proportion of patients (33-36). According to WHO 5th edition, accelerated phase is "irrelevant" in the era of TKI therapy, and therefore, it is replaced with the terminology "high-risk chronic phase" (3). The criteria to define the high-risk chronic phase or still now labeled "accelerated phase" based on ICC classification collectively include peripheral blood or marrow blast count of 10–19%, peripheral basophilia >= 20%, presence of additional clonal cytogenetic abnormalities in the cells harboring the *BCR::ABL1* translocation (Philadelphia chromosome), and clusters of small megakaryocytes associated with significant reticulin and/or collagen fibrosis. Those required to define the blast phase include peripheral blood or bone marrow blast count of >= 20%, extramedullary blast proliferation (myeloid sarcoma), or presence of abnormal lymphoblasts (> 5% based on ICC classification) as confirmed by immunophenotyping (e.g., by flow cytometry analysis). In addition, emerging resistance to TKI that may include "loss of prior responses, emergence of additional cytogenetic abnormalities, and *BCR::ABL1* kinase domain mutations" as specified by WHO classification constitutes increased risk of disease progression on therapy.

The classic *BCR::ABL1*-negative MPNs include polycythemia vera (PV), essential thrombocythemia (ET), and primary myelofibrosis (PMF) (Table 19.5). There is a significant clinical and morphological overlap among them, and their differential diagnosis is challenging but important since they have different risk of progression to acute leukemia and are thus managed differently. The majority of the classic MPNs harbor driver gene mutations in the JAK-STAT pathway. *JAK2*V617F is the most prevalent mutation associated with all three disorders and is present in about 95% of PVs. Mutations in exon 12 of *JAK2* are present in around 2% of PVs. Mutations in the thrombopoietin receptor (MPL) gene are mainly present in 5–10% of ET and PMF. The most frequent *MPL* mutation is W515L or W515K. Calreticulin (*CALR*) is mutated in 25–35% of ET and PMF, including both type 1 (insertion of 5 bp) and type 2 (deletion of 51 bp) mutations in exon 9. Mutations in other non-driver genes, such as *TET2*, *ASXL1*, and *DNMT3A*, are also frequently present in the classic MPNs. They are more commonly seen in PMF and advanced disease as compared to PV and ET, and some of them are known to be associated with a poorer prognosis. Other rare *BCR::ABL1*-negative MPNs include chronic neutrophilic leukemia (CNL), chronic eosinophilic Leukemia (CEL), juvenile myelomonocytic leukemia (JMML), and MPN, not otherwise specified (Table 19.5). CNL is characterized by persistent blood neutrophilia and frequent *CSF3R* gene mutations (37).

Targeted therapy for *BCR::ABL1*-negative MPNs is less well developed than their positive counterpart (27, 38-40). Ruxolitinib is the first JAK2 inhibitor that was approved by FDA to treat intermediate or high-risk PMF with improvement in survival. Unfortunately, chronic therapy with ruxolitinib has not led to pathologic or molecular remission in the majority of PMF patients in contrast to ABL TKIs for CML, and progression to acute leukemia was not significantly decreased. More recently, another JAK2 inhibitor pacritinib received FDA approval for the treatment of intermediate or high-risk primary or secondary myelofibrosis with low platelet counts with reduction of splenomegaly and improvement of marrow fibrosis (41). More experimental drugs targeting JAK2 are currently under investigation (Table 19.2).

19.4 Myelodysplastic/Myeloproliferative Neoplasms

Myelodysplastic/myeloproliferative neoplasms (MDS/MPNs) are a group of clonal myeloid disorders with both dysplastic and proliferative features that cannot be properly classified as either MDS or MPN. This category includes chronic myelomonocytic leukemia (CMML), MDS/MPN with thrombocytosis and *SF3B1* mutation, atypical CML or MDS/MPN with neutrophilia, and MDS/MPN not otherwise specified (42) (Tables 19.1 and 19.6).

CMML is the prototypic and most common MDS/MPN (42). It mainly affects older people with a median age of 65–75 years and a mild male predominance of 1.5–3.1. CMML is characterized by absolute (> 0.5 × 10^9/L) and relative (> 10%) persistent blood monocytosis (> 3 months) and fewer than 20% blasts in the blood or bone marrow. Anemia and thrombocytopenia are usually present. Recurrent somatic mutations have been identified in the genes of most CMML patients, which include genes of signal transduction pathways, such as *NRAS*, *KRAS*, *JAK2*, and *SETBP1*, genes of epigenetic regulators such as *TET2* and *ASXL1*, splicing factors, such as *SRSF2*, and genes of transcription factors such as *RUNX1* (42). The most detected mutations are *TET2*, *SRSF2*, *ASXL1*, and *RUNX1* (43). Some of these mutations are risk predictors (44).

There is little information about targeted therapy for patients with CMML. Hydroxyurea has been used to treat CMML patients with worsening leukocytosis, thrombocytosis, or splenomegaly. Azacitidine, inhibitor of the DNA methyltransferase, has also been approved by FDA for treatment of CMML largely based on clinical trials for MDS. Bone marrow or stem cell transplantation appears to be the only potential curative treatment for CMML. A few patients may respond to small molecule inhibitors targeting FLT3 and IDH (43).

MDS/MPN with thrombocytosis and *SF3B1* mutation frequently harbors *JAK2* V617F mutation. JAK2 inhibitor ruxolitinib may be of benefit. Recently, the FDA approved luspatercept to treat anemia in patients with MDS/MPN with ring sideroblasts and thrombocytosis (www.fda.gov/drugs/resources-

TABLE 19.5

Classification of Myeloproliferative Neoplasms

Classification	Driver Genes	Implicated Signaling Pathways
***BCR::ABL1*-positive myeloproliferative neoplasm**	*BCR::ABL1*	Tyrosine kinase
Chronic myeloid leukemia		
***BCR::ABL1*-negative myeloproliferative neoplasms**		
Polycythemia vera	*JAK2* V617F and exon 12	Tyrosine kinase
Essential thrombocythemia	*JAK2* V617F, *MPAL*, and *CALR*	Tyrosine kinase
Primary myelofibrosis	*JAK2* V617F, *MPAL*, and *CALR*	Tyrosine kinase
Chronic neutrophilic leukemia	*CSF3R*	Tyrosine kinase
Chronic eosinophilic leukemia	Not specified	Not specified
Juvenile myelomonocytic leukemia	*RAS*	RAS signaling pathways
Myeloproliferative neoplasm, not otherwise specified (WHO) or unclassifiable (ICC*)	Not specified	Not specified

*ICC, International Consensus Classification; WHO, World Health Organization classification 5th edition.

TABLE 19.6

Classification of Myelodysplastic/Myeloproliferative Neoplasms

Classification	Driver Genes	Implicated Signaling Pathways
Chronic myelomonocytic leukemia	*TET2, DNMT3A, ASXL1, EZH2, SRSF2, SF3B1, U2AF1, ZRSR2, NRAS, KRAS, CBL, PTPN11, JAK2, SETBP1, RUNX1*	Mutations affecting epigenetic regulation of transcription through DNA methylation (*TET2, DNMT3A*) and histone modification (*ASXL1, EZH2*), RNA splicing (*SRSF2, SF3B1, U2AF1, ZRSR2*), and signal transduction (*NRAS, KRAS, CBL, PTPN11, JAK2*), as well as transcription factors and nucleosome assembly (*SETBP1, RUNX1*).
MDS/MPN with neutrophilia (ICC* = atypical chronic myeloid leukemia)	*ETNK1* *SETBP1*	ETNK1 mutations result in relative depletion of phosphoethanolamine, a negative regulator of mitochondrial complex II, which causes increased reactive oxygen species (ROS) production and mutagenesis. SETBP1 mutations destroy a degron and stabilize the protein, which forms a multimeric complex (with HCF1/KMT2A/PHF8) to modulate gene transcription and histone modification.
MDS/MPN with *SF3B1* mutation and thrombocytosis	*SF3B1* Concurrent mutations include *JAK2* V617F in ~50% of cases, *TET2, ASXL1, DNMT3A, SETBP1, SRSF2, U2AF1, ZRSR2, EZH2, IDH2, ETV6, RUNX1, CBL, CALR*, and *MPL*	Spliceosome complex affecting RNA splicing along with many other pathways.
MDS/MPN, NOS	*JAK2* V617F, *MPL*, and *CALR*	Tyrosine kinase or tyroeine kinase receptor.

Note: *ICC, International Consensus Classification; WHO, World Health Organization 5th edition.

information-approved-drugs/fda-approves-luspatercept-aamt-anemia-adults-mds).

Atypical CML (ICC) or MDS/MPN with neutrophilia (WHO 5th edition) is characterized by dysplastic granulocytic proliferation without Philadelphia chromosome or *BCR::ABL1* gene fusion. No targeted treatment is available.

19.5 Acute Myeloid Leukemias

Acute myeloid leukemia (AML) represents a heterogeneous group of myeloid malignancies with maturation arrest and frequently increased blasts (3, 45) (Table 19.1). AML has been traditionally defined by establishing the myeloid lineage phenotype and further the resemblance to closest normal counterpart cell type (granulocytic, monocytic, erythroid, or megakaryocytic) if applicable. Immature cells (myeloblasts, monoblasts/promonocytes, and megakaryoblasts) must be >= 20% of nucleated marrow cells. However, this important but apparently subjective (based on visual inspection of blasts) morphologic criterion was first waived to be secondary to the presence of recurrent genetic abnormalities in WHO classification 2008. The following cytogenetic abnormalities, t(8;21), inv(16)/t(16;16), and t(15;17), were considered sufficient for the diagnosis of AML regardless of blast count. These cytogenetic abnormalities objectively establish the diagnosis of AML, and this list has been further expanded in the current WHO 5th edition and ICC classifications to include additional cytogenetic abnormalities and gene mutations (Table 19.7). The current WHO 5th edition and ICC classifications emphasize the importance of genetic abnormalities in AML. ICC went further to remove the various entities defined by morphology or differentiation, such as acute erythroid leukemia, since many of them could be classified based on the recurrent genetic abnormalities or as AML with myelodysplasia-related gene mutations or cytogenetic abnormalities, or AML, not otherwise specified.

These genetic abnormalities are not only important in the diagnosis and classification of AML, but also provide relevant prognostic information for risk stratification and disease management. According to the current European Leukemia Network (ELN) guidelines (46), t(8;21)(q22;q22.1)/*RUNX1::RUNX1T1*, inv(16)(p13.1q22) or t(16;16)(p13.1;q22)/*CBFB::MYH11*, bZIP in-frame mutated *CEBPA*, and mutated *NPM1* without *FLT3*-ITD are considered favorable genetic abnormalities. The presence of t(6;9)(p22.3;q34.1)/*DEK::NUP214*, t(v;11q23.3)/*KMT2A*-rearranged, t(9;22)(q34.1;q11.2)/*BCR::ABL1*, inv(3)(q21q26.2)/t(3;3)(q21;q26.2)/*MECOM* rearranged, -5 or del(5q), -7, -17/abnormal 17p, complex karyotype, monosomal karyotype and mutated *ASXL1, BCOR, EZH2, SF3B1, SRSF2, STAG2, U2AF1, ZRSR2, TP53* confers a poor prognosis. Mutated or wild-type *NPM1* with *FLT3*-ITD mutation is now considered an intermediate risk factor that also includes cytogenetic and/or molecular abnormalities not classified as either favorable or adverse , except for t(9;11)(p21.3;q23.3)/*MLLT3::KMT2A* that belongs to the intermediate risk category..

All trans retinoid acid (ATRA) and arsenic trioxide have been successfully used to treat acute promyelocytic leukemia with *PML::RARA*, an example of precise pathology in the targeted therapy for AML. With the discovery of driver mutations in AML, various small molecule inhibitors have been approved by FDA or are under investigation to treat newly diagnosed or relapsed refractory AMLs (4, 47, 48) (Table 19.2). Midostaurin was the first small molecule targeting *FLT3* mutation approved by the FDA in April 2017 to treat *FLT3*-mutated AML in combination with the standard chemotherapy. Subsequently, the FDA has approved a series of other drugs targeting IDH1/2, BCL2, SMO, and CD33 to treat newly diagnosed or relapsed refractory AMLs (49-51). It is

TABLE 19.7

Classification of Acute Myeloid Leukemia

AML with Defining Genetic Abnormalities (WHO)	Karyotype and/or Mutated Genes	Blast Count (WHO)	Blast Count (ICC*)
Acute promyelocytic leukemia (APL) with *PML::RARA* fusion (ICC*)	t(15;17)(q24.1;q21.2)	No cut-off (it could be < 20%)	≥ 10%
AML with *RUNX1::RUNX1T1* fusion	t(8;21)(q22;q22.1)	No cut-off (it could be < 20%)	≥ 10%
AML with *CBFB::MYH11* fusion	inv(16)(p13.1q22)/t(16;16)(p13.1;q22)	No cut-off (it could be < 20%)	≥ 10%
AML with *DEK::NUP214* fusion	t(6;9)(p22.3;q34.1)	No cut-off (it could be < 20%)	
AML (acute Megakaryoblastic leukemia) with *RBM15::MRTFA* fusion	t(1;22)(p13;q13)	No cut-off (it could be < 20%)	≥ 10%
AML with *BCR::ABL1* fusion	t(9;22)(q34.1;q11.2)	≥20%	≥ 20%
AML with *KMT2A* rearrangement	11q23.3 rearrangements. *KMT2A* with various fusion partners	No cut-off (it could be < 20%)	≥ 10%
AML with *MECOM* rearrangement	inv(3)(q21q26.2)/t(3;3)(q21;q26.2) [*RPN1::EVI1*]	No cut-off (it could be < 20%)	≥ 10%
AML with *NUP98* rearrangement	11p15.4 rearrangements. *NUP98* with various fusion partners	No cut-off (it could be < 20%)	≥ 10%
AML with *NPM1* mutation	Usually associated with normal karyotype	No cut-off (it could be < 20%)	≥ 10%
AML with *CEBPA* mutation	No specific abnormalities	≥ 20%	≥ 10%
AML, myelodysplasia-related (ICC*)	Complex karyotype (≥ 3 abnormalities), 5q deletion or loss of 5q, monosomy 7, 7q deletion, or loss of 7q due to unbalanced translocation, 11q deletion, 12p deletion or loss of 12p due to unbalanced translocation, monosomy 13 or 13q deletion, 17p deletion or loss of 17p due to unbalanced translocation, isochromosome 17q, and idic(X)(q13). Defining somatic mutations: *ASXL1*, *BCOR*, *EZH2*, *SF3B1*, *SRSF2*, *STAG2*, *U2AF1*, and *ZRSR2* (WHO) plus *RUNX1* (ICC)	≥ 20%	≥ 20%
AML with other defined genetic alterations (Emerging or provisional AML subtypes with distinct genetic features: AML with *RUNX1T3(CBFA2T3)::GLIS2*, AML with *KAT6A::CREBBP*, AML with *FUS::ERG*, AML with *MNX1::ETV6*, and AML with *NPM1::MLF1*	inv(16)(p13.3 q24), t(8;16)(p11.2;p13.3), t(16;21)(p11;q22), t(7;12)(q36;p13), t(3;5)(q25;q35)	≥ 20%	≥ 10%
AML, defined by differentiation			
AML with minimal differentiation	No defining genetic abnormalities mentioned above	≥ 20%	
AML without maturation		≥ 20%	
AML with maturation		≥20%	
Acute basophilic leukemia		≥ 20% with increased immature and mature basophils	
Acute myelomonocytic leukemia		≥ 20% (blasts and blast equivalents/promonocytes)	
Acute monocytic leukemia		≥ 20% (blasts and blast equivalents/promonocytes) and ≥ 80% of leukemic cells are monocytic	
Acute erythroid leukemia (ICC*)		≥ 80% erythroid cells with ≥ 30% erythroblasts	
Acute megakaryoblastic leukemia		≥ 20% blasts with megakaryocytic differentiation	
Myeloid sarcoma	Any	N/A	N/A

Note: APL with other *RARA* rearrangements (≥ 10%) including t(1;17)(q42.3;q21.2)/*IRF2BP2::RARA*; t(5;17) (q35.1;q21.2)/*NPM1::RARA*; t(11;17) (q23.2;q21.2)/*ZBTB16::RARA*; cryptic inv(17q) or del(17) (q21.2q21.2)/*STAT5B::RARA*, *STAT3::RARA*; other genes rarely rearranged with *RARA:TBL1XR1* (3q26.3), *FIP1L1* (4q12), *BCOR* (Xp11.4) (6). Acute erythroid leukemia is commonly associated with *TP53* mutation and therefore is classified according to ICC as AML with *TP53* mutation. Acute myeloid leukemia myelodysplasia-related is divided in ICC classification to AML with myelodysplasia-related gene mutations and myelodysplasia-related cytogenetic abnormalities.

*ICC, International Consensus Classification

now mandatory to test for these mutations or biomarker expression in the clinical laboratory for AML targeted therapy.

Morphological examination of blood and/or bone marrow aspirate smear is the initial step in the diagnostic workup for AML to enumerate blast percentage and detect clues for possible association with the recurrent genetic abnormalities or underlying gene mutations (Figures 19.4A and 19.5A). Multiparameter flow cytometry is essential to assign lineage of the blasts and to differentiate the morphologic mimics of myeloblasts (Figure 19.4B). It may also provide some clue to the underlying genetic abnormalities. However, various genetic and molecular tests are required to confirm the suspected chromosome abnormalities and/or gene mutations that are critical for genetic subclassification of AML (Figure 19.4C and Figures 19.5B and C). Figure 19.6 summaries the current approach to the diagnostic workup for AML according to WHO HAEM5.

19.6 Myeloid/Lymphoid Neoplasms with Eosinophilia and Tyrosine Kinase Gene Fusions

This category includes several entities with specific tyrosine kinase gene fusions involving *PDGFRA*, *PGDFRB*, *JAK2*, *FLT3*, *ABL1*, and other rare ones (52) (Table 19.8). These gene fusions result in constitutive activation of the specific tyrosine kinases, leading to cell signaling dysregulation and increased cell proliferation and survival. Eosinophilia is frequently but not invariably present. Their initial clinical and morphological presentations resemble a variety of reactive conditions and hematolymphoid neoplasms, such as MPN, MDS/MPN, CEL and lymphoblastic leukemia/lymphomas with or without eosinophilia. They should be differentiated from their morphologic mimics, particularly when eosinophilia is present (Figure 19.7) (3, 53).

Most myeloid/lymphoid neoplasms with *PDGFRA* have cytogenetically cryptic chromosome 4q12 deletion resulting in *FIP1L1::PDGFRA* gene fusion, evading its detection by routine chromosome analysis. Therefore, FISH or microarray should be performed to identify this abnormality in the diagnostic workup. The majority of myeloid/lymphoid neoplasms with *PDGFRB* have t(5;12)(q32;p13.2) leading to *ETV6::PDGFRB* gene fusion. Cases with *FGFR1* rearrangement typically have t(8;13)(p11.2;q12.1) with *ZMYM2::FGFR1* gene fusion and may present as chronic myeloid neoplasms or blast phase disease typically associated with eosinophilia.

Targeted therapy with TKIs, particularly imatinib, has dramatically altered the natural history of myeloid/lymphoid neoplasm with *PDGFRA/B* gene fusions, and most patients have excellent response (54). Patients with *FGFR1* gene fusion also respond well to FGFR inhibitors such as pemigatinib, which was approved by the FDA in August 2022.

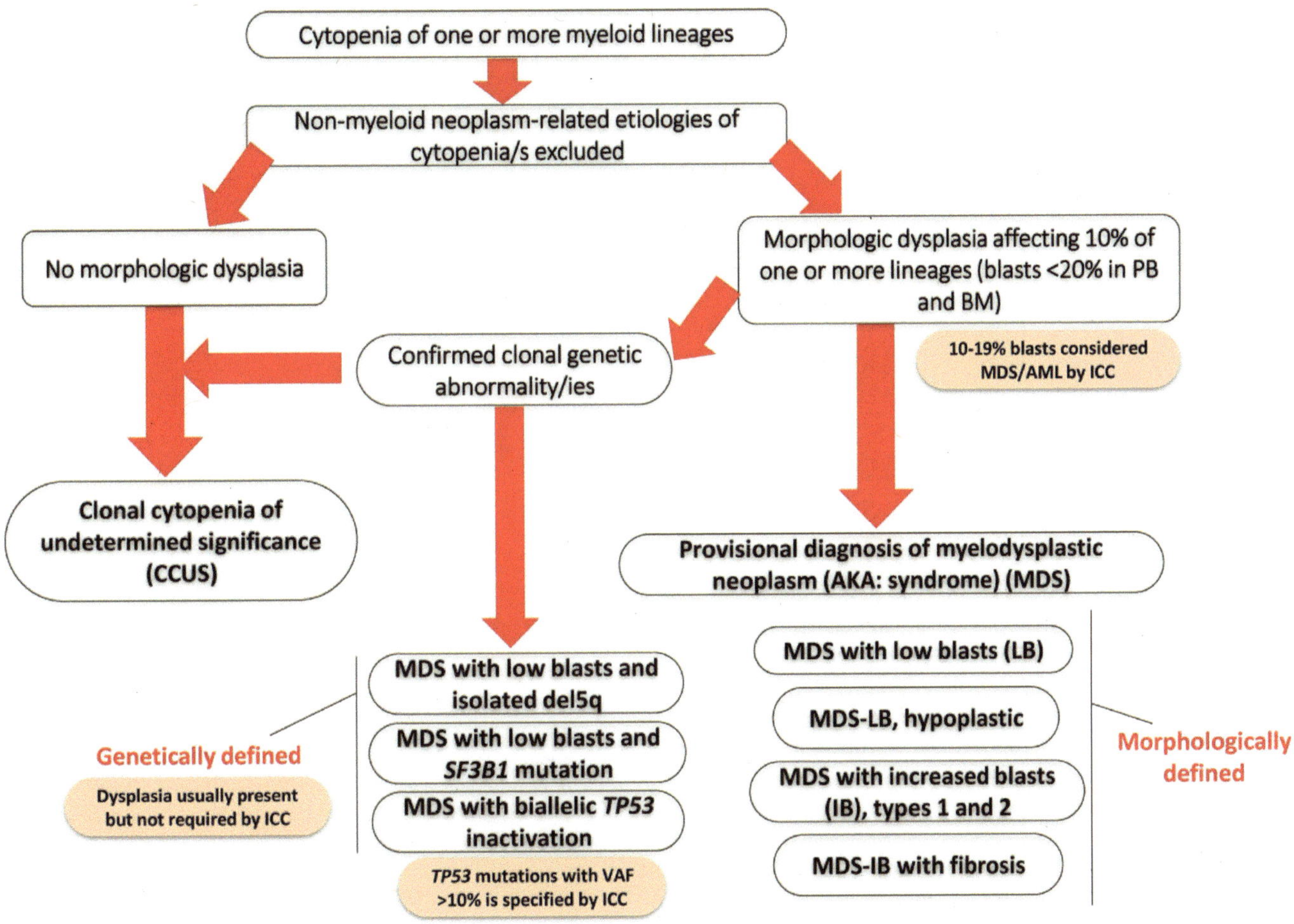

FIGURE 19.3 MDS diagnostic algorithm.

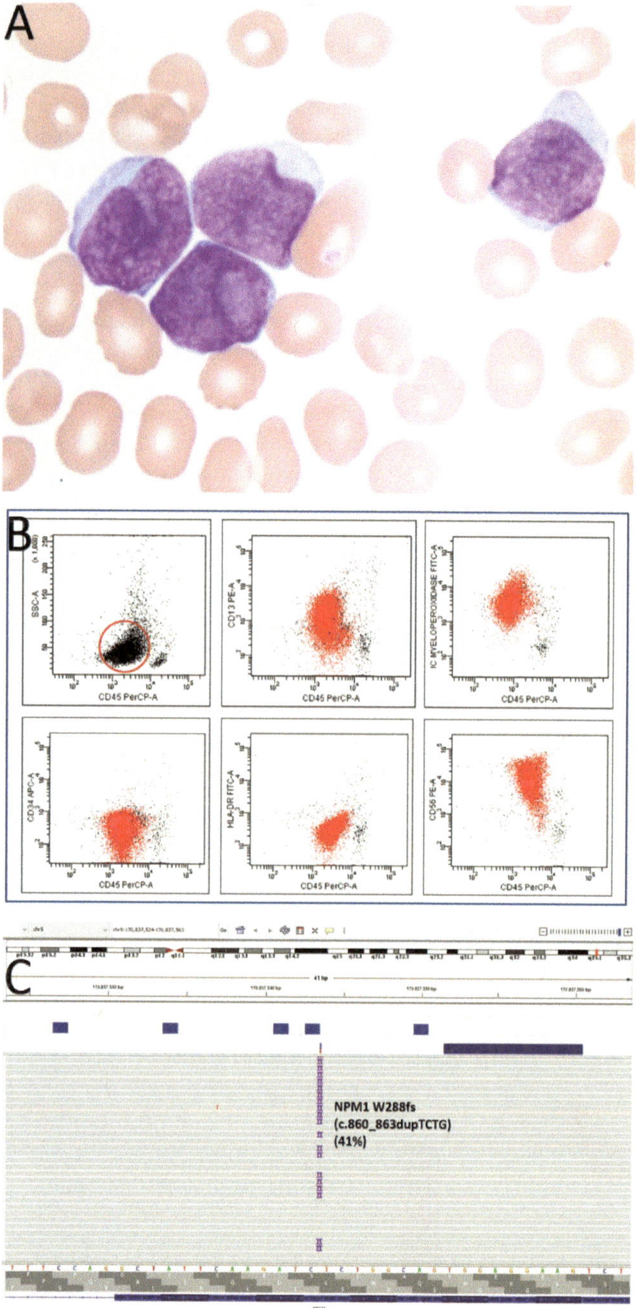

FIGURE 19.4 AML with normal cytogenetics and *NPM1* mutation. (A) Wright-Giemsa-stained blood smear shows myeloblasts with cup-like or fish-mouth-like nuclear morphology. (B) Flow cytometry shows a prominent population of myeloblasts that are negative for CD34 and HLA-DR with aberrant expression of CD56. (C) NGS analysis shows Type-A *NPM1* frameshift mutation.

Patients with other gene fusions have variable responses to TKIs and require bone marrow transplantation for long-term survival.

19.7 Mastocytosis

Mastocytosis encompasses a group of clonal and indolent to aggressive proliferation of mast cells with localized or systemic involvement, including bone marrow (52) (Figures 19.8A–C).

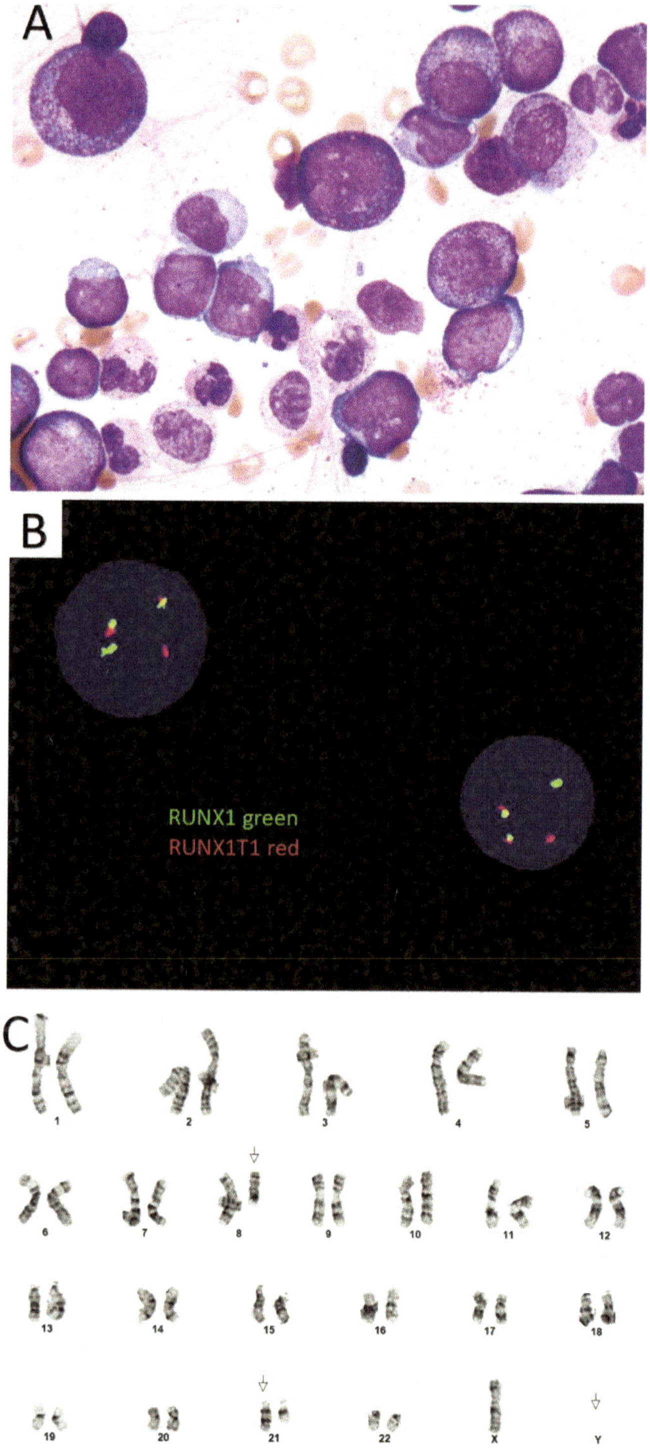

FIGURE 19.5 AML with t(8;21)/*RUNX1::RUNX1T1*. (A) Wright-Giemsa-stained bone marrow aspirate smear shows increased myeloblasts with maturation. (B) FISH shows the presence of *RUNX1::RUNX1T1* gene fusion. (C) Chromosome analysis shows the presence of a balanced translocation between the long arms of chromosomes 8 and 21 as well as loss of Y chromosome (arrows).

The mast cells may demonstrate degranulation and/or atypical spindle cell morphology and aberrant immunophenotype (Figures 19.8D–F). There are three disease types: systemic mastocytosis (SM), cutaneous mastocytosis (CM), and mast

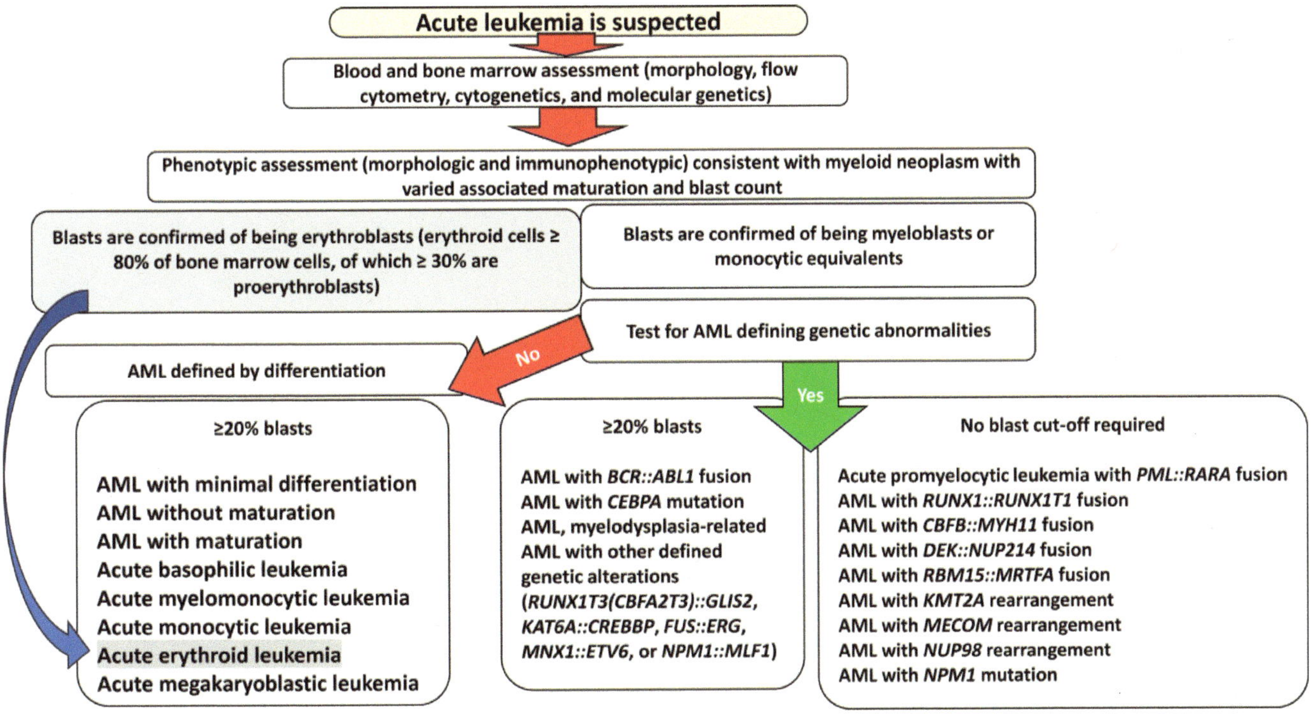

FIGURE 19.6 AML diagnostic algorithm.

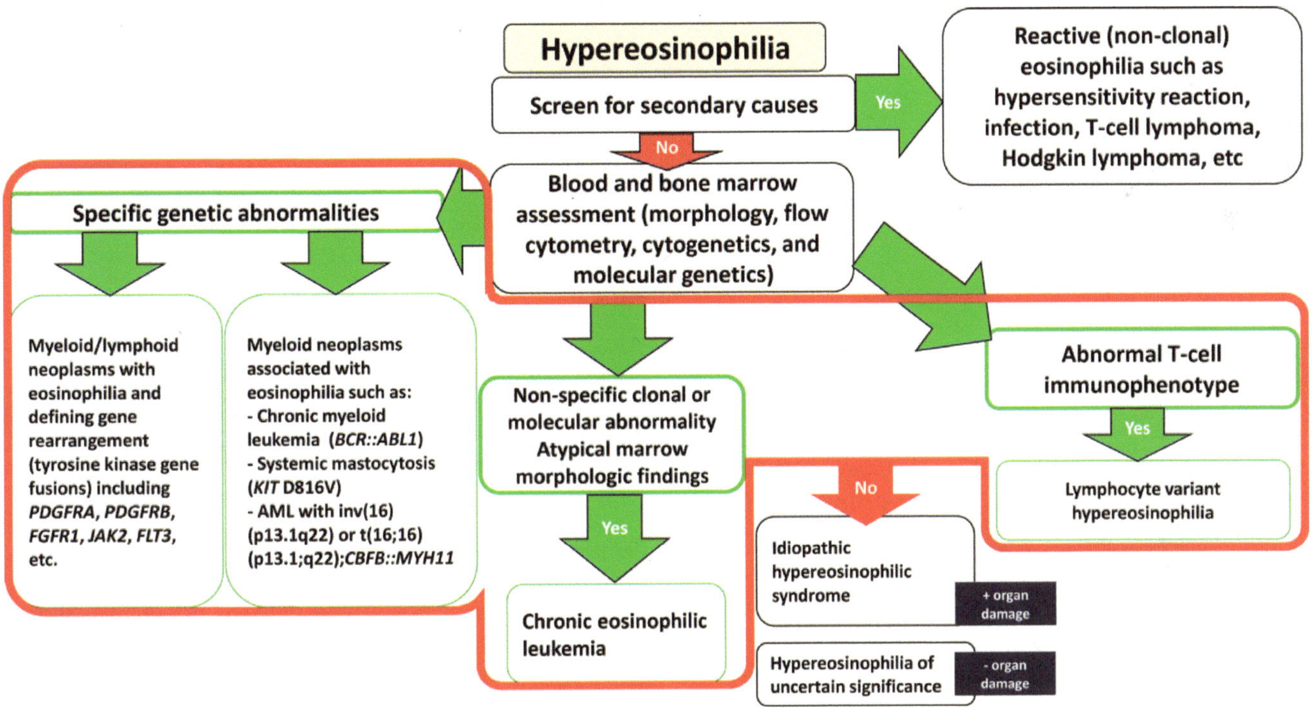

FIGURE 19.7 Hypereosinophilia workup algorithm.

cell sarcoma (MCS). There are five subtypes of SM: indolent, smoldering and aggressive SMs, mast cell leukemia, and SM with an associated myeloid neoplasm (2, 3).

Most SM cases contain a somatic point mutation in the *KIT* gene at codon 816. Other rare KIT mutations have also been identified (55). Avapritinib, a specific inhibitor of KIT with D816V mutation, has been approved by the FDA to treat indolent as well as aggressive SM (41, 56).

19.8 Histiocytic and Dendritic Cell Neoplasms

This disease category includes neoplasms derived from monocytic/histiocytic/dendritic cell lineages. The application of extensive immunophenotyping has reclassified many previously diagnosed histiocytic and dendritic cell neoplasm as either B-cell or T-cell lymphomas (57). Comprehensive

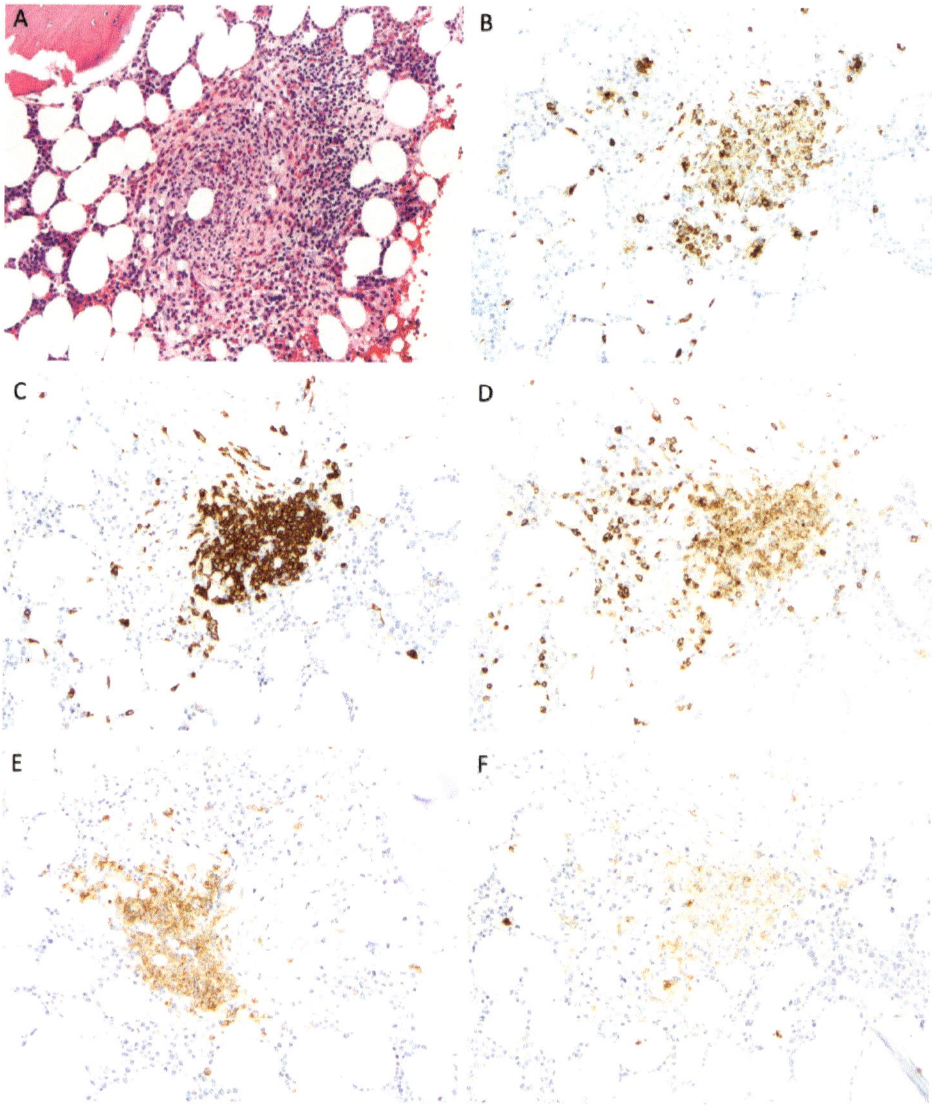

FIGURE 19.8 Systemic mastocytosis involving bone marrow. (A) Bone marrow trephine biopsy shows a large aggregate of typical mast cells with increased eosinophils (H&E stain). Immunohistochemical stains show the atypical mast cells positive for tryptase (B), CD117 (C), CD2 (D), CD25 (E), and CD30 (F).

molecular characterization of these rare tumors also revealed frequent activating mutations in the mitogen-activated protein kinase (MAPK) and the PI3K signaling pathways including *RAF*, *RAS*, *MEK*, and *MTOR* [57, 58]. Small molecule inhibitors targeting those mutations have shown efficacy in patients with these mutations (58, 59).

ALK-positive histiocytosis is a new entity in the current classifications (Figure 19.9A). The neoplastic cells have a mature histiocytic phenotype (Figure 19.9B) and often demonstrate foamy cytoplasm and overexpress ALK (Figure 19.9C) owing to *ALK* rearrangements. The most common fusion partner is the *KIR5B* (Figure 19.9D). Patients with ALK-positive histiocytosis respond well to ALK inhibitors such as lorlatinib or crizotinib, and some patients achieve long-term remission following crizotinib treatment (60, 61).

19.9 Testing Strategies

For precision diagnosis and classification of myeloid neoplasms and to provide prognostic and therapeutic target information, fresh blood, bone marrow, and/or tissue biopsy samples should be comprehensively analyzed using an integrated approach that includes morphology, immunophenotyping, and genetic/genomic testing. Cytomorphology and histomorphological examination should be performed on well-stained smear and tissue sections for assessment of dysplasia, blast count, and other features associated with the various myeloid neoplasms such as eosinophilia or basophilia. Comprehensive immunophenotyping should be performed using multiparameter flow cytometry if possible. Immunohistochemical and special stains are also important for assessment of immaturity and fibrosis, respectively, particularly when fresh sample is not available.

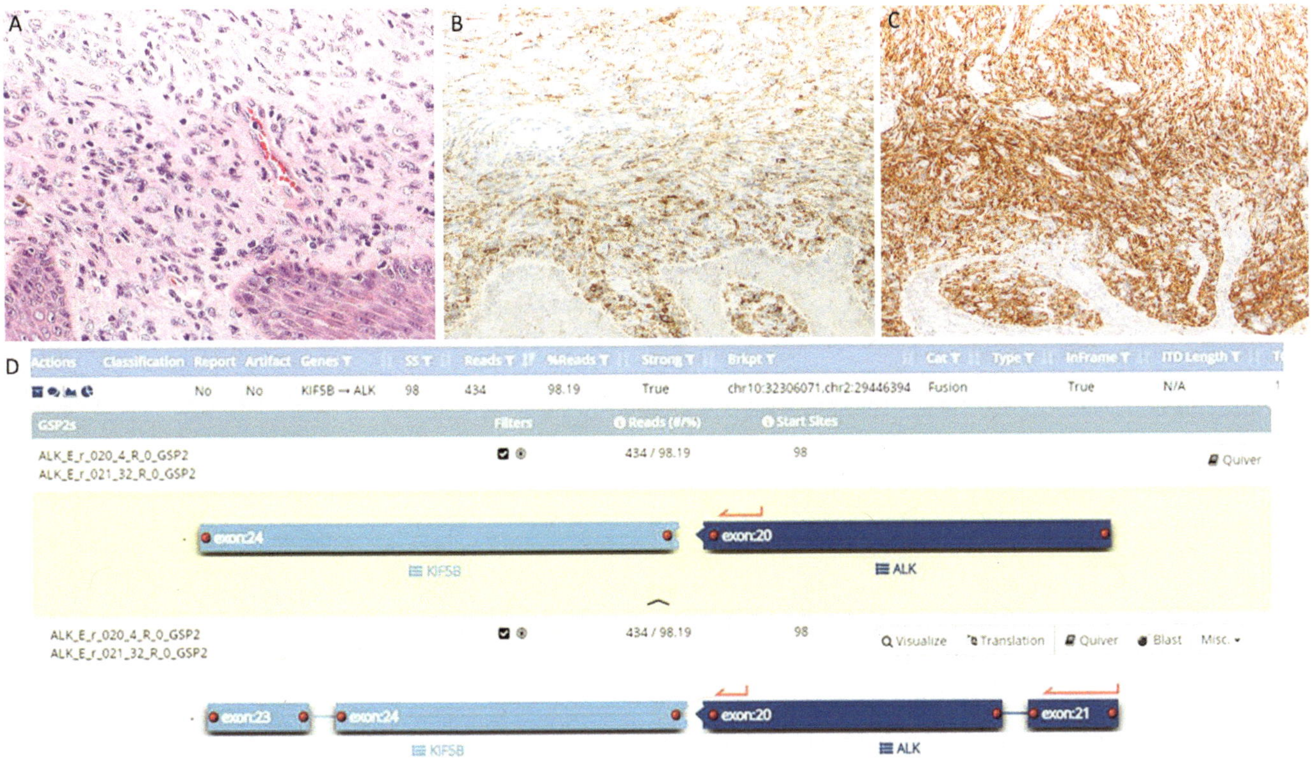

FIGURE 19.9 ALK-positive histiocytosis. (A) Skin biopsy section (H&E stain) shows a diffuse dermal infiltrate by atypical histiocytic cells that are positive for CD68 (B) and ALK(C) by immunohistochemical stains. NGS shows the classical *KIF5B::ALK* gene fusion (D).

TABLE 19.8

Classification of Myeloid/Lymphoid Neoplasms with Eosinophilia and Tyrosine Kinase Gene Fusions

Classification	Driver Genes	Implicated Signaling Pathways
Myeloid/lymphoid neoplasm with *PDGFRA* rearrangement	*PDGFRA*	Tyrosine kinase receptor
Myeloid/lymphoid neoplasm with *PDGFRB* rearrangement	*PDGFRB*	Tyrosine kinase receptor
Myeloid/lymphoid neoplasm with *FGFR1* rearrangement	*FGFR1*	Tyrosine kinase receptor
Myeloid/lymphoid neoplasm with *JAK2* rearrangement	*JAK2*	Tyrosine kinase receptor
Myeloid/lymphoid neoplasm with *FLT3* rearrangement	*FLT3*	Tyrosine kinase receptor
Myeloid/lymphoid neoplasm with *ETV6::ABL1* fusion	*ETV6::ABL1*	Tyrosine kinase receptor
Myeloid/lymphoid neoplasms with other tyrosine kinase gene fusions	*ETV6::FGFR2*; *ETV6::LYN*; *ETV6::NTRK3*; *RANBP2::ALK*; *BCR::RET*, and *FGFR1OP::RET*	Tyrosine kinases or tyrosine kinase receptors

Cytogenetics and FISH or PCR should be routinely performed to detect disease-defining cytogenetic abnormalities according to the current classifications. Targeted NGS with a panel of genes should also be routinely employed for analysis of the common driver gene mutations to provide diagnostic and prognostic information and state-of-the-art therapeutic targets. Other advanced molecular diagnostic technologies such as microarray, optical genome mapping, whole exome, transcriptome, or genome sequencing could be employed for rare difficult cases. An integrated pathology report should include the diagnostic, prognostic, and therapeutic information for the individual patient and the treating physician.

19.10 Summary

Myeloid neoplasms encompass a spectrum of hematopoietic stem cell disorders, ranging from precursor clonal hematopoiesis to myelodysplastic and/or myeloproliferative neoplasms to overt acute leukemias. In the last several decades, technological advances have greatly increased our knowledge of normal hematopoiesis and the understanding of the underlying pathobiology of myeloid neoplasms. These advancements have refined the diagnostic criteria and classification of myeloid neoplasms, provided biomarker information for prognosis and precise targeted therapy, and improved the treatment outcome of patients with these neoplasms.

REFERENCES

1. Solary E, Khoury JD and Campbell P. Myelodysplastic neoplasms. 5th ed. WHO Classification of Tumours Editorial Board. Haematolymphoid Tumours [Internet; beta version ahead of print]. Vol. 11. 2022, Lyon, France: International Agency for Research on Cancer.
2. Arber DA, Orazi A, Hasserjian RP, et al. International Consensus Classification of Myeloid Neoplasms and Acute Leukemias: Integrating Morphologic, Clinical, and Genomic Data. Blood. 2022; 140(11): 1200–1228.
3. Khoury JD, Solary E, Abla O, et al. The 5th Edition of the World Health Organization Classification of Haematolymphoid Tumours: Myeloid and Histiocytic/Dendritic Neoplasms. Leukemia. 2022; 36(7): 1703–1719.
4. Wang J, Tomlinson B and Lazarus HM. Update on Small Molecule Targeted Therapies for Acute Myeloid Leukemia. Curr Treat Options Oncol. 2023; 24(7): 770–801.
5. Bhansali RS, Pratz KW and Lai C. Recent Advances in Targeted Therapies in Acute Myeloid Leukemia. J Hematol Oncol. 2023; 16(1): 29.
6. Rodriguez-Sevilla JJ, Adema V, Garcia-Manero G, et al. Emerging Treatments for Myelodysplastic Syndromes: Biological Rationales and Clinical Translation. Cell Rep Med. 2023; 4(2): 100940.
7. Cazzola M. Myelodysplastic Syndromes. N Engl J Med. 2020; 383(14): 1358–1374.
8. Tefferi A and Vardiman JW. Myelodysplastic Syndromes. N Engl J Med. 2009; 361(19): 1872–1885.
9. Rotter LK, Shimony S, Ling K, et al. Epidemiology and Pathogenesis of Myelodysplastic Syndrome. Cancer J. 2023; 29(3): 111–121.
10. Valent P, Orazi A, Steensma DP, et al. Proposed Minimal Diagnostic Criteria for Myelodysplastic Syndromes (MDS) and Potential Pre-MDS Conditions. Oncotarget. 2017; 8(43): 73483–73500.
11. Porwit A, Béné, MC, Duetz C, et al. Multiparameter Flow Cytometry in the Evaluation of Myelodysplasia: Analytical Issues: Recommendations from the European LeukemiaNet/ International Myelodysplastic Syndrome Flow Cytometry Working Group. Cytometry B Clin Cytom. 2023; 104(1): 27–50.
12. Bejar R, Stevenson K, Abdel-Wahab O, et al. Clinical Effect of Point Mutations in Myelodysplastic Syndromes. N Engl J Med. 2011; 364(26): 2496–2506.
13. Papaemmanuil E, Gerstung M, Malcovati L, et al. Clinical and Biological Implications of Driver Mutations in Myelodysplastic Syndromes. Blood. 2013; 122(22): 3616–3627.
14. Haferlach T, Nagata Y, Grossmann V, et al. Landscape of Genetic Lesions in 944 Patients with Myelodysplastic Syndromes. Leukemia. 2014; 28(2): 241–247.
15. Beck DB, Ferrada MA, Sikora KA, et al. Somatic Mutations in UBA1 and Severe Adult-Onset Autoinflammatory Disease. N Engl J Med. 2020; 383(27): 2628–2638.
16. Shuai W, Zuo Z, Li N, et al. ETNK1 Mutation Occurs in a Wide Spectrum of Myeloid Neoplasms and Is Not Specific for Atypical Chronic Myeloid Leukemia. Cancer. 2023; 129(6): 878–889.
17. Sperling AS, Gibson CJ and Ebert BL. The Genetics of Myelodysplastic Syndrome: From Clonal Haematopoiesis to Secondary Leukaemia. Nat Rev Cancer. 2017; 17(1): 5–19.
18. Duncavage EJ, Bagg A, Hasserjian RP, et al. Genomic Profiling for Clinical Decision Making in Myeloid Neoplasms and Acute Leukemia. Blood. 2022; 140(21): 2228–2247.
19. Aguirre LE, Al Ali N, Sallman DA, et al. Assessment and Validation of the Molecular International Prognostic Scoring System for Myelodysplastic Syndromes. Leukemia. 2023; 37(7): 1530–1539.
20. Sauta E, Robin M, Bersanelli M, et al. Real-World Validation of Molecular International Prognostic Scoring System for Myelodysplastic Syndromes. J Clin Oncol. 2023; 41(15): 2827–2842.
21. Lee WH, Tsai M-T, Tsai C-H, et al. Validation of the Molecular International Prognostic Scoring System in Patients with Myelodysplastic Syndromes Defined by International Consensus Classification. Blood Cancer J. 2023; 13(1): 120.
22. Kewan T, Bahaj W, Durmaz A, et al. *Validation of the Molecular International Prognostic Scoring System in Patients with Myelodysplastic Syndromes*. Blood. 2023; 141(14): 1768–1772.
23. Hoff FW and Madanat YF. Molecular Drivers of Myelodysplastic Neoplasms (MDS)-Classification and Prognostic Relevance. Cells. 2023; 12(4): 627.
24. Zamanillo I, Poza M, Ayala R, et al. Impact of IPSS-M Implementation in Real-Life Clinical Practice. Front Oncol. 2023; 13: 1199023.
25. Sebert M. Next-Generation Therapy for Lower-Risk MDS. Hematology Am Soc Hematol Educ Prog. 2023; 2023(1): 59–64.
26. DiNardo CD, Venugopal S, Lachowiez C, et al. Targeted Therapy with the Mutant IDH2 Inhibitor Enasidenib for High-Risk IDH2-Mutant Myelodysplastic Syndrome. Blood Adv. 2023; 7(11): 2378–2387.
27. Pagliuca S, Gurnari C and Visconte V. Molecular Targeted Therapy in Myelodysplastic Syndromes: New Options for Tailored Treatments. Cancers (Basel). 2021; 13(4): 784.
28. Maggioni G and Della Porta MG. Molecular Landscape of Myelodysplastic Neoplasms in Disease Classification and Prognostication. Curr Opin Hematol. 2023. 30(2): 30–37.
29. Platzbecker U. Treatment of MDS. Blood. 2019; 133(10): 1096–1107.
30. Singh A, Al-Kali A, Foran JM, et al. Lenalidomide Therapy for Primary Myelodysplastic Syndromes with Isolated Del(5q): Determinants of Response and Survival in a Real-World Setting. Am J Hematol. 2022; 97(10): E377–E379.
31. Deeb G and Papadantonakis N. Immunotherapies for Myelodysplastic Syndromes: Current State and Future Developments. Erciyes Med J. 2022; 44(3): 245–251.
32. Thiele J, Kvasnicka HM, Orazi A, et al. The International Consensus Classification of Myeloid Neoplasms and Acute Leukemias: Myeloproliferative Neoplasms. Am J Hematol. 2023; 98(1): 166–179.
33. Mikhaeel S and Atallah E. SOHO State of the Art Updates and Next Questions | Update on Treatment-Free Remission in Chronic Myeloid Leukemia (CML). Clin Lymphoma Myeloma Leuk. 2023; 23(5): 333–339.
34. Hochhaus A, Larson RA, Guilhot F, et al. Long-Term Outcomes of Imatinib Treatment for Chronic Myeloid Leukemia. N Engl J Med. 2017; 376(10): 917–927.
35. Mobius S, Schenk T, Himsel D, et al. Results of the European Survey on the Assessment of Deep Molecular Response in Chronic Phase CML Patients During Tyrosine Kinase Inhibitor Therapy (EUREKA Registry). J Cancer Res Clin Oncol. 2019; 145(6): 1645–1650.
36. Lagana A, Pepe S, Scalzulli E, et al. One-Month qRT-PCR BCR::ABL1 Transcript Threshold to Predict Early Recurrence in Chronic Phase CML Patients Attempting First Treatment Free Remission. Eur J Haematol. 2023; 111(6): 970–972.

37. Szuber N, Finke CM, Lasho TL, et al. CSF3R-Mutated Chronic Neutrophilic Leukemia: Long-Term Outcome in 19 Consecutive Patients and Risk Model for Survival. Blood Cancer J. 2018; 8(2): 21.
38. Harrison N, Nangalia J, Boucher R, et al. Ruxolitinib Versus Best Available Therapy for Polycythemia Vera Intolerant or Resistant to Hydroxycarbamide in a Randomized Trial. J Clin Oncol. 2023; 41(19): 3534–3544.
39. Alvarez-Larran A, Garrote M, Ferrer-Marin F, et al. Real-World Analysis of Main Clinical Outcomes in Patients with Polycythemia vera Treated with Ruxolitinib or Best Available Therapy after Developing Resistance/Intolerance to Hydroxyurea. Cancer. 2022; 128(13): 2441–2448.
40. Chen EC, Johnston H and Patel AA. Targeted Therapy for MPNs: Going Beyond JAK Inhibitors. Curr Hematol Malig Rep. 2023; 18(3): 41–55.
41. Lamb YN. Pacritinib: First Approval. Drugs. 2022; 82(7): 831–838.
42. Patnaik MM and Tefferi A. Chronic Myelomonocytic Leukemia: 2022 Update on Diagnosis, Risk Stratification, and Management. Am J Hematol. 2022; 97(3): 352–372.
43. Castano-Diez S, López-Guerra M, Bosch-Castañeda C, et al. Real-World Data on Chronic Myelomonocytic Leukemia: Clinical and Molecular Characteristics, Treatment, Emerging Drugs, and Patient Outcomes. Cancers (Basel). 2022; 14(17): 4107.
44. Elena C, Galli A, Esperanza Such E, et al. Integrating Clinical Features and Genetic Lesions in the Risk Assessment of Patients with Chronic Myelomonocytic Leukemia. Blood. 2016; 128(10): 1408–1417.
45. Khoury JD, Solary E and Gujral S. Acute myeloid leukemia. 5th ed. WHO Classification of Tumours Editorial Board. Haematolymphoid tumours [Internet; beta version ahead of print]. Vol. 11. 2022, Lyon: International Agency for Research on Cancer.
46. Dohner H, Wei AH, Appelbaum FR, et al. Diagnosis and Management of AML in Adults: 2022 Recommendations from an International Expert Panel on Behalf of the ELN. Blood. 2022; 140(12): 1345–1377.
47. Lachowiez CA, DiNardo CD and Loghavi S. Molecularly Targeted Therapy in Acute Myeloid Leukemia: Current Treatment Landscape and Mechanisms of Response and Resistance. Cancers (Basel). 2023; 15(5): 1617.
48. Khanna V, Azenkot T, Liu SQ, et al. Outcomes with Molecularly Targeted Agents as Salvage Therapy Following Frontline Venetoclax + Hypomethylating Agent in Adults with Acute Myeloid Leukemia: A Multicenter Retrospective Analysis. Leuk Res. 2023; 131: 107331.
49. Pommert L and Tarlock K. The Evolution of Targeted Therapy in Pediatric AML: Gemtuzumab Ozogamicin, FLT3/IDH/BCL2 Inhibitors, and Other Therapies. Hematology Am Soc Hematol Educ Program. 2022; 2022(1): 603–610.
50. Kubicka E, Lum LG, Huang M, et al. Bispecific Antibody-Targeted T-Cell Therapy for Acute Myeloid Leukemia. Front Immunol. 2022; 13: 899468.
51. Chi SG and Minami Y. Emerging Targeted Therapy for Specific Genomic Abnormalities in Acute Myeloid Leukemia. Int J Mol Sci. 2022; 23(4): 2362.
52. Wang SA, Orazi A, Gotlib J, et al. The International Consensus Classification of Eosinophilic Disorders and Systemic Mastocytosis. Am J Hematol. 2023; 98(8): 1286–1306.
53. Reiter A and Gotlib J. Myeloid Neoplasms with Eosinophilia. Blood. 2017; 129(6): 704-714.
54. Zhang Y, Nguyen L, Lu CM, et al. Clinical Response to Upfront Targeted Tyrosine Kinase Inhibitors among Patients with Myeloid/Lymphoid Neoplasms with Eosinophilia and Tyrosine Kinase Gene Fusion. Clin Lymphoma Myeloma Leuk. 2023; 23(3): e150–e163.
55. Li JY, Ryder CB, Zhang H, et al. Review and Updates on Systemic Mastocytosis and Related Entities. Cancers (Basel). 2023; 15(23): 5626.
56. Gotlib J, Reiter A and DeAngelo DJ. Avapritinib for Advanced Systemic Mastocytosis. Blood. 2022; 140(15): 1667–1673.
57. Emile JF, Cohen-Aubart F, Collin M, et al. Histiocytosis. Lancet. 2021; 398(10295): 157–170.
58. Diamond EL, Durham BH, Ulaner GA, et al. Efficacy of MEK Inhibition in Patients with Histiocytic Neoplasms. Nature. 2019; 567(7749): 521–524.
59. Shanmugam V, Griffin GK, Jacobsen ED, et al. Identification of Diverse Activating Mutations of the RAS-MAPK Pathway in Histiocytic Sarcoma. Mod Pathol. 2019; 32(6): 830–843.
60. Kemps PG, Picarsic J, Durham BH, et al. ALK-Positive Histiocytosis: A New Clinicopathologic Spectrum Highlighting Neurologic Involvement and Responses to ALK Inhibition. Blood. 2022; 139(2): 256–280.
61. Chang KTE, Tay AZE, Kuick CH, et al. ALK-Positive Histiocytosis: An Expanded Clinicopathologic Spectrum and Frequent Presence of KIF5B-ALK Fusion. Mod Pathol. 2019; 32(5): 598–608.

20

Lymphoid Neoplasms

Xianfeng F. Zhao

20.1 Introduction

Lymphoid neoplasms originate from the lymphoid organs and tissues and are divided mainly into Hodgkin lymphomas (HLs) and non-Hodgkin lymphomas (NHLs) (Table 20.1) (1). Since nodular lymphocyte predominant Hodgkin lymphoma is a *bona fide* B-cell lymphoma, the 2022 International Consensus Classification renamed it "nodular lymphocyte predominant B-cell lymphoma" (2) as an NHL. NHLs consist of B-cell neoplasms, T-cell neoplasms, and NK-cell neoplasms. Compared to NHL, HL is less common and has a much better prognosis and survival rate with the current non-targeted therapies (3), whereas NHL cases are increasing with the escalating environmental risk factors. Based on the 2021 NCI Cancer Statistics, NHL is the sixth leading cause of death in the US and affect 81,560 patients per year (4). The mainstay standard treatment remains chemotherapy with/without radiotherapy or immunotherapy (5). In recent years, novel targeted therapies are playing increasing roles, and this chapter will focus on how pathology labs can assist with the more and more widely used precision therapies for various malignant lymphoid neoplasms.

TABLE 20.1

Simplified Classification of Malignant Lymphoid Neoplasms

Lymphoid Neoplasms	Differentiating Morphological Features
Hodgkin lymphoma (HL)	Rare large Hodgkin-Reed-Sternberg (prominently nucleated) cells in a reactive background and variable fibrosis
Non-Hodgkin lymphoma (NHL)	
B-cell neoplasms	Atypical lymphoid cells with pan-B cell markers
Lymphoblastic leukemia/lymphoma	Lymphoblasts with high N/C ratio, partially naked nuclei, and open chromatin
Indolent B-cell neoplasms	Small mature B-lymphocytes
Chronic lymphocytic leukemia/Small lymphocytic lymphoma	Diffuse with vaguely nodular pattern; soccer ball nuclei with clumped chromatin
Follicular lymphoma (grade 1–3A)	Back-to-back follicular/nodular pattern; loss of mantle zone and marginal zone
Marginal zone lymphoma	Expansion of marginal zone with infiltration of germinal center and disruption of follicular dendritic cell meshwork; has extranodal and splenic variants
Lymphoplasmacytic lymphoma	Diffuse infiltration of plasmacytoid lymphocytes and plasma cells
Hairy cell leukemia	Circulating atypical lymphocytes with enlarged nuclei and cytoplasmic projections
Plasma cell neoplasm	Atypical plasma cells with occasional plasmablasts
Aggressive B-cell neoplasms	Blastoid, pleomorphic (except for Burkitt) lymphoid cells
Mantle cell lymphoma	High N/C ratio with "squared-off" nuclei
Diffuse large B-cell lymphoma (DLBCL), NOS	Predominantly large atypical cells with various sizes, morphology and expression of B-cell markers
Large B-cell lymphoma variants	Large B cells with various expression of B-cell markers, locations, and unique genetic abnormalities
Burkitt lymphoma (BL)	Monotonous population of medium vacuolated lymphoma cells with germinal center B-cell phenotype
Grey zone lymphoma	B-cell lymphoma with overlapping features between HL and NHL, BL and DLBCL, and other different NHLs
T/NK-cell neoplasms	Atypical lymphoid cells with pan-T-cell or NK-cell markers
Indolent T/NK-cell neoplasm	T-cell lymphoproliferative diseases of GI tract

(Continued)

DOI: 10.1201/9781003513469-20

TABLE 20.1 (Continued)

Lymphoid Neoplasms	Differentiating Morphological Features
Aggressive T/NK-cell neoplasms	Medium to large atypical lymphoid cells
Anaplastic large cell lymphoma	Large atypical lymphoid cells with "hallmark" cells
Angioimmunoblastic T-cell lymphoma	Medium atypical lymphoid cells with clear cytoplasm; B immunoblasts often seen
Peripheral T-cell lymphoma, NOS	Not otherwise defined T-cell lymphoma
Adult T-cell leukemia	Circulating atypical lymphoid cells with florid or "butterfly-shaped" nuclei
Enteropathy-associated T-cell lymphoma	Atypical T cells with clear cytoplasm infiltrating small intestinal mucosa
Hepatosplenic T-cell lymphoma	Atypical T cells infiltrating the sinusoids of liver and spleen
Subcutaneous panniculitis T-cell lymphoma	Atypical T cells infiltrating subcutaneous adipose tissue with "rosette" formation
Primary cutaneous T-cell lymphoma	Atypical T cells infiltrating dermis and/or subcutaneous tissue
Aggressive NK-cell neoplasm	Morphologically similar to T-cell lymphoma, but with NK-cell immunophenotype

Source: compiled from refs. 2 and 47.

20.2 Hodgkin Lymphoma

Classic Hodgkin lymphoma is characterized by the proliferation of scattered large, atypical cells with a single to multiple prominent nucleoli, abundant cytoplasm (Hodgkin-Reed-Sternberg (HRS) cells) in a background of reactive small lymphocytes, granulocytes (eosinophils), plasma cells, and bands of sclerosis (Figure 20.1). The HRS cells invariably express CD30, MUM1, and PAX5 (weak). They can also express CD15, CD40, CD80, and CD25 (6). Although they are aborted developing B cells, CD20 expression only occurs in ~20% of the HRS cells and is often weak. These cells usually do not express CD45.

With the effective standardized regimen and good prognosis (3), targeted therapy seems not to be an urgent need for HL. Driven by a better understanding of its biology, targeted therapy becomes an option for HL, particularly in relapsed and refractory diseases (7, 8). As HL is a CD30+ lymphoma, targeting CD30 is a natural therapeutic option. Brentuximab vedotin is a monoclonal antibody against CD30 which may be used along with chemotherapy to treat advanced HL. It is also used to treat relapsed HL that does not respond to a standard regimen (9). HL growth is promoted by immunomodulation involving PD-1 and PD-L1 interaction (10). Therefore, disruption of this immunomodulation is another natural strategy to inhibit the growth of HL cells (8).

20.3 Non-Hodgkin Lymphoma

NHLs refer to all the other lymphoid leukemias/lymphomas except for HLs. Based on the lineages, NHLs are further divided into B-cell neoplasms, T-cell neoplasms, and NK-cell neoplasms (Table 20.1). B-cell lymphomas are classified largely following the ontogeny of B-cell maturation in the lymph node, whereas T-cell lymphomas are named after the organs and tissues where the neoplasms first developed. Compared to B and T cell neoplasms, NK cell neoplasms are much rarer.

20.3.1 B-Cell Neoplasms

B-cell neoplasms are characterized by expression of B-cell specific markers, such as CD19, CD20, CD22, CD79a, and PAX5. CD20 is considered a mature B-cell marker and is often absent on the precursor B cells. Other features include immunoglobulin light chain restriction or even absence of surface immunoglobulin (11). According to their ontogeny and clinical behavior, B-cell lymphomas are largely divided into B-lymphoblastic neoplasms, indolent mature B-cell neoplasms, and aggressive B-cell neoplasms (Figure 20.2).

20.3.1.1 B-lymphoblastic Neoplasms

Most of the B-lymphoblastic neoplasms present as acute lymphoblastic leukemias (80%); only a small fraction (20%) present as B-lymphoblastic lymphomas with a lymphoblastic morphology and precursor B-cell immunophenotype (Figure 20.2A). Both B-lymphoblastic leukemia and lymphoma invariably express at least one of the stem cell markers, such as CD10, CD34, and TdT (12); have a high proliferation index; and are associated with numerous genetic abnormalities (Figure 20.3) (13). Most of these genetic abnormalities make them liable to the current nonspecific chemotherapeutic agents and give them a high cure rate and excellent prognosis in children but not in adults (14). One exception is the B-lymphoblastic leukemia/lymphoma with *BCR::ABL1* genetic abnormalities (15), which can be specifically targeted by tyrosine kinase inhibitors, such as dasatinib. Humanized monoclonal antibodies or CAR-T cells targeting CD19, CD20, and CD22 recently became another option for relapsed diseases (Figure 20.4) (16).

20.3.1.2 Indolent B-Cell Neoplasms

Indolent B-cell neoplasms include biologically transformed immunoglobulin-producing mature B cell leukemias/lymphomas (Figure 20.2B), which include chronic lymphocytic leukemia/small lymphocytic lymphoma (CLL/SLL), non-nodal mantle cell lymphoma, follicular lymphoma including pediatric follicular lymphoma, marginal zone lymphoma, lymphoplasmacytic

A B C

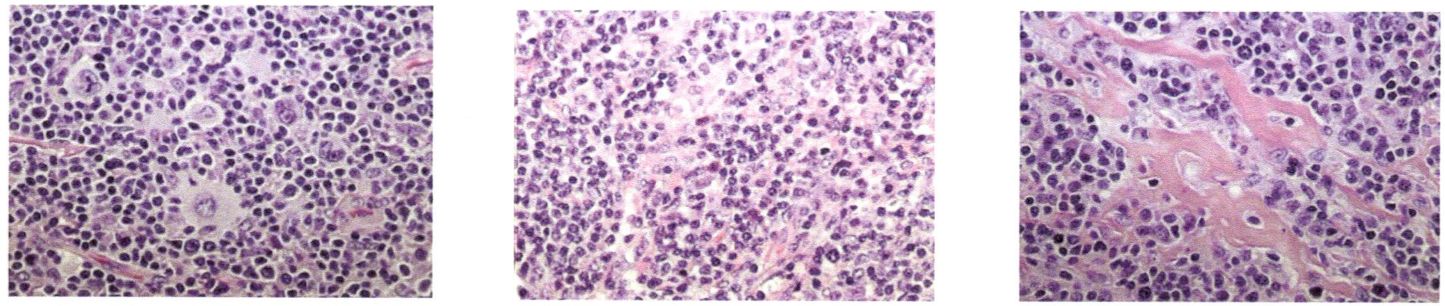

HRS cells | Reactive background | Fibrosis

	HRS cells	Reactive background
CD30	+	+ (rare immunoblasts and plasma cells)
CD15	+/-	+ (reactive granulocytes)
CD45	-	+ (reactive hematolymphoid cells)
PAX5	weak+	+ (reactive B cells)
CD3	-	+ (reactive T cells)
CD20	+/-	+ (reactive B cells)
CD138	-	+ (reactive plasma cells)
PD1	+	+ (reactive T cells)
PD-L1	+	+ (reactive lymphocytes and histiocytes)
OCT2	-/+	+ (reactive B cells)
BOB1	-/+	+ (reactive B cells)
MUM1	+	+ (reactive plasma cells)

FIGURE 20.1 Hodgkin lymphoma. It is characterized by the large atypical CD30+/CD15+/-/CD45- Hodgkin-Reed-Sternberg (HRS) cells (A) in a background of reactive B cells, T cells, granulocytes (particularly eosinophils), plasma cells (B), and bands of fibrosis (C). For immunomodulation therapy, PD1 and PD-L1 should always be investigated during the diagnostic workups. The biomarkers that can be used for therapeutic targets are in bold.

	A	B	C
	B-lymphoblastic leukemia/lymphoma	Indolent B-cell lymphoma	Aggressive B-cell lymphoma (BCL2/BCL6/MYC)
CD10	+	-/+	+/-
CD19	+	+	+
CD20	-/+	+	+
CD34	+	-	-
CD45	+/-	+	+
CD79a	+	+	+
PAX5	+	+	+
TdT	+	-	-

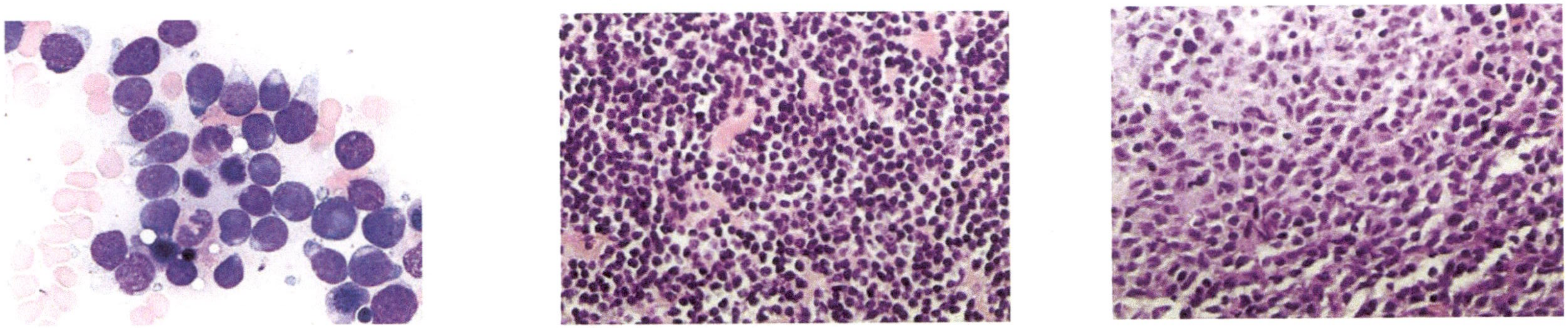

FIGURE 20.2 Three major clinical types of B-cell lymphomas. Based on the ontogeny and clinical behavior, the B-cell lymphomas can be largely divided into B-lymphoblastic leukemia/lymphoma (A), indolent (mature) B-cell leukemia/lymphoma (B), and aggressive (transformed mature) B-cell lymphoma (C). The B-lymphoblastic leukemias/lymphomas carry the precursor B-cell markers, whereas the mature B-cell lymphomas (indolent and aggressive) often do not express the precursor B-cell markers. The biomarkers that can be used for therapeutic targets are in bold.

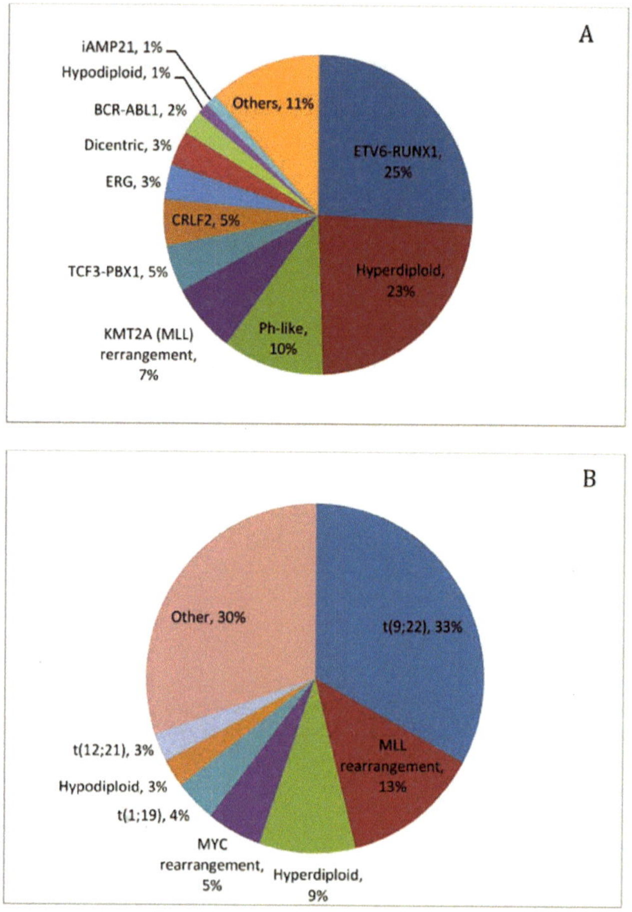

FIGURE 20.3 Frequency of cytogenetic and molecular genetic abnormalities in pediatric ALL (A) and adult ALL (B) (from ref. 13).

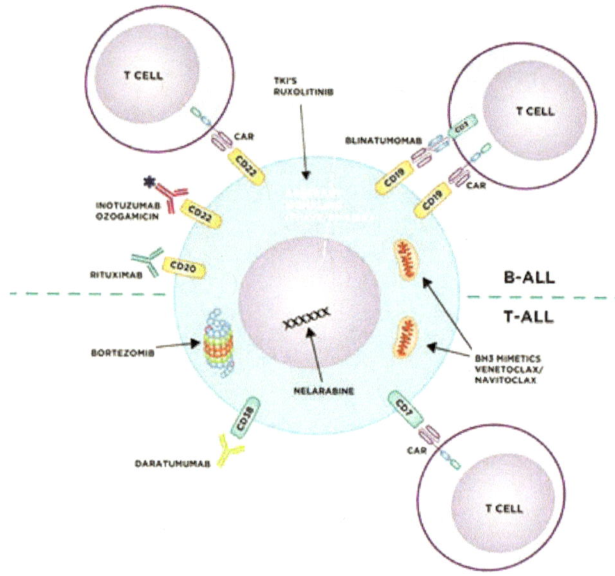

FIGURE 20.4 Targeted therapeutic strategies for acute lymphoblastic leukemia/lymphoma (ALL). Engagement of cytotoxic T cells either through a CAR T-cell directed against various cell surface receptors such as CD19, CD22, or CD7 or through the CD3/CD19 bispecific T-cell engager, blinatumomab; binding of monoclonal antibodies to induce antibody-dependent cellular cytotoxicity and complement-dependent cytotoxicity, or deliver a cytotoxic payload, via receptors such as CD22 (inotuzumab ozogamicin), CD20 (rituximab), or CD38 (daratumumab); blockade of aberrant cell proliferation signaling via JAK-activating lesions (ruxolitinib) or *ABL*-class fusions (TKIs); induction of apoptosis via BH3 mimetics (venetoclax, navitoclax); inhibition of DNA synthesis in leukaemic blasts and induction of apoptosis by nelarabine; regulation of protein homeostasis by the proteasome inhibitor bortezomib. CAR, chimeric antigen receptor (T cell therapy). TKIs, tyrosine kinase inhibitors. PH + ve, Philadelphia chromosome positive ALL. PH-LIKE, Philadelphia chromosome-like ALL (from ref. 16, CC BY 4.0).

lymphoma, and plasma cell neoplasms. Besides the common association with monoclonal gammopathy of undetermined significance (MGUS), they each have precursors in their clinical courses (Table 20.2).

CLL/SLL is the most common lymphoid neoplasm in the older population of the Western world. Patients are often asymptomatic when the disease is incidentally detected by a routine complete blood cell count (CBC) and blood smear review (Figure 20.5A). WHO classification uses 5,000/µL neoplastic B cells as the cutoff value between CLL/SLL and its precursor, monoclonal B-cell lymphocytosis, since they have the same immunophenotype: CD19+, CD20 dim+, CD22+, CD5+, CD23+, CD200+, CD38+/-, FMC7+/-, dim surface immunoglobulin light chain kappa or lambda restriction (17). CLL/SLL can be divided into pre-germinal center B-cell type and post-germinal center B-cell type based on the presence or absence of the *IGHV* somatic hypermutations. The paraprotein is associated with the post-germinal center B-cell type, which has a better prognosis (18). The pre-germinal center B-cell type clinically behaves like mantle cell lymphoma rather than post-germinal center CLL/SLL, except for the lack of t(11;14) and cyclin D expression (19, 20). Several genetic abnormalities, including 11q23, trisomy 12, and 17q(del), currently have only prognostic values rather than serving as molecular targets for therapy (17). For decades, CLL/SLL was managed with a cocktail of chemotherapy agents including fludarabine, bendamustine, and rituximab, a humanized monoclonal antibody that targets the surface CD20. Recently clinical trials with targeted

TABLE 20.2

Indolent B-cell Neoplasms and Their Precursors

Neoplasms	Precursor	Paraprotein
CLL/SLL	MBL, CLL-type	Yes
Non-nodal MCL	MBL, non-CLL-type	No
Follicular lymphoma	In situ follicular B cell neoplasm	No
Marginal zone lymphoma	MBL, non-CLL-type	Yes
Lymphoplasmacytic lymphoma	MBL, non-CLL-type	40%
Plasma cell neoplasm	Plasma cell dyscrasia (MGUS)	Yes

Abbreviations: MCL, mantle cell lymphoma; MBL, monoclonal B-cell lymphocytosis; MGUS, monoclonal gammopathy of unknown significance.

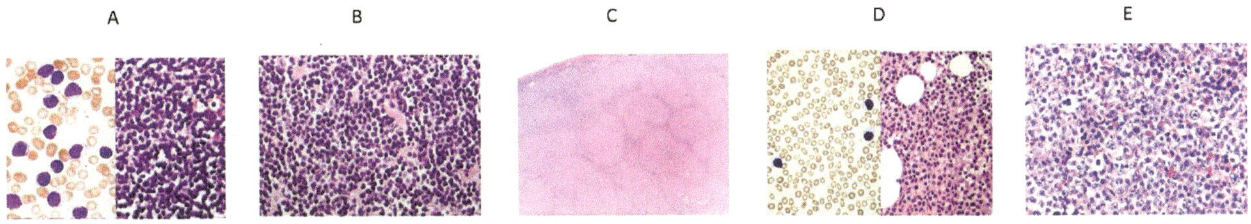

	CLL/SLL	Marginal zone/lymphoplasmacytic	Follicular	Hairy cell	Plasma cell neoplasm
CD5	+	-/+	-	-	-
CD10	-	-	+	+/-	-
CD11c	+/-	-	-	bright +	-
CD20	**dim+**	+	+	+	-/+
CD23	+	-	-/+	-	-
CD25	-	-	-	+	-
CD38	+/-	-	-	-	bright +
CD43	+	-/+	-	-	+/-
CD138	-	-	-	-	+
CD200	+	+/-	+/-	+/-	-
CD103	+	-/+	-	+	-

FIGURE 20.5 Representative indolent B-cell neoplasms/plasma cell neoplasm. This group all express pan B-cell markers (except for plasma cell neoplasm) and monotypic (or absent in some cases) immunoglobulin on their cell surface or in the cytoplasm. Indolent mature B-cell neoplasms often have a slow clinical progression. They are mainly named after their normal counterparts in the lymph node.

TABLE 20.3

Most Common MCRs in the Different Variants of MZL

Histotype	Lesion	Cytoband	Frequency %	Start	Size	Correlation with Gene Expression
MZL (unidentified location)	Gains	3q11.2-q29 (*NFKBIZ, BCL6*)	24	9.50×10^7	1.04×10^8	Yes
		6q27	16	1.70×10^8	1.01×10^6	
		13q11-q12.11	25	1.80×10^7	5.33×10^5	
		18q23 (*NFATC1*)	18	7.40×10^7	2.12×10^6	Yes
		21p	15			
	Losses	1p36.21-p36.13	12	1.51×10^7	1.62×10^6	Yes
		4p12-p11	13	4.82×10^7	5.72×10^5	
		6q23.2-q24.1 (*TNFAIP3*)	16	1.35×10^8	4.78×10^6	Yes
		7q31.31-q32.3	17	1.20×10^8	1.15×10^7	Yes
		17p13.3-p13.1 (*TP53*)	13	1.89×10^4	9.71×10^6	Yes
MALT lymphoma	Gains	3q (*NFKBIZ, BCL6*)	30			Yes
		3p (*FOXP1*)	26			Yes
		6p25.1-p21.32	14	4.35×10^6	2.85×10^7	
		7p15.1	14	3.15×10^7	1.78×10^4	
		7q11.22	18	6.88×10^7	5.68×10^5	
		8p21.2	14	2.72×10^7	1.36×10^5	
		18p	21			Yes
		18q (*BCL2, NFATC1*)	21			Yes
	Losses	1p36.21-p36.13	12	1.56×10^7	1.12×10^6	Yes
		4p11–12	14	4.81×10^7	6.81×10^5	
		6q23.3-q24.1 (*TNFAIP3*)	30	1.37×10^8	2.35×10^6	Yes
		13q32.1-q32.2	16	9.69×10^7	8.28×10^5	Yes

(Continued)

TABLE 20.3 (Continued)

Histotype	Lesion	Cytoband	Frequency %	Start	Size	Correlation with Gene Expression
Splenic MZL	Gains	3q13.13-q29 (*NFKBIZ, BCL6*)	20	1.10×10^8	8.89×10^7	Yes
		6q27	19	1.70×10^8	4.83×10^5	
		8p23.1-p22	15	1.23×10^7	5.08×10^5	Yes
		9q31.1	13	1.05×10^8	3.20×10^4	
		12q21.31	13	8.07×10^7	4.06×10^4	
		13q11-q12.11	28	1.80×10^7	5.33×10^5	
		18q23 (*NFATC1*)	15	7.35×10^7	2.57×10^6	Yes
		21p	17			
	Losses	1p36.21-p36.13	13	1.51×10^7	1.62×10^6	
		4p12-p11	13	4.82×10^7	5.72×10^5	
		7q31.31-q32.3	26	1.20×10^8	1.15×10^7	Yes
		8p	13			
		17p13.3-p13.1 (*TP53*)	17	1.89×10^4	9.71×10^6	Yes
Nodal MZL	Gains	2p16.3	20	4.95×10^7	2.11×10^6	
		3p25.3	24	1.04×10^7	6.06×10^5	
		3p14.3-q29 (*FOXP1, NFKBIZ, BCL6*)	24	5.46×10^7	1.45×10^8	Yes
		6p21.2-p21.1	16	4.01×10^7	1.46×10^6	
		6q27	16	1.70×10^8	1.04×10^6	
		18q23 (*NFATC1*)	24	7.42×10^7	1.95×10^6	Yes
	Losses	1p36.33-p36.22	16	7.76×10^5	9.76×10^6	Yes
		1p21.2	16	9.98×10^7	1.86×10^6	Yes
		6q23.3 (*TNFAIP3*)	16	1.37×10^8	1.44×10^6	Yes
		12q21.33-q23.1	16	9.07×10^7	4.81×10^6	Yes
		19p13.3-p12	16	2.12×10^5	1.98×10^7	Yes

Source: adapted from ref. 23

Abbreviations: MZL, marginal zone lymphoma; MCR, minimal common region.

agents ibrutinib (BTK inhibitor), venetoclax (BCL2 inhibitor), and obinutuzumab (CD20 inhibitor) showed promising clinical outcomes (21).

Marginal zone lymphoma (MZL) is the second most common indolent B-cell lymphoma in older adults and the only lymphoma that can be reversed by eliminating stimulatory factors (such as microorganisms) (22). This lymphoma can occur in lymph nodes, extranodal lymphoid tissues, or spleen. It usually infiltrates the nodal marginal zone and thus is so named (Figure 20.5B). It develops on the persistent activation of the normal signal transduction pathways; when a clone of the B cells gains a new hit by an activated oncogene, the B-cell progenies become neoplastic. No disease-specific genetic abnormalities have been identified, but there are shared genetic abnormalities among the three subtypes (Table 20.3) (23). Like CLL/SLL, MZL is currently managed with rituximab and chemotherapy, but the recently developed combination targeted agents for CLL/SLL (21) may also be effective for MZL. More investigations are required to evaluate the efficacy.

Lymphoplasmacytic lymphoma (LPL) resembles MZL morphologically, immunophenotypically, and genetically (24). It's not uncommon for some pathologists to use the IgM paraprotein to distinguish LPL from MZL (IgG, IgA) in difficult cases. NGS identified the *MYD88* mutation in ~90% of the LPL (25), which makes it much easier to separate LPL from MZL, and at the same time opened the door to targeted therapy using ibrutinib, a Bruton tyrosine kinase (BTK) inhibitor (26), with excellent clinical outcomes.

Except for grade 3B, follicular lymphoma (FL) is considered a low-grade (grade 1–3A) mature B-cell lymphoma. In the lymph node, FL proliferates in back-to-back follicular or nodular patterns with the loss of polarization and the mantle zone (Figure 20.5C). It commonly expresses CD10 and BCL2 with the characteristic t(14;18) in the lymphoma cells. The average 15 mitotic figures per high power field in the neoplastic follicles arbitrarily separate low-grade FL (=<15 mitotic figures/hpf) from high-grade FL (>15 mitotic figures/hpf), and this separation determines the therapeutic regimens to be used in the treatment of FL (27). Although the centroblast count is arbitrary and varies from pathologist to pathologist, it dictates the management plans (28). The low-grade was treated with alkylating agent-based chemotherapy plus rituximab, whereas the high-grade was managed similarly to DLBCL with RCHOP. The FDA newly approved venetoclax may be an ideal agent for both low-grade and aggressive FL.

Indolent mantle cell lymphoma does exist and presents as leukemic non-nodal mantle cell lymphoma (29). These cases all harbor the t(11;14) and aberrantly express cyclin D1 but have an indolent clinical course and limited nodal involvement and are usually negative for SOX11 and often positive for CD23 and CD200, with hypermutated *IGHV* (2). The clinical behavior resembles CLL/SLL more than MCL.

Hairy cell leukemia is a rare and indolent B-cell neoplasm which is characterized by the circulating atypical B cells with cytoplasmic projections (Figure 20.5D). Considered an indolent disease, it responds to chemotherapy and rituximab with an excellent prognosis (30). Recent identification of *BRAF* mutation provides a good target for precision therapy with higher efficacy and lower toxicity (31). The morphologic mimics without the *BRAF* V600E mutation, however, do not respond very well to chemotherapy or targeting BRAF, but ibrutinib is the first-line targeting agent (32).

Although classified as a distinct entity, plasma cell neoplasm can be regarded as end-stage mature B-cell neoplasm. Retaining most of the phenotypic features of mature B cells (CD20, CD79a, and immunoglobulin production), plasma cell neoplasm has acquired CD138, an adhesion molecule that helps plasma cells to communicate with the bone marrow environment and serves as a potential therapeutic target (33) (Figure 20.5E). It also has an indolent precursor lesion with extremely low plasma cell numbers and low levels of secreted immunoglobulins, so called MGUS (Table 20.2). The NCCN and International Myeloma Working Group have defined criteria for the diagnosis of MGUS, plasma cell dyscrasia, plasma cell myeloma, and the management guidelines (34). Owing to the prevalent expression of CD38 and B-cell maturation antigens (BCMAs) on neoplastic plasma cells (35), multiple clinical trials targeting CD38 and/or BCMAs are being carried out and have yielded impressive outcomes (36). Occasionally, targeted agents used for B-cell lymphoma can also be used for myeloma (6, 33).

Spontaneous regression of indolent B-cell lymphomas has been reported (37), whereas transformation from indolent to aggressive B-cell lymphomas is more frequent, often due to acquired additional genetic "hits", such as *MYC* (38). However, FL progression from low grade to grade 3A is still not well understood. Grade 3A FL may serve as the intermediate from the low-grade FL to diffuse large B-cell lymphoma (DLBCL). Combined PI3K inhibitor and rituximab therapy showed promising results in refractory and relapsed low-grade B-cell lymphomas (39).

20.3.1.3 Aggressive B-Cell Neoplasms

MCL infiltrates lymph nodes with an expansion of the mantle zone, shrunk lymphoid follicle, and atypical cytology with high N:C ratio and "squared" nuclei (Figure 20.6A). It characteristically harbors the t(11;14) with aberrant cyclin D1 (or D2/D3) expression. Almost all the MCLs originate from the pre-germinal center B cells, so they usually express CD5 and SOX11. CD5-negative and cyclin D1-negative MCL have been reported, but the t(11;14) genetic abnormality and SOX11 expression are required for the diagnosis (40). Indolent MCL is rarely reported, and it is often of post-germinal center B-cell origin (41). Except for the t(11;14) and aberrant cyclin D1 expression, indolent MCL has a similar clinical course as that of post-germinal center CLL/SLL. Therefore, the *IGHV* somatic hypermutations may be more biologically relevant in differentiating CLL/SLL and MCL, since both MCL and pre-germinal center CLL/SLL have a bad prognosis, while post-germinal center CLL/SLL and MCL have a better prognosis with the current chemotherapeutic regimens (19, 20). Due to its aggressiveness, MCL is currently treated with a RCHOP regimen like DLBCL (42). Although multiple clinical trials are being carried out, no definite answers have been obtained so far.

As the most common NHL, DLBCL is a heterogeneous group of lymphoid neoplasms (41). The most prominent feature of this neoplasm is "diffuse" infiltration of organs and tissues with "large" neoplastic cells of B-cell lineage (Figure 20.6B). In recent years, DLBCL was further classified into 15–17 distinct variants (42) under the umbrella of "large B-cell lymphoma": ALK+ large B-cell lymphoma, T cell/histiocyte-rich large B-cell lymphoma; primary DLBCL of the CNS; primary cutaneous DLBCL, leg type; EBV-positive DLBCL, NOS; DLBCL associated with chronic inflammation; primary mediastinal large B-cell lymphoma; and so on (Table 20.4).

The mainstay treatment for DLBCL remains rituximab + CHOP, with some variations (43). This regimen and dosage are based on numerous clinical trials; however, only 60–70% respond to the current chemotherapy, and 40–50% of patients relapse. Therefore, novel therapies are badly needed.

Although classification of DLBCL based on cell of origin has little value to therapy, both the WHO and ICC have kept this classification for prognostic purposes. Abramson (44) identified perturbations in the PI3K/AKT and JAK/STAT signaling pathways and a higher frequency of *BCL2* and *EZH2* mutations in the DLBCLs of the germinal center B-cell (GCB) subtype, whereas activated B-cell (ABC) DLBCLs are characterized by the activation of the NF-κB pathway and a higher frequency of *BCL6* rearrangements; *BCL2* amplifications; and recurrent mutations of *CD79B*, *MYD88*, and *PRDM1*. The NIH group (45) also mapped the key activated pathways in GCB DLBCL, which included PI3K/AKT/mTOR, BCL2, BCL6, and MYC, whereas in ABC DLBCL, the key pathways were BCR-mediated NF-κB as well as PI3K/AKT/mTOR pathways (Figure 20.7). Based on shared genetic abnormalities, DLBCL has recently been classified into four prominent genetic subtypes (46): 1) MCD (based on the co-occurrence of *MYD88*L265P and *CD79B* mutations), 2) BN2 (based on *BCL6* fusions and *NOTCH2* mutations), 3) N1 (based on *NOTCH1* mutations), and 4) EZB (based on *EZH2* mutations and *BCL2* translocations). However, this classification has not yet been accepted by WHO and ICC classifications (2, 47).

The recent breakthrough in DLBCL targeted therapy is the ibrutinib effect on DLBCL (48, 49). In combination with RCHOP, ibrutinib has gained a 100% response rate in a subgroup of young patients, and the response was highly dependent on the mutations fostering B-cell receptor (BCR) signaling and BTK dependence (48) (Figure 20.8). However, it is not known if ibrutinib by itself would gain a similar outcome. Another study by the same group found that the sole agent ibrutinib inhibitory effect on ABC DLBCL indeed depended on the activated BCR signaling rather than the *MYD88* mutation. When the mutated *MYD88* became independent of BCR activation, ibrutinib lost its inhibitory effect on the ABC DLBCL with NFκB pathway activation (49) (Figure 20.9).

Although the PI3K/AKT/mTOR/p70S6K pathway may be the most important signal transduction pathway in cancer and is activated in both GCB and ABC DLBCLs (46), its role in the

A B C D

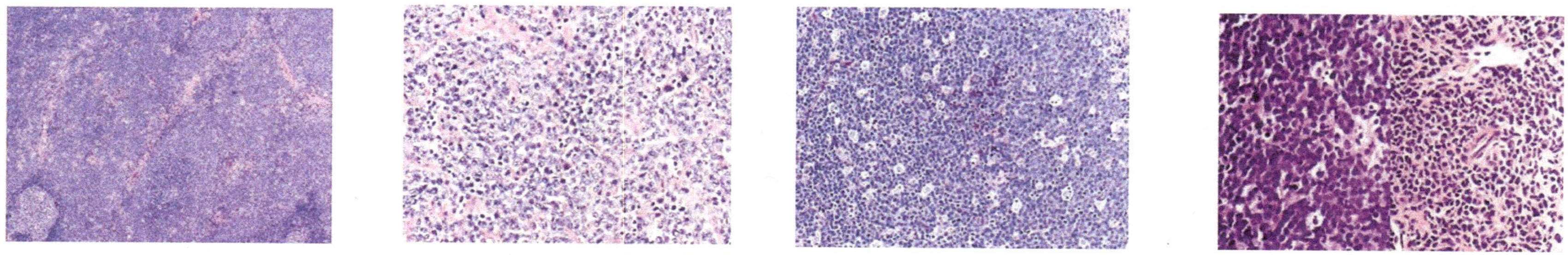

	Mantle cell lymphoma	DLBCL	Burkitt lymphoma	Grey zone lymphoma
CD5	+	-/+	-	-/+
CD10	-	+/-	+	+/-
CD20	+	+	+	+/-
CD79a	+	+	+	+
BCL2	+	+/-	-	+/-
BCL6	-	+/-	+	+/-
Cyclin D1/2/3	+	-/+	-	+/-
MYC	-	-/+	+	+/-
SOX11	+	-	-	+/-
CD200	-	+	+	+/-

FIGURE 20.6 Representatives of aggressive B-cell lymphoma. Besides CD20, CD79a is targeted for immunotherapy, and BCL2 is targeted by small molecules, BTK inhibitor ibrutinib, PI3K/AKT/MTOR pathway inhibitors, and RAS/MEK/ERK pathway inhibitors are also effective in targeted therapy for this group of neoplasms.

TABLE 20.4

Genetic Abnormalities of Aggressive Large B-Cell Lymphomas

Lymphoma	Subtype	Major Oncogene Alteration (mechanism of activation, % of DLBCL)
ALK+ large B-cell lymphoma		*ALK* (fusion)
DLBCL, NOS (42)	MCD	*MYD88*L265P (mut, 71.8%); *CD79B* (mut amp, 52.1%); *SPIB* (gain amp, 54.3%); *VMP1*(mut amp, 24.3%); *HASPIN* (mut, 11.6%)
	BN2	*BCL6* (fusion, 73.5%); *NOTCH2* (mut, 44.3%); *BCL10* (mut amp, 36.1%); *CCND3* (mut, 24.5%); *PRKCB* (mut amp, 13.5%); *TRRAP* (mut, 12.9%); *CXCR5* (trunc 12.2%)
	N1	*NOTCH1* (mut, 100%); *IRF4* (mut amp, 36.8%)
	EZB	*BCL2* (transloc, 68.1%); *EZH2* (mut, 43.5%); *REL* (amp, 42.9%); *IRF8* (mut amp, 28.8%); *MEF2B* (mut, 27.5%); *STAT6* (mut amp, 26.6%); *S1PR2* (mut, 17.4%); *MIR17HG* (amp, 14.3%); *MTOR* (mut, 11.6%)
EBV-associated large B-cell lymphoma		
Intravascular large B-cell lymphoma		Ch 1 (del/amp/rear, 72%), 6q (~58%), 14q32 (28%), +18 (38%), *PIM1* (mut, 67%), *MYD88* (mut, 44–59%), *CD79b* (mut, 26–67%), *PRDM1* (mut, 44%), *BTG2* (mut, 22%) and *EZH2* (mut, 4%)
Large B-cell lymphoma with 11q aberration		+11q/-11q
Large B-cell lymphoma with *IRF4* rearrangement		6p25/*IRF4* (rear), +7q32.1-qter, +11q22.3-qter, +Xq28, -6q13–16.1, -15q14–22.3, -17p
Plasmablastic lymphoma		*MYC* (transloc, 67%)
Primary cutaneous large B-cell lymphoma, leg type		*MYC* (rear, ~33%), *PD-L1/PD-L2* (transloc, 40%), 6q (del, >60%), 9p21.3 (del, >60%), *MYD88* (mut, 75%), *TNFAIP3* (mut, ~40%), BCR pathway (mut)
Primary large B-cell lymphoma of CNS		9p21.3(del), 6p21(del), 6q(del), +12q12-q24.33, 18q21.33–23(alt), 10q23.2(alt), *PIM1* mut, ~44%), *MYD88* (mut, 38–50%), *CD79B* (mut, ~44%), *TP53* (mut, 27–37%)
Primary large B-cell lymphoma of testis		3q27 (alt), 6q (alt), *MYD88* (mut), *CD79B* (mut), *BCL6* (rear, 50%), *BCL2* (rear, 10%), *MYC* (rear, 6–15%)
Primary mediastinal large B-cell lymphoma		*REL* (amp, <75%), *BCL11A* (amp, <50%), *NFKBIE* (del, <20%), *TNFAIP3* (mut, <60%), 9p24.1 (+/amp, 70%), *STAT6* (mut, 72%), *SOCS1* (mut, 45%), *PTPN1* (mut, 25%), *IL4R* (24%)
T cell/histiocyte-rich large B-cell lymphoma		Mutations in *JUNB*, *DUSP2*, *SGK1*, *SOCS1* and/or *CREBBP*
DLBCL associated with chronic inflammation		*MYC* (amp, 70%), *TP53* (mut, 70%)
Primary effusion lymphoma		Complex karyotypes
High-grade B-cell lymphoma with DH/TH		*BCL2*, *MYC* and/or *BCL2* (transloc), *MYC* (transloc), *BCL6* (transloc), *BCL6* (rear)
High-grade B-cell lymphoma, NOS		*MYD88* (mut), *CD79B* (mut), *TBL1XR1* (mut), *KMT2D* (mut, 43%), *TP53* (mut, 30%)
Burkitt lymphoma		*MYC* (fusion, 100%)

Source: summarized from refs. 2, 42, 46 and 47

Abbreviations: rear, rearrangement; mut, mutation; transloc, translocation; amp, amplification; Ch, chromosome; DH/TH, double-hit/triple-hit.

treatment of aggressive B-cell lymphomas was largely ignored (50). In the last 2 years, many clinical trials targeting PI3K, AKT, or mTOR have obtained some promising results (51). Our studies indicated that combined inhibition of PI3K/AKT/mTOR/p70S6K and CDC2 or RAS/RAF/MEK/ERK and CHK2 were effective strategies to inhibit the growth of DLBCL (52, 53). Furthermore, combined targeted therapies may also be an effective strategy to overcome drug resistance in targeted therapy for DLBCL (54). In addition, different DLBCLs may respond to the same therapy differently (52), suggesting that each DLBCL should be treated individually with precision therapy.

Burkitt lymphoma (BL) is a well characterized aggressive B-cell lymphoma composed of monotonous medium-sized lymphoma cells with *MYC* translocations (Figure 20.6C). Due to its excellent response to the hyperintensive chemotherapy (Hyper CVAD), targeted therapy is reserved only for the relapsed/refractory disease; targeting the PI3K/AKT/mTOR/p70S6K is a potential strategy (55).

20.3.2 T/NK-Cell Neoplasms

20.3.2.1 T-Lymphoblastic Neoplasms

As another malignancy derived from precursor lymphocyte, T-lymphoblastic leukemia/lymphoma (T-ALL) both morphologically and clinically resembles its precursor B-cell counterpart (Figure 20.10A). Numerous genetic abnormalities are also associated with T-ALL. Like B-ALL, it is mainly treated with hyper-intensive chemotherapy, and the survival is slightly worse than B-ALL. Targeted therapy is currently rare.

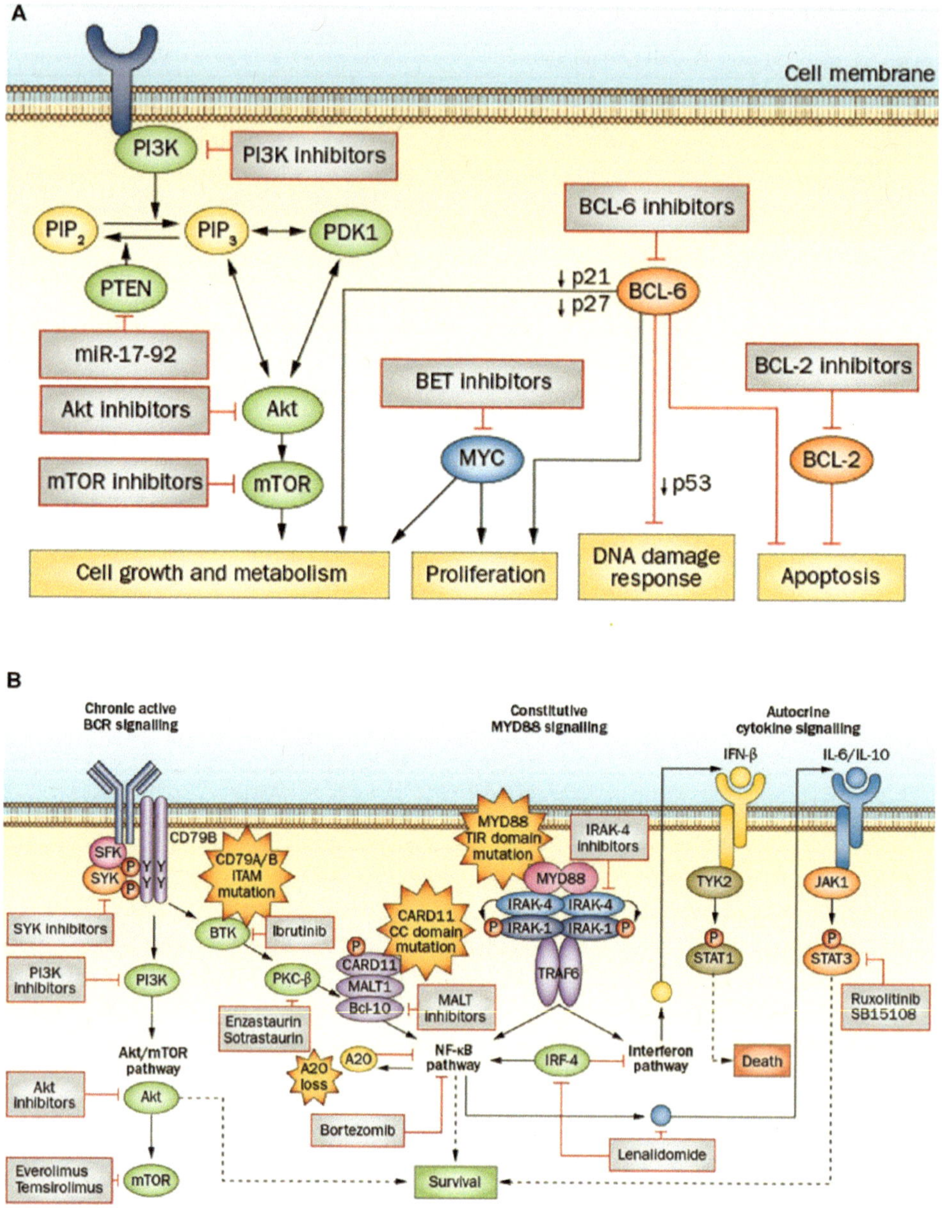

FIGURE 20.7 Activated pathways in diffuse large B-cell lymphomas with the novel target agents (adapted from ref. 45). (A) In germinal center B-cell (GCB) subtype. B-cell lymphoma 2, apoptosis regulator Bcl-2; BCL-6, B-cell lymphoma 6; DLBCL, diffuse large B-cell lymphoma; mTOR, mammalian target of rapamycin; PI3K, phosphatidylinositol 3-kinase. (B) In activated B-cell (ABC) subtype. BCR, B-cell receptor; DLBCL, diffuse large B-cell lymphoma; IRAK-4, interleukin-1 receptor-associated kinase 4; IRF-4, interferon regulatory factor 4; JAK, Janus activating kinase; mTOR, mammalian target of rapamycin; PMBL, primary mediastinal B-cell lymphoma; SYK, spleen tyrosine kinase.

20.3.2.2 Indolent T/NK-Cell Neoplasms

Indolent T/NK-cell lymphoproliferative disease (LPD)/neoplasm has been recognized as a provisional entity only recently, mainly in the gastrointestinal tract (2, 47). However, an indolent T-cell CLL (Figure 20.10B) remains controversial. Overall, diseases in this group have a tedious clinical course and do not respond to the current chemotherapeutic regimens. Immunosuppressants, such as cyclosporine and the mTOR inhibitor rapamycin, may be effective in treating these diseases.

20.3.2.3 Aggressive T/NK-Cell Lymphomas

Anaplastic large cell lymphoma (ALCL) (Figure 20.10C) is the most common aggressive peripheral T-cell lymphoma (PTCL) with at least three subtypes: ALK+ ALCL, ALK- ALCL, and primary cutaneous ALCL (56). ALK+ ALCL is characterized by the consistent expression of CD30 and ALK1 associated with the *ALK1* gene rearrangements (57). The most common *ALK1* rearrangement is the t(2;5) resulting in the production of NPM-ALK fusion oncoprotein. Truncated ALK1 expression

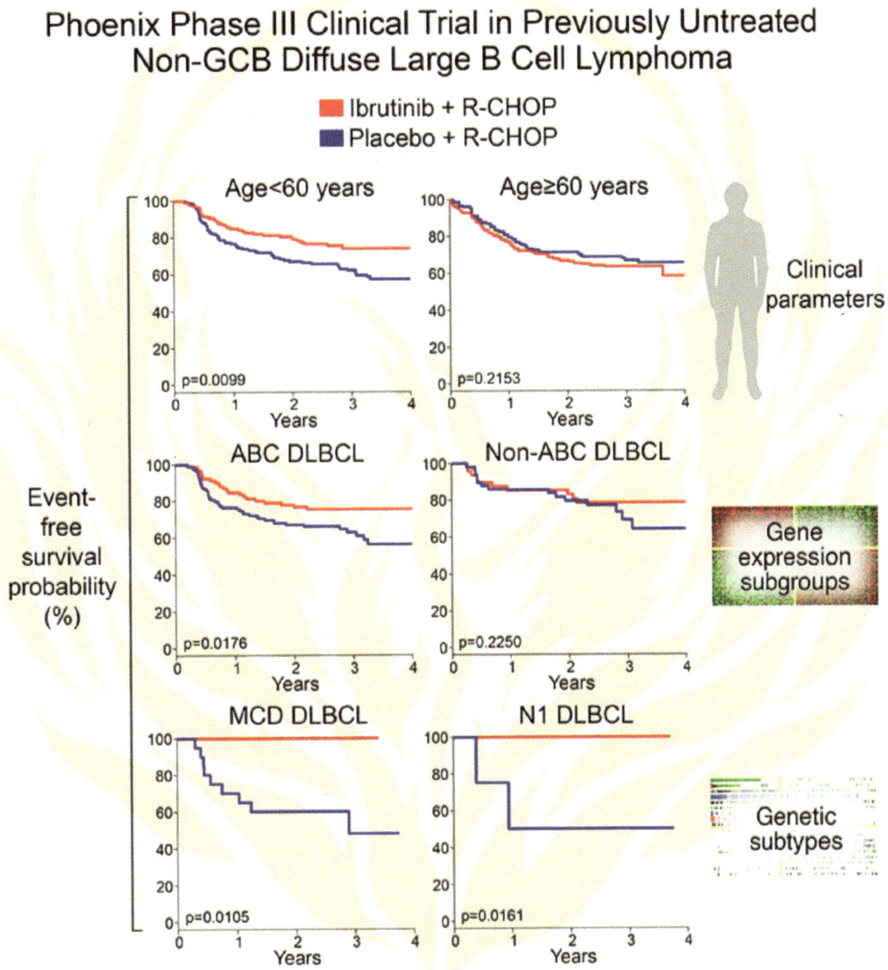

FIGURE 20.8 Ibrutinib + R-CHOP effects on diffuse large B-cell lymphomas in the young patients (adapted from ref. 48). Ibrutinib combined with R-CHOP achieved 100% event free survival in young (< 60 years old) patients of MCD and N1 genetic subtypes.

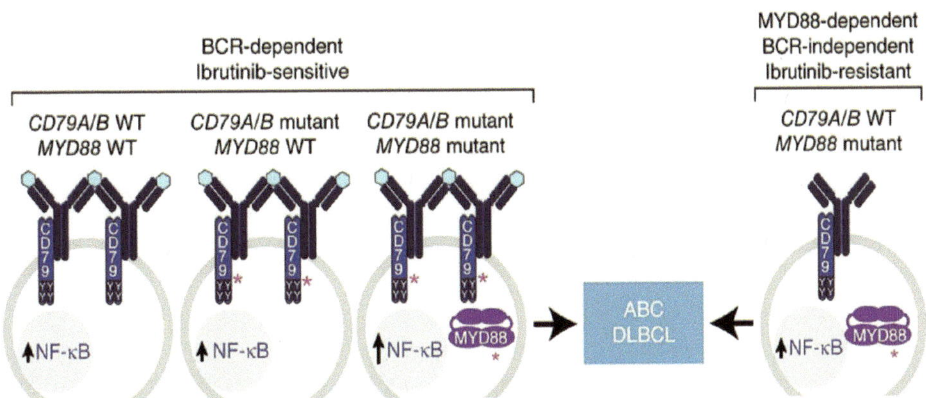

FIGURE 20.9 Ibrutinib effects on B-cell lymphomas are dependent on the activated B-cell receptor (BCR) (adapted from ref. 49). The inhibitory effect of ibrutinib on B-cell lymphomas depends on the activated BCR. When *MYD88* is mutated, the lymphoma cells are more sensitive to ibrutinib inhibition. However, when the mutated MYD88 activates NF-kB pathway independent of the BCR activation, the lymphoma cells become resistant to ibrutinib inhibition.

A B C D E

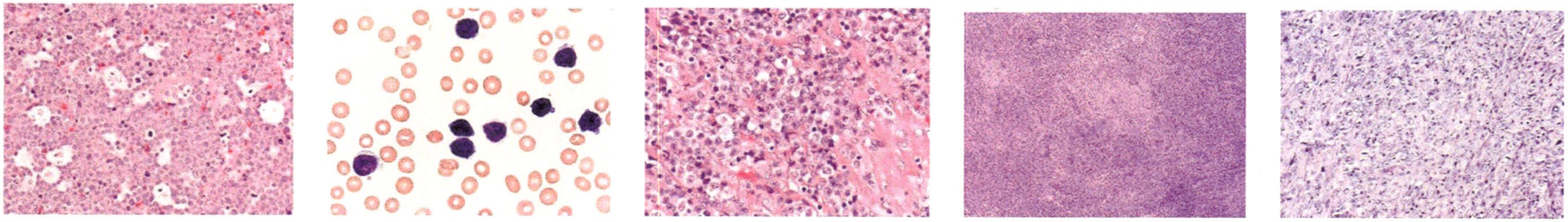

	T lymphoblastic lymphoma	Indolent T-cell leukemia	ALCL	AITL	Peripheral T-cell lymphoma
CD1a	+	-	-	-	-
CD2	+	+	+/-	+	+
CD3	s-/c+	+/-	-	+	+
CD4	+/-	+	+	+	+/-
CD5	+/-	+	+/-	+	-
CD7	+	+/-	-	-	-
CD8	+/-	-/+	-	-	-/+
CD10	+/-	-	-	+	-
CD30	-	-	**+**	-	-/+
CD34	+	-	-	-	-
ALK	-	-	**+/-**	-	-
BCL6	-	-	-	+	-
PD1	**-**	**+**	**+**	**+**	**+**
PD-L1	**-**	**-**	**-/+**	**+**	**-/+**
TdT	+	-	-	-	-

FIGURE 20.10 Representatives of T-cell lymphomas. Based on the ontogeny and clinical behavior, T-cell lymphomas can be largely divided into precursor T lymphoblastic leukemia/lymphoma (A), indolent (mature) T-cell leukemia/lymphomas (B), and aggressive (transformed mature) T-cell lymphomas (ALK+ ALCL (C), AILT (D), and PTCL (E) are presented here). The biomarkers that can be used for therapeutic targets are in bold.

is aberrantly activated by various chromosomal translocations and the full length of ALK1 can also acquire activating point mutations in the kinase domain. In addition to ALCL, aberrant *ALK1* expression has now been detected in multiple other malignancies, which include B-cell lymphoma, non-small cell lung cancer (NSCLC), and anaplastic thyroid carcinoma. All these aberrant ALK activities can be inhibited by various TKIs (Table 20.5).

As a tyrosine kinase, ALK1 can be either aberrantly expressed by persistent activation of the *NPM* promoter or constitutively activated by NPM domain-mediated oligomerization and ALK kinase domain-triggered autophosphorylation (57). Clinical trials confirmed the inhibitory effects of ALK inhibitors in both adult and pediatric patients. Due to the high efficacy, the FDA approved the first-generation ALK inhibitor crizotinib for ALK+ ALCL in January 2021. Unfortunately, drug resistance frequently develops, mainly through *ALK* mutations. New generations of ALK1 inhibitors have been produced and sequential treatment may be able to overcome the newly emerging drug-resistant mutations (Table 20.6). However, ALK-independent drug resistance remains a challenge, and novel multiagent combination therapy is an effective strategy to prevent the occurrence of drug resistance.

T-follicular helper (TFH) cell lymphoma united angioimmunoblastic T-cell lymphoma (AITL), follicular helper T-cell lymphoma, and PTCL with TFH phenotype in 2022 by a common genetic landscape in addition to a TFH immunophenotype (2, 47). AITL is characterized by proliferation of follicular helper T cells with clear cytoplasm, background small vascular proliferation, and scattered immunoblasts (Figure 20.10D). These diseases are invariably associated with a poor prognosis and genetic aberrations in epigenetic regulators such as TET2 (80%), RHOA (70%), and DNMT3A (30–40%) (2, 58). Common genetic abnormalities in AITL are summarized in Table 20.7 (58–60).

TABLE 20.5

ALK Inhibitors, Mechanisms, and Clinical Trials

Name	Mechanism	Generation	FDA Approval	Active ALCL Clinical Trials	Notes
Crizotinib/ Xalkori	Competitive binding to the ATP-binding site of ALK, HGFR, and RON	1st	Locally advanced and metastatic NSCLC (US)	NCT00939770	Phase I/II: pediatric ALCL, CNS tumors (monotherapy)
				NCT02487316	Phase IV: adult ALCL (+/- chemotherapy)
				NCT01606878	Phase I: pediatric ALCL (combination with chemotherapy)
				NCT02584634	Phase I: adult NSCLC (combination avelumab with crizotinib or lorlatinib)
Ceritinib/ LDK378/ Zykadia	Competitively inhibits autophosphorylation of ALK and phosphorylation of its downstream STAT3	2nd	Metastatic crizotinib-resistant NSCLC (US)		
Alectinib/ CH5424802/ AF802	Selectively block the kinase activities of ALK and RET	2nd	Crizotinib-resistant NSCLC (US); ALK+ NSCLC (Japan)	NCT01588028	Phase I: ALK+ NSCLC
ASP3026	ALK inhibitor that can overcome crizotinib resistance	2nd		NCT01284192	Phase I: adult refractory solid tumor or B cell lymphoma
Brigatinib/ AP26113	Inhibits attachment of phosphate to the ALK and results in inhibition of its downstream kinases	2nd		NCT01449461	Phase I/II: adult NSCLC, ALCL, DLCL, IMFT
				NCT02094573	Phase II: adult NSCLC
Lorlatinib/ PF-06463922	Competitively inhibits phosphorylation of ALK and ROS1 kinase	3rd		NCT01970865	Phase I/II: adult ALK+ and ROS1+ NSCLC
				NCT02584634	Phase I: adult NSCLC, avelumab (with crizotinib or lorlatinib)
				NCT02569554	Phase I: adult, healthy, PPI and food effect

Source: modified from ref. 57

Abbreviations: ALK (anaplastic lymphoma kinase), ALCL (anaplastic large-cell lymphoma), CNS (central nervous system), DLCL (diffuse large-cell lymphoma), HGFR (hepatocyte growth factor receptor), IMFT (inflammatory myofibroblastic tumor), NSCLC (non-small cell lung cancer), PPI (proton pump inhibitor), RON (recepteur d'Origine Nantais), US (United States).

TABLE 20.6

Resistant and Sensitive Mutations of ALK-TKIs

ALK-TKI	Crizotinib	Ceritinib	Alectinib	Brigatinib	Lorlatinib	Gilteritinib
Sensitive mutations	L1198F C1196Y+L1198F C1156Y+L1198F	G1269A/S I1171T/N L1196M S1206C/Y I1171S+G1269A	C1156Y/T F1174C/L/V G1269A/S I1151Tins L1196M L1256F L1152P/R S1206C/Y I1171N+L1256F	C1156Y/T E1210K F1174C/L/V F1245A G1202R(-) G1269A/S I1151tins L1152P/R L1196M I1171S + G1269A	C1156Y/T E1210K F1174C/L/V G1269A/S G1202R I1151Tins L1152P/R L1196M S1206C/Y	I1171N I1171N+F1174I I1171N+L1198H
Resistance mutations	C1156Y/T E1210K F1245V G1269A/S G1202R I1151Tins I1171N/S/T L1196M L1152P/R S1206Y/C V1180L E1210K +D1203N L1196M+G1202R	C1156Y/T F1174C/L/V I1151Tins G1202R V1180L I1171N+F1174I I1171N+L1198H L1196M+G1202R	G1202R I1171T/N/S V1180L L1196M+G1202R	D1203N G1202R(-) I1171T/N/S V1180L L1196M+G1202R	C1156F/Y L1198F L1256F G1202R+L1196M C1196Y+L1198F G1202R+T1151M G1202R+F1174C I1171N+F1174I I1171N+L1198H L1196M/D1203N F1174L/G1202R C1156Y/G1269A	

Source: adapted from ref. 57

TABLE 20.7

Genetic Abnormalities of AITL

Gene Fusion	Somatic Mutation	Variations	Frequency
ITK::SYK			Rare
CTLA4::CD28			50–60%
	TET2	Frameshift/nonsense	80–100%
	DNMT3A	Frameshift/nonsense	20–30%
	IDH2	R172X	20–30%
	RHOA	G17V	50–70%
	PLCG1	Missense	20–30%
	CD28	T195P	10–15%
	TNFRSF21	Frameshift deletion	10–20%
	CCND3	Premature stop codon	10–20%
	SAMSN1	Stop codon upstream of SH3	10–20%

Source: summarized from refs. 58–60.

Although still at the early stage, agents targeting histone acetylase and the CD30, PI3K/AKT/mTOR, and JAK/STAT pathways have yielded promising results (59).

PTCLs broadly include all the post-thymic T-cell neoplasms, including PTCL, NOS (Figure 20.10E). Except for the rarely reported indolent T-cell LPD, PTCL is considered phenotypically diverse and clinically aggressive. Although the JAK/STAT pathway is reportedly involved in the PTCL, whether this pathway serves as the oncogenic driver or therapeutic target remains to be defined. Recent gene expression profiling studies (61, 62) have identified PTCL molecular subgroups with differential expression of master T helper 1 (TH1) or TH2 cell-differentiation regulators (*TBX21* or *GATA3*) with corresponding target genes. The clinical significance of these subgroups is to be determined.

NK-cell neoplasms are rare, and the T/NK-cell lymphoma, nasal type, and aggressive NK-cell leukemia are invariably EBV driven (2, 47). Due to the scarcity, targeted therapy for NK-cell neoplasms is limited to immunotherapy and immunomodulation. More studies are required to identify the oncogenic drivers and therapeutic targets. Suppression of EBV activation may be useful in controlling these aggressive diseases.

20.4 Grey-Zone Lymphomas

Grey reflects the overlap between "black" and "white". Many cancers fall into the grey zone because of the overlapping features of some well-defined tumors (63–66), a characteristic feature of grey-zone lymphomas (Table 20.8). Due to the constant evolution, every lymphoma is unique, even with similar morphology, immunophenotypes, and gene expression profiles, since some small genetic changes often do not cause a change in the phenotype but determine the response to certain therapeutic drugs (49). With the current guidelines that therapies follow defined entities, lymphomas with grey zone features pose a challenge to the current phenotype-based diagnosis and treatment (67–69). However, precision pathology will avoid this dilemma due to its new concept of following specific molecular targets and pharmacomics, irrespective of the pathological diagnosis and classification (2, 47). For example, when a lymphoma harbors the BCR activated NF-κB pathway, ibrutinib will be effective regardless whether the lymphoma is DLBCL, BL, or B-cell lymphoma, unclassifiable, with features immediate between DLBCL and BL (70). If a lymphoma morphologically resembles both HL and large B-cell lymphomas, the lymphoma can be targeted with rituximab and brentuximab vedotin, as well as inhibitors of the PI3K/AKT/mTOR pathway. When PD-1 is activated, immunomodulation can also be effective in treating this lymphoma (64). On the other hand, one single mutation could also confer drug resistance even if everything else may look the same for the lymphomas (49). Therefore, rather than making serious efforts to classify them, it would be prudent to directly identify the therapeutic targets for precision therapy.

20.5 Testing Strategies

For precision diagnosis of malignant lymphomas, excisional biopsy is preferred because more tumor cells will be available for various studies (Figure 20.11). The specimen should be divided into at least three parts: 1) morphology and immunophenotyping for traditional pathological diagnosis; IHC testing for CD3, CD10, CD19, CD20, ALK, BCL2, BCL6, cyclin D1, and MYC should be routinely performed for B-NHL; CD3, CD7, CD10, CD20, CD30, ALK, BCL6, PD1, and PD-L1 should be routinely performed for T-NHL; biomarker testing for HL should include CD20, CD30, PD1, and PD-L1 for precision therapies. 2) NGS analyses of NHL should include *ALK1*, *BCL2*, *BCL6*, *BRAF*, *CCND*, *DNMT3A*, *IDH2*, *MYC*, *MYD88*, *NOTCH1*, *RHOA*, *SF3B1*, *SOCS1*, *TET2*, *TP53*, and components of BCR, NF-κB, JAK/STAT, PI3K/AKT/mTOR, and RAS/RAF/MEK/ERK pathways. 3) Lymphoma

TABLE 20.8

Characteristics of Grey Zone Lymphomas

Lymphoma	Morphology	Biomarkers	Gene Alterations
Mediastinal grey zone lymphoma	HRS-like cells in a background of delicate fibrosis	CD20, CD30, CD15, CD45, PAX5, cyclin E, p63, MAL, NFkB, PD1/PD-L1	*REL* (2p16.1, amp, 33%), *JAK2* (9p24.1, gains, 55%), *CIITA* (16p13.13, rear, 27%), *MYC* (8p24, gains, 27%) *SOCS1* (mut, 45%), *B2M* (mut, 45%), *TNFAIP3* (mut, 35%), *GNA13* (mut, 35%), *LRRN3* (mut, 32%), and *NFKBIA* (mut, 29%)
Lymphoma with overlapping features between NLPBL and T/HRLBCL	Large L&H cells and large high N/C B-cells coexist with small number of reactive background B cells	BCL6 (50–90%), c-MYC (65%), BCL2 (40%), EMA (30%), PD-L1	*JUNB* (mut, ~56%), *SOC1* (mut, ~45%), *DUSP2* (mut, ~33%), *SGK1* (mut, ~33%), *CREBBP* (mut, ~33%)
High-grade B-cell lymphoma with aberrant BCL2, MYC, and/or BCL6	Overlapping morphological features between BL and DLBCL	CD20, CD10, BCL2, BCL6, MYC, PAX5	*MYC* (transloc), and/or *BCL2* (transloc), and/or *BCL6* (transloc)
Lymphoma with overlapping features of ALK-ALCL and PTCL, NOS	Large atypical cells with rare "hallmark" cells	ALK1, CD3, CD4, CD7, CD30	*TET2* (mut), *DNMT3A* (mut)
Plasmablastic lymphoma	Large lymphoblastoid cells with overlapping features of BL and plasma cell myeloma	CD138, Ki67 (95–100%), IRF4/MUM1, EBV (60%)	*MYC* (transloc, 50%), *MCL1* (amp, 52%), *IRF4* (amp, 29%), *NRAS* (mut, 31%), *STAT3* (mut, 25%), *TP53* (mut, 14%), *ATN1* (mut, 12%), *TET2* (mut, 12%), *KRAS* (mut, 11%), *MYC* (mut, 9%), *BRAF* (mut, 6%)
DLBCL with plasmacytic differentiation	Large atypical B cells with abundant granular eosinophilic cytoplasm	CD20, CD45, CD138, cyclin D1, PAX5	ND

Source: summarized from refs. 63–66.

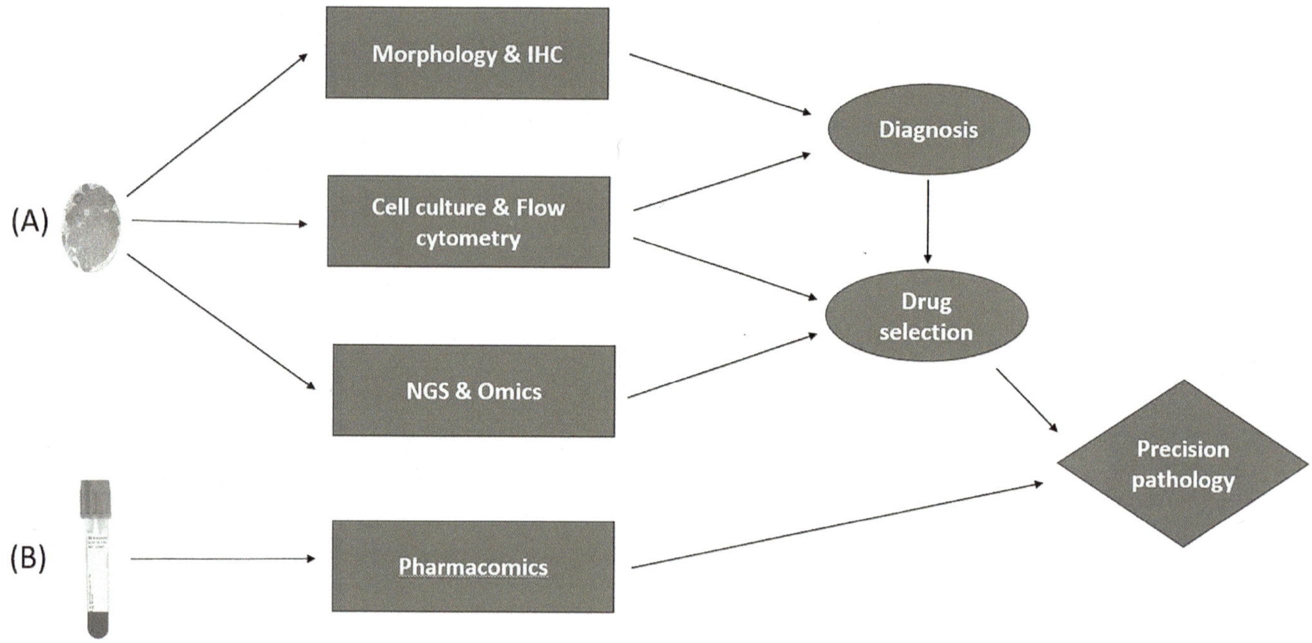

FIGURE 20.11 Testing strategies for malignant lymphomas. Lymph node biopsy specimen (A) is divided into three parts: 1) formalin fixed and paraffin embedded for H&E and IHC studies, 2) fresh tissue for flow cytometry and cell culture, and 3) preparation for molecular (NGS and omics) studies. Based on the diagnosis and molecular studies, drugs will be primarily selected and tested on the lymphoma cells. The target drugs with highest efficacy will be selected and analyzed with pharmacomics (B) to propose a regimen consisting of the drugs of appropriate dosage with the highest efficacy to the tumor and the minimal toxicity to the patient.

cell culture. Activated kinases of the pathways should be analyzed since they serve as the best targets for precision therapies. Once the mutations and/or activated kinases are identified, cultured lymphoma cells will be tested with selected drugs to target the oncoproteins/activated kinases; efficacy doses (EDs) will be defined for the lymphoma cells. Once the drugs are selected, draw the patient's blood for pharmacomics: 1) pharmacogenomics to determine metabolizing rate of therapeutic drugs, xenobiotic effects, and drug-drug interactions and 2) pharmacoproteomics and pharmacometabolomics to predict the half-life and adverse effects of the therapeutic drugs. All these information should be included in the comprehensive pathology report.

20.6 Summary

Lymphoid neoplasms are a heterogeneous group of malignancies derived from the lymphoid organs and tissues. Due to the traditionally effective combined radiotherapy/chemotherapy in lymphomas, targeted therapy has aroused enthusiasm only recently among clinicians. Molecular discoveries in recent years have identified dozens of oncogenic drivers in several important signal transduction pathways. New drugs have also been developed to target these driver oncogene products and obtained some promising results in clinical trials. Some disappointing clinical outcomes may be due to the lack of consideration of pharmacomics when patients were stratified in the clinical trials. As precision pathologists, we should provide as many therapeutic targets as possible to clinicians. At the same time, the lab also should provide as much pharmacomics information as possible for clinicians to design the proper regimens and dosages. The lab should also be able to test selected drugs on lymphoma cells first before they are tested directly on patients. All these efforts will lead to precise therapy and an optimal clinical outcome for patients.

REFERENCES

1. Lymphoma. Centers for disease control and preventions. May 29, 2018. Retrieved 3/15/2022. www.cdc.gov/cancer/lymphoma/index.htm
2. Campo E, Jaffe ES, Cook JR, et al. The International Consensus Classification of mature lymphoid neoplasms: A report from the Clinical Advisory Committee. Blood. 2022;140(11):1229–1253.
3. American Cancer Society. Survival rates for Hodgkin lymphoma. March 2, 2022. Retrieved on 3/15/2022. www.cancer.org/cancer/hodgkin-lymphoma/detection-diagnosis-staging/survival-rates.html
4. Cancer Stat Facts: Non-Hodgkin lymphoma. National Cancer Institute. Retrieved on 3/22/2022. https://seer.cancer.gov/statfacts/html/nhl.html
5. Maloney DG, Grillo-López AJ, White CA, et al. IDEC-C2B8 (Rituximab) anti-CD20 monoclonal antibody therapy in patients with relapsed low-grade non-Hodgkin's lymphoma. Blood. 1997;90(6):2188–2195.
6. Kim LH, Eow GI, Peh SC, Poppema S. The role of CD30, CD40 and CD95 in the regulation of proliferation and apoptosis in classical Hodgkin's lymphoma. Pathology. 2003;35(5):428–435.
7. Diefenbach C, Advani R. Customized targeted therapy in Hodgkin lymphoma: Hype or hope? Hematol Oncol Clin North Am. 2014;28(1):105–122.

8. Wang Y, Nowakowski GS, Wang ML, et al. Advances in CD30- and PD-1-targeted therapies for classical Hodgkin lymphoma. J Hematol Oncol. 2018;11(1):57.
9. Canadian Cancer Society. Targeted therapy for Hodgkin lymphoma. Retrieved on 3/23/2022. https://cancer.ca/en/cancer-information/cancer-types/hodgkin-lymphoma/treatment/targeted-therapy
10. Green MR, Monti S, Rodig SJ, et al. Integrative analysis reveals selective 9p24.1 amplification, increased PD-1 ligand expression, and further induction via JAK2 in nodular sclerosing Hodgkin lymphoma and primary mediastinal large B-cell lymphoma. Blood. 2010;116(17):3268–3277.
11. Li S, Eshleman JR, Borowitz MJ. Lack of surface immunoglobulin light chain expression by flow cytometric immunophenotyping can help diagnose peripheral B-cell lymphoma. Am J Clin Pathol. 2002;118(2):229–234.
12. Borowitz MJ, Chan JKC, Downing JR, et al. B-lymphoblastic leukaemia/lymphoma, not otherwise specified (NOS). In Swerdlow SH, Campo E, Harris HL, et al. (Eds.): WHO Classification of Tumours of Haematopoietic and Lymphoid Tissues (Revised 4th Edition). IARC: Lyon, 2017:200–202.
13. Zhang X, Rastogi P, Shah B, Zhang L. B lymphoblastic leukemia/lymphoma: New insights into genetics, molecular aberrations, subclassification and targeted therapy. Oncotarget. 2017;8(39):66728–66741.
14. Paul S, Kantarjian H, Jabbour EJ. Adult Acute Lymphoblastic Leukemia. Mayo Clin Proc. 2016;91(11):1645–1666.
15. Pui CH. Precision medicine in acute lymphoblastic leukemia. Front Med. 2020;14(6):689–700.
16. Salvaris R, Fedele PL. Targeted therapy in acute lymphoblastic leukaemia. J Pers Med. 2021;11(8):715.
17. Campo E, Ghia P, Montserrat E, et al. Chronic lymphocytic leukemia/small lymphocytic lymphoma. In Swerdlow SH, Campo E, Harris HL, et al. (Eds.): WHO Classification of Tumours of Haematopoietic and Lymphoid Tissues (Revised 4th Edition). IARC: Lyon, 2017:216–221.
18. Zhang S, Kipps TJ. The pathogenesis of chronic lymphocytic leukemia. Annu Rev Pathol. 2014;9:103–118.
19. Rotbain EC, Frederiksen H, Hjalgrim H, et al. IGHV mutational status and outcome for patients with chronic lymphocytic leukemia upon treatment: A Danish nationwide population-based study. Haematologica. 2020;105(6):1621–1629.
20. Navarro A, Clot G, Royo C, et al. Molecular subsets of mantle cell lymphoma defined by the IGHV mutational status and SOX11 expression have distinct biologic and clinical features. Cancer Res. 2012;72(20):5307–5316.
21. Davids MS, Lampson BL, Tyekucheva S, et al. Acalabrutinib, venetoclax, and obinutuzumab as frontline treatment for chronic lymphocytic leukaemia: A single-arm, open-label, phase 2 study. Lancet Oncol. 2021;22(10):1391–1402.
22. Fujimoto K, Endo T, Nishio M, et al. Complete remission of splenic marginal zone lymphoma after an acute flare-up of hepatitis B in a hepatitis B virus carrier. Int J Hematol. 2009;90(5):601–604.
23. Rinaldi A, Mian M, Chigrinova E, et al. Genome-wide DNA profiling of marginal zone lymphomas identifies subtype-specific lesions with an impact on the clinical outcome. Blood. 2011;117(5):1595–1604.
24. Braggio E, Dogan A, Keats JJ, et al. Genomic analysis of marginal zone and lymphoplasmacytic lymphomas identified common and disease-specific abnormalities. Mod Pathol. 2012;25(5):651–660.
25. Treon SP, Xu L, Yang G, et al. MYD88 L265P somatic mutation in Waldenström's macroglobulinemia. N Engl J Med. 2012;367(9):826–833.
26. Treon SP, Xu L, Hunter Z. MYD88 mutations and response to ibrutinib in Waldenstrom's macroglobulinemia. N Engl J Med. 2015;373(6):584–586.
27. NCCN. Follicular lymphoma. NCCN guidelines for patients®. Retrieved on 8/15/2019. https://daytonphysicians.com/wp-content/uploads/2021/11/Follicularlymphoma.pdf
28. Jaffe ES, Harris NL, Swerdlow SH, et al. Follicular lymphoma. In Swerdlow SH, Campo E, Harris HL, et al. (Eds.): WHO Classification of Tumours of Haematopoietic and Lymphoid Tissues (Revised 4th Edition). IARC: Lyon, 2017:266–273.
29. Royo C, Navarro A, Clot G, et al. Non-nodal type of mantle cell lymphoma is a specific biological and clinical subgroup of the disease. Leukemia. 2012;26(8):1895–1898.
30. Naik RR, Saven A. My treatment approach to hairy cell leukemia. Mayo Clin Proc. 2012;87(1):67–76.
31. Tiacci E, Trifonov V, Schiavoni G, et al. BRAF mutations in hairy-cell leukemia. N Engl J Med. 2011;364(24):2305–2315.
32. Kreitman RJ. Hairy cell leukemia: Present and future directions. Leuk Lymphoma. 2019;60(12):2869–2879.
33. Ren Z, Spaargaren M, Pals ST. Syndecan-1 and stromal heparan sulfate proteoglycans: Key moderators of plasma cell biology and myeloma pathogenesis. Blood. 2021;137(13):1713–1718.
34. Anderson KC, Alsina M, Atanackovic D, et al. National Comprehensive Cancer Network. Multiple Myeloma, Version 2.2016: Clinical practice guidelines in oncology. J Natl Compr Canc Netw. 2015;13(11):1398–1435.
35. Oracki SA, Walker JA, Hibbs ML et al. Plasma cell development and survival. Immunol Rev. 2010;237(1):140–159.
36. De Novellis D, Fontana R, Giudice V, et al. Innovative anti-CD38 and anti-BCMA targeted therapies in multiple myeloma: mechanisms of action and resistance. Int J Mol Sci. 2022;24(1):645.
37. Baird RD, van Zyl-Smit RN, Dilke T, et al. Spontaneous remission of low-grade B-cell non-Hodgkin's lymphoma following withdrawal of methotrexate in a patient with rheumatoid arthritis: Case report and review of the literature. Br J Haematol. 2002;118(2):567–568.
38. Wang L, Aghel A, Peterson B, et al. Richter transformation with c-MYC overexpression: Report of three cases. Int J Clin Exp Pathol. 2015;8(6):7540–7546.
39. Grunenberg A, Kaiser LM, Woelfle S, et al. A phase II study of the PI3K inhibitor copanlisib in combination with the anti-CD20 monoclonal antibody rituximab for patients with marginal zone lymphoma: Treatment rationale and protocol design of the COUP-1 trial. BMC Cancer. 2021;21(1):749.
40. Mozos A, Royo C, Hartmann E, et al. SOX11 expression is highly specific for mantle cell lymphoma and identifies the cyclin D1-negative subtype. Haematologica. 2009;94(11):1555–1562.
41. Ye H, Desai A, Zeng D, et al. Smoldering mantle cell lymphoma. J Exp Clin Cancer Res. 2017;36(1):185.
42. Sukswai N, Lyapichev K, Khoury JD, Medeiros LJ. Diffuse large B-cell lymphoma variants: An update. Pathology. 2020;52(1):53–67.

43. Rosenwald A, Wright G, Chan WC, et al. The use of molecular profiling to predict survival after chemotherapy for diffuse large-B-cell lymphoma. N Engl J Med. 2002;346(25):1937–1947.
44. Abramson JS. Hitting back at lymphoma: how do modern diagnostics identify high-risk diffuse large B-cell lymphoma subsets and alter treatment? Cancer. 2019;125(18):3111–3120.
45. Roschewski M, Staudt LM, Wilson WH. Diffuse large B-cell lymphoma-treatment approaches in the molecular era. Nature Rev Clin Oncol. 2014;11(1):12–23.
46. Schmitz R, Wright GW, Huang DW, et al. Genetics and pathogenesis of diffuse large B-cell lymphoma. N Engl J Med. 2018;378(15):1396–1407.
47. Alaggio R, Amador C, Anagnostopoulos I, et al. The 5th edition of the World Health Organization classification of haematolymphoid tumours: Lymphoid neoplasms. Leukemia. 2022;36(7):1720–1748.
48. Wilson WH, Wright GW, Huang DW, et al. Effect of ibrutinib with R-CHOP chemotherapy in genetic subtypes of DLBCL. Cancer Cell. 2021;39(12):1643–1653.
49. Wilson WH, Young RM, Schmitz R, et al. Targeting B cell receptor signaling with ibrutinib in diffuse large B cell lymphoma. Nature Med. 2015;21(8):922–926.
50. Mondello P, Nowakowski GS. Treatment of aggressive B cell lymphomas: updates in 2019. Curr Hematol Malig Rep. 2020;15(3):225–234.
51. Susanibar-Adaniya S, Barta SK. 2021 update on diffuse large B cell lymphoma: a review of current data and potential applications on risk stratification and management. Am J Hematol. 2021;96(5):617–629.
52. Zhao MY, Auerbach A, D'Costa AM, et al. Phospho-p70S6K/p85S6K and cdc2/cdk1 are novel targets for diffuse large B-cell lymphoma combination therapy. Clin Cancer Res. 2009;15(5):1708–1720.
53. Dai B, Zhao XF, Mazan-Mamczarz K, et al. Functional and molecular interactions between ERK and CHK2 in diffuse large B-cell lymphoma. Nature Com. 2011;2:402.
54. Zhao XF, Gartenhaus R. Phospho-p70S6K and cdc2/cdk1 as therapeutic targets for diffuse large B-cell lymphoma. Expert Opin Ther Targets. 2009;13(9):1085–1093.
55. Polaskova K, Merta T, Martincekova A, et al. Comprehensive molecular profiling for relapsed/refractory pediatric Burkitt lymphomas-Retrospective analysis of three real-life clinical cases-addressing issues on randomization and customization at the bedside. Front Oncol. 2020;9:1531.
56. Stein H, Foss HD, Dürkop H, et al. CD30(+) anaplastic large cell lymphoma: A review of its histopathologic, genetic, and clinical features. Blood. 2000;96(12):3681–3695.
57. Wasik M, Peker-Barclift D, Zhao XF. Precision pathology of lymphoid neoplasms. Hematopathology. 2022;7(1):11–22.
58. Wang M, Zhang S, Chuang SS, et al: Angioimmunoblastic T cell lymphoma: Novel molecular insights by mutation profiling. Oncotarget. 2017;8(11):17763–17770.
59. Moskowitz AJ: Practical treatment approach for angioimmunoblastic T-cell lymphoma. J Oncol Pract. 2019;15(3):137–143.
60. Yoo HY, Kim P, Kim WS, et al. Frequent CTLA4-CD28 gene fusion in diverse types of T-cell lymphoma. Haematologica. 2016;101(6):757–763.
61. Iqbal J, Wright G, Wang C, et al. Gene expression signatures delineate biological and prognostic subgroups in peripheral T-cell lymphoma. Blood. 2014;123(19):2915–2923.
62. Heavican TB, Bouska A, Yu J, et al. Genetic drivers of oncogenic pathways in molecular subgroups of peripheral T-cell lymphoma. Blood. 2019;133(15):1664–1676.
63. Hoeller S, Copie-Bergman C. Grey zone lymphomas: Lymphomas with intermediate features. Adv Hematol. 2012;2012:460801.
64. Schuhmacher B, Bein J, Rausch T, et al. JUNB, DUSP2, SGK1, SOCS1 and CREBBP are frequently mutated in T-cell/histiocyte-rich large B-cell lymphoma. Haematologica. 2019;104(2):330–337.
65. Sarkozy C, Hung SS, Chavez EA, et al. Mutational landscape of gray zone lymphoma. Blood. 2021;137(13):1765–1776.
66. Frontzek F, Staiger AM, Zapukhlyak M, et al. Molecular and functional profiling identifies therapeutically targetable vulnerabilities in plasmablastic lymphoma. Nat Commun. 2021;12(1): 5183.
67. Parker K, Venkataraman G. Challenges in the diagnosis of gray zone lymphomas. Surg Pathol Clin. 2019;12(3):709–718.
68. Rosales YMZ, Mesquita JL, Garcia YDO, et al. Use of checkpoint inhibitors in gray zone lymphoma. Hematol Oncol Stem Cell Ther. 2023;16(1):315–319.
69. Zhao XF. Editorial: Precision pathology: a new frontier. Hematopathology. 2018;3(2):24–25.
70. Burke GAA, Beishuizen A, Bhojwani D, et al. Ibrutinib plus CIT for R/R mature B-NHL in children (SPARKLE trial): Initial safety, pharmacokinetics, and efficacy. Leukemia. 2020;34(8):2271–2275.

Index

Note: Page numbers in *italics* indicate a figure and page numbers in **bold** indicate a table on the corresponding page.